THE
MD ANDERSON
MANUAL OF
MEDICAL
ONCOLOGY

NOTICE

Medicine is an ever-changing science. As new research and clinical experience broaden our knowledge, changes in treatment and drug therapy are required. The authors and the publisher of this work have checked with sources believed to be reliable in their efforts to provide information that is complete and generally in accord with the standards accepted at the time of publication. However, in view of the possibility of human error changes in medical sciences, neither the editors nor the publisher nor any other party who has been involved in the preparation or publication of this work warrants that the information contained herein is in every respect accurate or complete, and they disclaim all responsibility for any errors or omissions or for the results obtained from use of the information contained in this work. Readers are encouraged to confirm the information contained herein with other sources. For example and in particular, readers are advised to check the product information sheet included in the package of each drug they plan to administer to be certain that the information contained in this work is accurate and that changes have not been made in the recommended dose or in the contraindications for administration. This recommendation is of particular importance in connection with new or infrequently used drugs.

THE MD ANDERSON MANUAL OF MEDICAL ONCOLOGY

Hagop M. Kantarjian, MD

Professor of Medicine
Chairman, Department of Leukemia
The University of Texas MD Anderson Cancer Center
Houston, Texas

Robert A. Wolff, MD

Associate Professor of Medicine
Department of Gastrointestinal Medical Oncology
The University of Texas MD Anderson Cancer Center
Houston, Texas

Charles A. Koller, MD

Professor of Medicine
Department of Leukemia
The University of Texas MD Anderson Cancer Center
Houston, Texas

McGraw-Hill

MEDICAL PUBLISHING DIVISION

New York / Chicago / San Francisco / Lisbon / London / Madrid / Mexico City
Milan / New Delhi / San Juan / Seoul / Singapore / Sydney / Toronto

THE MD ANDERSON MANUAL OF MEDICAL ONCOLOGY

1234567890   DOW/DOW   09876

ISBN: 0-07-148497-3 (Book 4)
PART OF
ISBN 0-07-148493-0

This book was set in Times Roman by MidAtlantic Books & Journals, Inc.
The editors were Marc Strauss, Marsha S. Loeb, and Karen Edmonson.
The production supervisor was Sherri Souffrance.
The text designer was Marsha Cohen/Parallelogram
The cover designer was Aimee Nordin.
The indexer was Jerry Ralya.
RR Donnelley was printer and binder.

This book is printed on acid-free paper.

The authors wish to acknowledge the administrative and organizational
contributions of Judith A. Venoy, without whom this project would not
have been completed.

Library of Congress Cataloging-in-Publication Data

Kantarjian, Hagop, 1952–
    The MD Anderson manual of medical oncology /
Hagop M. Kantarjian, Robert A. Wolff, Charles A. Koller.
    p. ; cm.
ISBN 0-07-141499-1 (alk. paper)
    1. Cancer—Handbooks, manuals, etc. 2. Oncology—Handbooks,
manuals, etc. I. Title: Manual of medical oncology. II. Koller, Charles.
III. Wolff, Robert, 1957– IV. University of Texas MD Anderson Cancer
Center. V. Title.
    [DNLM: 1. Neoplasms. QZ 200 K175m 2006]
RC262.5.K36 2006
616.99'4—dc22   2004065572

CONTENTS

CONTRIBUTORS

James L. Abbruzzese, MD, FACP
Professor and Chair
Department of Gastrointestinal Medical Oncology
The University of Texas MD Anderson Cancer Center
Houston, Texas

Sridhar R. Allam, MD
Research Fellow
Department of Gastrointestinal Medical Oncology
The University of Texas MD Anderson Cancer Center
Houston, Texas

Jaffer A. Ajani, MD
Professor
Department of Gastrointestinal Medical Oncology
The University of Texas MD Anderson Cancer Center
Houston, Texas

Agop Y. Bedikian, MD
Professor
Department of Melanoma Medical Oncology
The University of Texas MD Anderson Cancer Center
Houston, Texas

L. Johnetta Blakely, MD
Clinical Fellow
Division of Cancer Medicine
The University of Texas MD Anderson Cancer Center
Houston, Texas

Gerald P. Bodey, MD, FACP, FCCP
Professor Emeritus
Department of Infectious Disease, Infection Control, and
   Employee Health
The University of Texas MD Anderson Cancer Center
Houston, Texas

Gautam Borthakur, MD
Assistant Professor
Department of Leukemia
The University of Texas MD Anderson Cancer Center
Houston, Texas

Aman U. Buzdar, MD
Professor
Department of Breast Medical Oncology
The University of Texas MD Anderson Cancer Center
Houston Texas

Carlos E. Bueso-Ramos, MD, PhD
Associate Professor
Department of Hematopathology
The University of Texas MD Anderson Cancer Center
Houston, Texas

Thomas W. Burke, MD
Professor
Department of Gynecologic Oncology
The University of Texas MD Anderson Cancer Center
Houston, Texas

Nita R. Burrer, RN, ANP, CNS
Department of Pediatrics – Patient Care
The University of Texas MD Anderson Cancer Center
Houston, Texas

Naifa L. Busaidy, MD
Assistant Professor
Department of Endocrine Neoplasia and Hormonal Disorders
The University of Texas MD Anderson Cancer Center
Houston, Texas

Richard E. Champlin, MD
Professor and Chair
Department of Blood and Marrow Transplantation
The University of Texas MD Anderson Cancer Center
Houston, Texas

Baochong B. Chang, MD
Clinical Fellow
Division of Cancer Medicine
The University of Texas MD Anderson Cancer Center
Houston, Texas

Roy F. Chemaly, MD, MPH
Assistant Professor
Department of Infectious Diseases, Infection Control, and
   Employee Health
The University of Texas MD Anderson Cancer Center
Houston, Texas

Jorge Cortes, MD
Professor
Department of Leukemia
The University of Texas MD Anderson Cancer Center
Houston, Texas

Bogdan Czerniak, MD
Professor
Department of Pathology
The University of Texas MD Anderson Cancer Center
Houston, Texas

Cesar de las Casas, MD
Assistant Professor
Department of Breast Medical Oncology
The University of Texas MD Anderson Cancer Center
Houston, Texas

Colin P. N. Dinney, MD
Professor and Chair
Department of Urology
The University of Texas MD Anderson Cancer Center
Houston, Texas

Ahmed Elsayem, MD
Assistant Professor
Department of Palliative Care and Rehabilitation Medicine
The University of Texas MD Anderson Cancer Center
Houston, Texas

Cathy Eng, MD
Assistant Professor
Department of Gastrointestinal Medical Oncology
The University of Texas MD Anderson Cancer Center
Houston, Texas

Maricer P. Escalón, MD, MS
Former Clinical Fellow
Division of Cancer Medicine
The University of Texas MD Anderson Cancer Center
Instructor
Division of Hematology/Oncology
University of Miami
Coral Gables, Florida

Elihu H. Estey, MD
Professor
Department of Leukemia
The University of Texas MD Anderson Cancer Center
Houston, Texas

Stefan Faderl, MD
Associate Professor
Department of Leukemia
The University of Texas MD Anderson Cancer Center
Houston, Texas

Michelle A. Fanale, MD
Assistant Professor
Department of Lymphoma and Myeloma
The University of Texas MD Anderson Cancer Center
Houston, Texas

Michael J. Fisch, MD, MPH
Associate Professor
Department of Gastroenterology Medical Oncology
Department of Palliative Care & Rehabilitation Medicine
The University of Texas MD Anderson Cancer Center
Houston, Texas

Dipak Ghelani, MD
Clinical Fellow
Division of Cancer Medicine
The University of Texas MD Anderson Cancer Center
Houston, Texas

Sergio Giralt, MD
Professor
Department of Blood and Marrow Transplantation
The University of Texas MD Anderson Cancer Center
Houston, Texas

Lawrence Ginsberg, MD
Professor
Department of Diagnostic Radiology
The University of Texas MD Anderson Cancer Center
Houston, Texas

Bonnie S. Glisson, MD, FACP
Professor
Department of Thoracic/Head and Neck Medical Oncology
The University of Texas MD Anderson Cancer Center
Houston, Texas

Mouhammed Amir Habra, MD
Clinical Fellow
Joint Program in Diabetes, Endocrinology and Metabolism
Baylor College of Medicine and the University of Texas MD Anderson
    Cancer Center
Houston, Texas

Fredrick B. Hagemeister, MD
Professor
Department of Lymphoma and Myeloma
The University of Texas MD Anderson Cancer Center
Houston, Texas

Karin Hahn, MD, MSc, MPH
Assistant Professor
Department of Breast Medical Oncology
Department of Epidemiology
The University of Texas MD Anderson Cancer Center
Houston, Texas

Bryan T. Hennessy, MD
Clinical Fellow
Division of Cancer Medicine
The University of Texas MD Anderson Cancer Center
Houston, Texas

Paulo M. Hoff, MD, FACP
Associate Professor
Department of Gastrointestinal Medical Oncology
The University of Texas MD Anderson Cancer Center
Houston, Texas

Sigmund Hsu, MD
Assistant Professor
Department of Neuro-Oncology
The University of Texas MD Anderson Cancer Center
Houston, Texas

Elias Jabbour, MD.
Clinical Fellow
Department of Leukemia
The University of Texas MD Anderson Cancer Center
Houston, Texas

Norman Jaffe, MD
Professor
Department of Pediatrics – Patient Care
The University of Texas MD Anderson Cancer Center
Houston, Texas

Faye M. Johnson, MD, PhD
Assistant Professor
Department of Thoracic/Head and Neck Oncology
The University of Texas MD Anderson Cancer Center
Houston, Texas

Eric Jonasch, MD
Assistant Professor
Department of Genitourinary Medical Oncology
The University of Texas MD Anderson Cancer Center
Houston, Texas

Hagop M. Kantarjian, MD
Professor and Chair
Department of Leukemia
The University of Texas MD Anderson Cancer Center
Houston, Texas

John J. Kavanagh, MD
Professor and Chair, ad interim
Department of Gynecologic Medical Oncology
The University of Texas MD Anderson Cancer Center
Houston, Texas

Merrill S. Kies, MD
Professor
Department of Thoracic/Head and Neck Medical Oncology
The University of Texas MD Anderson Cancer Center
Houston, Texas

Charles A. Koller, MD
Professor
Department of Leukemia
Medical Director, Leukemia Center
The University of Texas MD Anderson Cancer Center
Houston, Texas

Dimitrios P. Kontoyiannis, MD, ScD, FACP
Associate Professor
Department of Infectious Disease, Infection Control, and Employee Health
The University of Texas MD Anderson Cancer Center
Houston, Texas

Craig Kovitz, MD, FACP
Clinical Fellow
Division of Cancer Medicine
The University of Texas MD Anderson Cancer Center
Houston, Texas

Dax Kurbegov, MD
Clinical Fellow
Division of Cancer Medicine
The University of Texas MD Anderson Cancer Center
Houston, Texas

Guillermo Lazo, MD
Clinical Fellow
Division of Cancer Medicine
The University of Texas MD Anderson Cancer Center
Houston, Texas

Jan S. Lewin, PhD
Associate Professor
Department of Head and Neck Surgery
The University of Texas MD Anderson Cancer Center
Houston, Texas

Pei Lin, MD
Assistant Professor
Department of Hematopathology
The University of Texas MD Anderson Cancer Center
Houston, Texas

Scott M. Lippman, MD
Professor and Chair
Department of Clinical Cancer Prevention
The University of Texas MD Anderson Cancer Center
Houston, Texas

Nina S. Liu, MD
Clinical Fellow
Division of Cancer Medicine
The University of Texas MD Anderson Cancer Center
Houston, Texas

Christopher Logothetis, MD
Professor and Chair
Department of Genitourinary Medical Oncology
The University of Texas MD Anderson Cancer Center
Houston, Texas

Ellen Manzullo, MD, FACP
Professor
Department of General Internal Medicine, Ambulatory Treatment, and
    Emergency Care
The University of Texas MD Anderson Cancer Center
Houston, Texas

Surena F. Matin, MD, FACS
Assistant Professor
Departmentof Urology
The University of Texas MD Anderson Cancer Center
Houston, Texas

Eric C. McGary, MD, PhD
Clinical Fellow
Division of Cancer Medicine
The University of Texas MD Anderson Cancer Center
Houston, Texas

Peter McLaughlin, MD
Professor
Department of Lymphoma and Myeloma
The University of Texas MD Anderson Cancer Center
Houston, Texas

L. Jeffrey Medeiros, MD
Professor and Chair
Department of Hematopathology
The University of Texas MD Anderson Cancer Center
Houston, Texas

Randall E. Millikan, MD
Associate Professor
Department of Genitourinary Medical Oncology
The University of Texas MD Anderson Cancer Center
Houston, Texas

Alberto J. Montero, MD
Former Clinical Fellow
Division of Cancer Medicine
The University of Texas MD Anderson Cancer Center
Houston, Texas
Assistant Professor
Division of Hematology/Oncology
Medical University of South Carolina
Charleston, South Carolina

Stephanie B. Mundy, MD
Assistant Professor
Department of General Internal Medicine, Ambulatory Treatment, and
    Emergency Care
The University of Texas MD Anderson Cancer Center
Houston, Texas

Susan O'Brien, MD
Professor
Department of Leukemia
The University of Texas MD Anderson Cancer Center
Houston, Texas

Lance C. Pagliaro, MD
Associate Professor
Department of Genitourinary Medical Oncology
The University of Texas MD Anderson Cancer Center
Houston, Texas

Shreyaskumar Patel, MD
Professor and Deputy Chair
Department of Sarcoma Medical Oncology
The University of Texas MD Anderson Cancer Center
Houston, Texas

Alexandria T. Phan, M.D.
Assistant Professor
Department of Gastrointestinal Medical Oncology
The University of Texas MD Anderson Cancer Center
Houston, Texas

Katherine M. W. Pisters, MD
Professor
Department of Thoracic/Head and Neck Medical Oncology
The University of Texas MD Anderson Cancer Center
Houston, Texas

Naveen Ramineni, MD
Assistant Professor
Department of Palliative Care and Rehabilitation Medicine
The University of Texas MD Anderson Cancer Center
Houston, Texas

Pedro T. Ramirez, MD
Assistant Professor
Department of Gynecologic Oncology
The University of Texas MD Anderson Cancer Center
Houston, Texas

Ronald P. Rapini, MD
Professor and Chair
Department of Dermatology
The University of Texas MD Anderson Cancer Center
Houston, Texas

Suresh K. Reddy, MD, FFARCS
Associate Professor
Department of Palliative Care and Rehabilitation Medicine
The University of Texas MD Anderson Cancer Center
Houston, Texas

M. Alma Rodriguez, MD, FACP
Professor
Department of Lymphoma and Myeloma
The University of Texas MD Anderson Cancer Center
Houston, Texas

Kenneth V. I. Rolston, MD
Professor
Department of Infectious Diseases, Infection Control, and
  Employee Health
The University of Texas MD Anderson Cancer Center
Houston, Texas

Pamela N. Schultz, PhD, RN
Associate Professor
Department of Nursing
New Mexico State University
Las Cruces, New Mexico

Hui Ti See, MD
Clinical Fellow
Department of Gynecologic Medical Oncology
The University of Texas MD Anderson Cancer Center
Houston, Texas

Gregory Seymour, MD
Clinical Fellow
Division of Cancer Medicine
The University of Texas MD Anderson Cancer Center
Houston, Texas

Gary G. Shi, MD
Clinical Fellow
Division of Cancer Medicine
The University of Texas MD Anderson Cancer Center
Houston, Texas

Ki Y. Shin, MD
Associate Professor
Department of Palliative Care and Rehabilitation Medicine
The University of Texas MD Anderson Cancer Center
Houston, Texas

Arlene O. Siefker-Radtke, MD
Assistant Professor
Department of Genitourinary Medical Oncology
The University of Texas MD Anderson Cancer Center
Houston, Texas

Thomas B. Sneed, MD
Clinical Fellow
Division of Cancer Medicine
The University of Texas MD Anderson Cancer Center
Houston, Texas

Kay Swint, RN, MSN
Clinical Administrative Director
Department of Palliative Care and Rehabilitation Medicine
The University of Texas MD Anderson Cancer Center
Houston, Texas

Rudranath Talukdar, MD
Assistant Professor
Department of Palliative Care and Rehabilitation Medicine
The University of Texas MD Anderson Cancer Center
Houston, Texas

Siriwan Tangjitgamol, MD
Clinical Fellow
Department of Gynecologic Medical Oncology
The University of Texas MD Anderson Cancer Center
Houston, Texas

Melanie B. Thomas, MD
Assistant Professor
Department of Gastrointestinal Medical Oncology
The University of Texas MD Anderson Cancer Center
Houston, Texas

Jonathan C. Trent, MD, PhD
Assistant Professor
Department of Sarcoma Medical Oncology
The University of Texas MD Anderson Cancer Center
Houston, Texas

Anne S. Tsao, MD
Assistant Professor
Department of Thoracic/Head and Neck Medical Oncology
The University of Texas MD Anderson Cancer Center
Houston, Texas

Vicente Valero, MD, FACP
Professor
Department of Breast Medical Oncology
The University of Texas MD Anderson Cancer Center
Houston, Texas

Gauri R. Varadhachary, MD
Assistant Professor
Department of Gastrointestinal Medical Oncology
The University of Texas MD Anderson Cancer Center
Houston, Texas

Rena Vassilopoulou-Sellin, MD
Professor
Department of Endocrine Neoplasia and Hormonal Disorders
The University of Texas MD Anderson Cancer Center
Houston, Texas

Michael Wang, MD
Assistant Professor
Department of Lymphoma and Myeloma
The University of Texas MD Anderson Cancer Center
Houston, Texas

Donna Weber, MD
Associate Professor
Department of Lymphoma and Myeloma
The University of Texas MD Anderson Cancer Center
Houston, Texas

Robert A. Wolff, MD
Associate Professor
Department of Gastrointestinal Medical Oncology
The University of Texas MD Anderson Cancer Center
Houston, Texas

Christopher G. Wood, MD
Associate Professor
Department of Urology
The University of Texas MD Anderson Cancer Center
Houston, Texas

James C. Yao, MD
Assistant Professor
Department of Gastrointestinal Medical Oncology
The University of Texas MD Anderson Cancer Center
Houston, Texas

Sai-Ching Jim Yeung, MD, PhD
Assistant Professor
Department of Endocrine Neoplasia and Hormonal Disorders
Department of General Internal Medicine, Ambulatory Treatment and
    Emergency Care
The University of Texas MD Anderson Cancer Center
Houston, Texas

W.K. Alfred Yung, MD
Professor and Chair
Department of Neuro-Oncology
The University of Texas MD Anderson Cancer Center
Houston, Texas

PREFACE

The MD Anderson Manual of Medical Oncology has been designed to fill an important void in oncology reference material by serving as a hands-on resource for the practicing oncologist. It was written exclusively by our faculty and fellows, and we believe it presents a bird's eye view of medical oncology as it is currently practiced at our institution.

We planned the content with certain guiding principles in mind. First, although it was written primarily from the perspective of the medical oncologist, we have emphasized MD Anderson's multidisciplinary approach to cancer care. Some details of radiation therapy and surgery covered in other subspecialty textbooks, however, have not been included. Second, while this text demonstrates a rationale for patient care that is evidence-based, we make no apologies for articulating our unique perspectives and biases as they apply to cancer biology and therapy. We hope many readers find this refreshing. Third, we have tried to articulate the rationale for many of our ongoing clinical trials and the importance of continued clinical investigation.

Furthermore, one of the important goals we set for this reference was to make it visually stimulating, and it is therefore filled with tabulated data and graphics, pathology figures, and illustrative imaging. Moreover, the contributing authors have supplied algorithms in the form of flowcharts and diagrams to provide readers with a practical guide to the diagnostic and therapeutic strategies used at MD Anderson.

Finally, because we believe that palliative and supportive interventions are an integral component of all cancer care, we have included chapters that address MD Anderson's approach to oncologic emergencies, infections, palliation, and the long-term needs of cancer survivors.

We sincerely believe this book fulfills the important goals we set for it and that it will become an important resource for the oncologic community.

Hagop M. Kantarjian, MD
Robert A. Wolff, MD
Charles A. Koller, MD

FOREWORD

The MD Anderson Manual of Medical Oncology demonstrates the unique, multidisciplinary approach to cancer management pioneered by The University of Texas MD Anderson Cancer Center; an approach so effective that MD Anderson has been consistently ranked as one of the nation's top two cancer hospitals in the U.S. News & World Report's "America's Best Hospitals" survey every year. The MD Anderson approach has evolved from decades of clinical practice and research with more than 600,000 patients representing the full spectrum of metastatic diseases. This volume endeavors to bring an approach to cancer management that reaches well beyond the standard of care, to oncologists around the world—regardless of how remote or small their practice. Every one of the 44 chapters reflects how MD Anderson currently operates including many patient care practices that would not have been recognized by practitioners just a decade ago. This year alone, more than 70,000 people with cancer—25,000 of them new patients—will seek care at MD Anderson, and about one-third of them will come from outside Texas. They will participate in the largest clinical research program in the nation exploring novel therapies.

Discussion of epidemiologic issues in each chapter makes evident the burgeoning incidence rate of many cancer diseases over the past decade, with concomitant increases in mortality and an urgent need for more effective long-term management strategies. Some of these rising cancer incidence rates, beginning in 1990's, can be attributed to improved survival of patients with HIV infection. The incidence of other diseases, such as colorectal cancer, declined in the 1990's, with corresponding declines in mortality rates, possibly due to increased screening efforts, early intervention, and improved adjuvant therapies. Some, such as breast cancer, showed stable or increasing incidence, but steadily declining mortality rates since the 1990's. Overall, we have gotten better at finding biomarkers that are predictive for survival, a major triumph in medical oncology that is well-demonstrated throughout the text.

This volume emphasizes and discusses recent developments in more accurate diagnostic procedures, such as the ThinPrep liquid-based cervical cytology system, which improves the rate of detection of abnormal cells for detection of cervical cancer. The improved sensitivity and specificity of imaging studies has elevated them to standard of care status for diagnosing and staging cancer diseases at MD Anderson and rendered nearly obsolete many invasive surgical diagnostic and staging practices such as laparatomy or splenectomy, which were considered standard of care only a decade ago. Diagnostic procedures commonly conducted at other cancer centers are not performed at MD Anderson, and the text explains why while discussing preferred alternative techniques. Use of imaging studies becomes particularly important in diseases that are commonly misdiagnosed. When CT findings are equivocal, PDG-PET is a more sensitive technique that can spot malignancies less than 1 cm by detecting differences in glucose metabolism between normal cells and cancer cells. It is standard practice at MD Anderson to use objective radiographic criteria to define a potentially resectable primary tumor. This text also emphasizes how imaging can prevent administration of overly aggressive, toxic, or invasive surgical treatment regimens to superficial or indolent tumors.

Two major advances in therapeutic approach over the past decades are emphasized in The *MD Anderson Manual of Medical Oncology*: 1) better timing of therapeutic modalities to enhance response and 2) a growing capacity to individualize treatment and target specific patterns of genomics, protenomics, and cell signaling pathways identifiable through high-throughput microarray technology.

The MD Anderson Manual of Medical Oncology emphasizes new therapies that have changed the standard of care and outcomes for cancer diseases previously associated with a poor prognosis. For instance, due to the discovery of genetic and epigenetic events driving carcinogenesis, the development and testing of targeted molecules has mushroomed, resulting in a wider selection of therapeutic drug combinations to treat advanced metastatic disease.

While the Manual discusses special considerations in the treatment of populations such as the elderly and those with multiple co-morbidity, also stressed throughout the book are the many ways that recent progress in reducing treatment-associated toxicity has made aging less often an independent contraindication to many effective therapeutic regimens. Morbidity associated with radiation therapy has greatly decreased over the past decade as has morbidity associated with surgery.

This new era of novel therapeutics has also spearheaded the recent evolution of another crucial advancement in management of metastatic disease: the transition from a sequential care concept culminating in the sole delivery of palliative care, to the concept of integrating ongoing active disease treatment with simultaneous palliative care. Clinicians at MD Anderson no longer approach advanced metastatic disease management with palliative care goals alone; now these patients are often offered frontline cancer treatment and the opportunity to participate in clinical trials for investigational drugs.

To help clinicians quickly evaluate therapeutic regimen possibilities, every chapter includes abundant tables, diagrams, and imaging photos. For example:

- CT images of various solid tumors before and after treatment
- Gross pathology specimens from different types of cancer
- Pathogenesis of cancers, such as molar pregnancy
- Immunohistochemical stains illustrating cytologic and histologic features of various cancer diseases
- Common organ distributions of specific tumor classifications, for example, the carcinoid type of neuroendocrine tumor
- Risk factors for developing various cancer diseases and for shortened survival
- Incidence and five-year survival rates for different primary cancer sites
- Prognostic models, including prognostic indices, formulas, and hazard ratios
- Disease staging systems emphasizing recent changes in criteria based on tumor markers and latest research findings on prognosis
- Oncogenes commonly expressed in various cancer diseases
- Comparisons of the presence or absence of specific genetic lesions in different subsets of a cancer disease
- Common site of metastasis from various primary solid tumors

- Comparisons of chemotherapy regimen options
- Ongoing clinical trials of cancer therapies at MD Anderson
- New molecular therapies recommended to overcome resistance to previously effective therapies
- The MD Anderson approach to allogeneic transplantation for common hematologic diseases
- Indications for treatment decisions, such as when to use a sparing surgical procedure
- Treatment algorithms developed at MD Anderson for specific cancer diseases or disease subtypes
- Complex therapy schedules outlined by segment, with the appropriate dose and schedule for each regimen
- Comparisons of outcomes associated with various treatment strategies
- Comparative literature reviews of survival and other outcome studies
- Decision trees for management of recurrent cancers
- Guidelines for patient follow up
- Strategies for managing treatment-associated adverse events
- Recommendations for preventing and managing long-term complications

Chapters on long-term survival and follow up demonstrate the additional utility of this book for clinicians outside the specialty of oncology. A high proportion of the growing number of cancer survivors will end up being followed by a primary care physician, cardiologist, or other specialist. The text's description of the results from MD Anderson's survey of cancer survivors serves as an essential guide to typical long-term health problems both physicians and rehabilitation specialists can expect to manage.

Over the past decade and particularly in the current century, the practice of medical oncology at MD Anderson has truly evolved to epitomize the translational research concept of "bench to bedside and back," a paradigm shift that The MD Anderson Manual of Medical Oncology pertinently exhibits in every chapter.

Waun Ki Hong, MD
American Cancer Society Professor
Samsung Distinguished University Chair in Cancer Medicine
Division Head, Cancer Medicine
The University of Texas
MD Anderson Cancer Center
Houston, Texas
September 2005

Miscellaneous Tumors

CHAPTER
30

TUMORS OF THE CENTRAL NERVOUS SYSTEM

Sigmund Hsu
W.K. Alfred Yung

■ OVERVIEW

Brain tumors are a heterogeneous group of lesions that range from benign, slow-growing tumors found only incidentally on autopsy to malignant, rapidly growing tumors that cause death within months. The most common intracranial tumor is a brain metastasis from systemic cancer. The estimated number of new patients with brain metastases in the United States in 2003 was 130,000 to 200,000, based on a 10% to 15% incidence (1,2), whereas the expected number of all new cancer diagnoses was 1.33 million (3). In comparison, the incidence of primary brain tumors in 2002 was 39,550 new

cases (4). Because of the heterogenous histology and often refractory nature of these tumors, their management is complex, ideally requiring a multidisciplinary team effort and individualized treatment. Diagnosis is made on the basis of histology, so an accurate characterization of the lesion's pathology is crucial, often necessitating confirmation at a specialized cancer center. Optimal outcomes involve the coordination of neurosurgery, radiation oncology, and neuro-oncology, although low-grade tumors may not require initial therapy other than observation following optimal surgical resection. Despite advances in neurosurgical techniques, radiation therapy, and chemotherapy, the prognosis for patients with high-grade gliomas such as glioblastoma (GBM), the most common form of glioma, remains dismal. For patients with GBM, median survival is approximately 1 year. A recent review of eight consecutive phase II chemotherapy trials for recurrent GBM demonstrated only a 6% response rate [complete response (CR) and partial response (PR)], with a 6-month progression-free survival (PFS) of 15% and a 1-year overall survival of 21% (5). It is, however, important to consider patients with high-grade gliomas for entry into clinical trials at all stages of disease, not only at relapse, since new therapies target patients from initial diagnosis with presurgical protocols to salvage therapy at relapse. This chapter aims to provide basic principles that can be used for diagnosing and treating patients with brain tumors. Areas that present special challenges for the treating physician are highlighted, along with an introduction to the underlying molecular mechanisms of gliomagenesis.

■ CLASSIFICATION AND INCIDENCE

Brain tumors are either primary tumors that arise de novo or secondary brain metastases, the latter being far more common. The most common brain metastases result from lung cancer, followed by breast, melanoma, renal, and colorectal cancers (6). Most patients with brain metastases die from progression of their systemic cancer, although, because of improvements in systemic therapy, brain metastases are seen more frequently and produce escalating morbidity and mortality (1). On a more hopeful note, advances in treating brain metastasis with surgery and radiotherapy have elevated the prospects for improved survival when the patient's systemic disease is controlled. Primary brain tumors are classified by the World Health Organization (WHO) grading system (Table 30-1), which is based on the histologic pattern of cell differentiation in the tumor. Tumor grade is correlated with prognosis. The most common primary brain tumors are gliomas (all glial tumors), then meningiomas, followed by nerve sheath and pituitary tumors.

■ EPIDEMIOLOGY

BRAIN METASTASES

In 2003, the incidence of brain metastases was estimated to be 130,000 to 200,000 new cases per year, assuming a 10% to 15% incidence with 1.33 million new

TABLE 30-1	WORLD HEALTH ORGANIZATION (WHO) CLASSIFICATION OF TUMORS OF THE CENTRAL NERVOUS SYSTEM
WHO grade I	
Pilocytic astrocytoma	Meningioma
Myxopapillary ependymoma	Craniopharyngioma
Subependymoma	
WHO grade II	
Diffuse astrocytoma	Ependymoma
Pleomorphic	Pineocytoma
xanthoastrocytoma	Atypical meningioma
Oligodendroglioma	
Oligoastrocytoma	
WHO grade III	
Anaplastic astrocytoma	Anaplastic oligoastrocytoma
Anaplastic oligoden-	Anaplastic ependymoma
droglioma	
Anaplastic (malignant)	
meningioma	
WHO grade IV	
Glioblastoma	Pineoblastoma
Gliosarcoma	Medulloblastoma

diagnoses of cancer (3). Nearly any type of primary cancer can metastasize to the brain, including the hematologic malignancies (leukemia and lymphoma), carcinoma, and, rarely, prostate cancer (7).

The most common brain metastasis originates from lung cancer, which is also the most frequently occurring systemic cancer. The next most common brain metastasis–associated pathology is breast cancer, followed by melanoma, renal cancer, and colorectal cancer (6), with melanoma being the most likely tumor to metastasize to the brain. Based on autopsy findings, 40% to 60% of patients with melanoma develop brain metastases (8). Most brain metastases, particularly melanoma, present with multiple lesions (9); although when renal cancer metastasizes to the brain, it often results in only a single lesion. Overall, however, the pattern of distribution of metastases in the brain varies depending on the primary cancer (10).

The incidence of brain metastases appears to be rising, which may be a consequence of a greater degree of its recognition due to increasingly sensitive imaging modalities, most commonly magnetic resonance imaging (MRI), combined with the increased rate of survival, albeit not cure, of patients with cancer. The development of brain metastases usually occurs in the context of systemic relapse, although relapse can be isolated in the brain. The impermeability of the blood–brain barrier (BBB), which limits the penetration of many chemotherapy drugs into the brain, is thought to be a major factor when isolated brain metastasis is the recurrence.

PRIMARY BRAIN TUMORS

Gliomas are the most frequently occurring primary brain tumors and include all grades of astrocytoma, oligodendroglioma, and ependymoma. Combined, these histologies account for more than 40% of all primary brain tumors. The next most common tumor is meningioma, followed by nerve sheath tumor and pituitary tumor. The most recent data from the Central Brain Tumor Registry of the United States (4) report an incidence of all primary benign and malignant brain tumors of 14.0 cases per 100,000 person-years and a prevalence rate of 130.8 per 100,000 (4).

The incidence of primary brain tumors differs by age, with the incidence for all tumors peaking between the ages of 75 to 85 years. However, the peak incidence of gliomas is from ages 65 to 75. Low-grade glioma is more likely to occur in patients younger than 35 years. Unfortunately, after age 35, a diagnosis of GBM is much more common and accounts for more than half of all gliomas. In addition to the disparities of age, gender differences are seen in the incidence of primary brain tumors. The incidence of glioma in males is 8.0, compared with 5.6 for females per 100,000 person-years. In contrast, meningioma is more common in females, with an incidence of 5.2 per 100,000 person-years, compared with 2.7 for males (4).

Although an uncommon tumor, primary central nervous system (CNS) lymphoma has increased threefold in incidence from 1973 to 1984—a figure that continues to rise (11,12). This escalation is partly attributed to the effect of HIV infection in increasing immunosuppression, which is a strong risk factor for lymphoma (13). The incidence of CNS lymphoma is also rising in immunocompetent individuals (14). Limited studies have suggested that a history of autoimmune disease and/or of cancer are risk factors in developing primary CNS lymphoma (15,16).

Although many factors have been considered as putatively involved in gliomagenesis, therapeutic ionizing radiation is the strongest established causative agent underlying the development of brain tumors. Children with acute lymphoblastic leukemia (ALL), following prophylactic cranial irradiation, have a 27-fold increased risk of brain tumors (17). Increased risk of brain tumors has been seen following therapeutic irradiation for pituitary tumors, even with the low doses of radiation previously used to treat scalp ringworm, which has specifically increased the risk of developing nerve sheath tumors, meningiomas, and gliomas (18). Fortunately, diagnostic radiation does not appear to be strongly associated with the development of gliomas (19).

While brain tumors have been linked to chemical exposure, no specific agent has been identified with a link to brain tumors that can be validated with an exposure-disease correlation. Despite the fact that pesticides have been shown to cause tumors in experimental animal models and there is an association between the use of

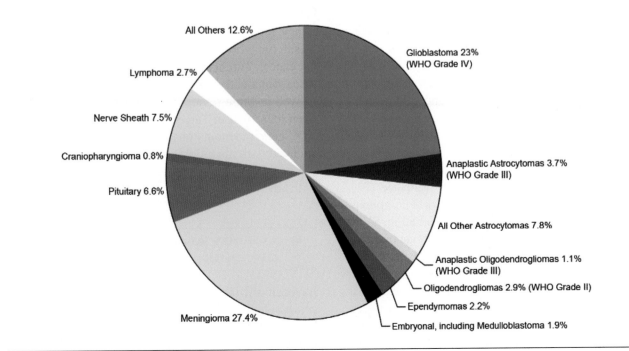

FIGURE 30-1 | Distribution of all primary brain and central nervous system tumors by histology, CBTRUS 1995 to 1999 (*n* = 37,788).

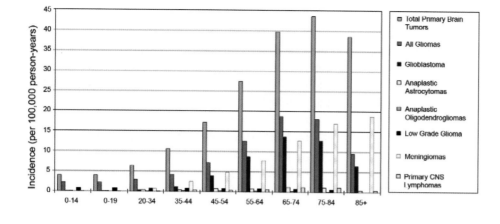

FIGURE 30-2 Age-specific incidence of primary brain and central nervous system tumors by selected histologies, CBTRUS 1995 to 1999.

pesticides and the development of tumors, no consistent link has been proven for the occurrence of cancer in agricultural workers (20). Positive correlations, but not proven, have been drawn between the occurrence of brain tumors and occupations involving exposure to synthetic rubber, vinyl chloride, and petroleum refining (21). Interestingly, however, whereas smoking is implicated in an increased risk for many cancers, it is not associated with an increased risk of brain tumors (22,23). On the other hand, *N*-nitroso compounds are neurocarcinogens in animals. They are highly ubiquitous, being found in endogenous sources when amino groups encounter a nitrosating agent as well as in exogenous sources such as cured foods, auto interiors, and cosmetics. Exposure to cured foods such as bacon has been linked to meningioma, and nitrosamines have been associated with glioma; however, exposure to cosmetics has not been clearly linked to the formation of brain tumors (19).

There has been concern, particularly in the popular press, about the relationship between exposure to cell phones and the risk for brain tumors. Thus far, several case control studies and a cohort study have failed to establish a link between brain tumors and cellular telephone usage.

Viral exposure has a suspected link to the formation of brain tumors. However, other than the increased incidence of primary CNS lymphoma in patients with HIV infection, the association has not been validated (24). The SV40 large T antigen is able to form complexes with the *p53* tumor suppressor gene. In addition, SV40 large T antigen has been isolated from human brain tumors (25), raising the hypothesis that the expression of SV40 large T antigen caused *p53* gene inactivation and favored gliomagenesis. There was also a concern that the contamination of polio vaccine with SV40 between 1955 and 1963 would result in an increased risk for brain tumors. However, two case control studies in the United States failed to validate this trepidation (26,27).

Although the etiologies of only a small proportion of brain tumors are attributed to heredity alone, cancer clearly has a genetic basis; this is increasingly being probed by researchers (28). The fraction of childhood brain tumors strictly due to heritable factors was, for example, only 2% in a national registry study in Great Britain (28). Brain tumors can arise as a component of familial tumor syndromes, such as neurofibromatosis (type 1), resulting in glioma and optic nerve glioma. Neurofibromatosis (type 1) is caused by a mutation of the *NF-1* gene and is also associated with leukemia and pheochromocytoma. Neurofibromatosis (type II) is marked by a mutation of the *NF-2* gene and is associated with bilateral vestibular schwannomas, meningioma, and glioma. The Li-Fraumeni syndrome results from an autosomal dominant mutation of the *p53* tumor suppressor gene, located on chromosome 17p (29). This *p53* mutation results in many types of malignancy, including glioma and medulloblastoma, as well as sarcoma, breast cancer, leukemia, and adrenocortical cancer. Turcot syndrome is an autosomal dominant disease characterized by multiple polyps of the GI tract as well as brain tumors. Two separate mutations have been identified in Turcot syndrome. One involves the *APC* gene (adenomatous polyposis coli), which is associated with medulloblastoma. A second mutation of the *hMLH1* DNA mismatch repair gene is associated with GBM (30).

■ BIOLOGY AND MOLECULAR GENETICS

Increasingly, the focus of understanding various cancers resides in a clear view of underlying molecular biologic mechanisms and signaling pathways. With the failure of high-grade tumors to markedly respond to chemotherapy and other treatment modalities, it is increasingly being thought that the only way to develop more effective treatments for brain tumors will be to understand these mechanisms. While delineating such mechanisms holds the ultimate promise for cure, they also confound the treatment of brain tumors by virtue of their tremendous molecular and histologic heterogeneity from tumor to tumor. Glial tumors can have areas composed both of low- and high-grade tissue in the same tumor. Additionally, tumor cells often have multiple genetic mutations. These can affect growth factor signaling, cell cycle events, apoptosis, cell survival pathways, and DNA repair mechanisms. The resulting multiple dysregulations have abrogated the effectiveness of therapies aimed at single genes. Drug delivery, a more common treatment approach, is affected by the BBB, especially when the focus of treatment involves areas of nonenhancing, infiltrating tumor. Meningiomas are typically slow-growing tumors that often become quite large before clinical diagnosis. These tumors are frequently managed with surgery alone. However, meningiomas also express receptors for growth factors, and they have the ability to progress to malignant tumors that are resistant to radiation and chemotherapy. The biology of brain metastasis has also been recently studied using animal modeling, and progress has been made in angiogenesis research. Understanding the distinction between the normal physiologic BBB and the neoplastic blood-tumor barrier is also important when chemotherapy is being considered for brain metastasis.

New classes of drugs that have recently been developed or are in development target specific extracellular receptors or block intracellular signal transduction systems. Owing to their specificity, these drugs often lack the side effects commonly associated with standard cytotoxic chemotherapy. If the therapeutic target is crucial for the cancer cell's continued viability, the drug can be especially effective. An example is the use of imatinib for chronic myelogenous leukemia (31,32). If the target is heterogeneous or is not critical for continued cell survival, the benefits can be more modest, such as the use of gefitinib in lung cancer (33). Technologic advances in the development of transgenic mice, cDNA microarrays, and protein analysis approaches are making possible a highly sophisticated and powerful molecular analysis of brain tumors. Molecular characterization of brain tumors using cDNA microarray technology has identified specific genetic profiles that are directly correlated with tumor grading and prognosis (34,35). Ultimately, tumors will be identified on the basis of their underlying molecular makeup and individual treatments will be targeted to these specific diseases rather than to broad categories such as glioma.

GLIAL TUMORS

Malignant glial tumors often exhibit significant histologic heterogeneity, which is reflected at the molecular level. One proposed explanation for this diversity hypothesizes an underlying genetic instability resulting in a progressive accumulation of mutations and leading to an increasingly malignant phenotype. Stem cells are increasingly becoming a focus of attention in regard to various cancers, and some researchers believe that cancer originates from progenitor cell populations becoming active in different locations in the body. The adult brain is one such organ that has a population of stem cells that could become targets for neoplastic transformation (36). Glial tumors have known mutations in critical cellular pathways, including cell cycle regulation, proliferation, cellular metabolism, cell death, and survival. Separate mutations may have an equivalent phenotypic effect if they are involved in the same signaling pathway. It is also becoming increasingly clear that intracellular signaling pathways are even more complicated than was originally hypothesized, due to crosstalk and interactions between pathways and the presence of redundant alternate pathways. These pathways can interact at multiple levels and can directly affect gene transcription, post-transcription processing, protein modification and transport, and protein-protein interactions.

Several growth factor pathways have been identified as being activated in glioma growth. The epidermal growth factor (EGF) pathway is overexpressed in GBM (37). It is estimated that the EGF receptor (EGFR) is amplified in 30% to 50% of GBM (38,39). An alternate mutation in the EGFR generates a truncated receptor, the EGFvIII mutant, which is constitutively activated in gliomas (40). Growth factors such as EGF and platelet-derived growth factor (PDGF) activate multiple signal transduction pathways that lead to cell survival and proliferation. EGFR can activate the PI3Kinase pathway, which is frequently mutated in glioma. When the PI3Kinase pathway is activated, the expression of *AKT* (protein kinase B) is triggered, in turn activating multiple prosurvival pathways such as NFkB, forkhead, and glycolysis (41). The activation of the PI3Kinase pathway has been associated with the reduced survival of glioma patients (42). Growth factors can also stimulate the *ras* pathway, which initiates a signal cascade through *Raf/MEK/Erk,* and also promotes cell survival and tumorigenesis (43).

The deletion of *MMAC/PTEN* is a key mutation in glioblastoma (44). PTEN has phosphatase activity that inhibits the PI3Kinase pathway. The deletion of *MMAC/PTEN* leads to *AKT* pathway amplification. One effector of the AKT signal involves mTOR. mTOR inhibitors are being investigated in clinical trials for GBM. The importance of these pathways has been shown in transgenic mouse-modeling studies; these have produced primary brain tumors that mimic many of the characteristics of human primary brain tumors (45,46) as well as allowing direct mapping of mutated pathways found in human tumor samples.

A commonly mutated gene in gliomas is *p53*, a transcription factor that, among other signals, is activated in response to DNA damage in an attempt to control the cell cycle. The activation of *p53* can result either in apoptosis or cell cycle arrest and initiation of DNA repair mechanisms (47). The functions of *p53* are complex and have been studied for many years. Initially, *p53* was thought to act mainly through *p21, BAX, GADD45,* and *MDM2.* Sequencing and scanning the promoter and enhancer regions of more than 2500 human genes has identified 300 genes that are putatively directly regulated by *p53* (48). An alternate mechanism that decreases *p53* pathway activity involves MDM2 protein, which binds to *p53* and inactivates it. Amplification of *MDM2,* seen in 10% of GBM that lack the mutant form of *p53,* decreases the activity of *p53* (49). The abrogation of *p53* activity would be expected to increase proliferation and accumulate mutations, leading to genetic instability, the prodrome of tumorigenesis.

The cell cycle represents stages of development via cell division that are necessary for cell replication, including DNA synthesis and the duplication of chromosomes (S phase), mitosis (M phase), and the intervals in between these events: cellular quiescence and differentiation (G0 phase), cell preparation and signaling to commit the cell to division (G1 phase), and cellular checks to DNA replication prior to cell division (G2 phase). Cell cycle regulation is a key target of carcinogenesis. The transition from each phase to the next phase is characterized by "checkpoints." These cell cycle checkpoints are affected by multiple proteins, acting either as accelerators or inhibitors of cell regulation. Important molecules in this process include *p53, p21,* and *MDM2,* which can both inhibit and accelerate the degradation of *p53.* Another cell cycle regulation pathway important for glial tumors involves the retinoblastoma (*RB*) gene. When the *RB* gene is phosphorylated, the E2F transcription factor is released and activates cellular proliferation. The regulation of *RB* activity is complex and involves multiple cyclins (cyclin D), cyclin-dependent kinases (CDK4/6), and cyclin-dependant kinase inhibitors (p16), whose activities continue to be investigated (50). A promising preclinical gene therapy takes advantage of the *RB* mutation to allow replication of a mutated adenovirus, which generates an oncolytic effect (51).

Apoptosis is genetically programmed cell death, an important process in embryogenesis, normal tissue turnover, ischemia, and degenerative disorders. Antiapoptotic proteins such as bcl-2 and proapoptotic proteins such as myc and bax are important regulators of this pathway. Apoptosis can be activated through binding of the fas/apo-1 receptor (CD95) by the fas ligand (tumor necrosis factor), which in turn activates caspases via proteolytic cleavage and ends in cell death. It is suspected that alterations in the regulation of apoptosis and response to apoptosis signals may be in part responsible for the resistance of glial tumors to chemotherapy.

The production of enzymes that repair the effects of chemotherapy is another mechanism of the resistance of cancer cells. O6-alkylguanine-DNA alkyltransferase (AGT) is expressed by glial tumors and removes the DNA adduct produced by nitrosourea compounds, the class of agents most widely used for brain tumor chemotherapy. Hypermethylation of the promoter region of the *AGT* gene, which inactivates *AGT* gene transcription, has been associated with response to alkylating agents and increased survival in glioma patients (52, 53). The mechanism of gene inactivation by hypermethylation can target other cellular pathways, including those involving DNA repair, cell cycle regulation, apoptosis, and tumor suppressor genes (54).

One of the hallmarks of glial tumors is their propensity to invade neighboring brain tissue, generally within 1 to 2 cm of the original tumor mass. Glial tumor cells can generate an extracellular matrix (ECM) that promotes migration through the production of tenascin, vitronectin, and fibronectin. Glial tumor cells can also express receptors for integrin, CD44 (a transmembrane glycoprotein), RHAMM (a hyaluronan-binding protein that regulates ras signaling), the ECM proteoglycan versican, and the neural cell adhesion molecule (NCAM). Glial tumors also secrete matrix metalloproteinases (MMPs) that degrade the adjacent ECM and facilitate invasion (55). Downregulation of MMP-2 activity by the *PTEN* gene has been shown to reduce invasion in glial tumor cell lines (56). These various molecules will hopefully be able to offer viable targets that will be instrumental in producing efficacious glioma therapies.

The molecular and cytogenetic characterization of brain tumors has suggested two models that can explain the development of GBM. One model, resting on the multi-hit hypothesis, attributes the development of GBM to a stepwise accumulation of mutations beginning in low-grade astrocytoma and progressing to high-grade astrocytoma. This process is marked by the presence of mutated *p53*. In this model, progression from a normal astrocyte to a low-grade astrocytoma is marked by *p53* mutation (>65%) and PDGF-A or PDGFR-alpha over-expression (60%). Progression from low-grade astrocytoma to anaplastic astrocytoma involves loss of heterozygosity (57) at 19q (50%) and alterations in the RB pathway (25%). Progression from anaplastic astrocytoma to GBM is marked by LOH at 10q/mutation of PTEN (5%), loss of expression of DCC [which induces apoptosis by a mechanism requiring receptor proteolysis (50%)], and amplification of PDGFR-alpha (<10%). A separate model has been proposed for primary de novo GBM, which is characterized by the lack of *p53* mutation, by EGFR amplification (40%) or overexpression (60%), MDM2 amplification (<10%) or overexpression (50%), *p16* deletion (30% to 40%), LOH at 10p and 10q/PTEN mutation (30%), and *RB* alterations (58,59). These models are, however, descriptive more than they are mechanistic and do not adequately take into account the genetic or histologic heterogeneity that is found even within a single tumor. The persistence of glioma is likely due to the fact that multiple mechanisms combine to generate a common tumor phenotype (38). Some speculate that this complexity involves genetic instability or cell fusion (60). Explication of the precise mechanisms involved has yet to be accomplished.

Increasing numbers of cytogenetic studies on direct patient tumor tissue are yielding intriguing evidence that a patient's response to chemotherapy might be correlated with his or her cytogenetic profile. Patients with anaplastic oligodendroglioma are generally considered to be more chemosensitive than those with other anaplastic gliomas. However, not all anaplastic oligodendrogliomas respond to standard alkylating agent chemotherapy. The allelic loss of chromosomes 1p and 19q has been linked to the response of oligodendroglioma and anaplastic oligodendroglioma to chemotherapy, and the presence of intact 1p, and 19q has been correlated with both lack of response and decreased survival (61–65). These results have not been validated prospectively in a large trial; however, they suggest that in the future, brain tumor oncology may be able to incorporate molecular markers to guide individualized therapy.

MENINGIOMAS

A mutation in the *NF2* gene, which is located on chromosome 22q12, has been closely associated with meningiomas. Germline mutations of this gene result in autosomal dominant neurofibromatosis type 2, a disorder that can manifest as multiple meningiomas, schwannomas, gliomas, and intracranial calcifications (66). Mutations of the *NF2* gene have also been detected in as many as 60% of sporadic meningiomas (67). How mer-

lin, the product of the *NF2* gene, functions as a tumor suppressor gene is, however, unclear. Merlin is a member of a family of cytoskeleton-associated proteins linked to receptor tyrosine kinase activity and ECM interactions (68). Merlin has also been reported to stabilize *p53* by inhibiting *MDM2*-mediated degradation of *p53* (69).

Cytogenetic alterations have similarly been described in higher-grade meningiomas. Atypical meningioma has been associated with chromosomal losses of 1p, 6q, 10q, 14q, and 18q and gains of 1q, 9q, 12q, 15q, 17q, and 20q. Malignant meningioma has been associated with these changes as well as losses of *9p*, rare mutations of *p53* and *PTEN,* and rare deletions of *CDKN2A* (70).

Several oncogenes and growth factor receptors have been identified in meningiomas. The oncogenes include *c-myc, n-myc, IGF-I,* and *IGF-II.* The growth factor receptors include EGF, interferon-α, PDGF-β, progesterone, somatostatin, and androgens (71). Meningiomas are sometimes associated with significant edema, which is unusual for a slow-growing tumor. This edema has been linked to the direct production of vascular endothelial growth factor (VEGF) by the tumor (72). EGF and basic fibroblast growth factor (bFGF) can induce VEGF secretion by meningioma cells, whereas the corticosteroid dexamethasone decreases VEGF secretion (73) and is often prescribed for patients with edema-causing brain tumors.

BRAIN METASTASES

The development of brain metastases is an intricate sequential process (74). In addition to proliferating, tumor cells must migrate and enter the systemic circulation, survive, be transported through the blood to the brain, adhere to and extravasate through the endothelium, invade the brain parenchyma, and proliferate, which requires the recruitment of a secondary blood supply. Failure at any of these steps will halt the metastatic process (75–77). Each of these steps requires complex interactions between the tumor cell and its changing microenvironment. The location of tumor metastases is not random and involves the interface between the tumor cell and tissue in a process that has been characterized as the "seed and soil" hypothesis, described by Stephen Paget more than 100 years ago (78–80). The primary tumor is regarded as biologically and molecularly heterogeneous, subject to a biological imperative favoring the selection of tumor cells that can survive the arduous process required for metastasis, i.e., the "seed." Experimentally, metastases arising from the same primary tumor can have different clonal origins and be traced back to different single cells (81). The local environment of the tumor cell greatly affects its success in proliferating and recruiting an adequate blood supply through angiogenesis, i.e., the "soil." The properties that allow success in producing tumor metastases are unrelated to the proliferative capacity of the cells at the primary site. In clinical practice, this is seen when distant metastases develop in the context of good local response of the tumor to treatment (82). The discovery of unique molecules expressed on endothelial cells that allow preferential targeting of tumor cells may also contribute to conditions that facilitate tumor metastases (83,84).

An understanding of the biological processes of brain metastases and the role of the BBB provides potential targets for intervention to improve treatment. There are multiple complex regulators of cell adhesion, including molecules such as integrins, cadherins, selectins, and heparin sulfate proteoglycans (82). Additionally, integrins can recruit intracellular signaling molecules such as focal adhesion kinase and src, which can lead to a cascade of cellular signaling that affects cell cycle control and proliferation (85,86). Integrins also play a part in regulating angiogenesis and tumor invasion (87). Other molecules that mediate invasion include the MMP family, serine proteases, and heparinase. The MMPs are proenzymes that degrade the ECM and basement membrane, promoting tumor invasion. The gelatinases (MMP-2 and MMP-9) are thought to have especially important roles in brain tumor invasion (88). Heparinase is an enzyme that degrades heparin sulfate chains, which are important components of the basement membrane (89), and heparinase activity has been detected in melanoma cells derived from brain metastasis (90). Tumor cells must generate their own blood supply if they are to grow successfully and remain viable. The regulation of such angiogenesis is influenced both by activators and inhibitors, which can be expressed either by tumor cells or other cells in the tumor's microenvironment. Important activators of angiogenesis include VEGF, angiopoietin, hypoxia-inducible transcription factor (HIF), cyclooxygenase 2 (COX 2), PDGF, integrins, MMPs, and others. Important inhibitors of angiogenesis include angiostatin, endostatin, tissue inhibitors of matrix metalloproteinases (TIMPs), interferons, and platelet factor 4 (91). Upregulation of activators or downregulation of inhibitors favor angiogenesis. As tumors grow, they begin to produce increasing numbers of angiogenic molecules that can participate in metastasis (91). Because a multitude of pathways are involved in tumor growth and invasion, it is likely that if one pathway is inhibited, cells may escape through alternate pathways.

The BBB is formed by tight junctions and nonfenestrated endothelial cells. The brain lacks lymphatic drainage and depends on the BBB to filter and block the entrance of macromolecules and invasion by microorganisms (92). Effective drug delivery through the BBB to tumor cells is a significant obstacle to chemotherapy, both for brain metastases and primary brain tumors. The blockade to charged hydrophilic molecules created by the BBB is passive, but it is also augmented by active transport from P-glycoprotein, which is expressed at high levels in the brain's endothelium (93). The P-glycoprotein family of transporters actively exports drugs such as anthracyclins, *Vinca* alkaloids, taxanes, and etoposide (94). The integrity of the BBB also depends on dynamic interactions between endothelial cells with astrocytes and oligodendrocytes (79,95).

The BBB can be breached by circulating cancer metastasis cells, a process that has been duplicated experimentally by direct carotid artery injection of tumor cell lines into nude mice (96). The selected tumor cells migrate across the BBB without degrading its permeability and proliferate. Once the tumor reaches a size that requires recruitment of new vessels, the BBB is disrupted, which allows imaging of brain tumors with contrast agents. In experimental models, brain metastases smaller than 0.25 mm in diameter are associated with an intact BBB, whereas larger tumors demonstrate BBB permeability (79). Despite the presence of the BBB, studies of drug levels in brain tumors from systemic delivery administered before surgery demonstrate pharmacologically relevant concentrations of drugs (97,98). Decreasing amounts of drug reach the tumor periphery and adjacent brain in animals, and comparatively lower drug levels are achieved in brain tumors compared to levels in subcutaneously implanted tumors (99). Measurements of drug levels in cerebrospinal fluid are not accurate indicators of tissue drug levels in tumor metastases and should not be assumed to predict activity (100).

■ CLINICAL PRESENTATION AND DIAGNOSIS

CLINICAL PRESENTATION (Figs. 30-3 to 30-10)

Brain tumors are usually diagnosed on presentation with symptoms such as seizure, headache, or focal neurologic deficits. High-grade, malignant tumors typically present with headache, which reflects elevated intracranial pressure, and focal neurologic signs, such as weakness or aphasia. Low-grade glial tumors often come to attention with seizure, while other slow-growing tumors, such as meningioma, may be clinically silent and incidentally detected during imaging for an unrelated problem. Contrast-enhanced MRI is the diagnostic standard for brain tumor imaging. In addition to its superior sensitivity, MRI provides more detailed anatomic as well as physiologic information that can contribute to a differential diagnosis. While contrast-enhanced CT is able to detect high-grade lesions that cause BBB breakdown, low-grade lesions may be detectable only on MRI, using sequences sensitive for edema and tissue changes (101). However, even in the case of known systemic primary cancer, contrast-enhanced CT may miss small foci of metastatic disease that are visible on MRI.

The brain tumor imaging characteristics seen in MRI are helpful in making a diagnosis. However, confirmation of the diagnosis with tissue pathology is necessary in nearly all cases. Noncancerous brain lesions that have been mistaken for malignancy include infection, demyelinating disease, vascular malformations, and stroke. A particular variant of brain demyelinating disease is known for having imaging characteristics resembling those of a malignant brain tumor (102). Unfortunately, some of these lesions have been irradiated, under the presumptive diagnosis of GBM, which only increases the severity of the demyelinating disease (103). Conversely, patients with primary brain tumors are sometimes initially diagnosed with stroke or demyelinating disease. Further complicating the picture are patients who have brain tumors in addition to stroke, which is far more prevalent with increasing age. Patients with systemic cancer, often in remission, or a stable condition, can present with brain lesions that are suspected to be brain metastases but turn out to be a second primary brain tumor. These types of cases often benefit from an interpretation by a specialized neuroradiologist who has been provided with a relevant patient history. A history of immunosuppression and multiple subcortical enhancing lesions may prompt the suspicion of a primary CNS lymphoma or infection with toxoplasmosis. In this case, further workup with brain thallium single photon emission computed tomography (SPECT) scanning or fluorodeoxyglucose positron-emission tomography (FDG-PET) imaging may serve to distinguish between these two possibilities.

There are several classic radiographic appearances of brain tumors that suggest malignancy. An irregular enhancing lesion with extensive edema following white matter pathways indicates a malignant glioma. Non-contrast-enhancing lesions with increased diffuse signals on FLAIR imaging suggest a low-grade astrocytoma. As a general rule for glial tumors, the presence of contrast enhancement suggests a high-grade malignancy. WHO grade IV tumors nearly always enhance, as opposed to grade II tumors, which are nonenhancing. Two notable exceptions to this guideline include pilocytic astrocytoma (WHO grade I) and pleomorphic xanthoastrocytoma (WHO grade II), which typically have an enhancing nodule and associated cyst. Meningiomas are typically homogeneously enhancing dural-based lesions, associated with calcification. The appearance of multiple enhancing subcortical lesions with a homogeneous enhancement suggests primary CNS lymphoma. However, the same lesions, if associated with a known primary malignancy, may indicate brain metastases.

DIAGNOSIS

The discovery of a brain lesion should prompt referral to a neurosurgeon for consideration of biopsy or resection. The management of brain tumors is crucially dependent on definitive pathology for diagnosis. Our institution insists on reviewing patient diagnostic slides prior to rendering a treatment recommendation, and it is not uncommon for our neuropathologists to disagree with the diagnosis provided by the referring physician. A referral to a specialized neuropathologist may be necessary for diagnosis of uncommon or rare tumors and also in cases where there is only limited biopsy tissue

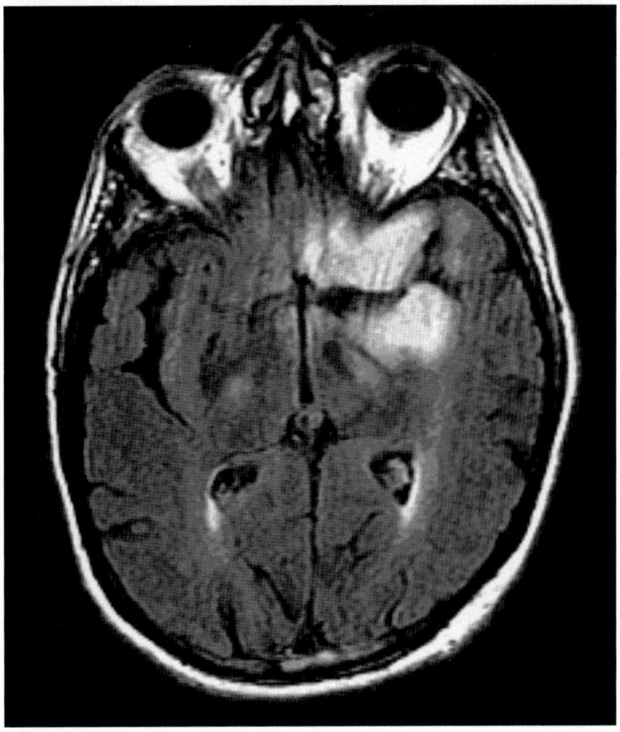

FIGURE 30-3 Low-grade glioma.

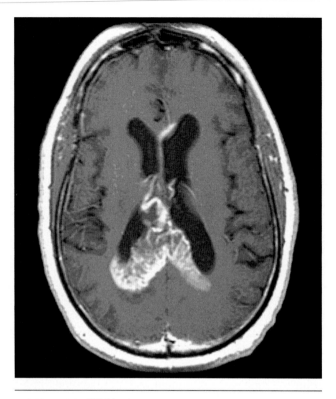

FIGURE 30-4 Glioblastoma.

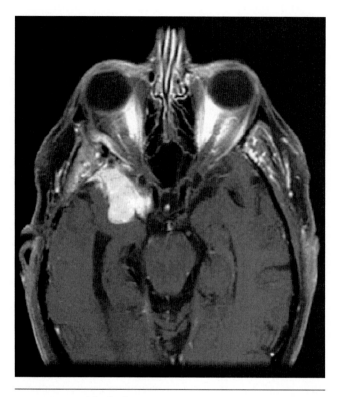

FIGURE 30-6 Meningioma.

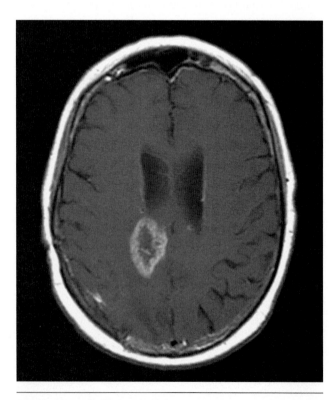

FIGURE 30-5 Radiation necrosis.

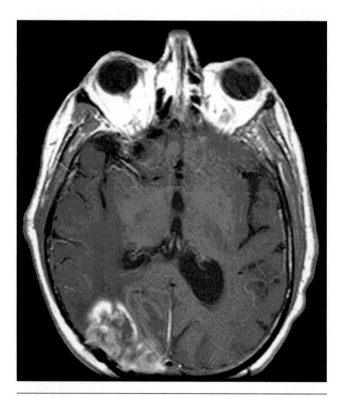

FIGURE 30-7 Malignant meningioma.

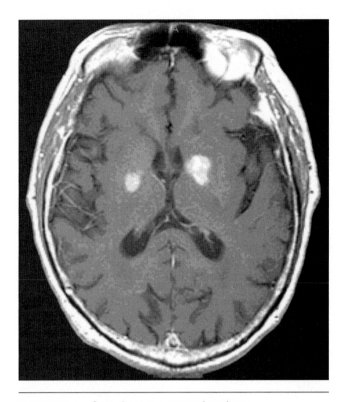

FIGURE 30-8   Central nervous system lymphoma.

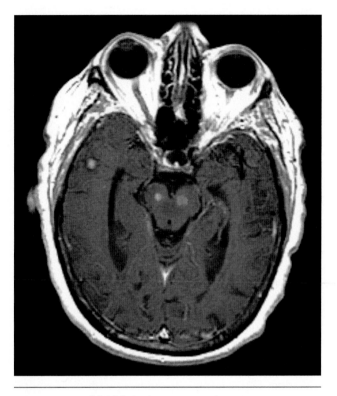

FIGURE 30-10   Multiple brain metastases, breast.

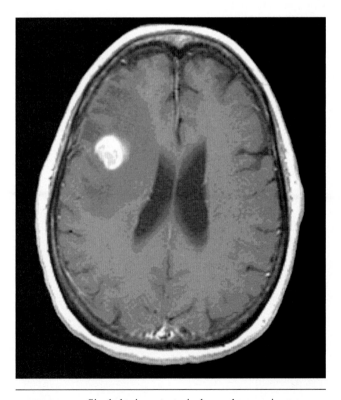

FIGURE 30-9   Single brain metastasis, lung adenocarcinoma.

available. Biopsies must be of adequate quality and be representative of the overall tumor to allow accurate diagnosis. Primary brain glial tumors are graded according to the most malignant portion of the tumor. A brain lesion that is predominantly grade III astrocytoma but has a few regions that meet the criteria for grade IV astrocytoma (GBM) is graded as a GBM. The tumor grade may be underestimated if the most malignant portion of the tumor is not sampled. Typically the most malignant region corresponds to an area of contrast enhancement. In the case of a non-contrast-enhancing tumor, the biopsy may be guided by MR spectroscopy or PET imaging (104). Clinically, this issue is critical in assessing a purported grade II astrocytoma in a patient who, because of his or her age, is more likely to have a grade III astrocytoma. With the former diagnosis, the patient might be followed by observation, whereas for the latter, the patient would require maximal resection, radiation therapy, and chemotherapy. If a patient is suspected of having primary CNS lymphoma, the use of corticosteroids should be avoided. Primary CNS lymphoma can be quite sensitive to steroids during initial presentation, and the preoperative use of even small doses of corti-

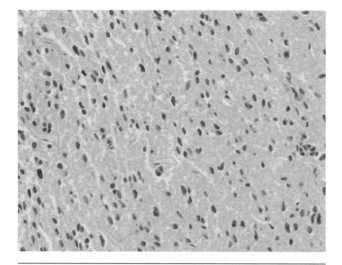

FIGURE 30-11 Low-grade astrocytoma, WHO grade II (×200). (*Pathology slides courtesy of Dr. Gregory N. Fuller.*)

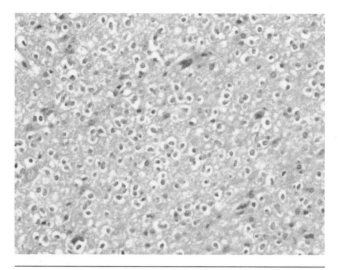

FIGURE 30-13 Oligodendroglioma, WHO grade II (×200).

costeroids can lead to a nondiagnostic biopsy. These patients usually require repeat biopsy after steroid discontinuation. Patients may also present with deep central lesions involving the brainstem or thalamus. These cases may require referral to a specialized neurosurgical center to evaluate whether open biopsy, resection, or stereotactic-guided biopsy is appropriate. In these cases close coordination with a department of neuropathology will be critical in obtaining adequate tissue for diagnosis.

Diffuse astrocytomas are characterized by well-differentiated astrocytes—either fibrillary, gemistocytic, or rarely protoplasmic—with mildly increased cellularity. The cellular morphology of the tumor cells may dif-

fer within the same tumor sample and show great variability between tumors. Necrosis and microvascular proliferation are absent. Rare mitotic figures may occur and nuclear atypia may be present, but not sufficiently to characterize the tumor as anaplastic astrocytoma. The typical MIB-1 labeling index is less than 4%. (See Figs. 30-11, 30-12.)

Oligodendrogliomas are characterized by moderately cellular tumor cells with rounded, homogenous nuclei, giving a "fried egg" artifactual appearance in fixed sections. Microcalcifications, microcyst formation, extracellular mucin deposition, and a dense network of branching capillaries are other oligodendroglioma features. Nuclear atypia may be seen, but significant mitotic activity or

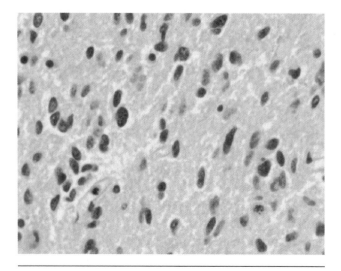

FIGURE 30-12 Low-grade astrocytoma, WHO grade II (×400). (*Pathology slides courtesy of Dr. Gregory N. Fuller.*)

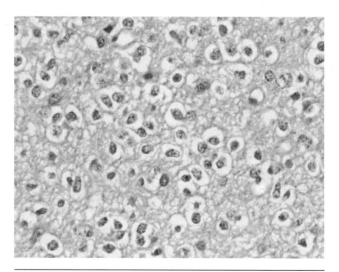

FIGURE 30-14 Oligodendroglioma, WHO grade II (×400).

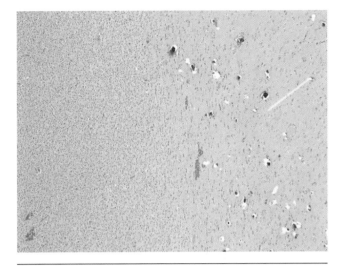

FIGURE 30-15 Anaplastic oligodendroglioma, WHO grade III (×40).

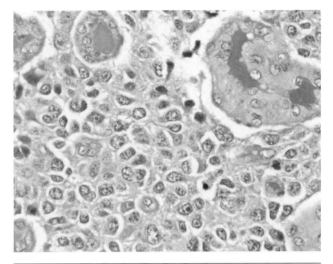

FIGURE 30-17 Anaplastic oligodendroglioma, WHO grade III (×400).

microvascular proliferation is suggestive of an anaplastic tumor. The MIB-1 index is typically less than 5%. (See Figs. 30-13 and 30-14.)

Anaplastic oligodendrogliomas are characterized by oligodendroglial cells, with signs of increased cellularity, nuclear atypia, and mitotic activity. Cellular pleomorphism may be present, with formation of multinucleated giant cells or spindle cells. Gliofibrillary oligodendrocytes and minigemistocytes are common. Although microvascular proliferation and necrosis may be present, their presence does not change the diagnosis to GBM. There is currently no designation for a WHO grade IV oligodendroglioma. The MIB-1 ratio is usually greater than 5%. (See Figs. 30-15 to 30-17.)

Anaplastic astrocytoma is characterized by diffusely infiltrating astrocytes with increased cellularity, nuclear atypia, and mitotic activity. They are more cellular than low-grade astrocytomas, and the nuclear atypia include formation of nuclear inclusions, multinucleated cells, and abnormal mitoses. Microvascular proliferation is absent; if present, it would upgrade the tumor to GBM. Previous classifications distinguished the presence of necrosis as a hallmark of GBM. Currently, microvascular proliferation is a sufficient criterion, so an anaplastic astrocytoma with necrosis is as valid a characterization as GBM without necrosis. The typical MIB-1 labeling index ranges from 5 to 10% and can occasionally overlap with index values

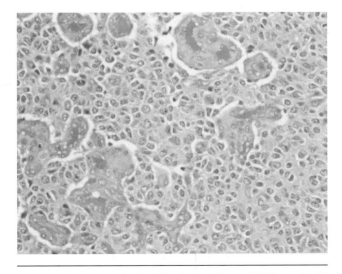

FIGURE 30-16 Anaplastic oligodendroglioma, WHO grade III (×200).

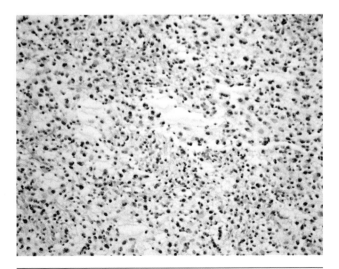

FIGURE 30-18 Anaplastic astrocytoma, WHO grade III (×100).

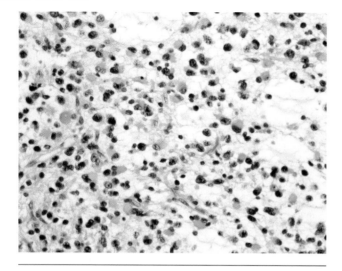

FIGURE 30-19   Anaplastic astrocytoma, WHO grade III (×200).

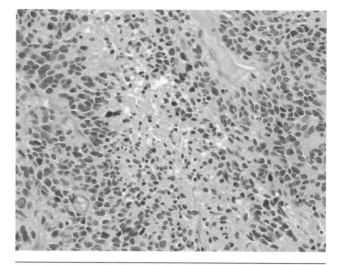

FIGURE 30-21   Glioblastoma, WHO grade IV (×200).

for low-grade astrocytoma and GBM. (See Figs. 30-17 to 30-19.)

Glioblastoma is an anaplastic cellular tumor with marked nuclear atypia and mitotic activity, often with marked regional heterogeneity and cellular polymorphism. Microvascular proliferation and often necrosis differentiate this lesion from anaplastic astrocytoma. Other features associated with GBM include formation of epithelial "adenoid" structures, multinucleated giant cells, granular cells, lipidized cells, perivascular lymphocytes, and metaplasia. Glioblastoma is associated with a high proliferative rate, and MIB-1 labeling typically ranges from 15 to 20%. (See Figs. 30-20 to 30-22.)

Meningiomas can have a wide range of appearances and are subtyped according to their appearance. The transitional variant has numerous concentric "onion-

bulb" structures. The psammomatous variant has calcified psammoma bodies. Pleomorphic nuclei and occasional mitoses are allowed, although four or more mitoses per 10 high-power fields would qualify in diagnosing atypical meningioma.(See Figs. 30-23 and 30-24).

■ TREATMENT AND PROGNOSIS

LOW-GRADE GLIOMA

Diffuse astrocytomas are disseminated, infiltrative low-grade brain tumors. Their peak incidence is in the third decade, followed by the second decade. Ten percent of diffuse astrocytomas occur in patients younger than 20 years of age and 30% in patients older than 45. Overall, these low-grade tumors represent 4% of glial tumors.

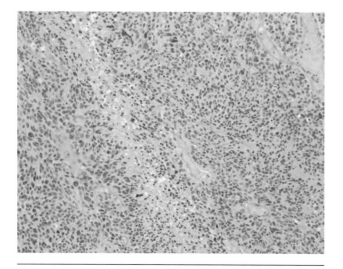

FIGURE 30-20   Glioblastoma, WHO grade IV (×100).

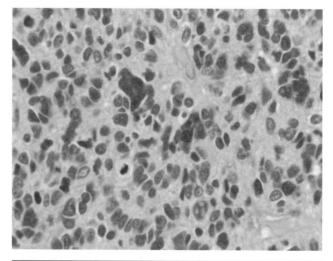

FIGURE 30-22   Glioblastoma, WHO grade IV (×400).

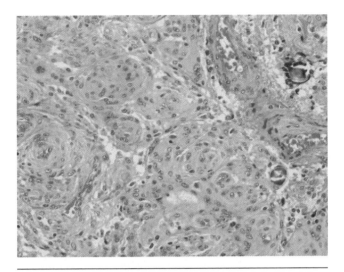

FIGURE 30-23 Meningioma ($\times$100).

Although these tumors are considered benign compared with malignant astrocytoma, they are still lethal. The median survival time of patients with diffuse astrocytoma is between 5 and 8 years (105). Variation in length of survival depends on patient age, performance status at diagnosis, and total versus partial tumor resection (106–108).

Oligodendroglioma is a diffusely infiltrative, well-differentiated tumor composed of oligodendrocytes. These tumors comprise 3 to 4% of all primary brain tumors and approximately 7% of glial tumors, with an incidence of 0.3 per 100,000 per year. The peak incidence is from the ages of 30 to 50. Children can be affected and represent approximately 6% of all patients with oligodendrogliomas. Tumors with pure oligodendroglioma differentiation behave more indolently than

astrocytomas. Oligodendrogliomas appear to be more sensitive to both chemotherapy and radiation therapy than astrocytomas, and the benefit from these therapies is more pronounced and durable. Median survival ranges from 4 to 12 years, and both oligodendroglioma and oligoastrocytoma have been included in the reported data (105).

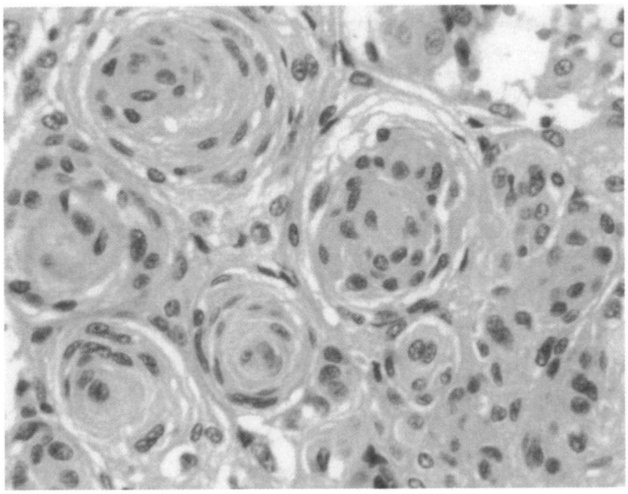

Oligoastrocytoma is a mixed tumor composed of cells that resemble both oligodendroglioma and diffuse astrocytoma. Based on only a few cytogenetic studies, these tumors are thought to be of monoclonal origin (109). Clinically, these tumors present in a similar fashion to other low-grade glial tumors, which are best imaged with MRI and have imaging characteristics that indicate a diffuse, nonenhancing tumor. There has been no demonstration of a better prognosis with an increased proportion of the oligodendroglioma component. Treatment is similar to that for other low-grade glial tumors. Median survival ranges from 3 to 6 years. In general, these mixed tumors behave more aggressively than pure oligodendrogliomas but are possibly less malignant than pure astrocytomas (110).

CLINICAL MANAGEMENT

Once a diagnosis of low-grade glioma is suspected, it is typical to probe this diagnosis with biopsy or resection so as to differentiate between a low-grade glioma and a nonenhancing anaplastic glioma (Tables 30-2 and 30-3).

In cases where gross total resection or a major resection is possible without significant morbidity, neuro-oncologists generally recommend a complete resection, which may obviate the need for irradiation and decrease the risk of malignant transformation from residual tumor cells. It has been shown in multiple retrospective series that a total resection of nonenhancing tumor improves survival (105), and a volumetric analysis of the preoperative tumor in addition to analysis of postoperative residual tumor showed a correlation with time to recurrence and the likelihood of malignant transformation (111). There are several low-grade tumors—such as pilocytic astrocytoma, ependymoma and subependy-

TABLE 30-2	INITIAL BRAIN TUMOR WORKUP

Contrast-enhanced MRI or MR spectroscopy may be helpful to diagnose nonenhancing tumors

Referral to neurosurgery for resection vs. biopsy for tissue diagnosis

Confirmation of pathology with second opinion

Postoperative MRI taken within 3 days of surgery

FIGURE 30-24 Meningioma ($\times$200).

MRI = magnetic resonance imaging.

TABLE 30-3	STAGING BY TUMOR TYPE
Astrocytoma, oligodendroglioma, anaplastic astrocytoma	
Anaplastic oligodendroglioma, glioblastoma	
MRI brain (with and without contrast)	
MRI spine (with and without contrast) only if patient is symptomatic	
Primary CNS lymphoma	
MRI brain and spine (with and without contrast)	
Lumbar puncture	
Ophthalmology evaluation including slit-lamp examination	
CT chest/abdomen/pelvis	

CNS = central nervous system; CT = computed tomography; MRI = magnetic resonance imaging.

moma, pleomorphic xanthoastrocytoma, ganglioglioma, and dysembryoplastic neuroepithelial tumor—that may be definitively treated by complete surgical resection alone. These patients may benefit from treatment at a specialized neurosurgical center that treats a large volume of brain tumors (Table 30-4).

In cases where a complete resection is not recommended, therapeutic options range from observation to treatment with focal brain irradiation. Older studies of low-grade astrocytomas suggested that irradiation improved survival. The 5-year survival rates ranged from 49% to 68% for irradiated tumors compared with 32% for nonirradiated tumors (112). However, an interim analysis has been published, with the preliminary results from a large prospective randomized trial of patients with low-grade glioma (290 patients) who were randomized to either upfront radiotherapy (54 Gy in 6 weeks) or delayed radiation therapy at progression. The

TABLE 30-4	MANAGEMENT OF LOW-GRADE GLIOMAS
Confirmation of diagnosis with biopsy is preferred, although observation is acceptable with close follow-up.	
Option for complete resection should be considered.	
Options after diagnosis include observation (especially if patient is at high risk for treatment morbidity) or treatment (especially if patient is symptomatic).	
Radiation therapy is the current standard of treatment (focal brain irradiation to 54 Gy), although the role of chemotherapy is being investigated.	
Formal serial neuropsychological testing is helpful in assessing cognitive function.	
Consider use of psychostimulants to improve cognitive function and quality of life.	
Consider biopsy/resection of progressive tumor to confirm diagnosis and consider same salvage regimens as for malignant glioma.	

patients were randomized and stratified to control for institution, tumor pathology, and amount of resection. The patients treated with radiation therapy had an improved time to progression (44% versus 37% in 5-year PFS) but not overall survival (63% versus 66% in 5-year overall survival) (113). The use of these data as a guide suggests that it is acceptable to delay radiation therapy until there are signs of tumor progression, especially for asymptomatic patients or patients who have had a complete tumor resection.

Patients with low-grade glioma should be carefully assessed to determine whether their symptoms are caused by the tumor. Formal neuropsychological testing may reveal cognitive deficits that are not apparent in the simple mental status screening used for dementia. In addition, these tests can be repeated to detect subtle cognitive decline, which may lead to a decision to alter a prescribed therapy. Patients who are symptomatic from their tumor from seizures, altered mental status due to tumor bulk or location, or who have other focal neurologic signs would be expected to improve with treatment of the tumor. Although there are concerns about the long-term effects of brain irradiation, radiation therapy is the current treatment standard (114). The dose of radiotherapy currently used by the Radiation Therapy Oncology Group (RTOG) for low-grade glioma is 54 Gy to localized treatment fields as defined by the tumor's appearance on T2-weighted MRI and including a 2-cm margin. A large European trial involving 379 patients with low-grade glioma did not demonstrate a benefit for higher radiation dose when comparing 45 Gy with 59.4 Gy (115). A second prospective study that randomized 203 patients with low-grade glioma to radiation therapy with either 50.4 or 64.8 Gy found a slightly lower survival (64% versus 72% at 5 years) and higher incidence of radiation necrosis in the group receiving the higher dose of 64.8 Gy (116).

Much less is known about the usefulness of chemotherapy for low-grade tumors. A small study of patients with incompletely resected tumors randomized to radiotherapy alone or radiotherapy with CCNU (lomustine) demonstrated a median survival time of 4.5 years with no difference between the two treatment arms (117). A RTOG trial (RTOG 98-02) that randomized patients with low-grade glioma and a high risk of recurrence (age ≥40 or subtotal resection/biopsy) to either radiation therapy alone or radiation therapy followed by six cycles of procarbazine, CCNU, and vincristine (PCV) was closed to accrual in 2002 and continues with followup. The usefulness of chemotherapy as an initial treatment for patients with low-grade gliomas is unproven (118). The rationale for using chemotherapy as an alternative to radiation therapy for these patients is that although radiation therapy has a proven record of treatment response, it does not improve survival and may be associated with the significant long-term side effect of cognitive decline. It is hoped that chemotherapy will delay the need for radiation therapy without reducing treatment efficacy or survival (119). Several limited studies have demonstrated an encouraging radiographic response by low-grade gliomas (primarily oligoden-drogliomas but also astrocytomas) after treatment with temozolomide and PCV (65,120–124). Patients who have residual tumor and would be at a high risk of cognitive side effects from radiation therapy may benefit from this strategy; however, there are no results from prospective randomized studies to recommend it. Patients with oligodendroglioma or oligoastrocytoma may be more attractive candidates for applying this strategy as they tend to have higher response rates to chemotherapy than patients with astrocytoma. The cytogenetic analysis of the tumor sample for LOH at 1p and 19q may predict patients who might benefit from this strategy.

The etiology of cognitive decline in primary brain tumor patients is multifactorial. The causes include direct tumor effects from invasion and destruction as well as side effects from radiation therapy, chemotherapy, and anticonvulsants (114). We have found the use of psycho-stimulants such as methylphenidate to be helpful in improving cognitive function, mood, and fatigue (125).

■ MALIGNANT GLIOMAS—
GRADES III AND IV

The survival of patients who have primary malignant brain tumors is unsatisfactory; it is particularly dismal for those with WHO grade IV tumors. The National Cancer Institute Surveillance, Epidemiology, and End Results (SEER) program reported a 32% 5-year survival from 1992 to 1998. These data include survival statistics for both WHO grade III and grade IV tumors (126). The median survival of patients with GBM, the most common primary glioma, has remained at approximately 12 months in recent clinical trials (127–129).

ANAPLASTIC OLIGODENDROGLIOMA

Anaplastic oligodendrogliomas comprise between 20% to 50% of all oligodendroglial tumors, approximately 5% of anaplastic tumors, and between 20% and 50% of all oligodendroglial tumors. The peak incidence is between ages 40 and 50. The clinical presentation of these tumors is similar to that of other anaplastic tumors, with focal neurologic signs, seizures, or symptoms of increased intracranial pressure. These lesions, which are usually contrast-enhancing, can show calcification on CT scans as well as cystic structures, necrosis, and hemorrhage. The standard therapy for anaplastic oligoden-droglioma does not significantly differ from that used for other anaplastic gliomas (WHO grade III). Initial therapy is surgery, with the goal of gross total resection, followed by radiation therapy. Anaplastic oligodendroglioma is more responsive to chemotherapy than anaplastic astrocytoma. Adjuvant chemotherapy is recommended, with PCV being the most studied regimen. However, due to a more favorable toxicity profile, temozolomide is increasingly being used, although prospective comparative data are not yet available for this type of tumor. Increasing evidence from multiple series suggests that analysis of cytogenetics predicts both survival and response to chemotherapy for patients with

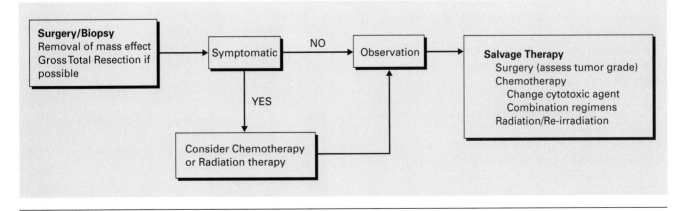

FIGURE 30-25 Treatment algorithm for low-grade glioma.

oligodendrogliomas and anaplastic oligodendrogliomas. Cytogenetic analysis indicates that patients who have oligodendrogliomas with codeletion of 1p and 19q are more sensitive to PCV chemotherapy and have significantly longer survivals than those with tumors without this deletion (61,64). This finding has been extended to predictions of response to temozolomide for patients with low-grade oligodendroglioma and oligoastrocytoma (65). The data suggest that in addition to age and Karnofsky performance status (KPS), the cytogenetic profile is predictive of survival for patients with oligodendroglioma and anaplastic oligodendroglioma, and clinical trials should take these factors into account in assessing survival and treatment response. Despite initially high response rates, these tumors usually recur. Median survival for anaplastic oligodendroglioma treated with surgery, irradiation, and chemotherapy ranges from 3 to 5 years, although some patients survive past 10 years (110,130). Recurrent tumors are treated with salvage regimens similar to those used for anaplastic astrocytoma and GBM (Tables 30-5 and 30-6).

TABLE 30-5 | MANAGEMENT OF MALIGNANT GLIOMAS

Consider clinical trials at all stages, especially up front, adjuvant, and at relapse (especially at first or second recurrence).

Multidisciplinary approach is necessary for optimal outcome:
 Neurosurgery
 Neuro-oncology
 Radiation therapy
 Psychiatry
 Neuropsychology
 Rehabilitation
 Social work

Maximal resection when possible.

Standard conformal radiation therapy—chemoirradiation (temozolomide) for glioblastoma.

Adjuvant chemotherapy for both anaplastic glioma (temozolomide or nitrosourea regimens) and glioblastoma (temozolomide).

Avoid use of anticonvulsants that induce cytochrome P-450 3A4 metabolism when possible (Table 30-7).

Progressive disease
 Consider clinical trials.
 Consider surgical resection at relapse (especially to rule out radiation necrosis).
 Salvage chemotherapy agents include single-agent and combination regimens incorporating temozolomide, nitrosoureas, retinoic acid, irinotecan, and platinum agents.
 Consider stereotactic radiotherapy.

TABLE 30-6 | CHEMOTHERAPY REGIMENS FOR GLIOMAS

Temozolomide
 75 mg/m^2/day PO days 1–42 during radiotherapy
 200 mg/m^2/day PO days 1–5 (patients with no prior chemotherapy)
  or
 150 mg/m^2/day PO days 1–5 (patients with prior chemotherapy)
Temozolomide and CRA (repeat every 28 days)
 200 mg/m^2/day PO days 1–5 (patients with no prior chemotherapy)
  or
 150 mg/m^2/day PO days 1–5 (patients with prior chemotherapy)
  with
 13-*cis*-retinoic acid 100 mg/m^2/days 1–21
Temozolomide and irinotecan
 Temozolomide 150 mg/m^2/day PO days 1–5 (patients with prior chemotherapy)
  with
 Irinotecan 200 mg/m^2/day IV days 1 and 14
  or
 Irinotecan 450 mg/m^2/day IV days 1 and 14 (if the patient is on a cytochrome P-450–inducing anticonvulsant)
Irinotecan (repeat every 3 weeks)
 300–350 mg/m^2/day IV day 1
  or
 700–750 mg/m^2/day IV day 1 (if patient receiving cytochrome P-450–inducing anticonvulsant)
PCV (repeat every 6 weeks)
 Procarbazine
 60 mg/m^2/day PO days 8–21
 Lomustine
 110 mg/m^2/day PO day 1
 Vincristine
 1.4 mg/m^2/day IV days 8 and 29 (maximum dose = 2 mg)
Carmustine (repeat every 6 weeks)
 80 mg/m^2/day IV days 1–3
6-Thioguanine and carmustine (repeat every 6 weeks)
 6-Thioguanine
 80–100 mg/m^2 PO every 6 h for 12 doses
  followed by
 Carmustine
 80 mg/m^2/day IV days 1–3
TPCH (repeat every 6 weeks)
 6-Thioguanine
 80–100 mg/m^2 PO every 6 h for 12 doses, days 1–4
 Procarbazine
 70 mg/m^2 PO every 6 h for 6 doses, days 4–6
 Lomustine
 130 mg/m^2 PO 6 h after third procarbazine dose on day 5
 Hydroxyurea
 600 mg/m^2 PO every 6 h for 11 doses, days 5–8
 except at time of lomustine dosing
CRA (repeat every 28 days)
 13-*cis*-retinoic acid
 100 mg/m^2/day PO in two divided doses, days 1–21

ANAPLASTIC ASTROCYTOMA

Anaplastic astrocytomas are diffusely infiltrating with nuclear atypia and anaplasia as well as marked proliferation, features that distinguish them from low-grade astrocytomas. The highest incidence of this tumor is in the fourth decade, followed by the third decade, with nearly equal incidence rates in the second, fifth, and sixth decades. These tumors account for approximately 36% of all glial tumors and have an incidence in the range of 2 per 100,000 per year (4).

Patients with anaplastic astrocytoma can present with seizures but are more likely to show signs of increased intracranial pressure and focal neurologic deficits. Some patients have a history of prior low-grade astrocytoma. Brain imaging shows diffuse hypointense tumor on CT scans and T1-weighted MRI. There is usually more mass effect and edema compared with low-grade astrocytomas and contrast enhancement is typical. However, since these tumors can occasionally be nonenhancing, neuroimaging alone is not sufficient to distinguish these lesions from low-grade astrocytomas. The median survival for patients with anaplastic astrocytoma ranges from 3 to 5 years; an increased survival is seen when chemotherapy is used in addition to radiotherapy. Optimal initial management begins with surgery with the goal of gross total resection, both to provide adequate tissue for accurate analysis of pathology and to improve survival. Following surgery, limited-field radiation therapy to a target dose of 60 Gy is commonly recommended. The target radiation field typically includes the contrast-enhancing region of the tumor as well as the surrounding edema or nonenhancing tumor plus a 2-cm margin. This size of this field is often reduced after a 46-Gy dose has been applied to the contrast-enhancing lesion alone plus a 2-cm margin. Chemotherapy has been used during irradiation in an effort to improve radiation sensitivity and efficacy. Hydroxyurea and bromodeoxyuridine have been used safely, but there is no randomized trial demonstrating benefit with this strategy compared to chemotherapy following standard radiation. Clinical trials using alternate radiation schemes of hyperfractionation or accelerated fractionation have not demonstrated an increased survival benefit over conventional fractionated conformal radiation therapy (130,131). Adjuvant chemotherapy following radiation therapy increases time to progression and survival. Standard agents include combination therapy composed of procarbazine/lomustine/vincristine (PCV) or another nitrosourea-based regimen of 6-thioguanine/bischloroethylnitrosourea (6TG +BCNU) (see Table 30-6). Temozolomide is the newest alkylating agent to show promising activity against anaplastic astrocytoma and GBM (127,132). Delivered via an oral route, it is better tolerated by patients than procarbazine. Temozolomide is approved for anaplastic astrocytoma in the United States and in Europe for GBM. Studies using this agent concurrently with radiation therapy, as well as in an adjuvant setting, are under way.

Patients with recurrent anaplastic astrocytoma should be considered for clinical trials. Surgical resection should also be considered to provide a palliative benefit, relieve

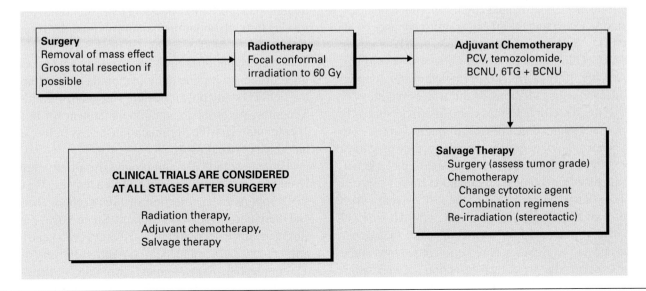

FIGURE 30-26   Treatment algorithm for anaplastic astrocytoma.

mass effect, and allow dose reduction of steroids, and confirm histology. The recurrent tumor may actually have progressed to GBM from anaplastic astrocytoma, and such patients are often eligible for a wider array of clinical trials than are available for recurrent anaplastic astrocytoma. Recent clinical trials have used temolozomide in combination with agents such as IFN-α, *cis*-retinoic acid, metalloproteinase inhibitors, carmustine, irinotecan, and thalidomide (133–135). Other agents that have been used for recurrent anaplastic astrocytoma include tamoxifen, carboplatin, etoposide, irinotecan, and combination chemotherapy. Stereotactic radiosurgery for recurrent tumors can also provide benefit if recurrence is local and if it can be targeted to limit dosage to the often previously irradiated tissue. (See Fig. 30-26.)

GLIOBLASTOMA

Glioblastoma is the most common and most malignant glial tumor of the brain and comprises approximately 50% of all glial tumors, with an incidence of approximately 2 to 3 per 100,000 per year (4). Glioblastomas are characterized by poorly differentiated astrocytes with cellular polymorphism, nuclear atypia, microvascular proliferation, and necrosis. The peak incidence is in the fifth decade, followed by the sixth and fourth decades. Glioblastoma is rare in children and young adults (4,136). Clinically, these tumors often present with signs of increased intracranial pressure such as headache. They also present with focal neurologic symptoms such as hemiparesis and aphasia, often with a short history of symptoms. Seizures are common. Imaging with CT or MRI usually reveals a contrast-enhancing lesion with irregular borders, frequently with a necrotic center. Vasogenic edema and nonenhancing tumor often surround the area of contrast enhancement, which is best seen on T2-weighted or FLAIR imaging on MRI. Glioblastomas commonly spread through white matter tracts across the corpus callosum, internal capsule, and optic radiations. Multifocal lesions are possible. If these multiple lesions truly arise independently as opposed to spreading diffusely through tracts that are not visualized by imaging or pathology, they may have a polyclonal origin. Glioblastoma is extremely lethal. Despite extensive clinical research, the rate of survival has not changed greatly during the last 20 years. Median survival is 9 to 14 months with a 5-year survival rate of approximately 3% (5). Prognostic factors include age and KPS. Surgical resection has shown some benefit, especially gross total resection (of enhancing tumor) or when 90% or more of the tumor is removed (137). There are also intriguing data indicating that the

volume of residual GBM tumor may correlate with subsequent response to chemotherapy, with a higher likelihood of response if the residual tumor volume is less than 10 cm^3 (138).

The current standard therapy for GBM is changing. The recent report of a large prospective randomized phase III trial from the EORTC supports the use of concurrent chemotherapy with temozolomide, with standard conformal radiotherapy followed by adjuvant temozolomide (139,140). This trial randomized 573 patients from 85 centers to receive either standard radiotherapy (60 Gy in 30 daily fractions) or concurrent temozolomide (75 mg/m^2/day) with radiotherapy followed by adjuvant temozolomide for 6 months (150 to 200 mg/m^2/day for 5 days every 28 days). Patients who had progressive disease after radiotherapy were allowed salvage therapy and 56% received temozolomide. The group receiving concurrent and adjuvant temozolomide had a significant improvement in PFS (7.2 versus 5.0 months), median survival (15 versus 12 months), and 2-year survival (26% versus 8%). Both groups had similar age, KPS, and surgical resection rates. Previously, although investigators had suspected that adjuvant chemotherapy could be of benefit, no phase III trials supported this strategy.

Our center continues to strongly recommend patient participation in clinical trials, which enroll patients from initial resection to radiation therapy and salvage therapy at relapse. If the patient is not enrolled in an upfront trial, we recommend evaluation by our neurosurgery service to explore the prospect of gross total resection. It is not unusual for our patients to have resection of tumor following outside biopsy or subtotal resection procedures. Following resection, we are now treating patients with concurrent temozolomide (75 mg/m^2/day through radiation therapy) and standard conformal radiation therapy (59.4 Gy in 1.8-Gy fractions). Following radiation therapy, we use adjuvant temozolomide or temozolomide combination therapy. Although the EORTC study only used adjuvant temozolomide for 6 months, we typically continue treatment for at least 1 year, and occasionally much longer, given the lethal natural history of GBM.

Patients with GBM and progressive disease are offered salvage therapy if their KPS is adequate. We consider options from resection of tumor, chemotherapy, and stereotactic radiation therapy. Some novel neurosurgical clinical trials offer local therapy with gene therapy using *p53* (141) and local convection delivery of IL-13–conjugated *Pseudomonas* exotoxin (142). One advantage of reresection of progressive disease is to confirm pathology and specifically to determine whether the progressive enhancement on MRI represents tumor or radiation necrosis. MRI dynamic contrast imaging, MR spectroscopy, FDG-PET scanning, and brain SPECT thallium imaging sometimes help to distinguish between these two possibilities. However, all of these modalities have limited sensitivity and specificity, and sometimes the pathology reveals both treatment-related necrosis and foci of active tumor. Patients with pathology-confirmed radiation necrosis are often treated with steroids and antiplatelet agents or anticoagulation, whose putative value is based on anecdotal case reports (143). Hyperbaric oxygen therapy has also been reported to produce a radiologic response (144,145).

Chemotherapy for recurrent disease typically produces response rates that are less than 10% and a 6-month PFS of 15% (5). Response rates that include stable disease and complete or partial responses are 40% at best, but as the 6-month progression-free survival value indicates, these responses are not durable. It is hypothesized that the multiple mutations and alterations in glioblastoma and the heterogeneity of the tumor cell population may partially explain the striking resistance of these tumors to therapy. Younger patients respond best to chemotherapy, although responses to nitrosourea-based therapy can be seen in patients older than 60 years of age. Long-term survivors of GBM (over 5 years) have typically had gross total resection, radiation therapy to a dose of 60 Gy, and chemotherapy, generally with a nitrosourea or other alkylating agent.

Salvage agents used for malignant glioma are identical to those used for recurrent anaplastic astrocytoma (see Table 30-6). After treatment failure with nitrosourea-based therapy (PCV, 6TG, and BCNU) and alkylating agents (temozolomide), switching to a biologic agent such as high-dose *cis*-retinoic acid may be helpful, especially as it does not cause myelosuppression (146). Other active agents include irinotecan (147), carboplatin, and etoposide (148). Clinical trials targeting angiogenesis are also under way, with the use of interferon, thalidomide, and epidermal growth factor–receptor tyrosine kinase antagonists, and integrin receptor

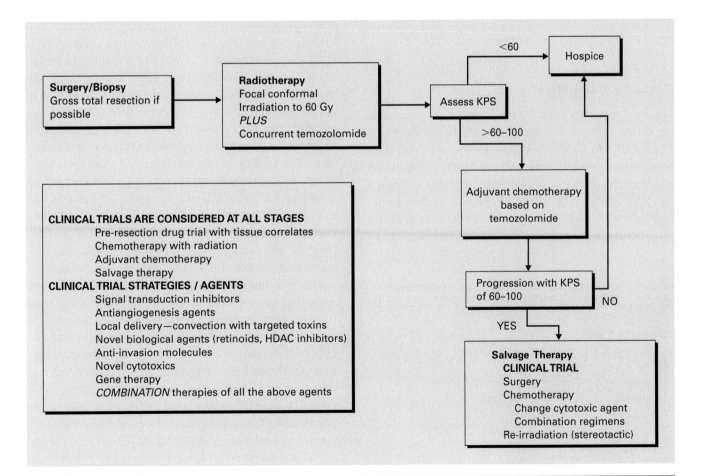

FIGURE 30-27 Treatment algorithm for glioblastoma.

antagonists. In general, many of these targeted therapies demonstrated only limited activity as single agents and efforts are under way to combine them with cytotoxic therapy (149,150). Other cellular pathways being investigated with small-molecule inhibitors include the *ras* pathway with farnesyl-transferase inhibitors and the PI3Kinase pathway with *mTOR* inhibitors. Other novel approaches to malignant brain tumor therapy include use of oncolytic adenovirus, vaccine and dendritic cell immunotherapy, and histone deacetylase inhibitors. (See Fig. 30-27.)

An important reaction has been discovered from the interaction between anticonvulsants that induce the hepatic cytochrome P-450 3A4 enzyme and other chemotherapy agents also metabolized by this same enzyme. Pharmacokinetic studies of patients with malignant glioma on single-agent irinotecan and sirolimus found significantly lower levels of active drug in patients on enzyme-inducing anticonvulsant drugs (151,152). In a phase I trial of irinotecan administered every 3 weeks, the recommended dose for patients not on enzyme-inducing agents was 350 mg/m^2, whereas the dose for patients on enzyme-inducing agents was 750 mg/m^2. We recommend that brain tumor patients on chemotherapy avoid use of anticonvulsants that induce the expression of the P-450 3A4 enzyme when possible (Table 30-7).

SEIZURE CONTROL

The management of seizures in brain tumor patients is important in order to improve patient functioning and quality of life. A degeneration of seizure control in brain tumor patients may indicate tumor progression and worsening edema. However, it may also indicate a systemic infection or a drug interaction leading to decreased anticonvulsant drug levels. In the case of tumor progression, a reduction in the amount of brain edema

TABLE 30-7	CYTOCHROME P-450 3A4-INDUCING AGENTS (ANTICONVULSANTS IN RED)
Carbamazepine	Phenytoin
Dexamethasone	Primidone
Ethosuximide	Progesterone
Glucocorticoids	Rifabutin
Griseofulvin	Rifampin
Nafcillin	Rofecoxib (mild)
Nelfinavir	St John's wort
Nevirapine	Sulfadimidine
Oxcarbazepine	Sulfinpyrazone
Phenobarbital	Troglitazone
Phenylbutazone	

through the use of high-potency corticosteroids (dexamethasone) may be sufficient to prevent further seizures. However, often a second anticonvulsant is necessary. It should also be noted that dexamethasone is a hepatic P-450 3A4–inducing agent. We often see a reduction in serum levels of phenytoin or carbamazepine (also enzyme inducers) when the dose of dexamethasone is increased. Similarly, patients can become symptomatic with toxic levels of anticonvulsants in the middle of a dexamethasone taper. It is important to follow serum anticonvulsant levels when using agents metabolized by the cytochrome P-450 system. Anticonvulsants that are highly protein-bound can demonstrate significant changes in levels of circulating free drug without significantly changing the total serum level. It is useful to check serum-free phenytoin or valproic acid levels when patients taking these agents have seizures or show signs of toxicity. Unfortunately, despite the numerous choices of anticonvulsants, it can be quite difficult to control seizures in brain tumor patients. Of the newer generation of anticonvulsants, we have had success using levtiracetam (Keppra), which is easily titrated without significant drug interactions, and topiramate (Topomax), which is one of the few anticonvulsants associated with weight loss and not weight gain. Phenobarbital and clonazepam can also be useful in resistant cases. Short-term use of lorazepam (Ativan) can be helpful to bridge changes in anticonvulsant regimens. Ultimately, if the tumor is successfully treated, the resulting reduction in mass effect and edema will improve seizure control.

It is critical to provide effective supportive care to brain tumor patients to improve their functional status, as well as quality of life for themselves and their caregivers. Unfortunately, this care is typically very labor-intensive and often beyond the means of patients and their families to provide. We involve social work and case management early in the treatment of brain tumor patients. They can provide interventions that may prevent a later breakdown in care. The incidence of depression is high among this population and should be treated early. The causes of depression are typically multifactorial and may include direct effects of the tumor, side effects of chemotherapy and radiation therapy, and side effects of steroids in addition to issues associated with a loss of independence and a diagnosis of cancer. We suggest referral to psychiatry to optimally address these issues. A related concern is the impact of fatigue in this population. A common side effect of brain radiation therapy is somnolence and fatigue. We advocate use of psychostimulants such as methylphenidate to treat both fatigue and cognitive side effects (125). Although there are theoretical concerns that the use of stimulants in this population may exacerbate seizures, we have not observed this in practice. Brain tumor patients often require high doses of steroids to manage edema, and they experience both acute and chronic toxicity from their administration. Acutely, the steroids may induce hyperglycemia requiring an insulin sliding scale. Patients often become agitated, irritable, suffer extreme mood swings, and even become psychotic when taking steroids. Low-dose standing neuroeleptics can be effective in treating these side effects. Clinicians should aim to taper steroid use to the lowest doses necessary. Patients typically tolerate initial steroid weaning but often experience fatigue or worsening of neurologic function as dexamethasone doses fall below 4 mg daily. This can be ameliorated somewhat by providing an extremely slow steroid taper and only lowering doses every week to 2 weeks by increments of 1 mg or even 0.5 mg. The use of psychostimulants can help treat the inevitable fatigue patients experience as they taper the steroid dose. There is no effective treatment for steroid myopathy other than tapering off steroids as soon as possible and prescribing physical therapy and rehabilitation as early as possible.

MENINGIOMA

Meningiomas comprise 29% of all primary brain tumors. The incidence of meningioma rises with age, with an incidence of 0.74 per 100,000 person-years from age 20 to 34, to a rate of 4.89 from age 45 to 54, to a rate of 12.79 from age 65 to 74 (4). The tumor is often discovered incidentally without any symptoms. Clinically, these tumors typically present with headache, cognitive or personality changes, persistent focal neurologic deficits, and sometimes seizure. The main treatment for these tumors is surgical resection, with the goal of complete resection when possible, accounting for relative risks and benefits depending on the patient's age and condition (153). Options for residual tumor include observation and radiation therapy, which can incorporate stereotactic delivery to minimize effects to local tissue (154–156).

Chemotherapy for meningioma has been used for patients who have progressive disease after resection and radiotherapy; it is sometimes used adjuvantly following radiotherapy when pathology indicates malignant meningioma. In general, response rates have been disappointing in small case series. Chemotherapy agents that have been used include hydroxyurea (157,158), IFN-α (159,160), and liposomal doxorubicin (161). Results using temozolomide have been discouraging, with no responders (162). Clinical trials are ongoing using the new generation of small-molecule signal transduction inhibitors such as erlotinib, gefitinib, and imatinib.

PRIMARY CNS LYMPHOMA

In contrast to most other brain tumors, chemotherapy is the initial treatment of choice for CNS lymphoma. The incorporation of high-dose methotrexate (greater than 1 g/m^2) has resulted in a significantly greater response and improved survival compared to previous regimens that used a CHOP regimen prior to whole-brain radiation therapy. Although 64% of patients in one study responded to CHOP prior to radiation therapy, their median survival was 9.6 months, but it was 20.7 months for those who were able to complete the entire regimen (163). The report by DeAngelis, incorporating methotrexate (1 g/m^2), followed by whole-brain irradiation and two cycles of high-dose cytarabine (ara-C) (3 g/m^2), demonstrated a median survival of 42.5 months (164). This strategy is the basis for current CNS lymphoma protocols that have increased the dose of methotrexate and incorporated agents that more easily cross the BBB, such as procarbazine. A follow-up clinical trial incorporating methotrexate at 3.5 g/m^2 with procarbazine and vincristine, followed by whole-brain irradiation and cytarabine demonstrated a median survival of 60 months (165). The improvement in patient survival has also brought to attention the significant rates of cognitive decline and radiation-induced dementia, especially in patients above age 60 (166,167). Current approaches to therapy of CNS lymphoma are investigating whether radiation therapy can be avoided or delayed in the hope of reducing rates of cognitive decline and dementia without adversely affecting survival. Preliminary results from a trial using single-agent methotrexate at 8 g/m^2 every 2 weeks demonstrated a PFS of 12.8 months. Median survival had not been reached at 22.8+ months (168). Many clinicians at our center are cautiously delaying radiation therapy until relapse and continuing to use high-dose–based methotrexate regimens. In hopes of improving the results of the single-agent methotrexate study (168), some regimens continue to incorporate procarbazine. Other agents that may be active in this setting include temozolomide and rituximab.

Patients with recurrent disease may respond to methotrexate a second time. Other regimens that have been used include PCV (169), high-dose cytarabine (166), temozolomide (170), rituximab (171), and the combination of temozolomide and rituximab (172).

BRAIN METASTASIS

To achieve optimal results, the treatment of brain metastasis involves taking into account the interaction between oncology, neurosurgery, and radiation therapy. Depending on the setting of relapse, patient survival may depend more on local tumor control in the brain or on systemic control for progressive metastasis. Advances in local brain tumor control with surgery and radiosurgery will not improve patient survival if the patient ultimately succumbs to progressive systemic disease or continues to develop new brain metastasis. Overall, the median survival of patients with brain metastases is 3 to 6 months (173). Local therapy and systemic chemotherapy will need further development to improve patient survival.

The options for therapy include surgical resection, whole-brain irradiation, stereotactic radiosurgery if the target is smaller than 3 cm, and systemic chemotherapy. The advantage of surgical resection is that mass effect can be immediately ameliorated and removal of the tumor decreases edema. Surgical resection also provides pathology confirmation of diagnosis. Surgery can be considered for large lesions that are not amenable to stereotactic radiosurgery. The drawback of surgery is the need for an invasive procedure that requires general anesthesia, especially in a patient who has additional sites of metastatic disease and who has an elevated medical risk for surgical complications.

Whole-brain radiation therapy (30 Gy in 10 fractions) is the standard therapy for brain metastasis, with an established body of literature supporting its use for multiple metastases. Whole-brain irradiation has the ability to eradicate micrometastatic disease to delay recurrence (173,174) and is often used in conjunction with surgical resection or radiosurgery. It is tolerated fairly well and can be very effective for radiosensitive tumors such as metastases from small cell lung cancer or germ cell cancer. However, whole-brain irradiation can be associated with cognitive loss and leukoencephalomalacia.

There is increasing evidence that radiosurgery can effectively achieve local control of a brain metastasis that is smaller than 3 cm. This modality is also less invasive than surgical resection and does not require the patient to undergo general anesthesia. The disadvantage of radiosurgery is that mass effect is not relieved and, in the short term, tumor edema may increase. There are no prospective randomized studies comparing radiosurgery to surgery. Retrospective comparative studies that match similar patient selection criteria have reached opposite conclusions (175,176).

We tend to treat patients at our institution with surgery if their lesions are greater than 3 cm and they are symptomatic. If the patient's medical condition makes a surgical procedure too risky, the patient may receive whole-brain radiation therapy. Patients who have lesions smaller than 3 cm can receive radiosurgery if they are asymptomatic or their lesion is in a deep region that is not amenable to resection. However, patients with symptoms resulting from their lesions more frequently receive surgery to remove mass effect as long as their medical condition permits. There is also debate over the role of whole-brain irradiation following surgery or radiosurgery to single lesions.

CHEMOTHERAPY FOR BRAIN METASTASIS

Several small clinical trials and case reports in the literature support the concept that systemic chemotherapy demonstrates activity in treating brain metastases. Chemosensitive tumor types include breast cancer, small cell lung cancer, and germ cell tumors. The primary consideration in choosing a given regimen of chemotherapy is to use agents with known activity in a given tumor type (177). A confounding problem in brain tumor chemotherapy is the use of corticosteroids, which are often necessary to control cerebral edema, but can reestablish disrupted BBB function, which may impair delivery of chemotherapy (178). A review of treatment with systemic chemotherapy of brain metastases from small cell lung cancer pooled data from five clinical trials. A 66% response rate was demonstrated (179). Unfortunately, this response is not durable when chemotherapy is used by itself, even in cases of complete response.

A trial using combination chemotherapy of cyclophosphamide, 5-fluorouracil, methotrexate, vincristine, and prednisone for treatment of breast cancer in patients who had not received prior chemotherapy demonstrated a greater than 50% response rate, although the median duration of response was only 7 months (180). In these trials, the response rate of brain metastases was comparable to the response rates of the systemic disease. Patients who had prior chemotherapy responded at lower rates. A recent small trial of first-line chemotherapy for brain metastases from non–small cell lung cancer demonstrated a response rate of 45%, with an equal number of minor responses and stable disease. The median time to response was 10 weeks and the median duration of response was 25 weeks. However, although the median survival was 33 weeks for the group, it was only 48 weeks for the responders (181). A trial of patients who had failed prior radiotherapy utilizing a multidrug regimen composed of 6-thioguanine, procarbazine, dibromodulcitol, lomustine, 5-flourouracil, and hydroxyurea demonstrated an overall (responders plus stable disease) response rates of 60% for breast cancer, 52% for non–small cell lung cancer, and 66% for small cell lung cancer. The disease-free period of survival for these patients was 27 weeks for breast cancer, 21 weeks for non–small cell lung cancer, and 133 weeks for small cell lung cancer (182). Temozolomide is an imidazotetrazine derivative of dacarbazine that has reasonable CNS penetration and is approved for use in malignant gliomas. This drug has been used as a single agent for recurrent brain metastases for a mixture of tumor types, predominantly non–small cell lung cancer. It demonstrated a modest response and disease control (partial response plus stable disease) in 41% of a small group of patients in one study. Overall median survival was 6.6 months (183). Capecitabine is an oral 5-fluorouracil prodrug that is approved for metastatic breast cancer. A case report demonstrated a response by brain metastases to capecitabine following failure of whole-brain irradiation, hormonal therapy, and systemic chemotherapy that included 5-fluorouracil (184). After demonstrating single-agent activity, the next step is to investigate combination therapy. A study of recurrent non–small cell lung disease investigated the combination of cisplatin, ifosfamide, and irinotecan in 121 patients. Thirty of these patients had brain metastases and had a 50% response rate without the use of radiotherapy (185). Other strategies for devising combination therapy have used novel biological agents combined with traditional cytotoxic agents. Temozolomide on a daily low-dose schedule combined with thalidomide was given to patients with metastatic melanoma in a small phase I trial. Five major responses were reported using a temozolomide daily dosing schedule of 75 mg/m^2/day, with a median duration of 6 months and median survival of 12.3 months (186). Patients with brain metastases were excluded from the trial because of concern of overlapping neurotoxicity from thalidomide; however, a case report from the same institution demonstrated a complete response of metastatic melanoma to brain and leptomeninges treated with temozolomide combined with thalidomide (187).

Chemotherapy produces a high response rate for brain metastases arising from germ cell tumors. A regimen of etoposide, methotrexate, dactinomycin, vincristine, cyclophosphamide, and cisplatin for gestational choriocarcinoma induced a 72% durable response rate (188). In a study of brain metastases from germinoma, 8 of 10 patients had a complete response to a combination regimen of cisplatin, vincristine, methotrexate, bleomycin, etoposide, dactinomycin, and cyclophosphamide (189).

Considering the widespread prevalence of brain metastases, relatively few clinical trials have addressed this issue. Most clinical trials of investigational agents for solid tumors explicitly exclude patients with brain metastases. Compounding this omission is their common inclusion into studies of a heterogeneous group of patients with mixed tumor types and differing prior exposure to chemotherapy. Patients might also be expected to be more resistant to treatment with chemotherapeutic agents if they have failed radiotherapy. If chemotherapy is given during and after radiotherapy, it may be difficult to separate efficacy due to radiotherapy and efficacy due to chemotherapy. These factors combined make it difficult to compare treatment regimens and meaningfully interpret studies (190). One approach to this problem is to stratify patients according to pretreatment factors. These can be analyzed to determine factors that have prognostic value. The RTOG analyzed a database of 1200 patients using differing radiation fractionation schemes or radiosenzitizers for brain metastasis treatment. First, a univariate analysis was performed, which considered 18 pretreatment factors, including age, tumor histology, control of systemic tumor, neurologic status, KPS, location of lesions, and three treatment-related variables, such as radiation dose. A recursive partitioning analysis (RPA) was performed to rank the significance of these factors. The study grouped patients into 3 classes. Class 1 patients had a KPS ≥70, age <65, a controlled primary tumor site, and no extracranial metastases. Class 3 patients had a KPS <70, and class 2 patients were all others. The median survival was 7.1 months for class 1, 4.2 months for class 2, and only 2.3 months for class 3 patients (173). The validity of this database was verified by a second RPA on a trial of 445 patients randomized to an accelerated hyperfractionation group or to an accelerated fractionation group. Class 1 patients had a median survival of 6.2 months, compared with 7.1 months for the database as a whole, and a 1-year survival of 29%, compared with 32% for the database (174). The use of RPA allows the most important pretreatment prognostic factors to be identified and provides a historic database against which to compare future studies.

Bioimmunotherapy is being assessed for the treatment of patients with malignant melanoma and a few responses have been demonstrated in a setting of brain metastases. A retrospective review at the National Cancer Institute of high-dose IL-2 in 36 patients with evaluable brain metastases found 2 patients with a regression of their brain lesions, a response that reflected the systemic response. The overall response rate for patients with previously untreated brain metastases demonstrated only a 5.6% response rate, compared with 19.8% for patients without brain metastases. The patients with brain metastases did not exhibit excess toxicity compared to the overall group (191). A study of interferon alpha with IL-2 following chemotherapy with cisplatin, dacarbazine, and carmustine included 15 patients with brain metastases. Seven (47%) of these patients had a partial response, with a median time to progression of 6 months and a median survival of 6.5 months (192).

The use of chemotherapy for brain metastases is faced with great challenges. The most important imperative is to discover new agents that can overcome the resistance of tumor cells to standard chemotherapy agents, whether through selection by prior pretreatment or inherent chemoresistance of tumor cell clones that metastasize from a primary site. Because most patients with brain metastases succumb to progressive systemic disease, improvement of local control in the brain will likely have a limited effect on survival. Conversely, development of agents that are effective in establishing durable tumor control, both systemically and in the brain, will improve survival, as in the unique case of germ cell tumors. If patients with a good performance status who have brain metastases are excluded from clinical trials of novel agents, it will be difficult to accurately determine the possible effectiveness of these agents against CNS disease. The use of RPA may help to identify patients who might benefit from chemotherapy as well as to design clinical trials that take into account specific tumor histology and prior exposure to chemotherapy. Improvement in patient survival will result from improved local control of CNS disease if the primary disease site remains dormant, illustrating the need for a multimodality approach to the treatment of the patient with brain metastases.

References

1. Posner JB, Chernik NL. Intracranial metastases from systemic cancer. *Adv Neurol* 1978;19:579–592.
2. Schouten LJ, Rutten J, Huveneers HA, et al. Incidence of brain metastases in a cohort of patients with carcinoma of the breast, colon, kidney, and lung and melanoma. *Cancer* 2002; 94(10):2698–2705.
3. American Cancer Society. *Cancer Facts and Figures 2003. Surveillance Research.* Atlanta: American Cancer Society; 2003.
4. CBTRUS. *Statistical Report: Primary Brain Tumors in the United States 1995–1999.* Central Brain Tumor Registry of the United States; 2002.
5. Wong ET, Hess KR, Gleason MJ, et al. Outcomes and prognostic factors in recurrent glioma patients enrolled onto phase II clinical trials [see comment]. *J Clin Oncol* 1999; 17(8):2572.
6. Sawaya R, Bindal RK, Lang FF, et al. Metastatic brain tumors. In: Kaye AH, Laws ER (eds): *Brain Tumors.* London: Churchill Livingstone; 2001:999–1026.
7. Tremont-Lukats IW, Bobustuc G, Lagos GK, et al. Brain metastasis from prostate carcinoma: The MD Anderson Cancer Center experience. *Cancer* 2003 98(2):363–368.
8. Patel JK, Didolkar MS, Pickren JW, et al. Metastatic pattern of malignant melanoma. A study of 216 autopsy cases. *Am J Surg* 1978;135(6):807–810.
9. Lang FF, Wildrick DM, Sawaya R. Metastatic brain tumors. In: Bernstein M (ed): *Neuro-Oncology: The Essentials.* New York: Thieme; 2000:329–337.
10. Delattre JY, Krol G, Thaler HT, et al. Distribution of brain metastases. *Arch Neurol* 1988;45(7):741–744.
11. Eby NL, Grufferman S, Flannelly CM, et al. Increasing incidence of primary brain lymphoma in the US. *Cancer* 1988; 62(11):2461–2465.
12. Corn BW, Marcus SM, Topham A, et al. Will primary central nervous system lymphoma be the most frequent brain tumor diagnosed in the year 2000? *Cancer* 1997;79(12):2409–2413.
13. Cote TR, Manns A, Hardy CR, et al. Epidemiology of brain lymphoma among people with or without acquired immunodeficiency syndrome. AIDS/Cancer Study Group. *J Natl Cancer Inst* 1996;88(10):675–679.
14. Olson JE, Janney CA, Rao RD, et al. The continuing increase in the incidence of primary central nervous system non-Hodgkin lymphoma: A surveillance, epidemiology, and end results analysis. *Cancer* 2002;95(7):1504–1510.
15. Tomlinson FH, Kurtin PJ, Suman VJ, et al. Primary intracerebral malignant lymphoma: A clinicopathological study of 89 patients. *J Neurosurg* 1995;82(4):558–566.
16. DeAngelis LM, Wong E, Rosenblum M, et al. Epstein-Barr virus in acquired immune deficiency syndrome (AIDS) and non-AIDS primary central nervous system lymphoma. *Cancer* 1992;70(6):1607–1611.
17. Nygaard R, Garwicz S, Haldorsen T, et al. Second malignant neoplasms in patients treated for childhood leukemia. A population-based cohort study from the Nordic countries. The Nordic Society of Pediatric Oncology and Hematology (NOPHO). *Acta Paediatr Scand* 1991;80(12):1220–1228.
18. Wrensch M, Bondy ML, Wiencke J, et al. Environmental risk factors for primary malignant brain tumors: A review. *J Neurooncol* 1993;17(1):47–64.
19. Preston-Martin S, Mack W. Neoplasms of the nervous system. In: (eds): *Cancer Epidemiology and Prevention.* New York: Oxford University Press; 1996:1231–1281.
20. Bohnen NI, Kurland LT. Brain tumor and exposure to pesticides in humans: A review of the epidemiologic data. *J Neurol Sci* 1995;132(2):110–121.
21. Wrensch M, Minn Y, Chew T, et al. Epidemiology of primary brain tumors: Current concepts and review of the literature. *Neurooncology* 2002;4(4):278–299.
22. Norman MA, Holly EA, Ahn DK, et al. Prenatal exposure to tobacco smoke and childhood brain tumors: Results from the United States West Coast childhood brain tumor study. *Cancer Epidemiol Biomarkers Prev* 1996;5(2):127–133.
23. Norman MA, Holly EA, Preston-Martin S. Childhood brain tumors and exposure to tobacco smoke. *Cancer Epidemiol Biomarkers Prev* 1996;5(2):85–91.
24. Wrensch MR, Minn Y, Bondy ML. Epidemiology. In: Bernstein M, Berger MS (eds): *Neuro-Oncology: The Essentials.* New York: Thieme; 2000:2–17.
25. Martini F, De Mattei M, Iaccheri L, et al. Human brain tumors and simian virus 40. *J Natl Cancer Inst* 1995;87(17):1331.
26. Strickler HD, Rosenberg PS, Devesa SS, et al. Contamination of poliovirus vaccines with simian virus 40 (1955–1963) and

subsequent cancer rates [see comment]. *JAMA* 1998;279(4): 292–295.

27. Rollison DE, Helzlsouer KJ, Alberg AJ, et al. Serum antibodies to JC virus, BK virus, simian virus 40, and the risk of incident adult astrocytic brain tumors. *Cancer Epidemiol Biomarkers Prev* 2003;12(5):460–463.

28. Narod SA, Stiller C, Lenoir GM. An estimate of the heritable fraction of childhood cancer. *Br J Cancer* 1991;63(6):993–999.

29. Malkin D, Li FP, Strong LC, et al. Germ line p53 mutations in a familial syndrome of breast cancer, sarcomas, and other neoplasms [see comment] [erratum appears in *Science* 1993 Feb 12;259(5097):878; PMID: 8438145]. *Science* 1990 250(4985):1233–1238.

30. Hamilton SR, Liu B, Parsons RE, et al. The molecular basis of Turcot's syndrome [see comment]. *N Engl J Med* 1995; 332(13):839–847.

31. Kantarjian H, Sawyers C, Hochhaus A, et al. Hematologic and cytogenetic responses to imatinib mesylate in chronic myelogenous leukemia [see comment] [erratum appears in *N Engl J Med* 2002 Jun 13;346(24):1923]. *N Engl J Med* 2002;346(9):645–652.

32. O'Brien SG, Guilhot F, Larson RA, et al. Imatinib compared with interferon and low-dose cytarabine for newly diagnosed chronic-phase chronic myeloid leukemia [see comment]. *N Engl J Med* 2003;348(11):994–1004.

33. Cohen MH, Williams GA, Sridhara R, et al. FDA drug approval summary: Gefitinib (ZD1839) (Iressa) tablets. *Oncologist* 2003;8(4):303–306.

34. Nutt CL, Mani DR, Betensky RA, et al. Gene expression–based classification of malignant gliomas correlates better with survival than histological classification. *Cancer Res* 200363(7):1602–1607.

35. Fuller GN, Hess KR, Rhee CH, et al. Molecular classification of human diffuse gliomas by multidimensional scaling analysis of gene expression profiles parallels morphology-based classification correlates with survival and reveals clinically-relevant novel glioma subsets. *Brain Pathol* 2002;12(1): 108–116.

36. Reynolds BA, Weiss S. Generation of neurons and astrocytes from isolated cells of the adult mammalian central nervous system [see comment]. *Science* 1992;255(5052):1707–1710.

37. Libermann TA, Nusbaum HR, Razon N, et al. Amplification, enhanced expression, and possible rearrangement of EGF receptor gene in primary human brain tumours of glial origin. *Nature* 1985;313(5998):144–147.

38. Louis DN, Gusella JF. A tiger behind many doors: Multiple genetic pathways to malignant glioma. *Trends Genet* 1995; 11(10):412–415.

39. Wong AJ, Bigner SH, Bigner DD, et al. Increased expression of the epidermal growth factor receptor gene in malignant gliomas is invariably associated with gene amplification. *Proc Natl Acad Sci USA* 1987;84(19):6899–6903.

40. Wong AJ, Ruppert JM, Bigner SH, et al. Structural alterations of the epidermal growth factor receptor gene in human gliomas. *Proc Natl Acad Sci USA* 1992;89(7):2965–2969.

41. Choe G, Horvath S, Cloughesy TF, et al. Analysis of the phosphatidylinositol 3′-kinase signaling pathway in glioblastoma patients in vivo. *Cancer Res* 2003;63(11):2742–2746.

42. Chakravarti A, Zhai G, Suzuki Y, et al. The prognostic significance of phosphatidylinositol 3-kinase pathway activation in human gliomas. *J Clin Oncol* 2004;22(10):1926–1933.

43. Guha A, Feldkamp MM, Lau N, et al: Proliferation of human malignant astrocytomas is dependent on Ras activation. *Oncogene* 1997;15(23):2755–2765.

44. Steck A, Lin H, Langford LA, et al. Functional and molecular analyses of 10q deletions in human gliomas. *Genes Chromosomes Cancer* 1999;24(2):135–143.

45. Holland EC, Celestino J, Dai C, et al. Combined activation of Ras and Akt in neural progenitors induces glioblastoma formation in mice. *Nat Genet* 2000;25(1):55–57.

46. Ding H, Shannon P, Lau N, et al Oligodendrogliomas result from the expression of an activated mutant epidermal growth factor receptor in a RAS transgenic mouse astrocytoma model. *Cancer Res* 2003;63(5):1106–1113.

47. Levine AJ. p53: The cellular gatekeeper for growth and division. *Cell* 1997;88(3):323–331.

48. Hoh J, Jin S, Parrado T, et al. The p53MH algorithm and its application in detecting p53-responsive genes. *Proc Natl Acad Sci USA* 2002;99(13):8467–8472.

49. Reifenberger G, Liu L, Ichimura K, et al. Amplification and overexpression of the MDM2 gene in a subset of human malignant gliomas without p53 mutations. *Cancer Res* 1993; 53(12):2736–2739.

50. Maher EA, Furnari FB, Bachoo RM, et al. Malignant glioma: Genetics and biology of a grave matter. *Genes Dev* 2001; 15(11):1311–1333.

51. Fueyo J, Alemany R, Gomez-Manzano C, et al. Preclinical characterization of the antiglioma activity of a tropism-enhanced adenovirus targeted to the retinoblastoma pathway. *J Natl Cancer Inst* 2003;95(9):652–660.

52. Esteller M, Garcia-Foncillas J, Andion E, et al. Inactivation of the DNA-repair gene MGMT and the clinical response of gliomas to alkylating agents [see comment] [erratum appears in *N Engl J Med* 2000;343(23):1740] *N Engl J Med* 2000; 343(19):1350–1354.

53. Paz MF, Yaya-Tur R, Rojas-Marcos I, et al. CpG island hypermethylation of the DNA repair enzyme methyltransferase predicts response to temozolomide in primary gliomas. *Clin Cancer Res* 2004;10(15):4933–4938.

54. Esteller M. CpG island hypermethylation and tumor suppressor genes: A booming present, a brighter future. *Oncogene* 2002;21(35):5427–5440.

55. Fillmore HL, VanMeter TE, Broaddus WC. Membrane-type matrix metalloproteinases (MT-MMPs): Expression and function during glioma invasion. *J Neurooncol* 2001;53(2): 187–202.

56. Koul D, Parthasarathy R, Shen R, et al. Suppression of matrix metalloproteinase-2 gene expression and invasion in human glioma cells by MMAC/PTEN. *Oncogene* 2001;20(46): 6669–6678.

57. Suh CO, Loh JJ, Kim GE, et al. Primary malignant lymphomas of the central nervous system: Radiotherapy results in 12 cases. *Yonsei Med J* 1989;30(1):54–64.

58. Kleihues P, Ohgaki H. Primary and secondary glioblastomas: From concept to clinical diagnosis. *Neurooncology* 1999; 1(1):44–51.

59. Watanabe K, Tachibana O, Sata K, et al. Overexpression of the EGF receptor and p53 mutations are mutually exclusive in the evolution of primary and secondary glioblastomas. *Brain Pathol* 1996;6(3):217–223; discussion 23–24.

60. Noble M, Dietrich J. The complex identity of brain tumors: Emerging concerns regarding origin diversity and plasticity. *Trends Neurosci* 2004;27(3):148–154.

61. Cairncross JG, Ueki K, Zlatescu MC, et al. Specific genetic predictors of chemotherapeutic response and survival in patients with anaplastic oligodendrogliomas. *J Natl Cancer Inst* 1998;90(19):1473–1479.

62. Jenkins RB, Curran W, Scott CB, et al. Pilot evaluation of 1p and 19q deletions in anaplastic oligodendrogliomas collected by a national cooperative cancer treatment group. *Am J Clin Oncol* 2001;24(5):506–508.

63. Ino Y, Betensky RA, Zlatescu MC, et al. Molecular subtypes of anaplastic oligodendroglioma: Implications for patient management at diagnosis. *Clin Cancer Res* 2001;7(4):839–845.

64. Smith JS, Perry A, Borell TJ, et al. Alterations of chromosome arms 1p and 19q as predictors of survival in oligodendrogliomas, astrocytomas, and mixed oligoastrocytomas. *J Clin Oncol* 2000;18(3):636–645.

65. Hoang-Xuan K, Capelle L, Kujas M, et al. Temozolomide as initial treatment for adults with low-grade oligodendrogliomas or oligoastrocytomas and correlation with chromosome 1p deletions. *J Clin Oncol* 2004;22(15):3133–3138.

66. Louis DN, Stemmer-Rachamimov AO, Wiestler OD. Neurofibromatosis type 2. In: Kleihues P, Cavenee WK (eds): *Pathology and Genetics of Tumors of the Nervous System.* Lyon, France: IARC Press; 2000:219–222.

67. Lee JH, Sundaram V, Stein DJ, et al. Reduced expression of schwannomin/merlin in human sporadic meningiomas. *Neurosurgery* 1997;40(3):578–587.

68. Xiao GH, Chernoff J, Testa JR. NF2: The wizardry of merlin. *Genes Chromosomes Cancer* 2003;38(4)389–399.

69. Kim H, Kwak NJ, Lee JY, et al. Merlin neutralizes the inhibitory effect of Mdm2 on p53. *J Biol Chem* 2004;279(9):7812–7818.

70. Louis DN, Scheithauer B, Budka H, et al. Meningiomas. In: Kleihues P, Cavenee WK (eds): *Pathology and Genetics of Tumors of the Nervous System.* Lyon, France: IARC Press; 2000:176–184.

71. McDermott M, Quinones-Hinosa A, Fuller GN, et al: Meningiomas. In: Levin VA (ed): *Cancer in the Nervous System.* New York: Oxford University Press; 2000:269–299.

72. Kalkanis SN, Carroll RS, Zhang J, et al. Correlation of vascular endothelial growth factor messenger RNA expression with peritumoral vasogenic cerebral edema in meningiomas. *J Neurosurg* 1996;85(6):1095–1101.

73. Tsai JC, Hsiao YY, Teng LJ, et al. Regulation of vascular endothelial growth factor secretion in human meningioma cells. *J Formosan Med Assoc* 1999;98(2):111–117.

74. Fidler IJ. The biology of brain metastasis. In: Sawaya R (ed): *Intracranial Metastases Current Management Strategies.* Malden, MA: Blackwell Futura; 2004:35–54.

75. Price JE, Aukerman SL, Fidler IJ: Evidence that the process of murine melanoma metastasis is sequential and selective and contains stochastic elements. *Cancer Res* 1986;46(10):5172–5178.

76. Posner JB. *Neurologic Complications of Cancer.* Contemporary neurology series no. 45. Philadelphia: FA Davis; 1995:77–110.

77. Fidler IJ. Host and tumour factors in cancer metastasis. *Eur J Clin Invest* 1990;20(5):481–486.

78. Kendal WS, Lagerwaard FJ, Agboola O: Characterization of the frequency distribution for human hematogenous metastases: Evidence for clustering and a power variance function. *Clin Exp Metastasis* 2000;18(3):219–229.

79. Fidler IJ, Yano S, Zhang RD, et al: The seed and soil hypothesis: Vascularisation and brain metastases. *Lancet Oncol* 2002;3(1):53–57.

80. Marchetti D, Li J, Shen R: Astrocytes contribute to the brain-metastatic specificity of melanoma cells by producing heparanase. *Cancer Res* 2000;60(17):4767–4770.

81. Fidler IJ, Kripke ML. Metastasis results from preexisting variant cells within a malignant tumor. *Science* 1977;197(4306):893–895.

82. Puduvalli VK. Brain metastases: Biology and the role of the brain microenvironment. *Curr Oncol Rep* 2001;3(6):467–475.

83. Pasqualini R, Arap W, McDonald DM. Probing the structural and molecular diversity of tumor vasculature. *Trends Mol Med* 2002;8(12):563–571.

84. Pasqualini R, Ruoslahti E. Organ targeting in vivo using phage display peptide libraries. *Nature* 1996;380(6572):364–366.

85. Felding-Habermann B, O'Toole TE, Smith JW, et al. Integrin activation controls metastasis in human breast cancer. *Proc Natl Acad Sci USA* 2001;98(4):1853–1858.

86. Cary LA, Han DC, Guan JL. Integrin-mediated signal transduction pathways. *Histol Histopathol* 1999;14(3):1001–1009.

87. Jin H, Varner J. Integrins: Roles in cancer development and as treatment targets. *Br J Cancer* 2004;90(3):561–565.

88. Stamenkovic I. Matrix metalloproteinases in tumor invasion and metastasis. *Semin Cancer Biol* 2000;10(6):415–433.

89. Marchetti D, Nicolson GL. Human heparanase: A molecular determinant of brain metastasis. *Adv Enzyme Regul* 2001;41:343–359.

90. Borsig L, Wong R, Feramisco J, et al. Heparin and cancer revisited: Mechanistic connections involving platelets, P-selectin, carcinoma mucins, and tumor metastasis. *Proc Natl Acad Sci USA* 2001;98(6):3352–3357.

91. Carmeliet P, Jain RK. Angiogenesis in cancer and other diseases. *Nature* 2000;407(6801):249–257.

92. Drewes LR. What is the blood-brain barrier? A molecular perspective: Cerebral vascular biology. *Adv Exp Med Biol* 1999;474:111–122.

93. Bendayan R, Lee G, Bendayan M. Functional expression and localization of P-glycoprotein at the blood brain barrier. *Microsc Res Tech* 2002;57(5):365–380.

94. Gottesman MM, Fojo T, Bates SE: Multidrug resistance in cancer: Role of ATP-dependent transporters. *Nat Rev Cancer* 2002;2(1):48–58.

95. Abbott NJ. Astrocyte-endothelial interactions and blood-brain barrier permeability. *J Anat* 2002;200(6):629–638.

96. Schackert G, Fidler IJ. Site-specific metastasis of mouse melanomas and a fibrosarcoma in the brain or meninges of syngeneic animals. *Cancer Res* 1988;48(12):3478–3484.

97. Savaraj N, Lu K, Feun LG, et al. Intracerebral penetration and tissue distribution of 25-diaziridinyl 36-bis(carboethoxyamino) 14-benzoquinone (AZQ NSC-182986). *J Neurooncol* 1983; 1(1):15–19.

98. Stewart DJ, Leavens M, Maor M, et al. Human central nervous system distribution of cis-diamminedichloroplatinum

and use as a radiosensitizer in malignant brain tumors. *Cancer Res* 1982;42(6):2474–2479.

99. Stewart A, Hayakawa K, Farrell CL. Quantitation of blood-brain barrier ultrastructure. *Microsc Res Tech* 1994;27(6): 516–527.

100. Stewart DJ, Lu K, Benjamin RS, et al. Concentration of vinblastine in human intracerebral tumor and other tissues. *J Neurooncol* 1983;1(2):139–144.

101. Graif M, Bydder GM, Steiner RE, et al. Contrast-enhanced MR imaging of malignant brain tumors. *AJNR* 1985;6(6):855–862.

102. Kepes JJ. Large focal tumor-like demyelinating lesions of the brain: Intermediate entity between multiple sclerosis and acute disseminated encephalomyelitis? A study of 31 patients [see comment]. *Ann Neurol* 1993;33(1):18–27.

103. Peterson K, Rosenblum MK, Powers JM, et al. Effect of brain irradiation on demyelinating lesions [see comment]. *Neurology* 1993;43(10):2105–2112.

104. Herminghaus S, Dierks T, Pilatus U, et al. Determination of histopathological tumor grade in neuroepithelial brain tumors by using spectral pattern analysis of in vivo spectroscopic data. *J Neurosurg* 2003;98(1):74–81.

105. Shaw E. Management of low-grade gliomas in adults. In: Prados M (ed): Brain Cancer. Hamilton, Ontario, Canada: BC Decker; 2002:279–302.

106. Westergaard L, Gjerris F, Klinken L: Prognostic parameters in benign astrocytomas. *Acta Neurochir (Wien)* 1993;123(1–2):1–7.

107. Philippon JH, Clemenceau SH, Fauchon FH, et al. Supratentorial low-grade astrocytomas in adults. *Neurosurgery* 1993; 32(4):554–559.

108. Piepmeier J, Christopher S, Spencer D, et al. Variations in the natural history and survival of patients with supratentorial low-grade astrocytomas. *Neurosurgery* 1996;38(5):872–878; discussion 878–879.

109. Kraus JA, Koopmann J, Kaskel P, et al. Shared allelic losses on chromosomes 1p and 19q suggest a common origin of oligodendroglioma and oligoastrocytoma. *J Neuropathol Exp Neurol* 1995;54(1):91–95.

110. Berger M, Leibel S, Bruner J, et al. Primary cerebral tumors. In: Levin V (ed): *Cancer in the Nervous System*. Oxford, UK: Oxford University Press; 2002:75–157.

111. Berger MS, Deliganis AV, Dobbins J, et al. The effect of extent of resection on recurrence in patients with low grade cerebral hemisphere gliomas. *Cancer* 1994;74(6):1784–1791.

112. Shaw EG, Daumas-Duport C, Scheithauer BW, et al. Radiation therapy in the management of low-grade supratentorial astrocytomas. *J Neurosurg* 1989;70(6):853–861.

113. Karim AB, Afra D, Cornu P, et al. Randomized trial on the efficacy of radiotherapy for cerebral low-grade glioma in the adult: European Organization for Research and Treatment of Cancer Study 22845 with the Medical Research Council study BRO4: An interim analysis. *Int J Radiat Oncol Biol Phys* 2002;52(2):316–324.

114. Taphoorn MJ. Neurocognitive sequelae in the treatment of low-grade gliomas. *Semin Oncol* 2003;30(6 suppl 19):45–48.

115. Karim AB, Maat B, Hatlevoll R, et al. A randomized trial on dose-response in radiation therapy of low-grade cerebral glioma: European Organization for Research and Treatment of Cancer (EORTC) Study 22844. *Int J Radiat Oncol Biol Phys* 1996;36(3):549–556.

116. Shaw E, Arusell R, Scheithauer B, et al. Prospective randomized trial of low- versus high-dose radiation therapy in adults with supratentorial low-grade glioma: Initial report of a North Central Cancer Treatment Group/Radiation Therapy Oncology Group/Eastern Cooperative Oncology Group study [see comment]. *J Clin Oncol* 2002;20(9):2267–2276.

117. Eyre HJ, Crowley JJ, Townsend JJ, et al. A randomized trial of radiotherapy versus radiotherapy plus CCNU for incompletely resected low-grade gliomas: A Southwest Oncology Group study. *J Neurosurg* 1993;78(6):909–914.

118. Stupp R, Baumert BG. Promises and controversies in the management of low-grade glioma. *Ann Oncol* 2003;14(12): 1695–1696.

119. van den Bent MJ. Can chemotherapy replace radiotherapy in low-grade gliomas? Time for randomized studies. *Semin Oncol* 2003;30(6 suppl 19):39–44.

120. Buckner JC, Gesme D Jr, O'Fallon JR, et al. Phase II trial of procarbazine lomustine and vincristine as initial therapy for patients with low-grade oligodendroglioma or oligoastrocytoma: Efficacy and associations with chromosomal abnormalities. *J Clin Oncol* 2003;21(2):251–255.

121. Diabira S, Rousselet MC, Gamelin E, et al. PCV chemotherapy for oligodendroglioma: Response analyzed on T2 weighted-MRI. *J Neurooncol* 2001;55(1):45–50.

122. Pace A, Vidiri A, Galie E, et al. Temozolomide chemotherapy for progressive low-grade glioma: Clinical benefits and radiological response. *Ann Oncol* 2003;14(12):1722–1726.

123. Sanson M, Cartalat-Carel S, Taillibert S, et al. Initial chemotherapy in gliomatosis cerebri. *Neurology* 2004;63(2):270–275.

124. Quinn JA, Reardon DA, Friedman AH, et al. Phase II trial of temozolomide in patients with progressive low-grade glioma. *J Clin Oncol* 2003;21(4):646–651.

125. Meyers CA, Weitzner MA, Valentine AD, et al. Methylphenidate therapy improves cognition mood and function of brain tumor patients. *J Clin Oncol* 1998; 16(7):2522–2527.

126. Ries L, Eisner M, Kosary C, et al. *SEER Cancer Statistics Review 1973–1999.* Bethesda, MD: National Cancer Institute; 2000.

127. Yung WK, Albright RE, Olson J, et al. A phase II study of temozolomide vs procarbazine in patients with glioblastoma multiforme at first relapse. *Br J Cancer* 2000;83(5): 588–593.

128. Brada M, Hoang-Xuan K, Rampling R, et al. Multicenter phase II trial of temozolomide in patients with glioblastoma multiforme at first relapse [see comment]. *Ann Oncol* 2001; 12(2):259–266.

129. Prados MD, Larson DA, Lamborn K, et al. Radiation therapy and hydroxyurea followed by the combination of 6-thioguanine and BCNU for the treatment of primary malignant brain tumors. *Int J Radiat Oncol Biol Phy* 1998;40(1):57–63.

130. Levin VA, Yung WK, Bruner J, et al. Phase II study of accelerated fractionation radiation therapy with carboplatin followed by PCV chemotherapy for the treatment of anaplastic gliomas. *Int J Radiat Oncol Biol Phys* 2002;53(1):58–66.

131. Prados MD, Wara WM, Sneed K, et al. Phase III trial of accelerated hyperfractionation with or without difluromethylornithine (DFMO) versus standard fractionated radiotherapy with or without DFMO for newly diagnosed patients with glioblastoma multiforme. *Int J Radiat Oncol Biol Phys* 2001; 49(1):71–77.

132. Yung WK, Prados MD, Yaya-Tur R, et al. Multicenter phase II trial of temozolomide in patients with anaplastic astrocytoma or anaplastic oligoastrocytoma at first relapse. Temodal Brain Tumor Group. *J Clin Oncol* 1999;17(9):2762–2771.

133. Jaeckle KA, Hess KR, Yung WK, et al. Phase II evaluation of temozolomide and 13-cis-retinoic acid for the treatment of recurrent and progressive malignant glioma: A North American Brain Tumor Consortium study. *J Clin Oncol* 2003; 21(12):2305–2311.

134. Groves MD, Puduvalli VK, Hess KR, et al. Phase II trial of temozolomide plus the matrix metalloproteinase inhibitor marimastat in recurrent and progressive glioblastoma multiforme. *J Clin Oncol* 2002;20(5):1383–1388.

135. Gilbert M. Phase I/II study of combination temozolomide (TMZ) and irinotecan (CPT-11) for recurrent malignant gliomas: A North American Brain Tumor Consortium (NABTC) study. *Proc Am Soc Clin Oncol* 2003;22:103 (abstr 410).

136. Dohrmann GJ, Farwell JR, Flannery JT. Glioblastoma multiforme in children. *J Neurosurg* 1976;44(4):442–448.

137. Lacroix M, Abi-Said D, Fourney DR, et al. A multivariate analysis of 416 patients with glioblastoma multiforme: Prognosis extent of resection and survival [see comment]. *J Neurosurg* 2001;95(2):190–198.

138. Keles GE, Lamborn KR, Chang SM, et al. Volume of residual disease as a predictor of outcome in adult patients with recurrent supratentorial glioblastomas multiforme who are undergoing chemotherapy. *J Neurosurg* 2004;100(1):41–46.

139. Stupp R, Mason WP, van den Bent MJ, et al. Concomitant and adjuvant temozolomide (TMZ) and radiotherapy (RT) for newly diagnosed glioblastoma multiforme (GBM). Conclusive results of a randomized phase III trial by the EORTC Brain & RT Groups and NCIC Clinical Trials Group. ASCO Annual Meeting Proceedings (Proc ASCO post-meeting ed). *J Clin Oncol* 2004;22(suppl 14S):2.

140. Stupp R, Dietrich Y, Ostermann Kraljevic S, et al. Promising survival for patients with newly diagnosed glioblastoma multiforme treated with concomitant radiation plus temozolomide followed by adjuvant temozolomide [see comment]. *J Clin Oncol* 2002;20(5):1375–1382.

141. Lang FF, Bruner JM, Fuller GN, et al. Phase I trial of adenovirus-mediated p53 gene therapy for recurrent glioma: Biological and clinical results. *J Clin Oncol* 2003;21(13):2508–2518.

142. Kunwar S. Convection enhanced delivery of IL13-PE38QQR for treatment of recurrent malignant glioma: Presentation of interim findings from ongoing phase 1 studies. *Acta Neurochir Suppl* 2003;88:105–111.

143. Glantz MJ, Burger C, Friedman AH, et al. Treatment of radiation-induced nervous system injury with heparin and warfarin. *Neurology* 1994;44(11):2020–2027.

144. Kohshi K, Imada H, Nomoto S, et al. Successful treatment of radiation-induced brain necrosis by hyperbaric oxygen therapy. *J Neurol Sci* 2003;209(1–2):115–117.

145. Chuba J, Aronin P, Bhambhani K, et al. Hyperbaric oxygen therapy for radiation-induced brain injury in children. *Cancer* 1997;80(10):2005–2012.

146. Yung WK, Kyritsis AP, Gleason MJ, et al. Treatment of recurrent malignant gliomas with high-dose 13-cis-retinoic acid. *Clin Cancer Res* 1996;2(12):1931–1935.

147. Reardon DA, Friedman HS, Powell JB Jr, et al. Irinotecan: Promising activity in the treatment of malignant glioma. *Oncology (Huntington)* 2003;17(suppl 5):9–14.

148. Franceschi E, Cavallo G, Scopece L, et al. Phase II trial of carboplatin and etoposide for patients with recurrent high-grade glioma. *Br J Cancer* 2004;91(6):1038–1044.

149. Reardon DA. A phase I/II trial of PTK787/ZK 222584 (PTK/ZK): A novel oral angiogenesis inhibitor in combination with either temozolomide or lomustine for patients with recurrent glioblastoma multiforme (GBM). ASCO Annual Meeting Proceedings (Proc ASCO post-meeting ed). *J Clin Oncol* 2004;22(suppl 14S):1513.

150. Conrad C, Friedman H, Reardon D, et al. A Phase I/II trial of single-agnet PTK 787/ZK 222584 (PTK/ZK) a novel oral angiogenesis inhibitor in patients with recurent glioblastoma multiforme (GBM). ASCO Annual Meeting Proceedings (Proc ASCO post-meeting ed). *J Clin Oncol* 2004;22(suppl 14S):1512.

151. Prados MD, Yung WK, Jaeckle KA, et al. Phase I trial of irinotecan (CPT-11) in patients with recurrent malignant glioma: A North American Brain Tumor Consortium study. *Neurooncology* 2004;6(1):44–54.

152. Chang SM, Kuhn J, Wen P, et al. Phase I/pharmacokinetic study of CCI-779 in patients with recurrent malignant glioma on enzyme-inducing antiepileptic drugs. *Invest New Drugs* 2004;22(4):427–435.

153. McDermott MW, Quinones-Hinojosa A, Bollen AW, et al. Meningiomas. In: Prados M (ed): *Brain Cancer.* Hamilton, Ontario, Canada: BC Decker; 2002:333–364.

154. Goldsmith BJ, Wara WM, Wilson CB, et al. Postoperative irradiation for subtotally resected meningiomas: A retrospective analysis of 140 patients treated from 1967 to 1990. *J Neurosurg* 1994;80(2):195–201.

155. Hakim R, Alexander E III, Loeffler JS, et al. Results of linear accelerator-based radiosurgery for intracranial meningiomas. *Neurosurgery* 1998;42(3):446–453; discussion 453–454.

156. Ojemann SG, Sneed K, Larson DA, et al. Radiosurgery for malignant meningioma: Results in 22 patients. *J Neurosurg* 2000;93(suppl 3):62–67.

157. Newton HB, Slivka MA, Stevens C. Hydroxyurea chemotherapy for unresectable or residual meningioma. *J Neurooncol* 2000;49(2):165–170.

158. Mason WP, Gentili F, Macdonald DR, et al. Stabilization of disease progression by hydroxyurea in patients with recurrent or unresectable meningioma. *J Neurosurg* 2002;97(2):341–346.

159. Kaba SE, DeMonte F, Bruner JM, et al. The treatment of recurrent unresectable and malignant meningiomas with interferon alpha-2B. *Neurosurgery* 1997;40(2):271–275.

160. Kyritsis AP. Chemotherapy for meningiomas. *J Neurooncol* 1996;29(3):269–272.

161. Travitzky M, Libson E, Nemirovsky I, et al. Doxil-induced regression of pleuro-pulmonary metastases in a patient with malignant meningioma. *Anticancer Drugs* 2003;14(3):247–250.

162. Chamberlain MC, Tsao-Wei DD, Groshen S. Temozolomide for treatment-resistant recurrent meningioma. *Neurology* 2004;62(7):1210–1212.

163. O'Neill BP, Wang CH, O'Fallon JR, et al. Primary central nervous system non-Hodgkin's lymphoma (PCNSL): Sur-

vival advantages with combined initial therapy? A final report of the North Central Cancer Treatment Group (NCCTG) study 86–72–52. *Int J Radiat Oncol Biol Phys* 1999;43(3): 559–563.

164. DeAngelis LM, Yahalom J, Thaler HT, et al. Combined modality therapy for primary CNS lymphoma. *J Clin Oncol* 1992;10(4):635–643.

165. Abrey LE, Yahalom J, DeAngelis LM. Treatment for primary CNS lymphoma: The next step. *J Clin Oncol* 2000; 18(17):3144–3150.

166. Abrey LE, DeAngelis LM, Yahalom J. Long-term survival in primary CNS lymphoma. *J Clin Oncol* 1998;16(3):859–863.

167. Harder H, Holtel H, Bromberg JE, et al. Cognitive status and quality of life after treatment for primary CNS lymphoma. *Neurology* 2004;62(4):544–547.

168. Batchelor T, Carson K, O'Neill A, et al. Treatment of primary CNS lymphoma with methotrexate and deferred radiotherapy: A report of NABTT 96–07. *J Clin Oncol* 2003; 21(6):1044–1049.

169. Herrlinger U, Brugger W, Bamberg M, et al. PCV salvage chemotherapy for recurrent primary CNS lymphoma. *Neurology* 2000;54(8):1707–1708.

170. Lerro KA, Lacy J. Case report: A patient with primary CNS lymphoma treated with temozolomide to complete response. *J Neurooncol* 2002;59(2):165–168.

171. Pels H, Schulz H, Schlegel U, et al. Treatment of CNS lymphoma with the anti-CD20 antibody rituximab: Experience with two cases and review of the literature. *Onkologie* 2003; 26(4):351–354.

172. Enting RH, Demopoulos A, DeAngelis LM, et al. Salvage therapy for primary CNS lymphoma with a combination of rituximab and temozolomide. *Neurology* 2004;63(5):901–903.

173. Gaspar L, Scott C, Rotman M, et al. Recursive partitioning analysis (RPA) of prognostic factors in three Radiation Therapy Oncology Group (RTOG) brain metastases trials. *Int J Radiat Oncol Biol Phys* 1997;37(4):745–751.

174. Gaspar LE, Scott C, Murray K, et al. Validation of the RTOG recursive partitioning analysis (RPA) classification for brain metastases. *Int J Radiat Oncol Biol Phys* 2000;47(4):1001–1006.

175. Bindal AK, Bindal RK, Hess KR, et al. Surgery versus radiosurgery in the treatment of brain metastasis. *J Neurosurg* 1996;84(5):748–754.

176. Auchter RM, Lamond JP, Alexander E, et al. A multi-institutional outcome and prognostic factor analysis of radiosurgery for resectable single brain metastasis. *Int J Radiat Oncol Biol Phys* 1996;35(1):27–35.

177. Yung WK, Kunschner LJ, Sawaya R, et al. Intracranial metastases. In: Levin V (ed): *Cancer in the Nervous System*, 2d ed. Oxford, UK: Oxford University Press; 2002:321–340.

178. Nakagawa H, Groothuis DR, Owens ES, et al. Dexamethasone effects on [^{125}I]albumin distribution in experimental RG-2 gliomas and adjacent brain. *J Cereb Blood Flow Metab* 1987;7(6):687–701.

179. Grossi, F Scolaro T, Tixi L, et al. The role of systemic chemotherapy in the treatment of brain metastases from small-cell lung cancer. *Crit Rev Oncol Hematol* 2001;37(1): 61–67.

180. Rosner D, Nemoto T, Lane WW. Chemotherapy induces regression of brain metastases in breast carcinoma. *Cancer* 1986;58(4):832–839.

181. Bernardo G, Cuzzoni Q, Strada MR, et al. First-line chemotherapy with vinorelbine gemcitabine and carboplatin in the treatment of brain metastases from non-small-cell lung cancer: A phase II study. *Cancer Invest* 2002;20(3):293–302.

182. Kaba SE, Kyritsis AP, Hess K, et al. TPDC-FuHu chemotherapy for the treatment of recurrent metastatic brain tumors. *J Clin Oncol* 1997;15(3):1063–1070.

183. Abrey LE, Christodoulou C. Temozolomide for treating brain metastases. *Semin Oncol* 2001;28(4 suppl 13):34–42.

184. Wang ML, Yung WK, Royce ME, et al. Capecitabine for 5-fluorouracil–resistant brain metastases from breast cancer. *Am J Clin Oncol* 2001;24(4):421–424.

185. Fujita A, Fukuoka S, Takabatake H, et al. Combination chemotherapy of cisplatin ifosfamide and irinotecan with rhG-CSF support in patients with brain metastases from non-small cell lung cancer. *Oncology* 2000;59(4):291–295.

186. Hwu WJ, Krown SE, Panageas KS, et al. Temozolomide plus thalidomide in patients with advanced melanoma: Results of a dose-finding trial. *J Clin Oncol* 2002;20(11):2610–2615.

187. Hwu WJ, Raizer J, Panageas KS, et al. Treatment of metastatic melanoma in the brain with temozolomide and thalidomide. *Lancet Oncol* 2001;2(10):634–635.

188. Rustin GJ, Newlands ES, Begent RH, et al. Weekly alternating etoposide, methotrexate, and actinomycin/vincristine and cyclophosphamide chemotherapy for the treatment of CNS metastases of choriocarcinoma. *J Clin Oncol* 1989;7(7):900–903.

189. Rustin GJ, Newlands ES, Bagshawe KD, et al. Successful management of metastatic and primary germ cell tumors in the brain. *Cancer* 1986;57(11):2108–2113.

190. Gilbert MR. Brain metastases: Still an "orphan" disease? *Curr Oncol Rep* 2001;3(6):463–466.

191. Guirguis LM, Yang JC, White DE, et al. Safety and efficacy of high-dose interleukin-2 therapy in patients with brain metastases. *J Immunother* 2002;25(1):82–87.

192. Richards JM, Gale D, Mehta N, et al. Combination of chemotherapy with interleukin-2 and interferon alfa for the treatment of metastatic melanoma. *J Clin Oncol* 1999;17(2): 651–657.

ENDOCRINE MALIGNANCIES

Naifa L. Busaidy
Mouhammed Amir Habra
Rena Vassilopoulou-Sellin

■ DIFFERENTIATED THYROID CARCINOMA

Carcinoma of the thyroid gland is the most common endocrine malignancy, accounting for 1.6% of all new malignant disease (1). It has a prevalence of 180,000, and approximately 22,000 new cases of thyroid carcinoma will be diagnosed in the United States in 2003 alone (1,2). Despite the generally good prognosis of thyroid carcinoma, 5 to 10% of patients will die of the disease (1,3,4). Differentiated thyroid carcinomas, those that derive from the follicular epithelial cells (papillary and follicular), account for 94% of these malignancies; 5% are medullary thyroid cancers, a neuroendocrine tumor derived from C cells in the thyroid gland; and the remaining 1% are anaplastic thyroid carcinoma.

Overall, papillary carcinoma is the most common type of thyroid carcinoma; however, in regions where there is an iodine insufficiency, the follicular type is more common. Follicular thyroid carcinoma occurs in older people, with a peak incidence in the fifth decade of life. Follicular thyroid malignancies have a worse prognosis than papillary tumors, especially in patients with fixed/invasive lesions. In one report from the Surveillance, Epidemiology, and End Results (SEER) database, of approximately 15,700 patients in the United States, overall survival rates corrected for age and sex were 98% for papillary, 92% for follicular, 80% for medullary, and 13% for anaplastic carcinoma (4). Worse prognoses are associated with increasing age at diagnosis and metastatic disease at presentation.

Women are affected twice as often as men, although the men die of the disease twice as often as women (1). Although the median age at diagnosis is 45 years, thyroid carcinoma can also affect children. In our institution, less than 10% of all patients with thyroid cancer were diagnosed before 20 years of age (6).

DIAGNOSTIC EVALUATION OF THE SOLITARY THYROID NODULE

The most common presentation of a patient with thyroid carcinoma is the presence of a solitary thyroid nodule found either on physical examination or discovered as an incidental nodule on imaging studies performed for other purposes. Cytologic examination of a fine-needle aspirate of a nodule more than 1 cm in diameter is the most appropriate first diagnostic procedure. Papillary, medullary, and anaplastic carcinomas can be readily diagnosed by fine-needle aspiration (FNA), but distinguishing benign from malignant follicular lesions proves more difficult. Histologic examination showing capsular or vascular invasion is necessary to classify a lesion as malignant. Because follicular adenoma and carcinoma cannot be differentiated cytologically, they are grouped as "indeterminate or suspicious follicular neoplasms." The false positive and false negative rates for all nodules categorized as malignant or benign, respectively, is less than 5% (7). The rate of carcinoma for suspicious follicular lesions is about 20%. The incidence of malignancy increases with larger nodule size, male sex, and increasing age. Some 15 to 25% of the time, the FNA will yield "inadequate diagnostic material," and this necessitates repeat aspiration. The availability of ultrasound guidance has increased the diagnostic yield.

The majority (85 to 95%) of thyroid nodules are benign. Radionuclide scans usually show malignant lesions as hypofunctioning or "cold," although 85% of cold nodules are still benign (Fig. 31-1). Radionuclide scanning is no longer advocated in the initial evaluation of thyroid nodules unless the concentration of thyroid-stimulating hormone (TSH) is suppressed; in this situation, a radioiodine scan is done to assess for a functioning ("hot") adenoma. The algorithm for evaluating the patient with a thyroid nodule is outlined in Table 31-1.

DIFFERENTIATED THYROID CARCINOMA

Etiology

External low-dose radiation therapy to the head and neck during infancy and childhood, used frequently from the 1940s to the 1960s to treat a variety of benign diseases, has been shown to predispose to thyroid cancer, specifically of the papillary type. The average time between irradiation and recognition of the tumor is 10 years, but it may be longer than 30 years (8). Patients exposed to

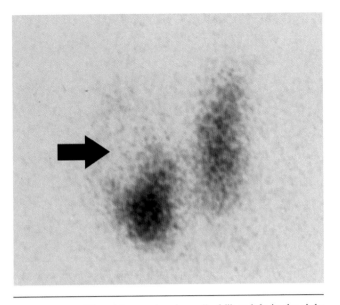

FIGURE 31-1 Thyroid scan showing a "cold" nodule in the right superior pole of the thyroid.

head or neck irradiation experience an increased frequency of benign tumors, but malignancy occurs in up to 30% of cases. Treatment of malignant diseases with higher radiation doses (more than 2000 cGy), especially at a young age, has also been associated with an increased risk of both benign and malignant neoplasms of the thyroid. Exposure to external sources of radiation after the Chernobyl nuclear accident led to a 3- to 75-fold increase in the incidence of papillary thyroid carcinoma in fallout regions, especially in younger children.

Except for reports of radiation-induced thyroid cancer, there is little information about the etiology of this malignancy. Prolonged TSH stimulation has been implicated as a potential risk factor; however, patients with primary hypothyroidism do not exhibit increased frequency of thyroid carcinoma. Thyroid-stimulatory immunoglobulins present in patients with Graves' disease have also been implicated, and associations between thyroid cancer and Hashimoto's thyroiditis, Graves'

TABLE 31-1	EVALUATION OF THE THYROID NODULE

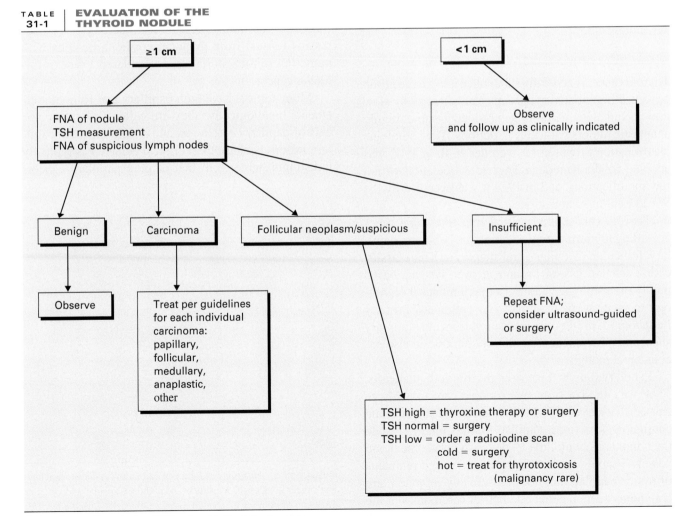

FNA = fine-needle aspiration; TSH = thyroid-stimulating hormone.

disease, and multinodular goiter have been reported. However, any causative relationship between these diseases remains poorly documented.

There are a few uncommon familial syndromes associated with differentiated thyroid carcinomas: familial adenomatous polyposis, Gardner's syndrome with polyposis of the large intestine, and Cowden's disease, which is characterized by inherited multiple hamartomas. Familial cases have been reported in 5% of all patients with papillary thyroid carcinoma and may portend a more aggressive disease course.

Follicular cell tumorigenesis pathways are receiving much attention of late. Chromosomal rearrangement of the gene encoding the transmembrane tyrosine kinase receptors *ret* and *trk* have been implicated as an early step in the development of these tumors. These genetic alterations have been found in 40 and 60% of papillary carcinomas in adults and children, respectively. Activating *ret* mutations may be the result of ionizing radiation (9). Other potential etiologic factors include DNA hypermethylation of the promoter region of the sodium-iodide symporter gene and constitutive activation of the MAP kinase cascade through activating mutations of *ras,* among others.

Pathology

Thyroid cancer is generally subdivided into a large group of well-differentiated neoplasms characterized by slow growth and high curability and a small group of highly anaplastic tumors with a bleak outlook. The pathologic classification proposed by Woolner et al. in 1961 was adopted by the American Thyroid Association with a few modifications, and in 1974 it was accepted by the World Health Organization.

Thyroid cancer is classified into four main types according to morphology and biologic behavior: papillary, follicular, medullary, and anaplastic. This classification scheme has an advantage over systems based purely on histologic patterns in that it relates morphology to methods of treatment and prognosis. Primary lymphoma of the thyroid, metastases from other primary sites, and other uncommon thyroid tumors are also encountered, though rarely.

Papillary tumors arise from thyroid follicular cells. They vary in size from microscopic cancers to large cancers that may invade the thyroid capsule and infiltrate contiguous structures. Papillary tumors tend to invade the lymphatics, with little tendency to invade the blood vessels. Psammoma bodies, calcified scarred remnants of tumor papillae that have presumably infarcted, are commonly seen in about one-half of carcinomas of the papillary type (Fig. 31-2). Follicular tumors, although

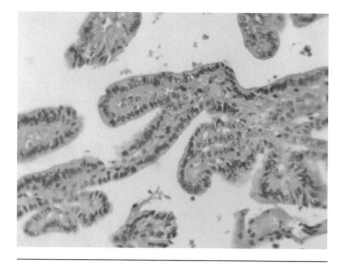

FIGURE 31-2   Classic histology for papillary thyroid carcinoma.

frequently encapsulated, commonly exhibit vascular and capsular invasion microscopically; it is this invasion that, when identified histopathologically, distinguishes benign neoplasms from malignant follicular neoplasms (Fig. 31-3). Cytology alone cannot be used to diagnose follicular carcinoma. Hurthle-cell carcinomas—neoplasms formed from granular, eosinophilic cells with numerous mitochondria—are considered a type of follicular cancer.

Many tumors have both papillary and follicular elements histologically; they are called follicular variants of papillary carcinoma and are classified as papillary lesions because their clinical behavior is typically indistinguishable from that of pure papillary cancers

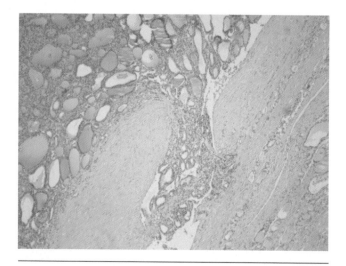

FIGURE 31-3   Histology of follicular carcinoma at the site at which the cancer invades the capsule of the nodule. Capsular and vascular invasion of nodules in a lesion that contains cells with the features of follicular neoplasm is follicular carcinoma by definition.

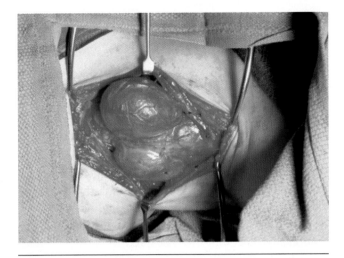

FIGURE 31-4 Intraoperative thyroid gland containing large foci of follicular variant of papillary thyroid carcinoma as seen on postoperative pathology.

(Fig. 31-4). Occasionally, both papillary and follicular tumors occur as small lesions surrounded by a dense fibrotic reaction; they are called occult sclerosing lesions and may be associated with lymph node metastases. Tall-cell variants, columnar-cell variants, and the Hurthle-cell variant are histologic subtypes that may portend a worse prognosis.

Staging

There are many clinicopathologic staging systems for differentiated thyroid carcinomas (2,10–13). The TNM (tumor, node, metastasis) method may be the most useful for predicting disease-free survival and it is generally used in our institution (14). Tumor size and the presence of extrathyroidal invasion carry prognostic importance and therefore should be reported by pathologists in every case. Anaplastic thyroid carcinoma is, by convention, always stage IV (Table 31-2).

Therapy

Surgical Management

Total thyroidectomy is the preferred initial surgical procedure for most patients with differentiated thyroid carcinoma at our institution. Arguments for total thyroidectomy rather than lobectomy are that (1) papillary foci are seen in bilateral lobes in 60 to 85% of patients (15) and (2) 5 to 10% of recurrences of papillary thyroid carcinoma after a unilateral lobectomy arise in the contralateral lobe (16). Whether the disease seen in the contralateral lobe is caused by tumor growth de novo or contralateral metastases is the subject of debate. Of the 1685 low-risk patients reviewed in a retrospective analy-

TABLE 31-2A	STAGING OF THYROID CARCINOMA

Primary Tumor (T)

Note: all categories may be subdivided into (a) solitary tumor and (b) multifocal tumor (the largest determines the classification).

TX	Primary tumor cannot be assessed
T0	No evidence of primary tumor
T1	Tumor 2 cm or less in greatest dimension limited to the thyroid
T2	Tumor more than 2 cm but not more than 4 cm in greatest dimension limited to the thyroid
T3	Tumor more than 4 cm in greatest dimension limited to the thyroid or any tumor with minimal extrathyroid extension (e.g., extension to sternothyroid muscle or perithyroid soft tissues)
T4a	Tumor of any size extending beyond the thyroid capsule to invade subcutaneous soft tissues, larynx, trachea, esophagus, or recurrent laryngeal nerve
T4b	Tumor invades prevertebral fascia or encases carotid artery or mediastinal vessels

All anaplastic carcinomas are considered T4 tumors

T4a	Intrathyroidal anaplastic carcinoma—surgically resectable
T4b	Extrathyroidal anaplastic carcinoma—surgically unresectable

Regional lymph nodes (N)

Regional lymph nodes are those of the central compartment as well as lateral cervical and upper mediastinal lymph nodes.

NX	Regional lymph nodes cannot be assessed
N0	No regional lymph node metastasis
N1	Regional lymph node metastasis
N1a	Metastasis to level VI (pretracheal, paratracheal, and prelaryngeal/Delphian lymph nodes)
N1b	Metastasis to unilateral, bilateral, or contralateral cervical or superior mediastinal lymph nodes

Distant metastasis (M)

MX	Distant metastasis cannot be assessed
M0	No distant metastasis
M1	Distant metastasis

SOURCE: Adapted from Greene FL, Page DL, Fleming ID, et al. *AJCC Cancer Staging Manual,* 6th ed. New York: Springer-Verlag; 2002:421.

sis of outcomes of patients with papillary carcinoma at the Mayo Clinic, the recurrence rate at 20 years after total thyroidectomy was 8 versus 22% after unilateral lobectomy, although there was no difference in cause-specific mortality rates (17). Other retrospective studies support these findings of lower recurrence and show only minimal improvement in survival (13,18,19). A

TABLE
31-2B | **STAGE GROUPING FOR
THYROID CARCINOMA**

Separate stage groupings are recommended for papillary or follicular, medullary, and anaplastic (undifferentiated) carcinomas.

PAPILLARY OR FOLLICULAR (<45 YEARS)

Stage I	Any T	Any N	M0
Stage II	Any T	Any N	M1

PAPILLARY OR FOLLICULAR (≥45 YEARS)

Stage I	T1	N0	M0
Stage II	T2	N0	M0
Stage III	T3	N0	M0
	T1/T2/T3	N1a	M0
Stage IVA	T4a	N0/N1a	M0
	T1/T2/T3/T4a	N1b	M0
Stage IVB	T4b	Any N	M0
Stage IVC	Any T	Any M	M1

MEDULLARY CARCINOMA

Stage I	T1	N0	M0
Stage II	T2	N0	M0
Stage III	T3	N0	M0
	T1/T2/T3	N1a	M0
Stage IVA	T4a	N0/N1a	M0
	T1/T2/T3/T4a	N1b	M0
Stage IVB	T4b	Any N	M0
Stage IVC	Any T	Any N	M1

ANAPLASTIC CARCINOMA

All anaplastic carcinomas are stage IV.

Stage IVA	T4a	Any N	M0
Stage IVB	T4b	Any N	M0
Stage IVC	Any T	Any N	M1

SOURCE: Adapted from Greene FL, Page DL, Fleming ID, et al. *AJCC Cancer Staging Manual,* 6th ed. New York: Springer-Verlag; 2002:421.

third reason that lends support to total thyroidectomy as the preferred surgical procedure is that treatment with radioiodine and the specificity of serum thyroglobulin (Tg) concentrations as a tumor marker become most efficacious after as much thyroid tissue as possible has been removed.

Some institutions still advocate unilateral surgery due to the lack of survival benefit with more extensive surgery and the apparent lower risk of hypoparathyroidism and recurrent laryngeal nerve injury (20); these two complications of thyroidectomy occur in 1% or less of total thyroidectomies when done by an experienced surgeon.

Many consensus guidelines state that a total thyroidectomy is indicated if the primary tumor is >1 cm, there is extrathyroidal invasion, or metastases are present. Patients with a history of head and neck irradiation should have the above preferred surgery, as they are at higher risk for multicentric disease and the subsequent higher recurrence risk that follows. For patients whose primary tumor is <1 cm, a unilateral lobectomy may be sufficient (5).

For patients with a cytologically suspicious follicular neoplasm, a unilateral lobectomy and isthmusectomy is the initial procedure of choice. If a malignant follicular lesion is confirmed on histopathology, then a completion thyroidectomy is warranted to allow for treatment with radioiodine therapy. Direct invasion of the strap muscles and trachea may occur and compromise resectability.

Microscopic regional nodal metastases are present in 80% of patients with papillary carcinoma. Only 35% of patients will have grossly detectable nodal (cervical or mediastinal) metastases (21). The presence of lymph node metastases increases risk of disease recurrence; however, unlike the case with other malignancies, it is only a minor risk factor for mortality. Nodal metastases represent an uncommon finding in follicular carcinoma; when they are present, however, they may indicate decreased survival.

It thus follows that neck dissection should be performed on patients with identifiable nodal disease, as its presence affects recurrence. Preoperative ultrasound of the entire neck (not just of the thyroid) is indicated to help identify the presence of nodal metastases and help the surgeon to perform a more focused operation in the hope that doing so will decrease both recurrence and complication rates. This modality is routinely applied at our institution.

Calcium and phosphorus levels should be monitored postoperatively owing to the distinct possibility of hypoparathyroidism due to either vascular damage intraoperatively or inadvertent removal.

Postoperative Iodine-131 Therapy (Radioactive Iodine Treatment)

Iodine 131 (^{131}I) has been advocated as adjuvant therapy for thyroid carcinoma; iodine is preferentially taken up and trapped by the thyroid follicular cells and malignant counterparts. It destroys cells of follicular origin by first becoming concentrated in the cell, where beta rays are released and their high-energy electrons induce radiation cytotoxicity; simultaneously, gamma rays are released that allow for detection of the emission by a camera. Postoperative examination with radioiodine scanning therefore allows the identification of residual regional or distant foci of disease, and radioiodine can be used therapeutically to ablate such tumor deposits.

The rationale for using ^{131}I as adjuvant therapy is that it (1) destroys any residual microscopic foci of disease, (2) increases specificity of subsequent ^{131}I scanning for the detection of recurrent or metastatic disease by eliminating uptake by residual normal tissue, and (3) improves the value of measurements of serum thyroglobulin (Tg) as a serum marker; hence, any elevation in Tg would be representative of recurrent or metastatic disease and not residual normal thyroid tissue (5). Combined retrospective data suggest that radioiodine ablation reduces long-term, disease-specific mortality in patients with primary tumors 1 cm or more in diameter, those with multicentric disease, or cases in which there is evidence of soft tissue invasion at presentation (13,22–24).

Patients with known residual disease, be it nodal disease or distant metastatic disease postoperatively, do have prolonged disease-free survival with postoperative radioiodine treatment. This patient population should be treated with radioactive iodine ablation as well. Radioactive iodine treatment is not recommended for solitary primary tumors <1 cm in size unless extrathyroid invasion is present or metastasis is known.

The efficacy of radioiodine depends on tumor characteristics, patient preparation, sites of disease, and radioiodine activity (21). Uptake of iodine by follicular cells (malignant and benign) is stimulated by TSH and is suppressed by increased iodide stores. For maximum uptake of radioiodine, thyroid hormone concentrations should be lowered sufficiently to allow the TSH to rise to above >25 mU/L. Postoperative hypothyroidism develops after 4 to 6 weeks. To help alleviate symptoms of hypothyroidism for the first 2 weeks, liothyronine (T3) may be administered at 25 μg twice a day. Lower doses are given to elderly patients and those with coronary artery disease. Two weeks prior to radioiodine scanning, the T3 is stopped; patients are also told to avoid foods with high iodine content for these 2 weeks. Administration of "cold" (nonradioactive) iodine, such as that found in contrast material routinely used for computed tomography (CT) imaging and various invasive procedures, should be avoided for at least 3 months prior to a radioactive iodine scan. This cold iodine will interfere with the therapeutic radioactive iodine and may make the radioiodine scans falsely "negative." Urinary concentrations of iodine can be checked to assess total body iodine content prior to scanning and treating a patient with ^{131}I. Using 2 to 5 mCi of either ^{123}I or ^{131}I, a radioiodine scan for localization of uptake prior to ab-

lation (pretreatment scan), is recommended. Some 24 to 96 h after dosing, whole-body scans and spot images of the neck are obtained using a gamma camera. After the thyroidectomy, most patients will demonstrate uptake of radioiodine in the thyroid bed (presumably normal residual tissue) of less than <5%. An uptake of more than 5% on a whole-body scan indicates that excessive thyroid tissue remains and that further surgical resection may be warranted. If extensive locoregional disease is seen, additional surgery should be considered. Once the decision is made to treat the patient with radioiodine, an empiric dose of radioactive iodine treatment is generally chosen, as follows: 75 to 150 mCi for adjuvant ablation, approximately 150 mCi for nodal disease, and 200 mCi or more for metastatic disease outside the lungs. Stricter dosing calculations using elaborate dosimetric techniques can be computed; however, these are not in routine clinical use at present.

A posttreatment scan is performed to assess for further uptake of radioiodine that was not previously seen on the pretreatment scan (i.e., regional or distant metastases). The post treatment scan is a more sensitive technique to detect metastatic disease, as the ability to demonstrate radioactive iodine avid lesions is directly proportional to amount of radioactive iodine given (Fig. 31-5).

Radioiodine treatment is usually administered in a hospital setting because of radiation safety issues. In most institutions and for most cases of thyroid cancer, treatment with high doses necessitates an inpatient stay.

Short-term complications, though rare, include radiation thyroiditis, neck edema, sialoadenitis, and tumor hemorrhage. These occur more often in the presence of bulky disease. Long-term complications, which increase with cumulative doses, include xerostomia, nasolacrimal duct obstruction (25,26), pulmonary fibrosis (if pulmonary metastasis is present and treated at high doses), and secondary malignant diseases, such as acute myelogenous leukemia. Patients treated with ^{131}I may be at a small but increased risk for other secondary malignancies such as bladder cancer, salivary gland tumors, colon cancer, and female breast carcinomas. Oligospermia and transient ovarian failure have also been described, but there is no definite dose relation.

There are no reports of congenital abnormalities in children conceived after radioiodine treatment; however, most physicians would recommend that women not conceive for at least 6 months after treatment. Radioiodine should not be given to a pregnant woman owing to the potential teratogenic effects on the fetus's growth and thyroid development; all women of childbearing age must have a negative pregnancy test prior to treatment.

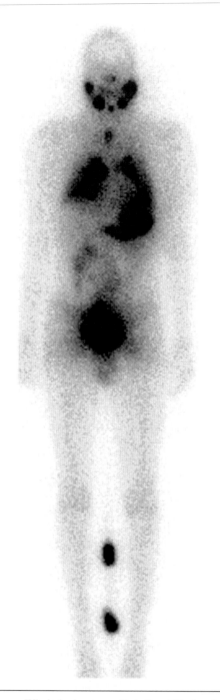

FIGURE 31-5 Whole-body scan with iodine 131 showing multiple metastatic deposits in the neck and lungs, with physiologic uptake in the salivary gland, stomach, intestines, and bladder.

Thyroid Hormone Therapy

After receiving radioactive ablation, patients are placed on thyroid hormone therapy for two reasons. The first and foremost reason is that it corrects the iatrogenic hypothyroidism and avoids all subsequent long-term complications. Second, it minimizes potential TSH-stimulated growth of thyroid cancer cells. TSH-suppressive therapy has been shown to increase disease-free sur-

vival two- to threefold, especially in high-risk patients. Oversuppression of TSH can lead to morbid consequences. Some of the complications of thyroid hormone suppression are osteopenia, atrial fibrillation, and possible cardiac hypertrophy. Enough thyroid hormone should be given to suppress TSH to 0.1 to 0.5 mU/L. In patients at higher risk of recurrence, TSH should be suppressed to less than 0.1 mU/L.

External-Beam Radiotherapy

External-beam radiotherapy (EBRT) has a role in the treatment of papillary thyroid carcinoma. Although the issue is controversial, two retrospective studies have shown that it may be an effective adjuvant therapy to prevent locoregional recurrence in patients 45 years of age and older with locally invasive papillary carcinoma (27,28). Ten-year local relapse-free rates (93 versus 78%) and disease-specific survival rates (100 versus 95%) were significantly improved in a subgroup of 155 patients with papillary histology and presumed microscopic disease (disease within 2-mm margin resections, tumor shaved off structures) treated with EBRT (27). Patients below 45 years of age are generally not treated with EBRT, both because of their good prognosis and the possible late side effects of such therapy, including secondary malignancies.

Doses in the range of 40 to 50 Gy may aid in locoregional control in patients with papillary thyroid carcinoma who are over 45 years of age and have incomplete resection near the aerodigestive tract and/or those with gross extrathyroidal invasion with presumed microscopic residual disease.

Long-Term Follow-Up

Imaging

After a total thyroidectomy followed by radioiodine ablation, patients need lifelong monitoring using both clinical and radiographic data. It is recommended that patients have a follow-up radioiodine scan 6 to 12 months after initial radioiodine ablation. The predictive value for 10-year disease-free survival is approximately 90% with one negative scan postablation (29). Recombinant human TSH (rhTSH) may be used in this follow-up scan at the clinician's discretion (a discussion of rhTSH follows). Scanning beyond this first follow-up must be individualized and is no longer routine for all thyroid cancer patients. Ultrasonography (US) of the neck (thyroid bed and cervical neck compartments) is used more in the preoperative and postoperative follow-up of these patients today. US can be used to accurately diagnose and identify lesions in the neck as small as 3 mm. Although US can aid in distinguishing benign lesions from malignant lesions, FNA (US-guided) is most helpful to definitively prove recurrent cancer. Routine use of US in the 3- to 12-month monitoring of patients with extrathyroidal invasion or locoregional nodal metastases is advocated in many consensus guidelines (30–32). As many as half the patients with findings of recurrence on US may have no uptake on radioiodine scanning or may have an undetectable serum Tg.

Other imaging techniques that can be used in individual cases of thyroid cancer follow-up include CT scan of the neck and chest, chest radiographs, fluorodeoxyglucose positron-emission tomography (FDG-PET or PET) and magnetic resonance imaging (MRI). MRI and CT scan of the neck play important roles in the detection of recurrent disease; they are not as sensitive as US but are much less operator-dependent. Chest radiographs may show macronodular pulmonary metastases that do not routinely take up iodine; however, they are less sensitive for micronodular metastases. CT scan of the chest may be more helpful in these situations. FDG-PET imaging has recently been approved for the follow-up of thyroid cancer patients who have a Tg greater than 20 and have negative radioiodine imaging. PET imaging is sensitive in detecting metastatic disease; however, it is not specific for thyroid cancer, and caution should be exercised in searching for recurrent disease. PET imaging is, therefore, not useful in the routine follow-up of patients with thyroid cancer, but may play a role in the less common radioiodine-negative, Tg-positive disease (Figs. 31-6 and 31-7). The latest technology in detection of recurrent thyroid cancer is PET/CT. This imaging technique takes advantage of both CT image technology and a PET image and fuses the two, making for more accurate localization and detection of both function (PET) and anatomy (CT). Many cases have been described in which imaging is convincingly positive (false positive); however, intra- and postoperative pathology is not consistent with thyroid carcinoma but rather confirms benign disease, such as scar.

Monitoring Serum Thyroglobulin

Tg is a protein synthesized only by the thyroid follicular cells (both benign and differentiated malignant tissue) and therefore is a good biochemical test to assess the presence of residual, recurrent, or metastatic disease. After total thyroidectomy and ablation, the Tg should be undetectable. The nadir should be reached within 3 months posttreatment but may take as long as 1 to 2 years. Tg should always be measured and recorded in the context of the TSH value because Tg production is

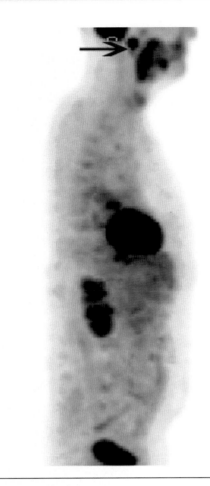

FIGURE 31-6 PET scan showing posterior pharyngeal metastatic papillary thyroid carcinoma. Thyroglobulin was 35 and radioiodine whole-body scan was negative for disease.

dependent on TSH secretion. The sensitivity of Tg measurements to detect cancer is increased to 85 to 95% during thyroid hormone withdrawal, with its subsequent elevated TSH levels, and is approximately 50% during TSH-suppressive therapy (33). When the tumor has dedifferentiated and no longer secretes the Tg protein, Tg levels will be falsely low and cannot be relied on.

Autoantibodies to Tg can falsely lower the reported Tg concentrations in immunometric assays, as the antibodies interfere with the assay's ability to bind to Tg. Tg antibodies are present in approximately 25% of patients with thyroid cancer, and the presence of antibodies in itself after total thyroidectomy and postradioactive ablation may be indicative of the presence of cancer. Sensitive methods to detect Tg mRNA are being developed and, if proven to be valid and useful, may circumvent the problem mentioned above. It is also important that the assay used for Tg measurement be repeated in the same laboratory to avoid erroneous misinterpretations of interassay variability.

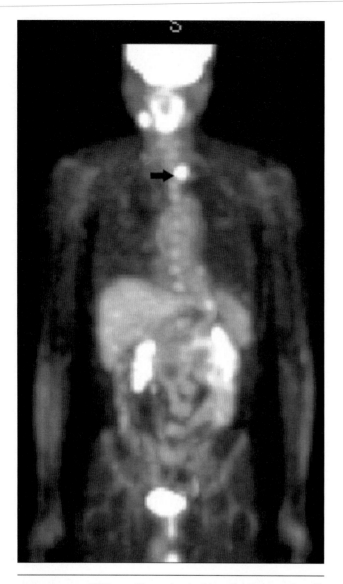

FIGURE 31-7   PET scan illustrating incidentally discovered papillary thyroid carcinoma during staging workup for lymphoma.

Recombinant Human TSH

Thyrotropin alpha, an rhTSH, may be used in lieu of standard thyroid hormone withdrawal to increase thyrotropin concentrations as needed for adequate stimulation of both radioiodine uptake for scanning and serum Tg concentrations. The use of rhTSH is of particular benefit in the patient in whom endogenous TSH levels cannot rise due to hypopituitarism or in whom the clinician prefers to avoid prolonged hypothyroidism and its resultant complications due to concurrent medical problems. Studies have shown that the accuracy of diagnostic radioiodine scanning and Tg measurement to detect residual thyroid tissue or carcinoma after two injections of thyrotropin alpha is almost as efficacious as thyroid hormone withdrawal. In general, patients who are at

lower risk of recurrence (stage I to II TNM) may be eligible for rhTSH-stimulated Tg measurement and scanning on their first follow-up scan. If there is evidence of abnormal uptake on this scan currently, the patient would have to be withdrawn from thyroid hormone to be treated with radioiodine ablation. An ongoing randomized multicenter trial will answer the question of whether rhTSH can be used for treatment with radioiodine as efficaciously as withdrawal in patients with evidence of radioiodine uptake.

Metastatic Disease

Gross nodal disease should be resected at the time of initial surgery or later at recurrence; this has been shown to increase relapse-free survival. Microscopic nodal metastases occur in up to 80% of cases at diagnosis, and their presence is associated with a high rate of recurrence. Resection of gross nodal disease and radioiodine treatment (approximately 150 mCi) should be performed for nodal metastases. Distant metastases are evident in less than 1% of patients at the time of presentation.

The most common sites of metastasis, in decreasing order of frequency, are the lungs, bones, and other soft tissues (Figs. 31-8 and 31-9). Older patients have a higher risk for distant metastases. The clinical course and prognosis of patients who have received head and neck irradiation predating the cancer is similar to that of random cases, even though the former group may present with more extensive disease.

Pulmonary metastases in differentiated thyroid carcinoma are often classified radiographically as either "micronodular" or "macronodular" disease. Micronodular metastases present a miliary, diffusely reticular pattern predominating in the lower lung fields and tend to concentrate radioiodine diffusely; this is the pattern of metastasis most often seen in children (Fig. 31-10) (6).

Macronodular (coarse) metastases with nodular masses of unequal size (varying between 0.5 and 3.0 cm) occur more frequently overall. Radioiodine incorporation is heterogeneous but often not present. The transition from micro- to macronodular metastasis may occur during the course of the disease.

In a review of 101 patients with differentiated thyroid carcinoma and pulmonary metastases, Samaan et al. (64) analyzed potential prognostic factors and the efficacy of radioiodine treatment over time. Uptake of radioiodine by lung metastases conferred a favorable prognosis, especially in patients with negative radiological findings. The probability of radioiodine uptake was related to the degree of differentiation of the primary tumor. Pulmonary metastases were least common in patients with papillary carcinoma and most common in those with

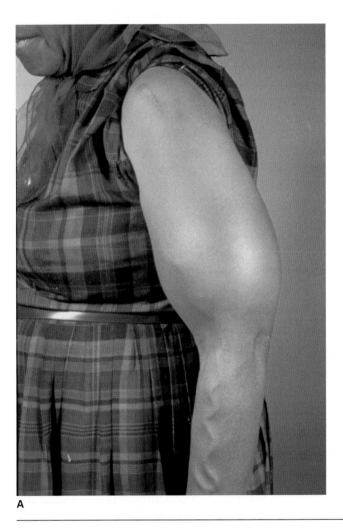

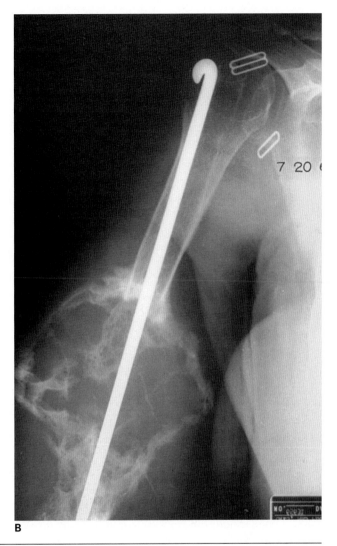

A   B

FIGURE 31-8 **A.** A woman with metastatic follicular thyroid carcinoma to left humerus. **B.** Radiograph of metastatic follicular thyroid carcinoma to left humerus in the same patient.

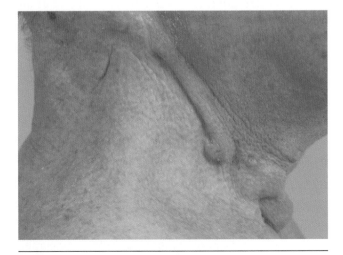

FIGURE 31-9 Patient with multiple metastatic deposits of papillary thyroid carcinoma to the skin.

Hurthle-cell carcinoma. Patients less than 40 years old had a better prognosis than those older than 40. Patients with radioiodine uptake in pulmonary metastases have a 5-year survival rate of 60%, compared with 30% in patients with no uptake in their lungs on radioiodine scanning. Radioiodine treatments in the range of 150 to 175 mCi are used to treat pulmonary metastases; higher doses are avoided to decrease the rare possibility of pulmonary fibrosis.

Median survival duration of patients with one or more brain metastases improves significantly from 4 to 22 months with surgical resection (34). Bone lesions tend to concentrate radioiodine as well as pulmonary metastases. Complete resolution is achieved in less than 10% of these cases. Follicular thyroid carcinoma tends to spread to bone (producing osteolytic lesions) and

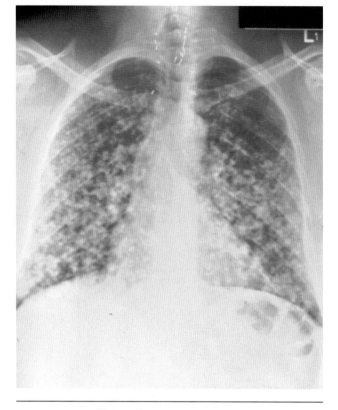

FIGURE 31-10 Chest radiograph showing classic miliary pattern of metastatic papillary thyroid carcinoma in the lungs.

lungs more readily than papillary carcinoma and may respond better to radioiodine treatment. Symptoms from painful bone lesions or spinal cord–compressing lesions may be relieved by surgical treatment. EBRT has also been used successfully to render bone lesions pain-free. In follicular thyroid carcinoma, where the lesions are highly vascular, arterial embolization has been used with successful reduction in pain at our institution. Intravenous bisphosphonates (pamidronate or zoledronic acid) are prescribed for painful bony metastases with some success as well.

Radioiodine treatment follows surgical resection of distant metastatic disease if the tumor takes up radioiodine. This represents a setting (especially with central nervous system lesions) where we are increasingly using rhTSH for the treatment of thyroid cancer in order to avoid potential complications such as edema, inherent in the prolonged hypothyroid state.

In general, doses of 200 mCi are used for the treatment of distant metastatic disease. This dose may then be repeated 6 to 12 months later. Radioiodine treatment should be used judiciously to avoid red marrow toxicity and pulmonary fibrosis.

EBRT may prove useful in patients with unresectable, grossly locally invasive or metastatic disease

to the neck. This may also help to control compressive symptomatology from residual/recurrent disease.

Systemic chemotherapy is used in certain cases of widespread disease, although available regimens have not been well studied and are not very effective to date. Doxorubicin is associated with a response rate of up to 40% for progressive differentiated cancers that do not respond to radioiodine. The recommended dosage is 60 to 75 mg/m^2 every 3 weeks. Combination therapies are also used, but data are limited because of the small number of patients in reported series.

Biological response modifiers are under investigation to determine whether dedifferentiated cancers can be modified to increase radioiodine uptake. These agents should be used within a clinical trial at this time.

Differentiated Thyroid Carcinoma in Children

Thyroid cancer rarely affects children; at our institution, less than 10% of all patients diagnosed with thyroid cancer were under the age of 20 years. Few data, therefore, exist regarding the optimal treatment in this population. Children with thyroid cancer generally have a good prognosis despite the initial extent of disease. In our review of outcomes of differentiated thyroid carcinoma in children, we found that 25% of patients diagnosed in childhood had recurrences, and 6% died of their disease. Three percent of patients died of late complications of EBRT, including tracheal necrosis and cervical sarcomas. Two patients treated with radioactive iodine and surgery died of breast carcinoma at young ages (35).

Cervical node involvement is more common in children than in adults. Up to 10% of children and adolescents may have lung involvement at the time of diagnosis (36). Regardless of the extent of disease, however, children with thyroid carcinoma live for many years after treatment.

In view of the high incidence of recurrence, multifocality, locoregional spread, and extracervical metastases, total thyroidectomy with nodal dissection and adjuvant radioiodine therapy is recommended for children with thyroid cancer. Lifelong surveillance, however, is of the utmost importance.

■ MEDULLARY THYROID CARCINOMA

Medullary thyroid carcinomas (MTC) represent 5% of all thyroid neoplasms. About 80% of patients with MTC have a sporadic form of the disease, and the remaining 20% inherit MTC as an autosomal dominant trait as part of the distinct clinical syndromes of multiple endocrine neoplasia (MEN) type 2A, type 2B, or familial MTC. In MEN 2A, MTC occurs in association with pheochromocytoma and multigland parathyroid tumors; MTC is usually the first manifested disease of the three aforementioned components of this syndrome. In MEN 2B, MTC occurs in association with pheochromocytoma and mucosal neuromas (Figs. 31-11A and B) or neurofibromas and marfanoid habitus.

Medullary thyroid carcinoma is derived from C cells (or calcitonin-secreting cells) that are of neural crest origin. MTC arises primarily in the upper two-thirds of the gland where the C cells are normally found (Fig. 31-12). C cells secret a 32-amino-acid peptide called calcitonin, which serves as a useful biochemical marker in patients with this cancer. MTC occurs as a solid mass or a cluster of C-cell hyperplasia interspersed between normal-appearing thyroid follicles. These can be visualized with calcitonin immunostaining, which shows variable amounts of fibrosis and deposits of amyloid in 60 to 80% of tumors. Even the smallest visible tumors can be associated with metastases.

The most common clinical presentation of sporadic medullary thyroid cancer is a solitary thyroid mass found incidentally during routine examination. Routine measurement of serum calcitonin concentrations is not recommended for the assessment of a thyroid nodule, as the results may be misleading and it is not cost-effective (37–40); there are other etiologies of elevated calcitonin levels that may make the level difficult to interpret. Most patients with sporadic MTC present in the fifth or sixth decade of life, with a male: female ratio of 1.4:1. Metastases to cervical and mediastinal lymph nodes are found in about 50% of the patients at the time of initial presentation (Fig. 31-13). Distant metastases to the lungs, liver, bones, and adrenal glands most commonly occur late in the course of the disease (Fig. 31-14).

Secretory diarrhea, often severe, is the most prominent hormone-mediated clinical feature of medullary carcinoma. Facial flushing is also a symptom commonly seen with hormone overproduction. Rarely, ectopic production of adrenocorticotropic hormone (ACTH) and/or corticotropin-releasing hormone (CRH) may cause paraneoplastic Cushing's syndrome.

INHERITED MEDULLARY THYROID CANCER

In kindreds with inherited MTC, prospective family screening is essential due to the 90 to 95% penetrance of the disease (41–43). MTC, in these cases, is usually pres-

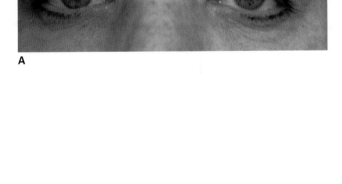

A

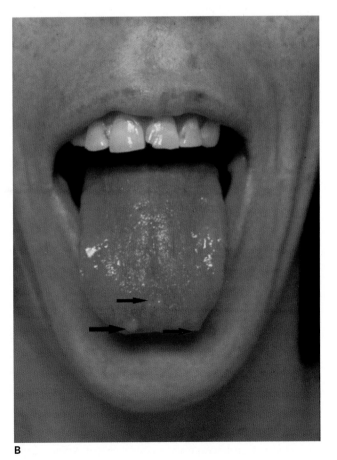

B

FIGURE 31-11   A. Patient with MEN 2B, with typical thickening of the palpebrum. Note also the ganglioneuroma on the left superior eyelid. **B.** Multiple ganglioneuromas on the tongue of a patient with MEN 2B.

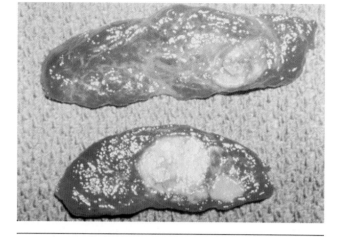

FIGURE 31-12   Gross specimen of thyroid gland containing medullary thyroid carcinoma.

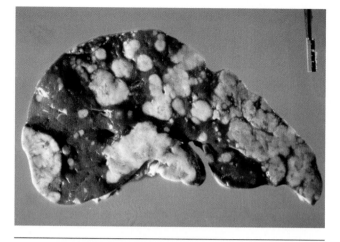

FIGURE 31-14   Gross specimen of liver containing metastatic lesions of medullary thyroid carcinoma.

ent by the third decade of life. Inherited syndromes of MTC are all transmitted in an autosomal dominant form. The mutation is detected in the tyrosine kinase proto-oncogene *ret* and can be identified in 98% of affected family members with appropriate screening (41,43–45). There is a 2 to 5% false-negative rate in patients known to have inherited medullary carcinoma (43). Six percent of patients with sporadic MTC carry a germline *ret* mutation (46). Genetic testing should thus be offered to all patients with newly diagnosed apparent sporadic disease. MEN 2B patients tend to exhibit more locally aggressive MTC (47); screening with *ret* testing is recommended at age 6 months or prior. For familial MTC and MEN 2A, screening is recommended by 5 years of age (30,32,43).

Analysis of the *ret* gene should include the most common sites of mutation, initially exons 10 and 11; if no mutation is found, testing should proceed with exons 13 to 16 (43). Appropriate genetic counseling must be a part of the initial evaluation, including the possibilities of errors in testing, the potential for discrimination, and changes that may occur in quality of life.

Five- and 10-year disease-specific survival rates of about 95 and 75%, respectively, for patients under 40 years contrast with rates of 65 and 50%, respectively, for those above 40 years of age (48).

THERAPY

Surgery

In MTC there is a high propensity for bilateral disease in both the sporadic and familial forms; therefore the usual treatment is total thyroidectomy with central neck compartment dissection in all patients. In unilateral sporadic disease, if the primary tumor is greater than 1 cm or central compartment disease is present, strong consideration should be given to ipsilateral modified radical neck or mediastinal dissections or both. Bilateral neck dissections are usually performed in many institutions, including our own, in patients with inherited disease (30,32,43,49). Radical neck dissections are not favored, as they cause major disfigurement without improving prognosis; rather, a function-preserving approach is preferred.

Patients should have a preoperative evaluation for possible coexisting pheochromocytoma via plasma or urine metanephrines and catecholamines and hyperparathyroidism via serum calcium testing. If the pheochro-

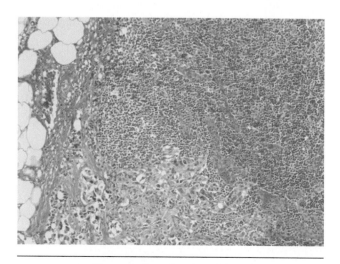

FIGURE 31-13   Hematoxylin and eosin staining of areas of lymph node containing metastasis from medullary thyroid carcinoma.

mocytoma is present, appropriate control of catechol-amine hypersecretion should precede thyroid surgery.

Hormone Replacement

Patients should be placed on thyroid hormone replace-ment therapy postoperatively. TSH has not been im-plicated in the growth or recurrence of MTC (as neuro-endocrine C cells are the cell of origin); therefore, unlike the case with differentiated thyroid carcinoma, there is no role for thyroid hormone suppression ther-apy; hence the goal should be to maintain the TSH and free T4 concentrations to within normal levels. There is also no role for radioiodine therapy in the treatment of MTC; therefore thyroid hormone replacement may be started immediately after surgery.

External Beam Radiotherapy

EBRT should be considered for patients who are at high risk for locoregional recurrence. In one study, the relapse-free rate at 10 years was 86% for patients with microscopic residual disease, extraglandular invasion, or lymph node metastases after optimal surgical exci-sion who were treated with EBRT compared with 52% for those not given adjuvant radiation therapy (50). In general, in MTC, 20 fractions totaling 40 Gy is given to the cervical, supraclavicular, and upper mediastinal lymph nodes over 4 weeks; subsequent booster doses of 10 Gy are then given to the thyroid bed, especially if there was gross residual disease (51). EBRT can also be given to treat painful skeletal metastases.

MONITORING AND FOLLOW-UP

Biochemical testing with serum calcitonin and carcino-embryonic antigen (CEA) is used in the routine fol-low-up of patients with MTC. Some 2 to 3 months post-operatively, these markers should be within the normal ranges (a nadir of 6 months has been reported). Sensi-tive detection of residual disease may be done by mea-suring calcitonin after calcium or pentagastrin stimu-lation tests when these tumor markers are within the normal range. Patients with palpable recurrent/residual disease in general will have stimulated calcitonin levels of at least 10 pg/mL, the exception being those tumors that are dedifferentiated and no longer secrete calcitonin (these tumors usually secrete CEA). Values of serum calcitonin greater than 100 pg/mL are indicative of resid-ual neck disease or distant metastases, and these patients should be aggressively assessed clinically and radio-graphically. Due to MTC's propensity for neck, medi-astinal, and liver metastasis, diagnostic imaging should

include ultrasound (US) of the neck, CT of the chest, and MRI of the liver. Routine use of positron emission tomography (PET), metaiodobenzylguanidine (MIBG) scintigraphy, and bone scans is not recommended. The liver should be the organ of highest suspicion for dis-tant metastases, for basal calcitonin levels greater than 1000 pg/mL and no obvious neck disease. Occasion-ally, venous catheterization is necessary to localize dis-tant metastases.

Postoperative hypercalcitonemia in one study was associated with 5- and 10-year survival rates of 90 and 86%, respectively (52); in other studies, high clinical recurrence rates are reported. Outcomes of hypercalci-tonemia in these patients correlate with their initial presentation of disease (5). Although there is a lack of long-term outcome studies, a few reports indicate nor-malization of calcitonin levels after surgical resection for nodal recurrences. The clinical significance of this remains to be elucidated.

PROPHYLACTIC SURGERY FOR KINDREDS WITH *RET* MUTATIONS

Carriers of a familial *ret* mutation are recommended to have prophylactic thyroidectomy; this is an area of much controversy. The controversy regards the age at which this should occur. The specifically mutated codon on the *ret* gene correlates with the MEN 2 variant and sub-sequently with the aggressiveness of MTC (43). The latest consensus guidelines (issued in December 2001) suggest risk stratification based on the three known levels of aggressiveness of the known codon mutation. MEN 2B patients and patients with codons known to have the highest risk (level 3) and most aggressive form of MTC are recommended to have prophylactic thy-roidectomy by the age of 6 months and preferably within the first month of life (43). It has been recommended that patients classified at level 2 or considered at high risk for MTC should have prophylactic thyroidectomy by age 5 years (78). There was no agreement as to whether routine lymph node dissections should be done. For pa-tients with level 1 risk, there was no consensus as to whether they should be treated by age 5, as level 2 pa-tients by age 10, or with periodic monitoring with pen-tagastrin stimulation testing.

ANAPLASTIC THYROID CARCINOMA

Anaplastic thyroid carcinoma is a locally and systemi-cally aggressive undifferentiated tumor derived from follicular cells. In fact, it has the poorest prognosis of all thyroid carcinomas, with a disease-specific mortality rate approaching 100% (53–56). More than 90% of patients with this disease are over the age of 50 years, and there is a male to female ratio of 2:3.

In sharp contrast with differentiated thyroid carcinomas, anaplastic thyroid carcinoma confers a dismal prognosis. Median survival duration after diagnosis ranges from 4 to 12 months; a long-term survival of more than 5 years is considered rare. Better survival rates are seen only in those patients with well-localized anaplastic tumors. Favorable prognostic features seem to be unilateral tumors, tumor size less than 5 cm, no invasion of adjacent tissue, and absence of nodal involvement or distant metastases.

PATHOLOGY

Anaplastic thyroid carcinoma most commonly presents as the rapid growth of a thyroid mass, frequently in a preexisting goiter. A history of a long-standing thyroid enlargement is noted in about 80% of these patients. FNA or surgical biopsy can usually establish the diagnosis. In 50% of cases, this disease arises from preexisting well-differentiated thyroid carcinoma (Fig. 31-15).

The presence of argyrophilic cytoplasmic granules distinguishes tumor of follicular origin from that of parafollicular origin and thus can differentiate anaplastic follicular thyroid lesions from undifferentiated variants of MTC. Tg, normally synthesized in the follicular epithelium of the thyroid, is present in well-differentiated papillary and follicular carcinomas and infrequently in anaplastic carcinomas. The absence of Tg immunoreactivity in anaplastic carcinomas does not exclude

follicular epithelial origin, because undifferentiated carcinoma cells may have lost the ability to synthesize this glycoprotein.

THERAPY

Treatment is generally palliative in nature, as anaplastic thyroid carcinoma is rarely cured and almost always fatal. Death occurs from upper airway obstruction and suffocation in half the patients and complications of therapy or distant metastases in the others. For resectable lesions (no extracervical disease) in anaplastic carcinoma, surgical excision with wide margins of adjacent soft tissue on the side of the tumor is appropriate, followed by adjuvant radiotherapy. Prolonged survival of 75 to 80% at 2 years has been reported for the 20% of patients whose tumor is confined to the neck and grossly resectable when treated by complete surgical resection followed by adjuvant radiotherapy and chemotherapy (53,56). Total thyroidectomy and radical neck dissection result in an increased complication rate and are not likely to increase survival time in patients in whom disease cannot be completely resected (53,56–58). Hyperfractionated radiotherapy and radiosensitizing doxorubicin may increase the local response rate. Paclitaxel has shown promise of late in newly diagnosed patients and may provide benefit (54,59). Radiotherapy and chemotherapy are important alternative approaches, but further evaluation is needed to optimize their effectiveness. Biological response modifiers aimed at restoring dedifferentiated functions of thyroid tissue may also be of some benefit in the future, but they are still under investigation at present.

■ PHEOCHROMOCYTOMA

Pheochromocytoma is a chromaffin-cell neoplasm that can arise as an adrenal (adrenal medulla) or extraadrenal tumor. Extraadrenal pheochromocytoma is also referred to as paraganglioma. Pheochromocytoma is an infrequent but potentially curable cause of secondary hypertension. If undiagnosed or improperly treated, it can lead to life-threatening complications that can be avoided by considering pheochromocytoma early in the differential diagnosis of symptomatic hypertension, which presents with headache, palpitations, or sweating.

These tumors are most often benign; in general, 10% are thought to be malignant, 10% extraadrenal, and 10% bilateral (most often in the setting of familial syndromes) (Fig. 31-16).

The incidence of reported pheochromocytomas depends on the screening method chosen. In the general

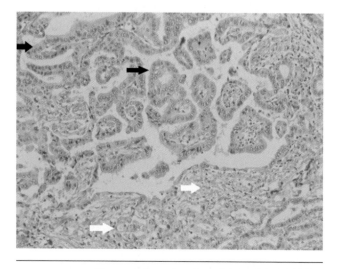

FIGURE 31-15 Hematoxylin and eosin staining of thyroid illustrating papillary thyroid carcinoma (*black arrows*) in transition to anaplastic thyroid carcinoma (*white arrows*).

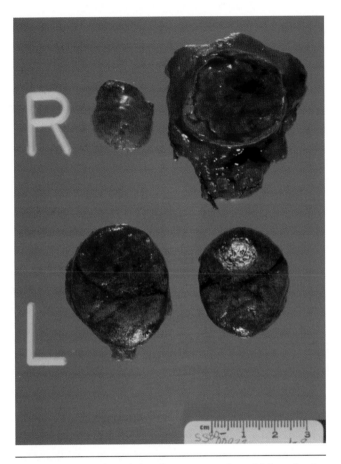

FIGURE 31-16 Bilateral pheochromocytoma in multiple endocrine neoplasia 2A.

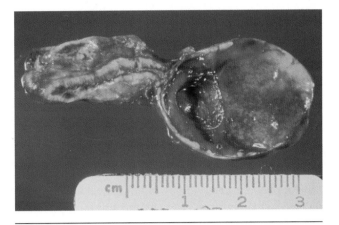

FIGURE 31-17 Adrenal gland with pheochromocytoma.

population, the incidence rate has been estimated at 0.95 per 100,000 person-years (60), whereas on autopsy series, the incidence rate was reported as 0.05% (one tumor per 2031 autopsies) (61). In one study, sporadic cases accounted for 84% of the patients and hereditary cases for the other 16% (62). Tumor is located in the adrenal gland in 81% of cases (Fig. 31-17) and is extraadrenal (Fig. 31-18) in 19% (63), with a slight female predominance (53.6% females and 46.4% males) (64).

CLINICAL FEATURES

The clinical presentation of pheochromocytoma is variable, ranging from asymptomatic to catastrophic sudden death. Hypertension is commonly reported with pheochromocytoma and has been reported to be paroxysmal in 48% of patients and persistent in 29%; 13% of patients were normotensive. Rarely, hypotension may occur with tumors that secrete mainly epinephrine. The symptomatic triad (headaches, palpitations, and sweating attacks) has a specificity of 93.8% and a sensitivity of 90.9% in the diagnosis of pheochromocytoma. The presence of the above symptoms in hypertensive patients justifies systematic assays of blood or urinary catecholamines; in their absence, the probability of pheochromocytoma is less than 1 in 1000 (65). Patients may have characteristic "spells" of paroxysmal headaches, pallor or flushing, hypertension, and diaphoresis that may persist anywhere from a few minutes to several hours. Attacks may be provoked by body position, straining, exercise, emotional stress, or voiding. Orthostatic hypotension in the presence of hypertension may be an additional clue to a diagnosis of pheochromocytoma; this may be due to the intravascular volume depletion associated with vasoconstriction. Patients may have impaired glucose tolerance from the suppressive effects of catecholamines on insulin secretion. Patients also may have constipation, cholelithiasis, or abdominal distention from the inhibitory effects of catecholamines on gut motility.

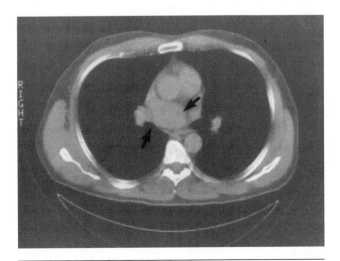

FIGURE 31-18 CT of the chest showing extraadrenal pheochromocytoma in the pericardium (*arrows*).

Rarely, pheochromocytoma can lead to the ectopic production of vasoactive intestinal polypeptide (VIP), growth hormone–releasing factor, adrenocorticotropin, and corticotropin-releasing hormone.

DIAGNOSIS

Laboratory Findings

There is ongoing discussion as to the optimal screening test for pheochromocytomas. Biochemical testing is indicated in the presence of (1) features or family history suggestive of syndromes associated with pheochromocytoma, including MEN 2A, MEN 2B, von Hippel–Lindau (VHL) disease, and neurofibromatosis 1 (NF-1); (2) clinical features of symptomatic pheochromocytoma (headache, diaphoresis, or palpitations), especially in the presence of hypertension; (3) adrenal incidentalomas; and (4) a hypertensive crisis at the time of delivery or induction of anesthesia (Table 31-3).

It is important to have chemical confirmation of pheochromocytoma before attempting costly localization procedures. Determination of catecholamines (norepinephrine, epinephrine, and dopamine) and their metabolites (metanephrine, normetaphrine, vanillylmandelic acid, and homovanillic acid) is the first step in the diagnosis of pheochromocytoma. Catecholamines and their metabolites can be measured in urine or plasma. Because pheochromocytomas can have intermittent catecholamine secretion, a 24-h collection of urine to measure catecholamines and their metabolites is usually ordered. Shorter periods of urine collection are less reliable but can still be done if a 24-h urine collection cannot be obtained. Urine should be acidified (with 30 mL 6N HCl preservative for a final pH of 1 to 3) and refrigerated during and after collection until the time at which an analysis is performed. Measurement of 24-h urine creatinine excretion is simultaneously ordered to ensure the adequacy of collection. Total plasma catecholamine levels greater than 2000 pg/mL are diagnostic of pheochromocytoma, while a level of less than 500 pg/mL during a symptomatic episode almost always rules out pheochromocytoma. Levels must be interpreted with caution because several medications (e.g., monoamine oxidase inhibitors, amphetamines, bromocriptine, buspirone, caffeine, levodopa, clonidine, diuretics, ethanol, nicotine, theophylline, tricyclic antidepressants, vasodilators, methyldopa, and labetalol) may affect the results. It is important to remember that normal plasma catecholamines while the patient is normotensive and asymptomatic do not rule out the diagnosis of pheochromocytoma. The glucagon stimulation test (1 mg IV

bolus) was previously performed in cases suspicious for pheochromocytoma and total catecholamine plasma levels are between 500 and 1000 pg/mL. This test has largely been abandoned as it carries significant risk for hypertensive crisis.

For baseline catecholamine plasma levels between 1000 and 2000 pg/mL, a clonidine suppression test may be helpful. A normal clonidine suppression test requires plasma catecholamines levels to drop more than 50% and be less than 500 pg/mL when measured 2 to 3 h after 0.3 mg of oral clonidine. In the presence of pheochromocytoma, the normal physiologic suppression of catecholamines is lost and plasma catecholamines levels remain elevated.

In a multicenter study (108), plasma free metanephrines were superior to plasma catecholamines in the diagnosis of pheochromocytoma. In hereditary pheochromocytoma, plasma-free metanephrines (with an upper reference limit of 0.9 nmol/L) had a sensitivity and specificity of 97 and 96% respectively; whereas in sporadic tumors, sensitivity and specificity were 99 and 82%, respectively.

In the same study, urinary fractionated metanephrines (with upper reference limit of 2.4 μmol/day for women and 4.2 μmol/day for men) had a sensitivity and specificity of 96 and 82% respectively in hereditary tumors and 97 and 45% in sporadic tumors. Vanillylmandelic acid (VMA) was the most specific test (99%) in hereditary pheochromocytoma, but its sensitivity was only 46% in this setting. The combination of various biochemical tests did not improve the diagnostic yield beyond that of a single test of plasma free metanephrines in this study (66). Practically, however, multiple and often repeated testing is done to enhance diagnostic accuracy and minimize the risk of sample errors.

Chromogranin A (CgA) is an acidic protein that is stored and released with catecholamines. It is nonspecific and widely distributed in neuroendocrine cells, particularly in chromaffin adrenal medullary cells. There is a significant concordance between CgA levels and ^{131}I MIBG imaging data (67). Elevated levels of serum CgA are not specific for the diagnosis of pheochromocytoma and may be of less benefit in patients with impaired renal function.

Genetic Testing

Pheochromocytoma is thought to be hereditary in about 10 to 16% of cases, although this maybe an underestimate. Multiple familial syndromes are associated with the development of pheochromocytoma, including MEN 2A and 2B, NF-1, and VHL disease. Routine genetic test-

**TABLE
31-3** | **ALGORITHM FOR CLINICAL APPROACH
AND MANAGEMENT OF PHEOCHROMOCYTOMA**

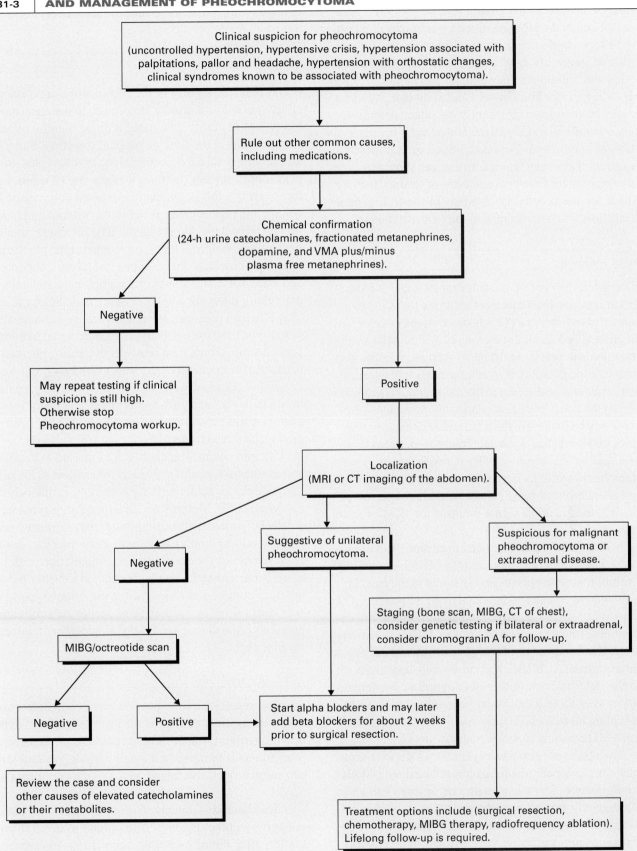

CT = computed tomography; MIBG = metaiodenzylguanidine; MRI = magnetic resonance imaging; VMA = vanillylmandelic acid.

ing in apparently sporadic pheochromocytomas is not widely practiced in the United States; but in the presence of any of the aforementioned syndromes or a family history suggestive of familial pheochromocytoma, multiple genes are now available in selected laboratories and should be analyzed. These include *ret* for MEN 2, *VHL* for Von Hippel-Lindau disease, *NF-1* for neurofibromatosis, and, recently, succinate dehydrogenase subunits B and D (*SDHB* and *SDHD*) for familial pheochromocytoma. Genetic counseling is imperative prior to and after any familial testing and should include an explanation of the pros and cons of testing, some of which are the possibility of errors in the test, genetic discrimination, and potential quality-of-life changes.

Imaging

Ninety-five percent of pheochromocytomas are intra-abdominal, and the majority of these are localized to the adrenal gland. When a pheochromocytoma is suspected on clinical and laboratory grounds, CT or MRI of the abdomen and pelvis can be performed as an initial step for tumor localization. If an adrenal mass is not seen, attention should be directed to the paraspinous region and urinary bladder; even less commonly, extraadrenal tumors may be located in the head and neck region. Pheochromocytoma has a characteristic hyperintense appearance on T2-weighted MRI scans; however, not all pheochromocytomas have this imaging characteristic, and pheochromocytoma cannot be excluded on the basis of a lack of high signal intensity on T2-weighted MRI scans.

MIBG scintigraphy has been used since 1981 to localize pheochromocytoma (68,69). MIBG structurally resembles norepinephrine and is stored in the catecholamine-storage vesicles. In a study of 284 patients, CT sensitivity was 98.9% for adrenal and 90.9% for extraadrenal tumors compared with an MIBG sensitivity of 87.4% for adrenal and 88.5% for extraadrenal pheochromocytomas. MIBG had an overall specificity of 98.9% (64,70). Some authorities suggest a complementary role of these localization procedures, with MIBG providing more specific functional information and CT and MRI providing superior anatomic detail.

The results of fluorodeoxyglucose (FDG) PET scanning were compared with images obtained with MIBG scintigraphy in 29 patients with one or more known or subsequently proved pheochromocytomas. Tumor uptake of FDG was detected in 22 of 29 patients. In 4 patients in whom the pheochromocytomas failed to accumulate MIBG, uptake of FDG in the tumors was intense, suggesting that FDG-PET is especially useful in pheochromocytomas that fail to concentrate MIBG (71).

Therapy

Medical

Blood pressure control in the preoperative and perioperative period is of utmost importance to decrease morbidity and mortality associated with a potential hypertensive crisis at the time of surgical resection. Patients are usually given a long acting alpha blocker (phenoxybenzamine) starting at 10 mg twice a day (2 weeks before surgery); this is gradually increased until adequate control of hypertension is achieved without inducing severe orthostatic hypotension. Beta blockers should not be added before achieving adequate alpha blockade; lone beta blockade leaves alpha receptors unopposed and open for activation by circulating catecholamines potentially inducing a hypertensive crisis. Selective alpha$_1$ blockers (e.g., prazosin, terazosin, and doxazosin) can also be used to control hypertension in patients with pheochromocytoma. In a retrospective study, phenoxybenzamine (21 patients), prazosin (11 patients), and doxazosin (17 patients) were used in preoperative preparation. There was no significant difference in operative or postoperative blood pressure or plasma-volume control among the three groups (72).

Calcium channel blockers were reported to be safer and as effective as alpha blockers when used as the primary mode of antihypertensive therapy in pheochromocytoma (73). Metyrosine (alpha-methyl-p-tyrosine), a catecholamine synthesis inhibitor, was evaluated retrospectively in combination with alpha blockers (prazosin or phenoxybenzamine). The combination of alpha metyrosine and alpha blockade resulted in better blood pressure control and less need for use of antihypertensive medication or vasopressors during surgery compared with the classic method of single-agent adrenergic blockade (74).

Surgical

Surgical resection of the pheochromocytoma after appropriate medical therapy is the primary mode of definitive treatment. Laparoscopic resection of pheochromocytomas is preferred for small tumors (<6 cm) and can reduce operative blood loss and shorten hospital stay.

Close hemodynamic monitoring with pre- and intraoperative volume repletion is important to avoid hypotension after tumor resection. Short-acting intravenous vasodilators (e.g., nitroprusside, nitroglycerine, phentolamine) may be needed intraoperatively to decrease the chances of precipitating a hypertensive crisis during tumor manipulation. Intravenous fluids should contain dextrose, as patients are prone to develop hypoglycemia due to rebound insulin secretion with the precipitous drop in catecholamine levels after successful tumor resection.

In patients with MEN 2 and VHL disease with bilateral pheochromocytomas, cortical-sparing adrenalectomy is the procedure of choice to avoid lifelong adrenal insufficiency, but this requires long-term follow-up, as recurrence may develop many years after operation.

EXTRAADRENAL PHEOCHROMOCYTOMA (PARAGANGLIOMA)

Extraadrenal pheochromocytomas probably represent 15 to 19% of adult and 30% of childhood pheochromocytomas (63,75,76). Extraadrenal pheochromocytomas frequently occur below the diaphragm; these are most commonly found in the superior paraaortic region between the diaphragm and lower renal poles, followed closely by the urinary bladder. Less often, extraadrenal pheochromocytoma can be found in the chest or head and neck region. It is believed that extraadrenal pheochromocytomas are more likely to be malignant than adrenal tumors and they carry a poorer prognosis (77).

MALIGNANT PHEOCHROMOCYTOMA

The exact prevalence of malignant pheochromocytoma is not well known. Pheochromocytoma has been reported to recur at intervals from 5 to 13 years following initial resection of a benign-appearing tumor (78); thus, after seemingly successful resection of benign tumor, lifelong follow-up is mandated in these patients (62). The malignancy rate is estimated to be 9.9 to 14% of all pheochromocytomas (64,76). The presence of familial syndromes (MEN 2 and VHL) is associated with bilateral pheochromocytomas, though these are rarely malignant (63,79). The axial skeleton is the most common site of metastases (Fig. 31-19), followed by the liver, lymph nodes, lung, and peritoneum.

Diagnosis

As in the case of many endocrine tumors, in the absence of clinically evident metastases or recurrences, there are no reliable histologic features that can distinguish benign from malignant pheochromocytoma. A recent study tried to create a scoring system to address this problem. This

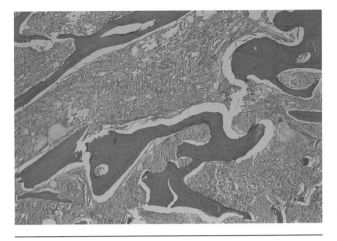

FIGURE 31-19 Histopathologic picture of metastatic pheochromocytoma to a rib.

included 50 histologically malignant tumors (including 17 clinically benign pheochromocytomas) and 50 histologically benign tumors. A pheochromocytoma of the adrenal gland scaled score (PASS) was suggested to separate tumors with a potential for a biologically aggressive behavior (PASS $\geq$ 4) from tumors that behave in a benign fashion (PASS $<$ 4) (129). The cases of malignant pheochromocytomas more frequently demonstrated invasion [vascular (PASS = 1), capsular (PASS = 1), periadrenal adipose tissue (PASS = 2); large nests or diffuse growth (PASS = 2); focal or confluent necrosis (PASS = 2); high cellularity (PASS = 2); tumor cell spindling (PASS = 2); cellular monotony (PASS = 2); increased mitotic figures ($>$3 of 10 high-power fields; PASS = 2), atypical mitotic figures (PASS = 2); profound nuclear pleomorphism (PASS = 1); and hyperchromasia (PASS = 1)] than the benign tumors. It is still premature to apply this scoring system to everyday practice, as this study included 17 clinically benign tumors that were histologically classified as malignant. This scoring system should be validated in a large-scale study.

Various markers have been proposed to differentiate benign from malignant pheochromocytomas. These include chromagranin A (CgA), secretogranin II-derived peptide EM66, neuron-specific enolase (NSE), and neuropeptide Y (NPY) (80–83). In most studies these markers have been shown to be higher in malignant pheochromocytomas as compared to benign ones.

Inhibin/activin beta B subunit is expressed in normal adrenal medullary cells. Strong staining was found in most benign adrenal pheochromocytomas, whereas malignant tumors were almost negative. This suggests that loss of inhibin/activin beta B subunit expression in pheochromocytomas may be used as an indicator of malignant potential (84).

Flow cytometry data and immunohistochemistry for markers of cell proliferation [proliferating cell nuclear antigen (PCNA) and MIB-1 (Ki-67)] were studied in 51 pheochromocytomas, including 6 malignant and 45 benign tumors, in order to aid in diagnosis. There was no correlation between DNA ploidy, S-phase fraction by flow cytometry, or PCNA with malignancy. Staining for the MIB-1 nuclear proliferation marker was positive (at least 10% expression) in 3 (50%) of 6 malignant pheochromocytomas and negative (<1% expression) in all 45 benign tumors ($p < 0.01$). However, other reports have suggested that a nuclear DNA ploidy pattern can be an independent prognostic variable for patients with pheochromocytoma and paraganglioma (85).

Therapy

In the few selected cases of malignant pheochromocytoma with limited disease, surgery can be attempted in conjunction with other therapeutic measures. The role of debulking surgery is more controversial in cases where total resection is deemed impossible.

^{131}I MIBG therapy has been suggested as a useful palliative adjunct in selected patients with malignant pheochromocytoma. In a review of 116 patients with malignant adrenal pheochromocytomas or extraadrenal pheochromocytoma treated with ^{131}I MIBG, the cumulative dose ranged from 96 to 2322 mCi (3.6 to 85.9 GBq), with a mean ($\pm$standard deviation) of 490 ± 350 mCi (18.1 ± 13.0 GBq). Initial symptomatic improvement was achieved in 76% of patients, tumor responses in 30%, and hormonal responses in 45%. Five patients (4.3%) had complete response, ranging from 16 to 58 months. Patients with metastases to soft tissue had more favorable responses to treatment than those with metastases to bone. Adverse effects (in 41% of patients) were generally mild except for one fatality from bone marrow aplasia. Forty-five percent of the responders relapsed after a mean interval of 29.3 ± 31.1 months (median 19 months) (86). High-dose ^{131}I MIBG (the median single-treatment dose was 800 mCi or 11.5 mCi/kg with a median cumulative dose of 1015 mCi) used following debulking surgery and stem cell harvest in 12 patients with malignant pheochromocytomas. Three patients had a complete response, including 2 who had soft tissue and skeletal metastases; 7 patients had a partial response; and 2 patients without a response died with progressive disease. Patients with massive hepatic metastases were excluded due to concerns of hepatic necrosis after high-dose ^{131}I MIBG (87).

Streptozocin-based regimens were used in metastatic pheochromocytoma with variable results ranging from no response to partial response (88–90). Combination chemotherapy has also been tried in this disease. In a study of 14 patients with metastatic pheochromocytoma, combination chemotherapy of cyclophosphamide (750 mg/m^2 body-surface area on day 1), vincristine (1.4 mg/m^2 on day 1), and dacarbazine (600 mg/m^2 on days 1 and 2) every 21 days was used in all (141). Complete and partial tumor responses were achieved in 57% of patients; 79% of patients had a complete or partial response biochemically. All responding patients had objective improvement in performance status and blood pressure (91). At MDACC the most commonly used regimen for metastatic pheochromocytoma is CVAD [cyclophamide, vincristine, Adriamycin (doxorubicin), and dacarbazine].

Fractionated EBRT is mainly used for symptomatic relief of bony metastases. It can lead to short-lived reduction in catecholamine production and reduced need for analgesics (92). Radiofrequency ablation (RFA) has been attempted in a very limited number of patients with metastatic pheochromocytoma and proposed as a potential treatment modality (93,94).

Prognosis

In a series of 86 patients with 85 benign and 10 malignant pheochromocytomas, the 5-year survival rate for malignant pheochromocytomas was reported at 20%, and all patients with malignant pheochromocytomas died within 10 years (63).

■ ADRENOCORTICAL CARCINOMA

Adrenocortical carcinoma (ACC) is a rare malignancy with significant morbidity and mortality. The increasing use of body imaging techniques (e.g., US, CT, and MRI) has led to the discovery of silent adrenal tumors that may have malignant potential. The earlier identification of ACC by such detection methods facilitates earlier intervention and may translate into improved survival rates.

The incidence of ACC is approximately two cases per million population per year. It can occur at any age with reported bimodal age incidence in the first and fourth decades of life with near equal sex distribution. The normally functioning adrenal cortex produces a variety of hormones, namely mineralocorticoids, glucocorticosteroids, and sex steroids. Functional tumors are

TABLE 31-4	CLINICAL SYNDROMES ASSOCIATED WITH FUNCTIONAL ADRENOCORTICAL CARCINOMA		
Clinical Syndrome	**Suggestive Clinical Features**	**Suggested Laboratory Workup**
Cushing's syndrome	Obesity, moon face, purple striae, cervical fat pads, easy bruising, myopathy, hypertension, diabetes mellitus	Plasma electrolytes, plasma glucose, ACTH, cortisol, 24-h urine-free cortisol
Virilizing syndrome	Hirsutism, clitoromegaly, temporal balding, increased muscle mass, amenorrhea, male precocious puberty, advanced bone age in children.	DHEA sulfate, testosterone, 17-OH progesterone
Feminizing syndrome	Gynecomastia, loss of libido	Estradiol, prolactin, testosterone
Hyperaldosteronism	Hypertension, hypokalemia	Plasma renin activity, plasma aldosterone concentration, plasma electrolytes, 18-OH corticosterone
Mixed syndromes		

ACTH = adrenocorticotropic hormone; DHEA = dihydroepiandrosterone.

found in 34 to 62% of adrenocortical carcinoma cases (95,96), with variable clinical signs and symptoms based on the predominantly produced hormone. The various syndromes seen with functioning adrenal cancers are presented in Table 31-4 (Figs. 31-20, 31-21, and 31-22).

Adrenocortical tumors may also present as nonfunctioning tumors, with nonspecific symptoms of abdominal discomfort or pain, indigestion, or site-specific symptoms based on the location of the metastatic disease (see Figs. 31-23 and 31-24).

PATHOLOGY

ACC can arise from either adrenal gland. Some series have reported a higher prevalence of left-sided ACC while others have reported an equal prevalence of right- and left-sided ACC (97). In another study, ACC was bilateral in 4% of cases (98).

Adrenal tumor size has been suggested as a predictor of malignancy. ACCs are usually large (>5 to 6 cm), whereas benign adenomas are usually small (<5 cm); however, there is remarkable overlap, and tumor size

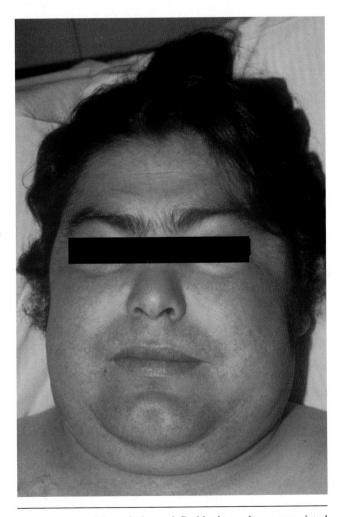

FIGURE 31-20 Moon facies and Cushing's syndrome associated with adrenocortical carcinoma.

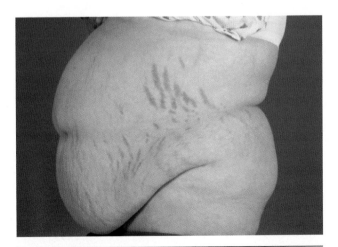

FIGURE 31-21 Purple striae on the abdomen associated with Cushing's syndrome.

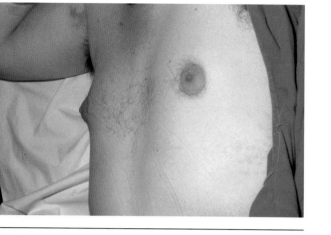

FIGURE 31-22   Gynecomastia associated with feminizing adrenocortical carcinoma.

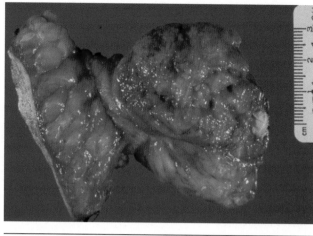

FIGURE 31-24   Adrenocortical carcinoma invading the abdominal wall.

cannot be used as a sole pathologic criterion for predicting malignancy (99).

ACCs, especially the nonfunctioning tumors, are often large at diagnosis. They are commonly encapsulated and lobulated and can be solid or cystic, with areas of necrosis and hemorrhage evident on gross sections.

Microscopically, it can be hard to differentiate ACC from benign adenomas based on histologic features alone. ACC is described as polygonal cells arranged in sheets, nests, trabeculae, or ribbons and at times contains anaplastic features. Cells are usually eosinophilic, in contrast to the clear cells of normal adrenals or benign adenomas, although clear cells can be found in some ACCs. Increased mitotic figures and vascular and capsular invasion are other signs that suggest a diagnosis of ACC. Weiss proposed a scoring system consisting of nine criteria to aid in the diagnosis of adrenal can-

cer (100). The criteria are (1) mitotic rate greater than five mitoses per 50 high-power fields in the most active areas of the tumor, (2) atypical mitoses, (3) venous invasion, (4) clear cells comprising 25% or less of the tumor, (5) tumor necrosis, (6) nuclear grade III or IV tumor according to Fuhrman's method for renal carcinoma, (7) diffuse (solid) architecture in more than one-third of the tumor, (8) invasion of sinusoidal structures, and (9) capsular invasion. The presence of three or more of these nine features is highly suggestive of ACC (101).

Despite this system, there are still borderline cases in which a systematic approach is needed to make a definitive diagnosis. ACC usually spreads early by direct invasion, hematogenous spread, and lymphatic channels. Liver, lungs, bones, and regional lymph nodes are the main sites for metastases. Table 31-5 summarizes the staging system used at MDACC (102); it is modified from the earlier accepted system proposed by MacFarlane in 1958 (103).

PATHOGENESIS

ACC is considered a monoclonal disease in contrast to benign adrenal adenomas. ACC may present in the setting of inherited cancer syndromes. Li-Fraumeni syndrome, one such example, is a constellation of diseases that all have a *p53* germline mutation in common; this raises the possibility that loss of *p53* tumor suppressor activity can lead to the development of ACC (104). Loss of heterozygosity (LOH) at 11p, 13q, and 17p is also found in ACC but not adenomas or hyperplastic lesions (105). ACC frequently show loss of heterozygosity (LOH) of 11q13 (the gene locus for MEN 1) but do not contain point mutations within the MEN 1 coding region (106). The Beckwith-Wiedemann syndrome

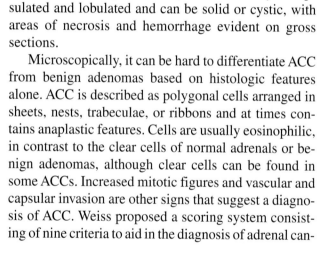

FIGURE 31-23   Liver metastases from adrenocortical carcinoma.

Stage	MacFarlane (103)	Lee et al. (102)
I	T1 (≤5 cm), N0, M0	T1 (≤5 cm), N0, M0
II	T2 (>5 cm), N0, M0	T2 (>5 cm), N0, M0
III	T3 (local invasion without involvement of adjacent organs) or mobile positive lymph nodes, M0	T3/T4 (local invasion as shown by histologic evidence of adjacent organ invasion, direct tumor extension to IVC, or tumor thrombus within IVC (or renal vein), and/or N1 (positive regional lymph nodes), M0
IV	T4 (invasion of adjacent organs) or fixed positive lymph nodes or M1 (distant metastases)	T1–4, N0–1, M1 (distant metastases)

TABLE 31-5 | STAGING OF ADRENOCORTICAL CARCINOMA

IVC = inferior vena cava.

(BWS) is characterized by somatic overgrowth and a predisposition to tumors, including ACC. BWS results from mutations or epimutations affecting imprinted genes on chromosome 11p15.5.

DIAGNOSIS

Laboratory Findings

In patients found to have an adrenal mass, it is necessary to obtain a complete blood count and serum chemistries. Hormonal evaluation includes random plasma renin activity; plasma aldosterone concentration; ACTH; serum cortisol; and 24-hour urine collection for creatinine, free cortisol, catecholamines, fractionated metanephrines, and VMA. Total testosterone, dehydroepiandrosterone sulfate (DHEAS), and estradiol can be obtained if there is a clinical suspicion of increased sex-hormone secretion (i.e., virilizing or feminizing features).

Radiologic Findings

The expanding use of body imaging methods has led to the increasing discovery of adrenal masses. Radiologic studies play a critical role in detecting adrenal masses and characterizing malignant potential. Numerous imaging modalities—including CT, MRI, US, and nuclear medicine imaging—can be used to evaluate the adrenal gland.

Benign adrenal adenomas are usually smaller than the malignant variety and have a higher lipid content, giving them characteristic features on imaging. CT scanning with 3-mm cuts targeted to the adrenal gland is a useful tool for both the detection and characterization of adrenal masses. A nonenhanced examination should initially be performed, followed by a contrast-enhanced study if necessary (Figs. 31-25 and 31-26).

Benign adenomas usually have low attenuation on nonenhanced CT scans; using a threshold of 10 Houns-

field units (HU), the sensitivity of nonenhanced CT for characterizing adrenal adenomas was 79%, with a specificity of 96% (107). However, 30% of adenomas do not contain sufficient lipid to have low attenuation at CT. On the other hand, benign adenomas enhance rapidly with intravenous contrast media and wash out rapidly. More than 50% washout between the dynamic phase of contrast enhancement and the 10-min delayed images is highly diagnostic of benign adenoma and confirms the finding on the low attenuation on nonenhanced CT scan.

When results of CT examinations are equivocal, MRI is another good study of choice for characterizing adrenal lesions. Chemical-shift imaging is an MRI technique used to detect lipid within an organ and is the most sensitive method for differentiating benign adeno-

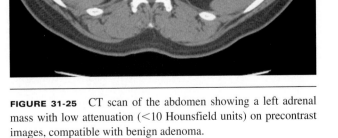

FIGURE 31-25 CT scan of the abdomen showing a left adrenal mass with low attenuation (<10 Hounsfield units) on precontrast images, compatible with benign adenoma.

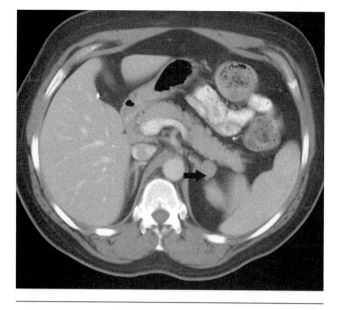

FIGURE 31-26 Postcontrast CT scan images showing enhancement of the left adrenal mass, but these images still have lower attenuation than those of the normal right adrenal gland.

mas from metastases of nonadrenal cancers. Tissues with higher lipid content (benign adenomas) show loss of signal intensity (i.e., appear darker) on out-of-phase images on chemical-shift MRI. MRI with T2-weighted imaging is also a useful modality when the adrenal gland is being evaluated because in addition to the heterogenous characteristics of ACC due to hemorrhage or tumor necrosis typically seen on other radiographic studies, malignant adrenal masses usually have higher signal intensity with this modality than benign adrenal adenomas in addition to the heterogeneity of ACC be-

cause of hemorrhage or tumor necrosis. [131]I 6-beta-iodomethyl-19-norcholesterol (NP-59) scintigraphy can be used to detect aldosteronomas and other hyperfunctioning cortical tumors (Fig. 31-27).

PET shows promise in differentiating benign from malignant masses. In small series studies, FDG-PET had 100% sensitivity and 80 to 100% specificity for differentiating malignant masses versus benign adrenal masses (108–110). In a prospective study in 10 patients with ACC, FDG-PET had a sensitivity and specificity of 100 and 95% respectively based on the number of PET-detected lesions. PET-FDG also modified tumor staging in 3 of 10 patients and affected management in 2 of 10 (111).

Although FDG-PET scans seem to be a sensitive tool for detecting malignant tissue, the false-positive results, together with the small number of patients studied so far, make it premature to recommend the routine use of this modality in patients with adrenal cancer.

Larger adrenal lesions have a greater likelihood of being malignant; an increase in the size of the lesion is a useful indicator of malignancy, as adenomas in general tend to grow slowly and often do not change in size over time. An adrenal tumor diameter of 5 cm identifies ACC with a sensitivity of 93% and a specificity of 64% (112). Other radiologic features suggestive of malignancy include heterogeneity, irregular shape, irregular margins, or hemorrhage (Figs. 31-28 and 31-29). Although these findings are helpful in differentiating a benign from a malignant adrenal mass, they are not specific.

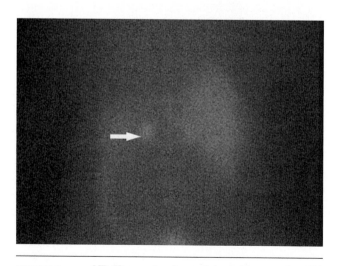

FIGURE 31-27 NP-59 scan showing activity (*white arrow*) at 120 h after injection in the left adrenal gland (posterior view), compatible with functioning adenoma.

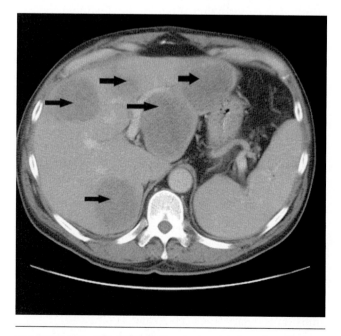

FIGURE 31-28 CT of the abdomen showing hepatic metastases from adrenocortical carcinoma (*black arrows*).

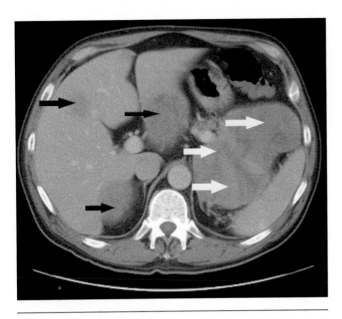

FIGURE 31-29 Left-sided adrenocortical carcinoma (*white arrows*) with liver metastases (*black arrows*).

Fine-Needle Aspiration

Adrenal incidentalomas are relatively common, whereas occult metastatic cancers only rarely present as isolated asymptomatic adrenal masses. An adrenal mass may also represent pheochromocytoma, and performing FNA may therefore precipitate a hypertensive crisis. For these reasons, the routine FNA of asymptomatic adrenal masses is not indicated unless a patient has a known primary malignant tumor with possible metastases to the adrenal gland (i.e., small cell lung cancer). In this instance, FNA may be considered if the result seems to affect the management plan. In a study of 1639 patients found to have cancer, the adrenal gland was involved at diagnosis in 95 patients (5.8%), and only one patient had ACC. In 4 patients (0.2%), the disease was limited to the adrenal gland at presentation, with tumor size ≥6 cm (113).

THERAPY

Surgery

At our institution, adrenalectomy is performed for adrenal masses that are either functional or have suspicious radiologic features. For benign-appearing nonfunctional tumors, surgery is considered if the tumor is ≥4 cm and the patient is a good surgical candidate (112); however, the National Institutes of Health (NIH) consensus guidelines for adrenal nonfunctional incidentalomas currently state that all tumors greater than 6 cm should be surgically resected, whereas surgical decisions should be individualized for tumors between 4 and 6 cm (114).

Complete surgical resection is the mainstay of therapy for ACC and offers the best chance for prolonged disease-free survival (102). Subcostal transabdominal or thoracoabdominal incision is the preferred approach at our institution; if ACC is suspected, laparoscopic adrenalectomy is not recommended, as it can result in early locoregional recurrence through tumor spillage and seeding and decreases the ability to achieve tumor-free margins. Occasionally, en bloc resection sacrificing adjacent organs is performed with the aim of complete resection of tumor and invaded structures. In locally invasive right-sided ACC, complete mobilization of the liver combined with proximal and distal control of the inferior vena cava (IVC) should routinely be performed at the time of right ACC resection (112). The surgeon should be prepared to perform hepatic and IVC resection with the possibility of venovenous bypass or even cardiac bypass when the tumor extends into the IVC. In locally invasive left-sided ACC, tumor encasement of the celiac axis, aorta, or proximal superior mesenteric artery (SMA) may make tumor unresectable (102). The presence of tumor thrombus in the IVC, or renal vein, or tumor invasion of the pancreas, spleen, or kidney is not a contraindication for complete resection in select patients. Although there is limited evidence of benefit from resection of the primary tumor in the presence of metastatic disease, there might still be a role for resection of primary tumor and all visible metastases in an otherwise young, healthy patient, especially in cases of functioning tumors (102).

In corticosteroid-producing ACC, preoperative blockade of steroid production using agents such as ketoconazole or metyrapone reduces postoperative morbidity. In these cases, the contralateral adrenal gland is usually atrophic and the patient requires peri- and postoperative corticosteroid replacement. This relative adrenal insufficiency may last for months after successful resection.

Chemotherapy

In 1949, it was found that oral administration of insecticide (DDD, or Rothane) to dogs induced selective necrosis of zona fasciculata and zona reticularis of the adrenal cortex. Mitotane (o,p′-DDD) has been used to treat ACC since 1960.

Until now, o,p′-DDD has been considered an efficacious agent in treating patients with cancer, especially when its plasma levels exceed 14 mg/L (115–117) (Fig. 31-30).

Mitotane blocks adrenal 11β hydroxylase and cholesterol side-chain cleavage, alters zona fasciculata mitochondrial morphology, and destroys the adrenal cortex. Treatment starts with 1 g twice daily and increases

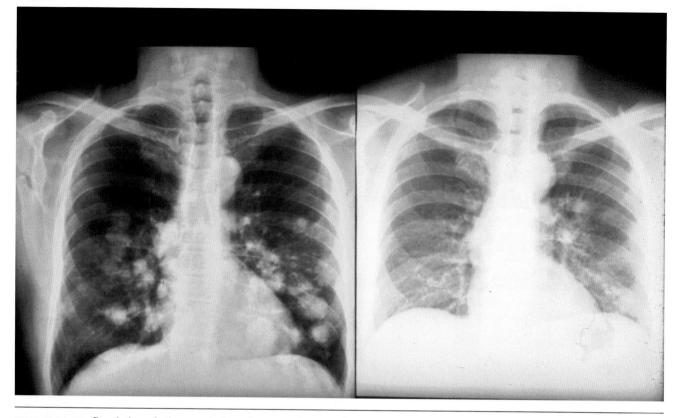

FIGURE 31-30   Resolution of adrenocortical carcinoma metastases with mitotane therapy (before mitotane on the left and after mitotane on the right).

to 9 to 10 g/day, depending on clinical response, plasma levels, and adverse effects. Clinical monitoring, including neurologic assessment, should be combined with plasma-level monitoring to keep levels between 14 to 20 mg/L. In addition, patients receiving mitotane should receive glucocorticosteroid replacement, as they may develop adrenal insufficiency. Mitotane increases corticosteroid binding globulin and enhances dexamethasone clearance. These effects of mitotane may provide an explanation for the increased corticosteroid requirements during mitotane therapy. Steroid replacement can be potentially guided by ACTH monitoring for two reasons: to ensure adequate replacement and to probably suppress endogenous ACTH production in a manner similar to thyroxine-suppression therapy in differentiated thyroid cancer. Side effects of mitotane include nausea, vomiting, anorexia, diarrhea, lethargy, confusion, depression, ataxia, skin rash, and visual disturbances as well as hypercholesterolemia (117–119). Mitotane is mainly used for inoperable and metastatic disease. The use of adjuvant mitotane is still discussed but has not been shown to be effective (120). In metastatic ACC, the achievement of mitotane plasma levels greater than 14 mg/L resulted in objective tumor response in 4 of 6 patients (31%): one patient had a complete response and three

had objective hormone responses. In contrast, no response was observed among the 7 patients with plasma mitotane levels that remained consistently low. When mitotane was used as adjuvant therapy, 8 of 11 patients who received mitotane had disease recurrence, although the plasma mitotane level was 14 mg/L in 6 patients. Remarkable neurotoxicity was associated with plasma levels >20 mg/L. Other chemotherapeutic agents have been used with mixed results.

A combined regimen of cyclophosphamide, doxorubicin, and cisplatin was used in 11 patients and was of some benefit, mainly in disease stabilization (121). Adjuvant etoposide (165 mg/m^2) and cisplatin (90 mg/m^2) over 8 h on the same day, with hydration and mannitol diuresis continuing to day 2, was used in 5 children with ACC. All 5 were reported to be in complete remission at least to 29 months of follow-up (122).

Irinotecan (CPT-11) was studied in 12 patients with metastatic ACC and no objective or complete responses were observed (123).

The combination of mitotane with etoposide, doxorubicin, and cisplatin (EDP) (etoposide 100 mg/m^2 on days 5 to 7, doxorubicin 20 mg/m^2 on days 1 and 8, and cisplatin 40 mg/m^2 on days 1 and 9 intravenously every 4 weeks) in the treatment of patients with advanced inoperable ACC was tested in 28 patients (186). Complete response was achieved in 2 patients and partial response in 13; stable disease was observed in 8 patients, and progressive disease in 5. The EDP regimen was well tolerated. Only 4 patients received reduced doses, whereas 3 discontinued chemotherapy early due to toxicity. The addition of mitotane increased neurologic and gastrointestinal side effects, and only 9 patients consistently took the drug at the planned dose (4 g/day) (124).

Suramin has a narrow therapeutic window. In patients with metastatic disease, it has been shown to produce transient tumor response with serious side effects, including coagulopathy, thrombocytopenia, polyneuropathy, and allergic skin reactions. Two fatalities possibly related to suramin therapy have been reported (125).

Gossypol, a male contraceptive derived from cotton seeds, has been shown to have antiproliferative activity in a variety of human cancer cell lines, including ACC. It was studied in 21 patients with metastatic ACC at doses of 30 to 70 mg/day (189). Eighteen patients completed at least 6 weeks of gossypol treatment. Three of these patients, whose tumors were refractory to other chemotherapeutic agents, had partial tumor responses that lasted from several months to over 1 year. One patient had a minor response followed by resection of her remaining disease, 1 patient had stable disease, and 13 patients had disease progression. Gossypol was well tolerated; the only serious side effect was abdominal ileus, which resolved when the treatment was interrupted and restarted at a lower dose (126).

Radiation Therapy and Radiofrequency Ablation

ACC is considered a radioresistant tumor. There is limited evidence for using adjuvant radiation therapy (127). Currently, radiation treatment is mainly used for palliative purposes in metastatic ACC. Percutaneous image-guided radiofrequency ablation has been attempted in the treatment of unresectable primary or metastatic adrenocortical carcinoma. The procedure was effective for the short-term local control of small adrenal tumors, especially for tumors less than 5 cm (128); however, further data are needed to examine its long-term efficacy and its effect on survival.

PROGNOSIS

Adrenal cancer remains a tumor with high morbidity and mortality. Long-term survival is possible in these patients if complete resection with tumor-free margins can be achieved (102). Survival is inversely correlated with disease stage at diagnosis.

High mitotic figures, but not DNA aneuploidy, have been associated with reduced survival and hence proposed as a prognostic factor. Younger age may portend a better prognosis, as children, when adjusted for stage, seem to have improved outcomes compared with adults (129). At our institution, the 5-year survival rate improved from 30% in 1983 (97) to 60% in 2001, which is likely secondary to the improvement in supportive measures (95).

■ PARATHYROID CARCINOMA

Parathyroid carcinoma is the least common endocrine malignancy, with a prevalence of 0.005% of all cancers (130). It is a rare cause of primary hyperparathyroidism, accounting for 0.4 to 5% of all cases.

The etiology of parathyroid carcinoma remains obscure. Radiation exposure has been implicated in a number of reports of carcinoma occurring within an adenoma, hyperplastic gland, or even normal glands; however, overall, head and neck irradiation does not seem to be as significant a factor in malignant parathyroid disease as it is in the genesis of parathyroid adenomas and benign hyperparathyroidism (131). Parathyroid carcinoma has been reported in families with isolated familial hyperparathyroidism, in patients with MEN types 1 and 2A, and in hereditary hyperparathyroidism jaw tumor syndrome. Thus it may be prudent to screen the relatives of certain patients with parathyroid carcinoma for hypercalcemia to improve the chance of early diagnosis of parathyroid disease. Parathyroid carcinoma has also been described in patients with chronic renal failure and dialysis, raising the possibility of malignant transformation of benign hyperplastic parathyroid glands.

CLINICAL PRESENTATION

Patients with parathyroid carcinoma tend to be approximately a decade younger than those with benign hyperparathyroidism. The disease occurs with similar frequency in both sexes. Most patients with malignant disease are symptomatic and have moderate to severe hypercalcemia (serum calcium greater than 12), although patients with parathyroid carcinoma can present anywhere along the calcemic spectrum, including asymptomatic and mild hypercalcemia. Parathyroid hormone (PTH) levels are generally five times normal. Rare cases of nonfunctioning parathyroid carcinoma have been described; their clinical course is similar to that in patients with functioning tumors.

Unlike patients with benign disease, patients with parathyroid carcinoma are more likely to have a palpable mass in the neck. Manifestations of hypercalcemia in peripheral target organs, such as kidneys or bone, are no longer considered characteristic of benign hyperparathyroidism but are rather common in patients with functioning parathyroid cancer (Fig. 31-31). This is probably related to the generally more severe hypercalcemia at presentation in the malignant disease.

DIAGNOSIS

The diagnosis of parathyroid carcinoma in the absence of regional or distant metastases is a challenging issue. Differentiating benign adenoma from a malignant parathyroid carcinoma on the basis of pathology alone can be difficult. Palpable neck masses, high calcium values (greater than 13.5 mg/dL), and high intact parathyroid hormone (iPTH) values raise the suspicion for this disease (132,133). Gross invasion and adherence at the time of surgery, recurrences, or the classic histopathologic criteria are other clues that may assist in diagnosis (Fig. 31-32).

PATHOLOGY

Pathologic criteria may not definitively differentiate parathyroid carcinoma from the more common adenoma. The classic histopathologic criteria initially described by Schantz and Castleman (134) are still used

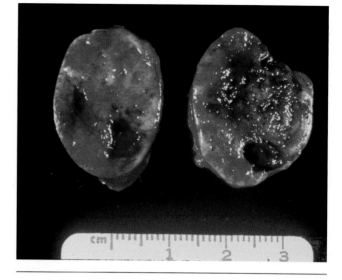

FIGURE 31-32 Gross specimen of a parathyroid gland containing a focus of parathyroid carcinoma.

today. These include the presence of a trabecular or lobular pattern, mitotic figures, thick fibrous bands, and capsular or blood vessel invasion (Fig. 31-33).

Although cytologic evidence of mitoses is generally necessary to confirm malignancy, mitotic activity alone is an unreliable indicator of such malignancy. The likelihood of malignancy increases as more of the aforementioned histologic features appear in the tumor. DNA aneuploidy determined by flow cytometry is a valuable adjunct marker in the diagnosis of malignancy and is associated with a poor prognosis (135,136). Aneuploid parathyroid carcinomas are likely to show more malignant behavior than those with a diploid DNA pattern. It should be pointed out, however, that DNA aneu-

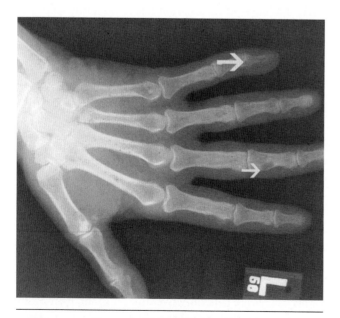

FIGURE 31-31 X-ray of of the left hand of a patient with parathyroid carcinoma. Cystic bone changes are seen in the third middle phalanx; typical resorption of the terminal phalanges is also seen.

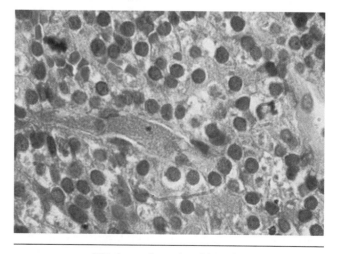

FIGURE 31-33 Histology of parathyroid carcinoma with numerous mitotic figures.

ploidy may be found in some benign lesions. Therefore this feature should be interpreted with caution (137). Immunohistochemical staining for various markers, including tumor suppressor genes, retinoblastoma, *p53*, and others, may, perhaps in the future, help differentiate benign from malignant parathyroid disease. Other important distinguishing features include metastases and gross or histologic evidence of tumor infiltration into the surrounding tissues (including macroscopic adherence or vocal cord paralysis).

On occasion, some highly differentiated tumors without distinct nuclear atypia or classic histopathologic criteria are initially considered to be adenomas but are later reclassified when recurrence is found or metastases appear. On the other hand, a few parathyroid tumors may be classified as malignant because of their atypia, but neither metastasis nor relapse develops. One view is that the only reliable microscopic findings of malignancy are invasion of surrounding structures or metastasis. Thus, the ultimate diagnosis of parathyroid carcinoma can be made with confidence only after recurrence or metastatic spread occurs. Local invasion (micro- or macroscopically) of adjacent structures may be present at initial operation. This malignancy rarely metastasizes to lymph nodes. The thyroid gland is the most common site of involvement, but any of the following may be involved: recurrent laryngeal nerve, strap muscles, esophagus, and trachea. Distant metastases to the lung, bone, and liver can be present at initial presentation or may develop later in the disease. Parathyroid carcinomas are most often found to originate from the inferior parathyroid glands (138); rarely are they found in the mediastinum. To improve the accuracy of diagnosis of malignant parathyroid disease, pathologic specimens of suspected cases should be reviewed by experienced pathologists.

STAGING

There are no accepted staging criteria for parathyroid carcinoma. The standard TNM staging system cannot be applied to this disease for two reasons: first, parathyroid carcinoma is not a disease that frequently metastasizes to lymph nodes; second, tumor size does not seem to play a role in prognosis (130). No current staging system can be used to determine prognosis in this rare disease.

THERAPY

Preoperative suspicion and intraoperative identification of malignancy and appropriate initial surgery are critical in the therapy for parathyroid carcinoma. Compre-

hensive resection of the tumor along with the ipsilateral lobe of the thyroid and abnormal or involved adjacent tissues ("en bloc" resection) is indicated (139). Ideally, these tumors should be identified and removed by experienced parathyroid surgeons. A gray, dark, husky, gross appearance on intraoperative examination may be one indication for performing the more comprehensive resection required of malignant parathyroid disease. Every effort should be made to maintain the integrity of the capsule so as to prevent seeding of tumor, as this will contribute to recurrence. Because this tumor does not typically metastasize to lymph nodes, routine lymph node dissection is not indicated unless the nodes are involved by tumor (130,139).

For recurrences, a wide excision of locally recurrent tumor and an aggressive surgical resection of metastases whenever possible are recommended (Figs, 31-34 and 31-35). Although these repeat operations are not always curative, they usually offer palliation of the marked hypercalcemia (the cause of true morbidity in these patients) for a considerable although variable period.

As of yet, chemotherapeutic agents do not seem to be efficacious in this disease.

The role of radiation therapy for this malignancy has been the subject of much debate. Select patients treated in the Princess Margaret Hospital and our institution have benefited from radiotherapy (138,140,141). It seems to effectively decrease the local relapse rate in patients at high risk for recurrence. Radiotherapy has not become the standard of care in patients with parathyroid carcinoma because, with such small numbers of patients being treated in reported series, it is difficult to prove its efficacy. We recently presented data about the potential benefit of adjuvant radiation therapy after initial surgery in 6 patients, of whom only 1 later had a recurrence of

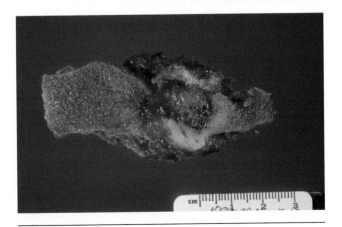

FIGURE 31-34 Section of resected rib containing parathyroid carcinoma metastases.

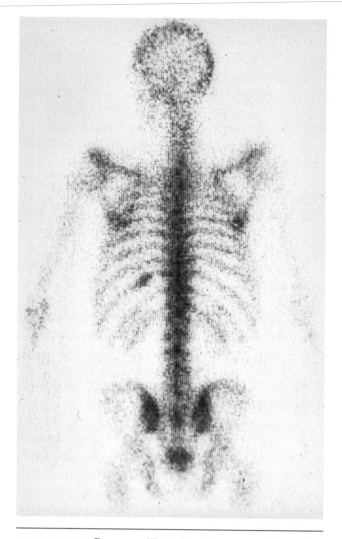

FIGURE 31-35 Bone scan illustrating rib metastases in a patient with parathyroid carcinoma.

disease (142). Radiation therapy should be considered in select patients at high risk of local relapse (those with gross or local invasion or tumor spillage intraoperatively) or those left with gross disease.

Morbidity and mortality are generally caused by the effects of unremitting hypercalcemia rather than tumor growth. Medical treatments, especially in patients with unresectable disease—such as intravenous fluids, diuretics, calcitonin, plicamycin (Mithracin), and bisphosphonates—offer only temporary and palliative control of hypercalcemia. However, therapies such as calcimimetic agents that focus on decreasing PTH secretion may better prevent complications and improve survival in patients whose disease is not curable (143). Because of the variable clinical course of this disease, it is important to individualize therapeutic strategies. Nevertheless, surgical resection where possible remains the most effective treatment for both local and metastatic disease.

Parathyroid carcinoma is a slow-growing but tenacious malignancy, and the hypercalcemia it engenders may have catastrophic consequences. Recurrences usually appear regionally within the neck and may be seen anywhere from 1 to 20 years after the initial diagnosis. Therefore, because of the protracted and unpredictable course of malignant parathyroid disease, regular lifetime surveillance of serum calcium and PTH levels is essential. The 5-year survival rate of this disease has improved over the years to approximately 85%, and the 10-year survival rate is approximately 70 to 77% (138, 140). Death usually results from hypercalcemia and its associated complications.

Because of the rarity and unpredictable clinical course of parathyroid carcinoma, an individualized, multidisciplinary approach to caring for such patients—which involves the endocrinologist, surgeon, oncologist, and radiotherapist—offers the best chance of cure.

References

1. Jemal A, Murray T, Samuels A, et al. Cancer statistics. *CA Cancer J Clin* 2003;53(1):5–26.
2. Sherman SI, Brierley JD, Sperling M, et al. Prospective multicenter study of thyroid carcinoma treatment: Initial analysis of staging and outcome. National Thyroid Cancer Treatment Cooperative Study Registry Group. *Cancer* 1998;83(5):1012–1021.
3. Robbins J, Merino MJ, Boice JD Jr, et al. Thyroid cancer: A lethal endocrine neoplasm. *Ann Intern Med* 1991;115(2):133–147.
4. Gilliland FD, Hunt WC, Morris DM, Key CR. Prognostic factors for thyroid carcinoma. A population-based study of 15,698 cases from the Surveillance, Epidemiology and End Results (SEER) program 1973–1991. *Cancer* 1997;79(3):564–573.
5. Sherman SI. Thyroid carcinoma. *Lancet* 2003;361(9356):501–511.
6. Vassilopoulou-Sellin R. *Thyroid Cancer.* In press.
7. Gharib H, Goellner JR. Fine-needle aspiration biopsy of the thyroid: An appraisal. *Ann Intern Med* 1993;118(4):282–289.
8. DeGroot L, Paloyan E. Thyroid carcinoma and radiation. A Chicago endemic. *JAMA* 1973;225(5):487–491.
9. Bounacer A, Wicker R, Caillou B, et al. High prevalence of activating ret proto-oncogene rearrangements, in thyroid tumors from patients who had received external radiation. *Oncogene* 1997;15(11):1263–1273.
10. Hay ID, Grant CS, Taylor WF, McConahey WM. Ipsilateral lobectomy versus bilateral lobar resection in papillary thyroid carcinoma: A retrospective analysis of surgical outcome using a novel prognostic scoring system. *Surgery* 1987;102(6):1088–1095.
11. Cady B, Rossi R. An expanded view of risk-group definition in differentiated thyroid carcinoma. *Surgery* 1988;104(6):947–953.

12. Byar DP, Green SB, Dor P, et al. A prognostic index for thyroid carcinoma. A study of the EORTC Thyroid Cancer Cooperative Group. *Eur J Cancer* 1979;15(8):1033–1041.

13. Mazzaferri EL, Jhiang SM. Long-term impact of initial surgical and medical therapy on papillary and follicular thyroid cancer. *Am J Med* 1994;97(5):418–428.

14. Sherman SI. Toward a standard clinicopathologic staging approach for differentiated thyroid carcinoma. *Semin Surg Oncol* 1999;16(1):12–15.

15. Katoh R, Sasaki J, Kurihara H, et al. Multiple thyroid involvement (intraglandular metastasis) in papillary thyroid carcinoma. A clinicopathologic study of 105 consecutive patients. *Cancer* 1992;70(6):1585–1590.

16. Silverberg SG, Hutter RV, Foote FW Jr. Fatal carcinoma of the thyroid: Histology, metastases, and causes of death. *Cancer* 1970;25(4):792–802.

17. Hay ID, Grant CS, Bergstralh EJ, et al. Unilateral total lobectomy: Is it sufficient surgical treatment for patients with AMES low-risk papillary thyroid carcinoma? *Surgery* 1998; 124(6):958–964; discussion 964–966.

18. Samaan NA, Schultz PN, Hickey RC, et al. The results of various modalities of treatment of well differentiated thyroid carcinomas: A retrospective review of 1599 patients. *J Clin Endocrinol Metab* 1992;75(3):714–720.

19. DeGroot LJ, Kaplan EL, Straus FH, Shukla MS. Does the method of management of papillary thyroid carcinoma make a difference in outcome? *World J Surg* 1994;18(1):123–130.

20. Cady B. Papillary carcinoma of the thyroid gland: Treatment based on risk group definition. *Surg Oncol Clin North Am* 1998;7(4):633–644.

21. Sherman SI, Gillenwater A. Neoplasms of the thyroid. In: Bast RJ, Kufe D, Pollock R (eds): *Cancer Medicine.* Hamilton, Ontario, Canada: BC Decker; 2000:1105–1114.

22. DeGroot LJ, Kaplan EL, McCormick M, Straus FH. Natural history, treatment, and course of papillary thyroid carcinoma. *J Clin Endocrinol Metab* 1990;71(2):414–424.

23. Taylor T, Specker B, Robbins J, et al. Outcome after treatment of high-risk papillary and non-Hurthle-cell follicular thyroid carcinoma. *Ann Intern Med* 1998;129(8):622–627.

24. Wong JB, Kaplan MM, Meyer KB, Pauker SG. Ablative radioactive iodine therapy for apparently localized thyroid carcinoma. A decision analytic perspective. *Endocrinol Metab Clin North Am* 1990;19(3):741–760.

25. Shepler T, Sherman S, Faustina M, et al. Nasolacrimal duct obstruction associated with radioactive iodine therapy for thyroid carcinoma. *J Ophthalm Plast Reconstr Surg* 2003; 19(6):479–481.

26. Kloos RT, Duvuuri V, Jhiang SM, et al. Nasolacrimal drainage system obstruction from radioactive iodine therapy for thyroid carcinoma. *J Clin Endocrinol Metab* 2002;87(12):5817–5820.

27. Tsang RW, Brierley JD, Simpson WJ, et al. The effects of surgery, radioiodine, and external radiation therapy on the clinical outcome of patients with differentiated thyroid carcinoma. *Cancer* 1998;82(2):375–388.

28. Farahati J, Reiners C, Stuschke M, et al. Differentiated thyroid cancer. Impact of adjuvant external radiotherapy in patients with perithyroidal tumor infiltration (stage pT4). *Cancer* 1996;77(1):172–180.

29. Grigsby PW, Baglan K, Siegel BA. Surveillance of patients to detect recurrent thyroid carcinoma. *Cancer* 1999;85(4): 945–951.

30. AACE/AAES medical/surgical guidelines for clinical practice: Management of thyroid carcinoma. American Association of Clinical Endocrinologists. American College of Endocrinology. *Endocr Pract* 2001;7(3):202–220.

31. Singer PA, Cooper DS, Daniels GH, et al. Treatment guidelines for patients with thyroid nodules and well-differentiated thyroid cancer. American Thyroid Association. *Arch Intern Med* 1996;156(19):2165–2172.

32. Sherman S. *NCCN Practice Guidelines for Thyroid Cancer.* Dec 2001.

33. Haugen BR, Pacini F, Reiners C, et al. A comparison of recombinant human thyrotropin and thyroid hormone withdrawal for the detection of thyroid remnant or cancer. *J Clin Endocrinol Metab* 1999;84(11):3877–3885.

34. Chiu AC, Delpassand ES, Sherman SI. Prognosis and treatment of brain metastases in thyroid carcinoma. *J Clin Endocrinol Metab* 1997;82(11):3637–3642.

35. Vassilopoulou-Sellin R, Goepfert H, Raney B, Schultz PN. Differentiated thyroid cancer in children and adolescents: Clinical outcome and mortality after long-term follow-up. *Head Neck* 1998;20(6):549–555.

36. Vassilopoulou-Sellin R, Klein MJ, Smith TH, et al. Pulmonary metastases in children and young adults with differentiated thyroid cancer. *Cancer* 1993;71(4):1348–1352.

37. Horvit PK, Gagel RF. The goitrous patient with an elevated serum calcitonin—What to do? *J Clin Endocrinol Metab* 1997;82(2):335–337.

38. Hahm JR, Lee MS, Min YK, et al. Routine measurement of serum calcitonin is useful for early detection of medullary thyroid carcinoma in patients with nodular thyroid diseases. *Thyroid* 2001;11(1):73–80.

39. Bennedbaek FN, Perrild H, Hegedus L. Diagnosis and treatment of the solitary thyroid nodule. Results of a European survey. *Clin Endocrinol (Oxf)* 1999;50(3):357–363.

40. Redding AH, Levine SN, Fowler MR. Normal preoperative calcitonin levels do not always exclude medullary thyroid carcinoma in patients with large palpable thyroid masses. *Thyroid* 2000;10(10):919–922.

41. Gagel RF, Cote GJ. Pathogenesis of medullary thyroid carcinoma. In: Fagin J (ed): *Thyroid Cancer.* Boston: Kluwer; 1998:85–103.

42. Ponder BA, Ponder MA, Coffey R, et al. Risk estimation and screening in families of patients with medullary thyroid carcinoma. *Lancet* 1988;1(8582):397–401.

43. Brandi ML, Gagel RF, Angeli A, et al. Guidelines for diagnosis and therapy of MEN type 1 and type 2. *J Clin Endocrinol Metab* 2001;86(12):5658–5671.

44. Niccoli-Sire P, Murat A, Rohmer V, et al. Familial medullary thyroid carcinoma with noncysteine *ret* mutations: Phenotype-genotype relationship in a large series of patients. *J Clin Endocrinol Metab* 2001;86(8):3746–3753.

45. Hansford JR, Mulligan LM. Multiple endocrine neoplasia type 2 and RET: From neoplasia to neurogenesis. *J Med Genet* 2000;37(11):817–827.

46. Wohllk N, Cote GJ, Bugalho MM, et al. Relevance of RET proto-oncogene mutations in sporadic medullary thyroid carcinoma. *J Clin Endocrinol Metab* 1996;81(10):3740–3745.

47. O'Riordain DS, O'Brien T, Weaver AL, et al. Medullary thyroid carcinoma in multiple endocrine neoplasia types 2A and 2B. *Surgery* 1994;116(6):1017–1023.

48. Saad MF, Ordonez NG, Rashid RK, et al. Medullary carcinoma of the thyroid. A study of the clinical features and prognostic factors in 161 patients. *Medicine (Baltimore)* 1984;63(6):319–342.

49. Hyer SL, Vini L, A'Hern R, Harmer C. Medullary thyroid cancer: Multivariate analysis of prognostic factors influencing survival. *Eur J Surg Oncol* 2000;26(7):686–690.

50. Brierley J, Tsang R, Simpson WJ, et al. Medullary thyroid cancer: Analyses of survival and prognostic factors and the role of radiation therapy in local control. *Thyroid* 1996;6(4): 305–310.

51. Brierley J, Maxon HR. Radioiodine and external radiation therapy in the treatment of thyroid cancer. In: Fagin J (ed): *Thyroid Cancer*. Boston: Kluwer; 1998:285–317.

52. van Heerden JA, Grant CS, Gharib H, et al. Long-term course of patients with persistent hypercalcitoninemia after apparent curative primary surgery for medullary thyroid carcinoma. *Ann Surg* 1990;212(4):395–400; discussion 400–401.

53. Pierie JP, Muzikansky A, Gaz RD, et al. The effect of surgery and radiotherapy on outcome of anaplastic thyroid carcinoma. *Ann Surg Oncol* 2002;9(1):57–64.

54. Xu G, Pan J, Martin C, Yeung SC. Angiogenesis inhibition in the in vivo antineoplastic effect of manumycin and paclitaxel against anaplastic thyroid carcinoma. *J Clin Endocrinol Metab* 2001;86(4):1769–1777.

55. McIver B, Hay ID, Giuffrida DF, et al. Anaplastic thyroid carcinoma: A 50-year experience at a single institution. *Surgery* 2001;130(6):1028–1034.

56. Haigh PI, Ituarte PH, Wu HS, et al. Completely resected anaplastic thyroid carcinoma combined with adjuvant chemotherapy and irradiation is associated with prolonged survival. *Cancer* 2001;91(12):2335–2342.

57. Venkatesh YS, Ordonez NG, Schultz PN, et al. Anaplastic carcinoma of the thyroid. A clinicopathologic study of 121 cases. *Cancer* 1990;66(2):321–330.

58. Junor EJ, Paul J, Reed NS. Anaplastic thyroid carcinoma: 91 patients treated by surgery and radiotherapy. *Eur J Surg Oncol* 1992;18(2):83–88.

59. Ain KB, Egorin MJ, DeSimone PA. Treatment of anaplastic thyroid carcinoma with paclitaxel: Phase 2 trial using ninety-six-hour infusion. Collaborative Anaplastic Thyroid Cancer Health Intervention Trials (CATCHIT) Group. *Thyroid* 2000; 10(7):587–594.

60. Beard CM, Sheps SG, Kurland LT, et al. Occurrence of pheochromocytoma in Rochester, Minnesota, 1950 through 1979. *Mayo Clin Proc* 1983;58(12):802–804.

61. McNeil AR, Blok BH, Koelmeyer TD, et al. Phaeochromocytomas discovered during coronial autopsies in Sydney, Melbourne and Auckland. *Aust N Z J Med* 2000;30(6):648–652.

62. Goldstein RE, O'Neill JA Jr, Holcomb GW III, et al. Clinical experience over 48 years with pheochromocytoma. *Ann Surg* 1999;229(6):755–764; discussion 764–766.

63. John H, Ziegler WH, Hauri D, Jaeger P. Pheochromocytomas: Can malignant potential be predicted? *Urology* 1999; 53(4):679–683.

64. Mannelli M, Ianni L, Cilotti A, Conti A. Pheochromocytoma in Italy: A multicentric retrospective study. *Eur J Endocrinol* 1999;141(6):619–624.

65. Plouin PF, Degoulet P, Tugaye A, et al. [Screening for phaeochromocytoma: In which hypertensive patients? A semi-ological study of 2585 patients, including 11 with phaeo-

chromocytoma (author's transl)]. *Nouv Presse Med* 1981; 10(11):869–872.

66. Lenders JW, Pacak K, Walther MM, et al. Biochemical diagnosis of pheochromocytoma: Which test is best? *JAMA* 2002; 287(11):1427–1434.

67. d'Herbomez M, Gouze V, Huglo D, et al. Chromogranin A assay and (131)I-MIBG scintigraphy for diagnosis and follow-up of pheochromocytoma. *J Nucl Med* 2001;42(7): 993–997.

68. Sisson JC, Frager MS, Valk TW, et al. Scintigraphic localization of pheochromocytoma. *N Engl J Med* 1981;305(1): 12–17.

69. Valk TW, Frager MS, Gross MD, et al. Spectrum of pheochromocytoma in multiple endocrine neoplasia. A scintigraphic portrayal using ^{131}I-metaiodobenzylguanidine. *Ann Intern Med* 1981;94(6):762–767.

70. Shapiro B, Copp JE, Sisson JC, et al. Iodine-131 meta-iodobenzylguanidine for the locating of suspected pheochromocytoma: Experience in 400 cases. *J Nucl Med* 1985;26(6): 576–585.

71. Shulkin BL, Thompson NW, Shapiro B, et al. Pheochromocytomas: Imaging with 2-[fluorine-18]fluoro-2-deoxy-D-glucose PET. *Radiology* 1999;212(1):35–41.

72. Kocak S, Aydintug S, Canakci N. Alpha blockade in preoperative preparation of patients with pheochromocytomas. *Int Surg* 2002;87(3):191–194.

73. Ulchaker JC, Goldfarb DA, Bravo EL, Novick AC. Successful outcomes in pheochromocytoma surgery in the modern era. *J Urol* 1999;161(3):764–767.

74. Steinsapir J, Carr AA, Prisant LM, Bransome ED Jr. Metyrosine and pheochromocytoma. *Arch Intern Med* 1997;157(8): 901–906.

75. Whalen RK, Althausen AF, Daniels GH. Extra-adrenal pheochromocytoma. *J Urol* 1992;147(1):1–10.

76. van Heerden JA, Sheps SG, Hamberger B, et al. Pheochromocytoma: Current status and changing trends. *Surgery* 1982; 91(4):367–373.

77. O'Riordain DS, Young WF Jr, Grant CS, et al. Clinical spectrum and outcome of functional extraadrenal paraganglioma. *World J Surg* 1996;20(7):916–921; discussion 922.

78. van Heerden JA, Roland CF, Carney JA, et al. Long-term evaluation following resection of apparently benign pheochromocytoma(s)/paraganglioma(s). *World J Surg* 1990; 14(3):325–329.

79. Kebebew E, Duh QY. Benign and malignant pheochromocytoma: Diagnosis, treatment, and follow-up. *Surg Oncol Clin North Am* 1998;7(4):765–789.

80. Rao F, Keiser HR, O'Connor DT. Malignant pheochromocytoma. Chromaffin granule transmitters and response to treatment. *Hypertension* 2000;36(6):1045–1052.

81. Yon L, Guillemot J, Montero-Hadjadje M, et al. Identification of the secretogranin II-derived peptide EM66 in pheochromocytomas as a potential marker for discriminating benign versus malignant tumors. *J Clin Endocrinol Metab* 2003; 88(6):2579–2585.

82. Grouzmann E, Gicquel C, Plouin PF, et al. Neuropeptide Y and neuron-specific enolase levels in benign and malignant pheochromocytomas. *Cancer* 1990;66(8):1833–1835.

83. Helman LJ, Cohen PS, Averbuch SD, et al. Neuropeptide Y expression distinguishes malignant from benign pheochromocytoma. *J Clin Oncol* 1989;7(11):1720–1725.

84. Salmenkivi K, Arola J, Voutilainen R, et al. Inhibin/activin betaB-subunit expression in pheochromocytomas favors benign diagnosis. *J Clin Endocrinol Metab* 2001;86(5):2231–2235.

85. Nativ O, Grant CS, Sheps SG, et al. The clinical significance of nuclear DNA ploidy pattern in 184 patients with pheochromocytoma. *Cancer* 1992;69(11):2683–2687.

86. Loh KC, Fitzgerald PA, Matthay KK, et al. The treatment of malignant pheochromocytoma with iodine-131 metaiodobenzylguanidine (131I-MIBG): A comprehensive review of 116 reported patients. *J Endocrinol Invest* 1997;20(11):648–658.

87. Rose B, Matthay KK, Price D, et al. High-dose ^{131}I-metaiodobenzylguanidine therapy for 12 patients with malignant pheochromocytoma. *Cancer* 2003;98(2):239–248.

88. Hamilton BP, Cheikh IE, Rivera LE. Attempted treatment of inoperable pheochromocytoma with streptozocin. *Arch Intern Med* 1977;137(6):762–765.

89. Feldman JM. Treatment of metastatic pheochromocytoma with streptozocin. *Arch Intern Med* 1983;143(9):1799–1800.

90. Bukowski RM, Vidt DG. Chemotherapy trials in malignant pheochromocytoma: Report of two patients and review of the literature. *J Surg Oncol* 1984;27(2):89–92.

91. Averbuch SD, Steakley CS, Young RC, et al. Malignant pheochromocytoma: Effective treatment with a combination of cyclophosphamide, vincristine, and dacarbazine. *Ann Intern Med* 1988;109(4):267–273.

92. Edstrom Elder E, Hjelm Skog AL, et al. The management of benign and malignant pheochromocytoma and abdominal paraganglioma. *Eur J Surg Oncol* 2003;29(3):278–283.

93. Pacak K, Fojo T, Goldstein DS, et al. Radiofrequency ablation: A novel approach for treatment of metastatic pheochromocytoma. *J Natl Cancer Inst* 2001;93(8):648–649.

94. Ohkawa S, Hirokawa S, Masaki T, et al. [Examination of percutaneous microwave coagulation and radiofrequency ablation therapy for metastatic liver cancer]. *Gan To Kagaku Ryoho* 2002;29(12):2149–2151.

95. Vassilopoulou-Sellin R, Schultz PN. Adrenocortical carcinoma. Clinical outcome at the end of the 20th century. *Cancer* 2001;92(5):1113–1121.

96. Ng L, Libertino JM. Adrenocortical carcinoma: Diagnosis, evaluation and treatment. *J Urol* 2003;169(1):5–11.

97. Nader S, Hickey RC, Sellin RV, Samaan NA. Adrenal cortical carcinoma. A study of 77 cases. *Cancer* 1983;52(4):707–711.

98. Samaan NA, Shultz PN, Hickey RC. Adrenocortical carcinoma. In: Samaan Ma (ed): *Endocrine Tumors*. Cambridge, MA: Blackwell; 1993:422–425.

99. Barnett CC Jr, Varma DG, El-Naggar AK, et al. Limitations of size as a criterion in the evaluation of adrenal tumors. *Surgery* 2000;128(6):973–982; discussion 982–983.

100. Weiss LM. Comparative histologic study of 43 metastasizing and nonmetastasizing adrenocortical tumors. *Am J Surg Pathol* 1984;8(3):163–169.

101. Weiss LM, Medeiros LJ, Vickery AL Jr. Pathologic features of prognostic significance in adrenocortical carcinoma. *Am J Surg Pathol* 1989;13(3):202–206.

102. Lee JE, Berger DH, el-Naggar AK, et al. Surgical management, DNA content, and patient survival in adrenal cortical carcinoma. *Surgery* 1995;118(6):1090–1098.

103. MacFarlane D. Cancer of the adrenal cortex: The natural history, prognosis, and treatment in a study of fifty-five cases. *Ann R Coll Surg Engl* 1958;23:155–186.

104. Reincke M, Karl M, Travis WH, et al. p53 mutations in human adrenocortical neoplasms: Immunohistochemical and molecular studies. *J Clin Endocrinol Metab* 1994;78(3):790–794.

105. Yano T, Linehan M, Anglard P, et al. Genetic changes in human adrenocortical carcinomas. *J Natl Cancer Inst* 1989;81(7):518–523.

106. Zwermann O, Beuschlein F, Mora P, et al. Multiple endocrine neoplasia type 1 gene expression is normal in sporadic adrenocortical tumors. *Eur J Endocrinol* 2000;142(6):689–695.

107. Lee MJ, Hahn PF, Papanicolaou N, et al. Benign and malignant adrenal masses: CT distinction with attenuation coefficients, size, and observer analysis. *Radiology* 1991;179(2):415–418.

108. Boland GW, Goldberg MA, Lee MJ, et al. Indeterminate adrenal mass in patients with cancer: Evaluation at PET with 2-[F-18]-fluoro-2-deoxy-D-glucose. *Radiology* 1995;194(1):131–134.

109. Erasmus JJ, Patz EF Jr, McAdams HP, et al. Evaluation of adrenal masses in patients with bronchogenic carcinoma using 18F-fluorodeoxyglucose positron emission tomography. *AJR Am J Roentgenol* 1997;168(5):1357–1360.

110. Maurea S, Mainolfi C, Bazzicalupo L, et al. Imaging of adrenal tumors using FDG PET: Comparison of benign and malignant lesions. *AJR Am J Roentgenol* 1999;173(1):25–29.

111. Becherer A, Vierhapper H, Potzi C, et al. FDG-PET in adrenocortical carcinoma. *Cancer Biother Radiopharm* 2001;16(4):289–295.

112. Dackiw AP, Lee JE, Gagel RF, Evans DB. Adrenal cortical carcinoma. *World J Surg* 2001;25(7):914–926.

113. Lee JE, Evans DB, Hickey RC, et al. Unknown primary cancer presenting as an adrenal mass: Frequency and implications for diagnostic evaluation of adrenal incidentalomas. *Surgery* 1998;124(6):1115–1122.

114. Grumbach MM, Biller BM, Braunstein GD, et al. Management of the clinically inapparent adrenal mass ("incidentaloma"). *Ann Intern Med* 2003;138(5):424–429.

115. Baudin E, Pellegriti G, Bonnay M, et al. Impact of monitoring plasma 1,1-dichlorodiphenildichloroethane (o,p'DDD) levels on the treatment of patients with adrenocortical carcinoma. *Cancer* 2001;92(6):1385–1392.

116. Haak HR, Hermans J, van de Velde CJ, et al. Optimal treatment of adrenocortical carcinoma with mitotane: Results in a consecutive series of 96 patients. *Br J Cancer* 1994;69(5):947–951.

117. van Slooten H, Moolenaar AJ, van Seters AP, Smeenk D. The treatment of adrenocortical carcinoma with o,p'-DDD: Prognostic implications of serum level monitoring. *Eur J Cancer Clin Oncol* 1984;20(1):47–53.

118. Hogan TF, Citrin DL, Johnson BM, et al. o,p'-DDD (mitotane) therapy of adrenal cortical carcinoma: Observations on drug dosage, toxicity, and steroid replacement. *Cancer* 1978;42(5):2177–2181.

119. Vassilopoulou-Sellin R, Samaan NA. Mitotane administration: An unusual cause of hypercholesterolemia. *Horm Metab Res* 1991;23(12):619–620.

120. Vassilopoulou-Sellin R, Guinee VF, Klein MJ, et al. Impact of adjuvant mitotane on the clinical course of patients with adrenocortical cancer. *Cancer* 1993;71(10):3119–3123.

121. van Slooten H, van Oosterom AT. CAP (cyclophosphamide, doxorubicin, and cisplatin) regimen in adrenal cortical carcinoma. *Cancer Treat Rep* 1983;67(4):377–379.

122. Hovi L, Wikstrom S, Vettenranta K, et al. Adrenocortical carcinoma in children: A role for etoposide and cisplatin adjuvant therapy? Preliminary report. *Med Pediatr Oncol* 2003; 40(5):324–326.

123. Baudin E, Docao C, Gicquel C, et al. Use of a topoisomerase I inhibitor (irinotecan, CPT-11) in metastatic adrenocortical carcinoma. *Ann Oncol* 2002;13(11):1806–1809.

124. Berruti A, Terzolo M, Pia A, et al. Mitotane associated with etoposide, doxorubicin, and cisplatin in the treatment of advanced adrenocortical carcinoma. Italian Group for the Study of Adrenal Cancer. *Cancer* 1998;83(10):2194–2200.

125. Arlt W, Reincke M, Siekmann L, et al. Suramin in adrenocortical cancer: Limited efficacy and serious toxicity. *Clin Endocrinol (Oxf)* 1994;41(3):299–307.

126. Flack MR, Pyle RG, Mullen NM, et al. Oral gossypol in the treatment of metastatic adrenal cancer. *J Clin Endocrinol Metab* 1993;76(4):1019–1024.

127. Markoe AM, Serber W, Micaily B, Brady LW. Radiation therapy for adjunctive treatment of adrenal cortical carcinoma. *Am J Clin Oncol* 1991;14(2):170–174.

128. Wood BJ, Abraham J, Hvizda JL, et al. Radiofrequency ablation of adrenal tumors and adrenocortical carcinoma metastases. *Cancer* 2003;97(3):554–560.

129. Mendonca BB, Lucon AM, Menezes CA, et al. Clinical, hormonal and pathological findings in a comparative study of adrenocortical neoplasms in childhood and adulthood. *J Urol* 1995;154(6):2004–2009.

130. Hundahl SA, Fleming ID, Fremgen AM, Menck HR. Two hundred eighty-six cases of parathyroid carcinoma treated in the U.S. between 1985–1995: A National Cancer Data Base Report. The American College of Surgeons Commission on Cancer and the American Cancer Society. *Cancer* 1999; 86(3):538–544.

131. Cohn K, Silverman M, Corrado J, Sedgewick C. Parathyroid carcinoma: The Lahey Clinic experience. *Surgery* 1985;98(6): 1095–1100.

132. Shane E, Bilezikian JP. Parathyroid carcinoma: A review of 62 patients. *Endocr Rev* 1982;3(2):218–226.

133. Shane E. Clinical review 122: Parathyroid carcinoma. *J Clin Endocrinol Metab* 2001;86(2):485–493.

134. Schantz A, Castleman B. Parathyroid carcinoma. A study of 70 cases. *Cancer* 1973;31(3):600–605.

135. Obara T, Fujimoto Y, Kanaji Y, et al. Flow cytometric DNA analysis of parathyroid tumors. Implication of aneuploidy for pathologic and biologic classification. *Cancer* 1990;66(7): 1555–1562.

136. Obara T, Fujimoto Y, Hirayama A, et al. Flow cytometric DNA analysis of parathyroid tumors with special reference to its diagnostic and prognostic value in parathyroid carcinoma. *Cancer* 1990;65(8):1789–1793.

137. Joensuu H, Klemi PJ. DNA aneuploidy in adenomas of endocrine organs. *Am J Pathol* 1988;132(1):145–151.

138. Busaidy N, Jimenez C, Habra M, et al. Parathyroid carcinoma: A 22-year experience. *Head Neck* 2004;26(8):716–726.

139. Grau AM, Evans D, Hoff AO. Carcinoma of the parathyroid glands. In: Pellitteri P, McCaffrey T (eds): *Endocrine Surgery of the Head and Neck.* New York: Delmar Learning; 2003: 429–440.

140. Anderson BJ, Samaan NA, Vassilopoulou-Sellin R, et al. Parathyroid carcinoma: Features and difficulties in diagnosis and management. *Surgery* 1983;94(6):906–915.

141. Chow E, Tsang RW, Brierley JD, Filice S. Parathyroid carcinoma—The Princess Margaret Hospital experience. *Int J Radiat Oncol Biol Phys* 1998;41(3):569–572.

142. Jimenez C, Busaidy N, Habra M, et al. Parathyroid Carcinoma. Two Decades Experience at MD Anderson Cancer Center. In: Chicago: American Society of Clinical Oncology; 2003.

143. Collins MT, Skarulis MC, Bilezikian JP, et al. Treatment of hypercalcemia secondary to parathyroid carcinoma with a novel calcimimetic agent. *J Clin Endocrinol Metab* 1998; 83(4):1083–1088.

CHAPTER
32

MALIGNANT MELANOMA

Eric C. McGary
Agop Y. Bedikian
Ronald P. Rapini

■ EPIDEMIOLOGY

In the United States, malignant melanoma is the sixth most prevalent cancer (1). Melanoma is predominantly diagnosed in the third and fourth decades of life; thus the disease is a significant public health concern. In women in the 25 to 29 age group, melanoma is the most common cancer. In women between 30 and 34 years of age, it is the second most common type of malignancy, breast cancer being the most common (2). In 1998, the age-adjusted rate for invasive cutaneous malignant melanoma was 18.3 per 100,000 males and 13.0 per 100,000 females in the United States (3). The high rate of malignant melanoma in this county is surpassed only by Australia, New Zealand, Norway, and Israel. Although the incidence of melanoma in the United States rose dramatically from the 1970s through the 1990s, this trend appears to be slowing for those born after 1945 (4). The cause for the slowing trend is multifaceted, including reduced exposure to ultraviolet rays, widespread use of sunscreen, and improvements in community-based education and screening.

Malignant melanoma is largely curable if identified at an early stage. Therefore understanding the host and environmental factors that predispose individuals to an increased risk of having the disease is of paramount importance. Those individuals at increased risk of developing melanoma benefit from regular screening examinations and education regarding the warning signs of melanoma.

Commonly acquired nevi (benign nevi) typically appear after the first year of life. Although nevi are benign in and of themselves, several studies have demonstrated that higher numbers of nevi are directly related to an increased risk of developing melanoma. Swerdlow et al. demonstrated a relative risk of 12.1 in patients with 50 or more nevi (5). Similarly, studies by Weiss et al. demonstrated a relative risk of 14.9 in patients with greater then 50 benign nevi (6).

Irregular borders, contour, and color characterize dysplastic or atypical nevi. In contrast to benign nevi, these tend to start to appear in the second decade of life and continue developing throughout adulthood. These nevi can occur sporadically or can be inherited in a familial pattern; this has been given several names, including "the B-K mole syndrome," "familial atypical mole and melanoma syndrome," and the "dysplastic nevus syndrome." The familial syndrome is characterized by the occurrence of melanoma in at least one first- or second-degree relative; the presence of a large number of acquired nevi, some of which are atypical; and nevi that demonstrate specific histologic features. The risk of eventually developing melanoma in these patients is increased 184-fold compared to the general population (7). Studies have demonstrated that the occurrence of malignant melanoma is significantly increased in patients with atypical nevi but who do not meet the criteria for the familial syndrome. Tucker et al. demonstrated a twofold increase in the risk of developing melanoma in patients with even just one atypical nevus. The risk increased to 12-fold in patients with at least 10 dysplastic nevi (8).

Congenital nevi present at birth are divided into groups according to size: small (<1.5 cm), medium (1.5 cm), and large (>20 cm). Only patients with large nevi have been shown to be at increased risk of developing melanoma (9).

■ CELLULAR AND MOLECULAR BIOLOGY

Melanocytes, the precursor cells to melanoma, are distributed as single cells scattered throughout the epidermis. The growth of a melanocyte is dependent on other cells in the local environment, including dermal fibroblasts, inflammatory cells, endothelial cells, and epidermal keratinocytes. Of these cells, the keratinocytes are perhaps the most important with regard to maintaining normal homeostasis by inhibiting the continuous proliferation of melanocytes (10,11).

Tumor progression and metastasis depend on factors intrinsic to the tumor cell, including but not limited to growth factors and their cognate receptors, extracellular matrix proteins, proteases, chemokines, and cellular adhesion molecules. The expression of these factors is influenced by the environment, microenvironment, epistasis, and genetic/epigenetic factors. Malignant melanoma has served as an excellent model to study the expression of many of these factors, partly due to the well-described sequential progression of the disease and characterization of these factors at each step.

Melanoma cells have both radial and vertical growth phases. The radial growth phase encompasses horizontal growth in the epidermis. These lesions represent early-stage disease and may be curable with surgical excision. When the lesion enters the vertical growth phase, however, the repertoire of the many factors that influence tumorigenicity and metastasis changes as the tumor proliferates, enters the dermis, and acquires the capacity to metastasize (Fig. 32-1).

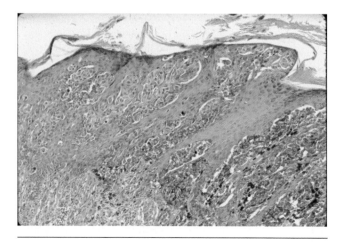

FIGURE 32-1 Melanoma pathology (superficial spreading melanoma). Atypical pagetoid melanocytes are seen within the epidermis, invading the dermis.

CELLULAR ADHESION MOLECULES

Cellular adhesion molecules play an important role in various biological processes, including organogenesis, tissue homeostasis, wound healing, and inflammatory/ immune responses (12). Cellular adhesion molecules of the cadherin, integrin, and immunoglobulin superfamilies are important to both the growth and metastasis of many cancers, including malignant melanoma.

The cellular adhesion molecule MCAM/MUC18 confers metastatic potential and increased tumorigenicity to melanoma cells (13,14). MCAM/MUC18 mediates homotypic and heterotypic adhesion between melanoma cells and endothelial cells, respectively (15–17). Both types of interaction have been shown to promote melanoma growth and metastasis. A fully human monoclonal antibody against MCAM/MUC18 was recently developed. It was shown that this monoclonal antibody inhibits both tumorigenicity and metastasis of melanoma cells in vivo (18).

During melanoma progression, the loss of E-cadherin expression disrupts normal homeostasis in the skin by freeing melanoma cells from structural and functional regulation by keratinocytes (19–22). The loss of functional E-cadherin is paralleled by a gain in N-cadherin function that mediates homotypic interaction between melanoma cells, facilitates gap-junctional formation with fibroblasts and endothelial cells, and promotes melanoma cell migration and survival (23–27). In addition, loss of E-cadherin may affect the β-catenin/wnt signaling pathways, resulting in deregulation of genes involved in growth and metastasis (28).

The integrin family member $\alpha_v\beta_3$ is widely expressed on melanoma cells in the vertical growth phase. When $\alpha_v\beta_3$ is expressed in melanoma cells in the radial growth phase, this integrin is associated with increased tumor growth in vivo; $\alpha_v\beta_3$ may also promote melanoma invasion through an interaction with MMP-2, and transendothelial migration via a heterotypic melanoma-endothelial cell interaction (reviewed in 29).

GROWTH FACTORS

Melanocytes respond to a host of growth factors. Many of these growth factors have been shown to play an important role in promoting the growth of melanoma cells. Co-expression of the growth factors and their cognate receptors suggests their role in autocrine or paracrine growth mechanisms. For example, fibroblast growth factor promotes autocrine and paracrine growth of melanoma cell through binding its cognate receptor, fibroblast growth factor receptor 1. Inhibition of this receptor leads to cell death and inhibition of tumor growth (30,31).

As melanoma cells acquire a more malignant phenotype as determined by the extent of local tumor growth, invasion, and the ability to metastasize, there is a corresponding decrease in the expression of the tyrosine kinase receptor c-Kit (32–34). Both c-Kit and its ligand play important roles in the normal growth and differentiation of embryonic melanoblasts. Mutations in the c-Kit receptor have been identified in human piebald patients (35), suggesting that normal function of c-Kit is required for human melanocyte development. These observations suggest that the malignant transformation of melanocytes may be associated with the loss of c-Kit expression.

Recently, Gleevec (Novartis) has been approved for the treatment of chronic myelogenous leukemia and gastrointestinal stromal tumors (GISTs). Although it was originally designed to inhibit the ABL tyrosine kinase, it also inhibits other tyrosine kinase receptors, including the platelet-derived growth factor (PDGF) receptor and c-Kit (36). Melanomas express high levels of PDGFR-α and PDGFR-β, suggesting their role in autocrine growth. At present, several clinical studies are in progress to determine the effect of Gleevec on tumor growth in patients with malignant melanoma.

GENETICS

Several genes are either lost or mutated in human melanomas. Many of these genes control vital cellular functions such as transcription, cell cycle regulation, regulatory channels, and signal transduction. However, unlike somatic mutations, which are often pathognomonic in other cancers such as the leukemias, the occurrence of genetic changes is somewhat less common in malignant melanoma and demonstrates low correlation with malignant transformation. Mutations in the *p53* gene, *ras* oncogene, and the tumor suppressor *p16INK4A* are present in 5, 21, and 25% of all melanomas, respectively (37,38). Germline mutations or deletions in the 9p21 chromosome are present in 20 to 40% of familial melanoma cases. This chromosomal region contains cell cycle inhibitors as well as tumor suppressors (p16INK4A and p15INK4B) (39). Loss of crucial genes in this region may indirectly target *p53* for degradation.

As melanomas take on a more malignant phenotype, expression of the activator protein-2 (AP-2) transcription factor is lost. AP-2 regulates not only c-Kit (40) and MCAM/MUC18 (41) expression on melanomas but also other genes involved in the progression of human melanoma, such as *E-cadherin, p21/WAF-1, HER-2, Bcl-2, IGF-R1,* and *FAS/APO-1* (42). In contrast to the loss of AP-2 expression, the progression of human melanoma from the radial growth phase to the vertical growth phase is associated with the overexpression of the transcription factors CREB and ATF-1. It has been shown that CREB/ATF-1 acts as a survival factor for melanoma cells (43–47).

Vast advances in our understanding of gene regulation in melanoma have had an important impact on the identification of target genes for drug development. Overexpression of the antiapoptotic *Bcl-2* gene in human melanoma underscores this (48). Inhibition of this gene has been shown to make tumor cells more susceptible to undergoing apoptosis (49). This effect may be especially pronounced in tumor cells treated with chemotherapeutic agents. Today, antisense molecules that inhibit the expression of *Bcl-2* are being studied in clinical trials for the management of this disease (50).

■ CLINICAL-PATHOLOGIC SUBTYPES

MAJOR SUBTYPES

There are four major clinical-pathologic subtypes of cutaneous melanoma. Distinctions among the groups are primarily based on anatomic site.

Superficial Spreading Melanoma

Superficial spreading melanoma is the most common subtype of malignant melanoma, comprising approximately 70% of cases (51) (Figs. 32-2 through 34-4). These lesions can occur anywhere on sun-protected skin and often occur on the upper back in both sexes and the lower extremities in women. The lesions demonstrate irregular and asymmetrical borders. Their size is typically

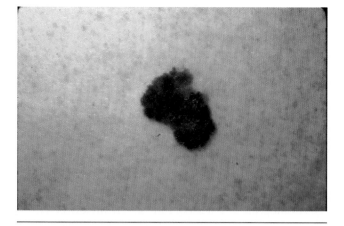

FIGURE 32-3 Melanoma of the trunk with notched borders and variegated blue, black, and brown pigmentation.

greater than 6 to 8 mm, with notable color variegation. These lesions are often confused with traumatized nevi, commonly acquired nevi, and seborrheic keratoses.

Nodular Melanoma

The second most common melanoma subtype, nodular melanoma, accounts for between 15 and 30% of cases (51). Unlike the other three major subtypes, nodular melanoma lacks a preceding radial growth phase. Thus, these melanomas are characterized by rapid growth over weeks to months. The lesions, which typically occur on the trunk or legs, appear as raised dark brown to black nodules. Ulceration and bleeding are common. For this reason amelanotic variants may mimic squamous or basal cell carcinomas.

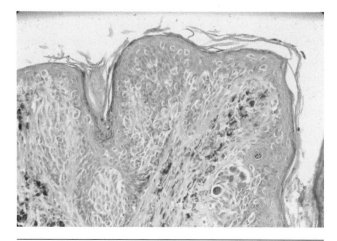

FIGURE 32-2 Superficial spreading melanoma. Note the variegated color and irregular border.

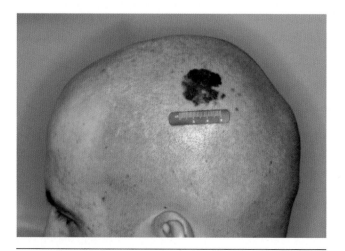

FIGURE 32-4 This melanoma of the scalp did not become apparent until the patient developed alopecia from chemotherapy for another primary cancer.

Lentigo Maligna Melanoma

Lentigo maligna melanoma accounts for 4 to 15% of cutaneous melanomas (52). This subtype typically appears on the head, neck, and arms (Fig. 32-5). Like other skin cancers, lentigo maligna melanoma is linked to cumulative sun exposure. The precursor lesion, lentigo maligna, may be present for up to two decades and grow to sizes greater than 3 cm in diameter before being transformed into lentigo maligna melanoma. Clinically, these lesions appear as flat tan to brown macules with areas that appear hypopigmented. Approximately 5 to 8% of them will transform to invasive melanoma; clinically, this is often heralded by the development of a nodule within the flat precursor lesion (52).

Acral Lentiginous Melanoma

Acral lentiginous melanoma is the least common subtype of malignant melanoma, accounting for 2 to 8% of cases in Caucasians (53). However, among African Americans, Asians, and Hispanics, this subtype accounts for 29 to 72% of cases (53). Typically occurring on the palms or soles or beneath the nail plate, these melanoma tend to be large (>3 cm in diameter) and irregularly pigmented (Figs. 32-6 and 32-7). The presence of pigmentation in the proximal or lateral nail fold (Hutchinson's sign) is diagnostic of subungual melanoma. These lesions may be mistaken for pyogenic granuloma, subungual hematoma, or a bacterial or fungal infection.

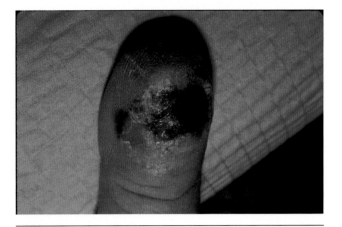

FIGURE 32-6   Melanoma of the toe.

LESS COMMON SUBTYPES

Amelanotic, desmoplastic, mucosal, and uveal melanomas are less common subtypes of malignant melanoma. Although a discussion of their management is beyond the scope of this chapter, they deserve mention because of their distinct clinical presentations and relatively poor prognoses.

Amelanotic melanomas lack the typical pigment expected to be present in most melanomas (Fig. 32-8). These lesions are notorious for resembling other lesions, such as inflammatory conditions, basal cell carcinoma, and pyogenic granuloma. The pathologist sometimes has to perform immunostaining for antigens such as S-100, HMB-45, or MART-1 to make the diagnosis.

Desmoplastic melanoma is a rare subtype that is locally aggressive and tends to have a high rate of local reoccurrence. This subtype has a male predominance (2:1) and typically develops on the sun-exposed area of the head and neck in the elderly. Most are deeply invasive at

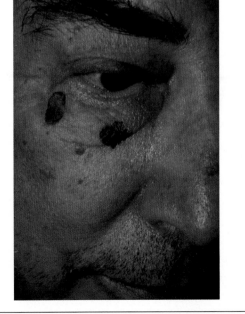

FIGURE 32-5   Melanoma of the face. Lentigo maligna (melanoma in situ) of the eyelid. The lateral lesion was a seborrheic keratosis.

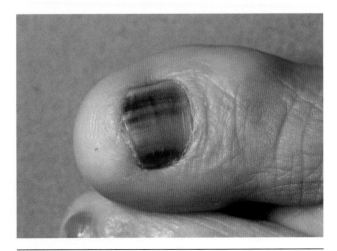

FIGURE 32-7   Acral lentiginous melanoma of the nail.

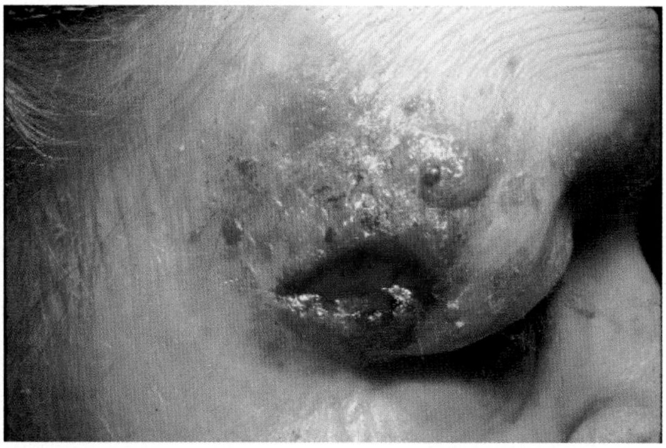

FIGURE 32-8 An amelanotic melanoma that was initially thought to be a basal cell carcinoma.

the time of diagnosis (>5 mm) and tend to invade perineurally, which may cause the patient significant discomfort (54). The lesion may appear as a nodule or pigmented macule with or without an associated nodule.

Frequently desmoplastic melanomas develop in association with lentigo maligna.

Mucosal melanomas can arise in the head and neck, anus, genital tract, respiratory tract, or the gastrointestinal tract (55). This melanoma subtype tends to present at an advanced stage with a very aggressive natural history. Mucosal melanomas tend to be less responsive to conventional therapy, portending a poor prognosis.

PATTERN OF SPREAD OF MALIGNANT MELANOMA

Despite the differences in the appearance of the four subtypes of cutaneous melanoma, they have similar patterns of metastatic spread. Cutaneous and mucosal melanomas tend to spread to regional lymph nodes through the lymphatic channels at an early stage of progression. Spread to distal organs occurs through invasion of local capillaries at the later stage of progression. Lymph node, lung, liver, and brain are the common metastatic sites of spread for cutaneous melanoma (Fig. 32-9).

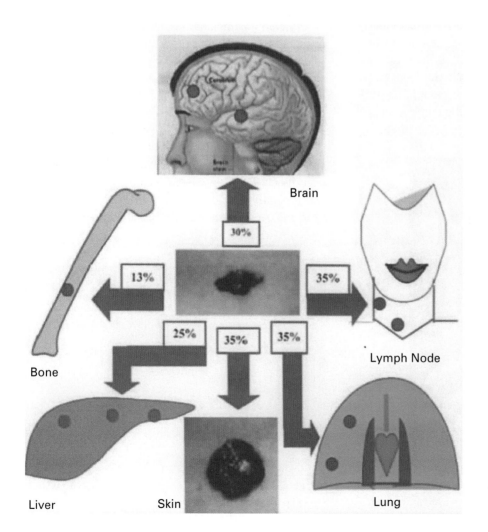

FIGURE 32-9 Pattern of systemic spread of skin melanoma.

Uveal melanomas may involve the iris, ciliary body, or, most frequently, the choroids. Localized disease is often treated with local excision, photocoagulation, external-beam radiotherapy, or enucleation (56). The uveal tract is poor in lymphatics; therefore metastasis is typically hematogenous in origin. The pattern of spread of the choroidal melanoma is significantly different from that of cutaneous melanoma (Fig. 32-10). The rate of metastasis to the liver and brain differs significantly in patients with skin and choroidal melanoma. By far, the liver is the most common site of metastasis for choroidal melanoma (57). In our review, over 95% of the patients had liver metastasis. About half of the patients had the disease confined in the liver; another third have liver and other organ involvement (see Fig. 32-2). Brain involvement with metastasis, which occurs in 20 to 40% of patients with metastatic skin melanoma, occurred in less than 3% patients with choroidal melanoma. In contrast

to patients with cutaneous melanoma, none of the patients with choroidal melanoma had tumor spread to the regional lymph nodes. Four percent of patients had metastasis to distant lymph node basins, most commonly in the abdomen. The median time from diagnosis of primary choroidal melanoma to discovery of metastatic disease was 36 months. The median of survival from date of detection of metastatic disease was 8 months.

■ SURGICAL THERAPY FOR LOCALIZED MELANOMA

In the early 1900s, Handley described the existence of a satellite lesion as far as 3 to 5 cm from the primary melanoma lesion (58) (Fig. 32-11). For that reason, for much of the twentieth century, surgeons typically

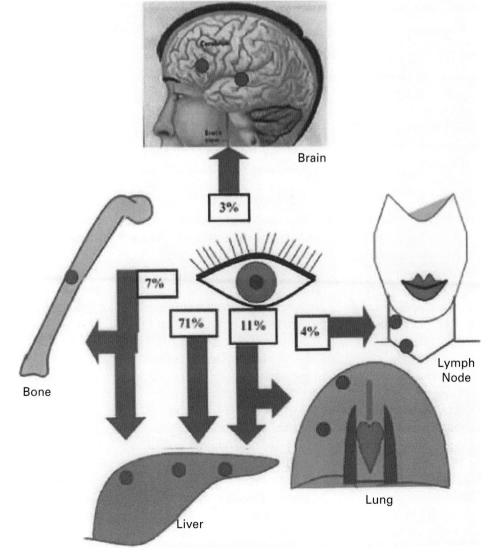

Brain

3%

7%

71%   11%   4%

Bone

Lymph Node

Liver

Lung

FIGURE 32-10 Pattern of systemic spread of choroidal melanoma.

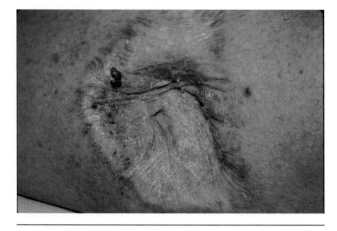

FIGURE 32-11 Metastatic melanoma appearing within and around a graft site.

resected melanomas with 5-cm margins. Data to support more conservative resection margins have come from the World Health Organization Melanoma Programme Trial and the Intergroup trial as well as many studies conducted in the 1970s and 1980s. Today, surgeons in the United States generally follow the guidelines proposed during the 1997 World Health Organization (WHO) Melanoma Programme meeting (59). Those guidelines recommend more conservative surgical margins that are based on tumor thickness. Lesions more than 2 mm thick require a 2-cm margin, those less than 2 mm thick require a 1-cm margin, and excision of melanoma in situ requires a 0.5-cm margin (59).

MOHS SURGERY

The role of Mohs micrographic surgery in the management of cutaneous malignant melanoma remains controversial. Findings from one study in 1997 support the efficacy of the Mohs technique for the treatment of melanoma versus wide local excision (60). Furthermore, the local recurrence rate was lower in the Mohs group in comparison to the group that underwent conventional surgery (61). The margins required to remove the tumor averaged 6 mm in 83% of the cases (61). At present Mohs surgery is not widely used in the management of melanoma. It is labor-intensive, time-intensive, and costly. Furthermore, no randomized prospective studies have been conducted comparing this technique to conventional surgery. Results of such a study would, of course, be dependent on the experience of the Mohs surgeon. Finally, cutting part of the tumor in an attempt to obtain a strict margin is a risk that is not deemed acceptable by

most surgeons. Others have advocated its use in areas where tissue conservation is desired, such as on the face.

ELECTIVE LYMPH NODE DISSECTION

As in the case of other tumors, lymph node metastasis remains the most important predictor of survival in patients with malignant melanoma (62,63). Studies have shown that the number of lymph nodes bearing cancer, rather than their size, is the most important prognostic feature in this disease (64). Ten-year survival for patients with one, two to four, or five or more lymph nodes involved with melanoma are approximately 40, 26, and 15%, respectively (64). Therefore many believe that elective lymph node dissection (ELND) is important not only for staging but also for potential cure through removal of disseminated tumor foci. Indeed, many studies have shown a survival advantage for patients who undergo ELND as part of staging compared to those who wait until the development of clinically evident metastases (65–67). However, the WHO trial concluded that ELND offered no survival benefit over delayed lymph node dissection (68).

SENTINEL LYMPH NODE BIOPSY

ELND carries risks of morbidity. These include lymphedema, nerve damage, and wound complications. To circumvent these problems, intraoperative lymphatic mapping and sentinel lymph node (SLN) biopsy have now become the standard of care in most institutions for staging the lymphatic basin. The indication for SLN is the presence of primary melanoma without clinical, radiographic, or histologic evidence of distant metastases. At present, there is still disagreement as to when to perform SLN biopsy. Many surgeons feel that this procedure is appropriate for melanomas at least 0.75 mm thick, whereas others would argue that it should be employed only for lesions at least 1 mm thick.

Morton et al. have published one of the first clinical studies demonstrating the efficacy of SLN biopsy (69). In this study they identified the SLN(s) in 82% of lymphatic basins. Metastases were present in approximately 18% of the SLNs identified (69). This correlates well with prior studies indicating metastases in 12 to 15% of SLNs (70,71). Combinations of blue dye and radiocolloid-guided lymphatic mapping are accurate in determining the SLN. This accuracy is reduced, however, in patients who have previously had surgical disruption of their tumor site. This is most problematic if the primary site was resected with large margins or a rotational flap was used for closure. For this reason, it is preferred that SLN biopsies occur at the time of excision. Techniques to further enhance the histopathologic analysis of SLNs are under investigation. These include immunohistochemistry for the S-100 protein and the HMB-45 antigen and RT-PCR to detect the tyrosinase gene mRNA (72,73). If there is histopathologic evidence of metastasis in the SLN, it is standard to proceed with lymphadenectomy.

Although ELND and SLN biopsies may not increase survival in patients with regional lymph node involvement, they clearly provide accurate staging informa-

tion, which may help guide the clinician's decision as to whether or not to offer adjuvant therapy.

■ REVISED STAGING INFORMATION

The American Joint Committee on Cancer (AJCC) staging system for cutaneous melanoma has recently been revised to more accurately reflect variables of prognostic significance. Revisions in the tumor microstaging, nodal staging, and metastasis staging were published in 2001 (74) and have replaced the prior staging system in the sixth edition of the *AJCC Staging Manual* (see Figs. 32-3 and 32-4 and Tables 32-1 and 32-2) (75).

Tumor staging (T) in the old system was based on both the Clark's level and Breslow thickness. The new staging system focuses on melanoma thickness and ulceration, two parameters that are strong predictors of outcome as determined by Cox regression analysis (75). Clark's level thickness is used in further staging only of T1 tumors (<1 mm) because it is an independent predictor of outcome in that subgroup.

The major revision to nodal staging (N) places an emphasis on the number of involved lymph nodes. Cox regression analysis has demonstrated that the number, not the size, of metastatic lymph nodes was the strongest predictor of outcome (75). N1, N2, and N3 include patients with one involved lymph node, two to three involved lymph nodes, and four or more involved lymph nodes, respectively. The next most important predictor of outcome is the tumor burden within the involved lymph nodes (75). N groups are further characterized as having microscopic metastases or macroscopic metastases that are clinically or radiographically apparent and confirmed pathologically. Both satellite lesions and in-transit metastases involve the lymphatics and

TABLE 32-1	THE NEW AMERICAN JOINT COMMITTEE ON CANCER STAGING SYSTEM FOR MELANOMA	
Classification		
T classification		
T1	< or = 1.0 mm	a: without ulceration
T1		b: with ulceration or level IV or V
T2	1.01–2.0 mm	a: without ulceration
T2		b: with ulceration
T3	2.01–4.0 mm	a: without ulceration
T3		b: with ulceration
T4	>4.0 mm	a: without ulceration
T4		b: with ulceration
N classification		
N1	One lymph node	a: micrometastasis*
		b: macrometastasis†
N2	2–3 lymph nodes	a: micrometastasis*
		b: macrometastasis†
		c: in-transit met(s)/ satellite(s) *without* metastatic lymph nodes
N3	4 or > metastatic lymph nodes, matted lymph nodes, or combinations of in-transit met(s)/ satellite(s), or ulcerated melanoma *and* metastatic lymph node(s)	
M classification		
M1	Distant skin, SQ, or lymph node mets	Normal LDH
M2	Lung mets	Normal LDH
M3	All other visceral or any distant mets	Normal LDH Elevated LDH

mets: metastases

* Micrometastases are diagnosed after elective or sentinel lymphadenectomy.

† Macrometastases are defined as clinically detectable lymph node metastases confirmed by therapeutic lymphadenectomy or when any lymph node metastasis exhibits gross extracapsular extension.

SOURCE: Balch CM, Buzaid AC, Atkins MB, et al. A new American Joint Committee on Cancer staging system for cutaneous melanoma. *Cancer* 2000;88:1484–1491.

| TABLE 32-2 | AJCC STAGING SYSTEM FOR MELANOMA |

Clinical Staging*				Pathologic Staging†			
0	Tis	N0	M0	0	Tis	N0	M0
IA	T1a	N0	M0	1A	T1a	N0	M0
IB	T1b	N0	M0	1B	T1b	N0	M0
	T2a	N0	M0		T2a	N0	M0
IIA	T2b	N0	M0	IIA	T2b	N0	M0
	T3a	N0	M0		T3a	N0	M0
IIB	T3b	N0	M0	IIB	T3b	N0	M0
	T4a	N0	M0		T4a	N0	M0
IIC	T4b	N0	M0	IIC	T4b	N0	M0
IIIA	any T1-4a	N1b	M0	IIIA	T1-4a	N1a	M0
IIIB	any T1-4a	N2b	M0	IIIB	T1-4a	N1b	M0
			M0		T1-4a	N2a	M0
IIIC	any T	N2c	M0	IIIC	any T	N2b, N2c	M0
	any T	N3	M0		any T	N3	M0
IV	any T	any N	any M	IV	any T	any N	any M

* Clinical staging includes microstaging of the primary melanoma and clinical/radiologic evaluation for metastases; by convention, it should be used after complete excision of the primary melanoma with *clinical* assessment for regional and distant metastases.
† Pathologic staging includes microstaging of the primary melanoma and pathologic information about the regional lymph nodes after partial or complete lymphadenectomy, except for *pathologic Stage 0 or Stage IA patients, who do not need pathologic evaluation of their lymph nodes.*

portend a poor prognosis. These were grouped separately in the old staging system but are now grouped together as N2c disease in the revised AJCC staging system. The presence of satellite lesions or in-transit metastases in patients with nodal metastasis represents N3 disease. Finally, in patients with lymph node metastasis, ulceration of the primary tumor was the feature that independently predicted an adverse outcome among stage III patients. In the revised AJCC staging system, all stage III patients whose primary tumor is ulcerated are staged upward by one substage.

In patients with metastasis, the metastases (M) staging has been broken down into three subgroups (M1a, M1b, and M1c) in the revised AJCC staging system. The subgroups reflect the site of metastasis and whether or not lactate dehydrogenase (LDH) is elevated.

■ ADJUVANT THERAPY FOR STAGES II AND III MELANOMA

The risk of melanoma recurrence and death is closely related to Breslow thickness and the number of regional lymph nodes involved. Surgery can be curative in more than 90% of low-risk patients with stage I disease (Breslow thickness <1.5 mm) and 70% of intermediate-risk patients with stages IIA disease (Breslow thickness 1.5 to 4 mm) at presentation (Fig. 32-12). In contrast, patients with stage IIB disease (Breslow thickness >4 mm) have a 5-year survival of about 30 to 50% despite surgical excision. Recurrence of disease lowers the survival rates to 30% at 5 years for locoregional recurrences

and to less than 5% for patients with systemic metastases. The pretreatment work-up and management of patients with local/regional melanoma depend on thickness of primary and status of regional lymph nodes (Fig. 32-12), which in turn determines risk of tumor recurrence. Adjuvant therapies are prescribed following surgery to patients at high risk for tumor recurrence with the hope that such treatments might be most successful in patients with micrometastasis. Patients with clinically detectable metastatic melanoma have a median survival of 7 to 9 months, depending on the bulk of the disease at the time of recurrence. These patients are more intensely evaluated before treatment and more closely monitored following start of systemic therapy (Fig. 33-13).

A number of modalities of treatments have been tested to reduce the risk of recurrence in high-risk patients through eradication of occult micrometastases. Chemotherapy, nonspecific immune response modifiers, hormonal agents, and lymphokines have been tried. Unfortunately, despite the promising results from pilot studies, none of these therapies have proved consistently to be beneficial in prospectively randomized clinical trials when compared to observation or placebo. The current status of randomized systemic adjuvant clinical trials is discussed below.

Chemotherapy outcomes in adjuvant settings were recently reviewed (76). The following general conclusions were reached. First, dacarbazine (DTIC), the only cytotoxic drug approved by the U.S. Food and Drug Administration (FDA) specifically for the treatment of metastatic melanoma, has been most widely evaluated

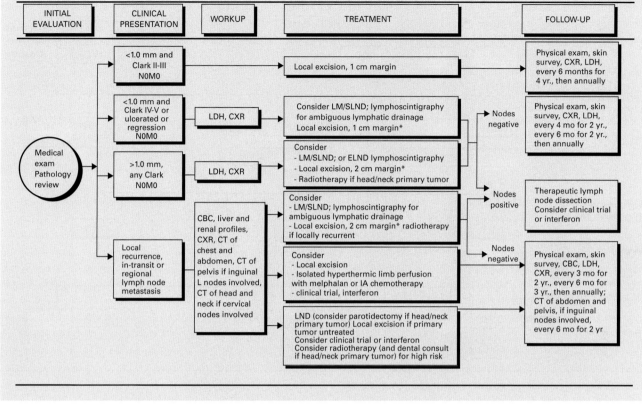

FIGURE 32-12   Management of local/regional melanoma.

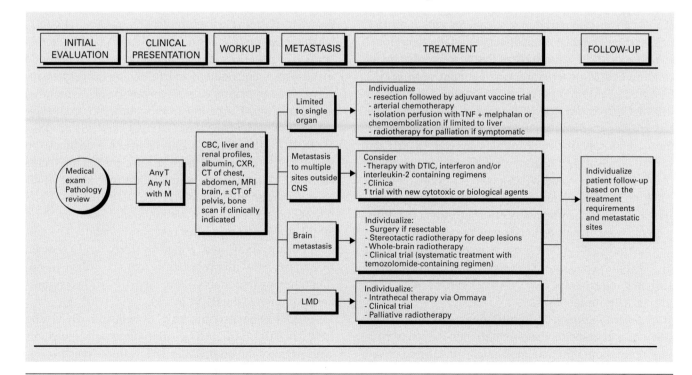

FIGURE 32-13   Management of melanoma metastatic to the organs.

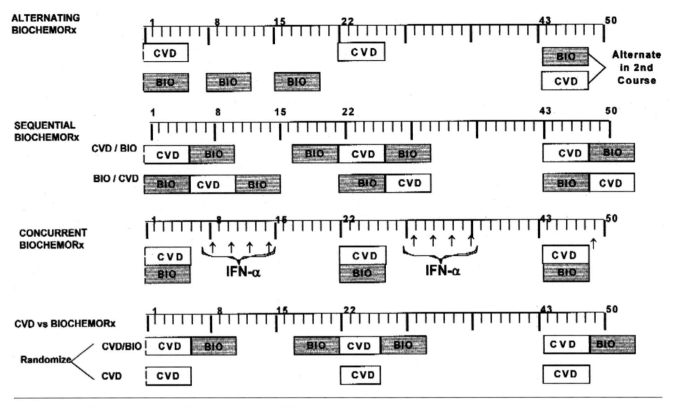

FIGURE 32-14 Treatment schema of biochemotherapy trials.

in adjuvant settings. The overall results have revealed no significant benefit. Two of the large number of studies evaluated the efficacy of DTIC alone or in combination in an adjuvant setting. The Central Oncology Group (COG) conducted a trial in 174 patients with high-risk primary melanoma or melanoma metastatic to regional lymph nodes (77). After surgery, they were prospectively randomized to observation or treatment with DTIC. The treated group were given four courses of DTIC at 4.5 mg/kg per day for 10 days, repeated every four weeks. At a median follow-up of 2.5 years, the control group had superior relapse-free survival (RFS) and overall survival (OS) than the DTIC-treated group. In another study, the Southwest Oncology Group (SWOG) randomized 123 patients with resected primary melanoma to either chemotherapy or observation (78). Fifty patients were given a chemotherapy regimen containing carmustine (150 mg/m^2 every 8 weeks), hydroxyurea (1500 mg/m^2 per day × 5 every 4 weeks) and DTIC (150 mg/m^2 per day × 5 every 4 weeks) for 1 year. Both groups had similar OS: 65% at 6 years.

Immunotherapy trials of melanoma got started four decades ago based on the observation that objective tumor regression of human melanoma could be achieved with the administration of bacillus Calmette-Guérin (BCG) (79). Observation of positive results from BCG in pilot studies led to several prospectively randomized studies comparing BCG with observation in patients with stage I to III melanoma who were rendered free of disease by surgery. One of the large studies was conducted by Eastern Cooperative Oncology Group (ECOG) and has been reported by Cunningham et al. (80). In this study, 474 patients with primary or regional lymph node metastases were randomized following surgery to receive immunotherapy with Tice strain BCG (18 months) or observation. The results of this study showed no statistically significant benefit with BCG in RFS and OS.

In 1975, the National Cancer Institute conducted a study in 181 patients at high risk for melanoma recurrence (81). The patients were randomly assigned to receive either methyl-lomustine (CCNU), BCG, or BCG plus allogeneic cultured melanoma cells, or observation after being rendered free of disease surgically. The outcome of the study, as reported by Terry et al., showed that compared with observation, neither of the two immunotherapy treatments nor methyl-CCNU had significantly improved the RFS and OS.

ECOG evaluated the role of adjuvant BCG and DTIC in Trial E1673 (82). After surgery, 471 patients with primary melanoma and 181 with in-transit or regional lymph node metastases were randomly assigned to one of three study groups: (1) treatment with immunotherapy with BCG, (2) DTIC plus BCG, or (3) observation. Cunningham et al. reported that there were no significant differences in RFS and OS among the treatment groups and the control arm.

The WHO conducted a large multi-institutional trial in patients with histologically confirmed regional lymph node metastasis or with Clark's level III to V skin melanoma of the trunk with negative regional nodes (83). In this trial, 761 patients were prospectively randomized to one of four groups: (1) 185 patients to surgery alone; (2) 192 to surgery plus DTIC at 200 mg/m^2 per day $\times$ 5 every 4 weeks; (3) 203 to surgery plus BCG; and (4) 181 to surgery plus DTIC and BCG. Veronisi reported in 1982 that over 70% of these patients experienced tumor recurrence. There was no significant difference in RFS and OS among the four groups.

In a similar chemoimmunotherapy trial conducted by Group Inter France in 1975, a total of 284 melanoma patients with either Clark's level $\geq$III or with positive regional lymph nodes were randomly assigned to either BCG, for 2 years or adjuvant chemotherapy with DTIC, CCNU and VM26 for 6 months followed by BCG after surgery (84). Of the total, 136 patients received BCG and 148 received the chemoimmunotherapy. After a median follow-up of 3 years, Misset et al. reported in 1984 that there was no difference among the groups for RFS. However, there was a significant difference in overall survival in favor of immunotherapy alone ($p = 0.03$).

Levamisole trials in melanoma were initiated after the discovery of its immuno-modulating activity. The European Organization for Research on the Treatment of Cancer (EORTC) evaluated its role in adjuvant therapy of patients with melanoma. After surgical resection, more than 200 patients with melanoma Clark levels $\geq$III and Breslow thickness $>$1.5 mm were randomized to receive either DTIC (250 mg/m^2 per day $\times$ 5 days monthly for 6 months), levamisole, or placebo (85). Czarnetzki et al. reported that no significant difference was found in RFS and OS among the three groups. Similarly, in a randomized double-blind trial comparing levamisole with placebo as adjuvant therapy for surgically treated patients with melanoma, Spitler and Sagebiel found no difference between levamisole and placebo with regard to RFS and OS and time to appearance of visceral metastases (86).

A phase III study conducted by the National Cancer Institute of Canada compared the roles of BCG and levamisole to observation in 543 poor-prognosis melanoma patients. Following complete resection, the patients were randomized to treatment in one of four groups: (1) levamisole for 3 years, (2) BCG for 3 years, (3) BCG alternating with levamisole for 3 years, and (4) observa-

tion (87). At the median follow-up of 8.5 years, there was a trend toward a significant reduction in mortality as well as of recurrence rates in patients treated with levamisole alone ($p = 0.08$ and 0.09, respectively) compared to those in observation. However, patients treated with BCG-containing regimens did not have improvement in RFS and OS. Further investigation is needed to define the role of levamisole as adjuvant treatment of melanoma.

Melanoma vaccines—including whole cell, cell lysate, or shed antigen vaccines as well as ganglioside vaccines—have been evaluated in intermediate- and high-risk patients with melanoma. These vaccines were reported to result in significantly prolonged survival when administered as a surgical adjuvant compared with historical controls. However, the initial promising results could not be confirmed with these agents when used alone or in combination in the few prospectively randomized adjuvant studies designed to compare them to placebo or observation in stages III and IV in the postoperative settings.

Vaccinia melanoma oncolysates (*VMO*) showed significant improvement in survival relative to historical controls in the pilot clinical trial. In the subsequent randomized clinical trial using a VMO derived from four melanoma cell lines infected with vaccinia virus, 215 patients with stage III melanoma were randomized to VMO or vaccinia alone. There was no evidence of RFS and OS benefit (88). In another trial, 700 patients with high-risk (66% with clinically detectable regional lymph node metastasis) melanoma, after definitive surgery, were prospectively randomized either to therapy with VMO for 2 years or to observation. At a median follow-up of 8 years, statistically significant prolongation of RFS and OS was not observed (89).

Allogeneic melanoma vaccine (Melacine) was evaluated by the SWOG in patients with stage II melanoma. Six hundred patients with intermediate-thickness (1.5 to 4.0 mm or Clark's level IV) melanoma and without clinical or histologic evidence of lymph node metastasis were randomized after surgery to treatment with Melacine for 2 years or to observation. After follow-up of 5.6 years, no improvement in RFS or OS with adjuvant vaccine was found (90).

G_{M2} *ganglioside* vaccine was found to induce antibody responses in a study conducted by Livingston et al. They postulated that T cells infiltrating melanoma lesions recognized specific tumor antigens located on the surface of melanoma cells. The presence of IgM antibody against G_{M2} ganglioside was associated with prolonged survival in patients with melanoma (91). In a randomized phase III trial, 122 patients who had undergone resection of regional node metastases were assigned to receive either G_{M2}/BCG vaccine or BCG alone (92). The patients with no pretreatment anti-G_{M2} antibodies who had IgM antibody production in response to administration of G_{M2}/BCG had improvement in RFS and OS, but only the improvement in RFS was statistically significant ($p = 0.02$).

In a subsequent study, the efficacy of the combination of G_{M2}, KLH, and QS21 adjuvant was compared to that of standard high-dose interferon (IFN)-α2b (Intergroup Trial E1694) (93). The primary objective of this trial was to determine whether GMK, a ganglioside vaccine, was superior to high-dose IFN-α2b with respect to RFS and OS, with early stopping rules in case IFN proved superior. An interim analysis demonstrated a highly significant RFS and OS improvement in favor of the patients treated with IFN. The trial was closed to further patient entry. Patients randomized to receiving the vaccine were offered IFN treatment instead. A Cox regression analysis showed statistically significant improvement in RFS and OS with IFN after adjusting for age, gender, performance status, and nodal status.

Interferon alpha (IFN-α) induces immune modulation and tumor regression in patients with metastatic melanoma. The antiviral and immunomodulatory properties of IFN could stimulate host rejection of tumor cells and induction of MHC antigens. The IFNs may inhibit angiogenesis and may have direct growth-inhibitory effects. A series of clinical trials were initiated to examine the role of IFN in the treatment and prevention of melanoma. Despite the clinical research over the past two decades, the optimum dose and schedule of IFN remain unsettled to date. The significant toxicity and cost associated with the higher-dose schedules and the marginal antitumor efficacy of IFN have been important factors in the decision to adopt different dose schedules as standard in Europe and the United States. In western Europe, the low-dose chronic (1 to 3 years) IFN administration schedule was preferred by the European Medicine Evaluation Agency as standard over the high-dose IFN schedule approved by the FDA in the United States. The outcomes of the adjuvant clinical trials with IFN are summarized in Tables 32-1 and 32-2.

STAGE II

Despite the justification for the use of high-dose adjuvant IFN for high-risk melanoma, its use in separate clinical trials conducted in the United States in patients without lymph node metastasis has been limited (Table 32-3). Most often these patients were treated on protocols designed for stage III patients rendered free of disease surgically, and a smaller number of such patients were accrued in these trials than in the European trials. While significant improvement in RFS has been demonstrated in high-risk patients without lymph node metastasis in a few of these trials, similar improvement in overall OS could not be confirmed.

STAGE III

The data from high-dose IFN adjuvant trials in patients with lymph node metastasis at high risk for melanoma recurrence quite often showed an improvement in RFS (Table 32-4). However, the only clinical trial that showed significant OS benefit with IFN compared to observation was that of the ECOG study E1684 (95). In that study, patients treated with high-dose IFN had a median RFS that was prolonged by about 9 months, and their 5-year RFS rate was increased to 37%, compared to the 26% observed in control group. The corresponding improvements in OS were about 1 year for median survival and 9% improvement in 5-year survival. These results led the FDA in 1996 to recommend the approval of this IFN regimen as standard therapy for patients with high-risk melanoma. However, an updated analysis by Kirkwood et al. indicated that, at median follow-up of 12.6 years, there was no significant survival benefit with IFN (103). IFN therapy was associated with considerable but generally manageable toxicity. Side effects included flu-like symptoms (fever, fatigue, nausea), depression, neutropenia, and reversible hepatotoxicity. Despite these problems, over 60 percent of patients were able to complete a year of therapy without serious toxicity. Contraindications to high-dose IFN-α2b adjuvant therapy include recent history of myocardial infarction or arrhythmias, preexisting liver or central nervous system disorders, and overall debility. The importance of dose and schedule in the use of IFN is still under investigation.

Results of the confirmatory Intergroup trial E1690, a three-arm trial comparing the IFN high-dose IV/SC regimen or low-dose subcutaneous regimen for 2 years with observation, confirmed the RFS advantage of the high-dose therapy but not the OS advantage, suggesting that the low-dose chronic regimen was less effective. The observation group of this trial did significantly better than the E1684 trial group. One possible cause for this finding was the crossover effect made possible by the FDA's approval of IFN during the life of the trial. Other randomized trials of adjuvant IFN in high-risk patients employed lower doses; differing doses, durations, and routes of administration showed no significant survival benefit.

TABLE 32-3 | ADJUVANT THERAPY OF PATIENTS WITH PRIMARY MELANOMA AT INTERMEDIATE OR HIGH RISK FOR TUMOR RECURRENCE

Trial, Year of Publication	Breslow Thickness	No. of Patients	Interferon	Control	Outcome*	Ref.
SWOG 8642, Meykens et al, 1995	T ≥ 1.5 mm	73	IFN-γ 0.2 mg SC 3 × per week for 1 year	Observation	No significant RFS or OS benefit	93
NCCTG, Creagan et al, 1995	T ≥ 1.7 mm	102	IFN-α2a 20 MU/m² IM 3 × per week for 3 months	Observation	No significant RFS or OS benefit	94
ECOG 1684, Kirkwood et al, 1996	T > 4.0 mm	31	IFN-α2b 20 MU/m²/day IV × 5 q 7 days for 4 weeks then 10 MU/m² SC 3 × per week for 11 months	Observation	IFN has significant RFS or OS benefit	95
French Multicenter Trial, Grob et al, 1998	T > 1.5 mm	489	IFN-α2a 3 MU/m² SC 3 × per week for 18 months	Observation	Significant RFS but no OS benefit	96
Austrian Malignant Melanoma Co-op. Group Pehamberger Kirkwood et al, 1998	T ≥ 1.5 mm	311	IFN-α2a 3 MU SC daily for 3 weeks then 3 × per week for 12 months	Observation	Significant RFS but no OS benefit	97
ECOG 1690, Kirkwood et al, 2000	T > 4 mm	163	IFN-α2b 20 MU/m²/day IV × 5 q 7 days for 4 weeks then 10 MU/m² SC 3 × per week for 11 months vs 3 MU SC 3 × per week for 2 years	Observation	No significant RFS or OS benefit	98
ECOG 1694, Kirkwood et al, 2001	T ≥ 4 mm	202	IFN-α2b 20 MU/m²/day IV × 5 q 7 days for 4 weeks then 10 MU/m² SC 3 × per week for 11 months	G$_{M2}$ ganglioside vaccine	IFN has significant DFS and OS benefit	99
EORTC18871, Eggermont et al, 2001	T > 3 mm	340	IFN-α2b 1 MU 3 × per week for 1 year	IFN-γ 0.2 mg SC 3 × per week for 1 year	No significant RFS or OS benefit	100
UKCCCR study, Hancock et al, 2001	T ≥ 4 mm	125	IFN-α2a 3 MU SC 3 × per week for 2 years	Observation	No significant RFS or OS benefit	101

OS = overall survival; RFS = relapse-free survival.

In the E1694 clinical trial, 1 year of high-dose IFN was compared with 2 years of GMK. In an earlier study, GMK was found to induce the production of IgM antibodies, a finding associated with better prognosis. In this study, the IFN arm had significantly better RFS and OS than the vaccine arm. It is still uncertain whether the difference in efficacy is related to a possible negative impact of GMK vaccine or the superiority of IFN.

Thus, although data from high-dose IFN clinical trials consistently demonstrated RFS benefit when IFN was given as surgical adjuvant to patients with stage III melanoma after lymphadenectomy, its impact on OS has been less clear. The limited benefit from IFN should be considered in light of the considerable toxicity associated with it when given at high doses.

The results of the adjuvant IFN trials reported to date indicate that a few of the regimens give at least an RFS advantage for patients with both stages II and III disease. It appears that high-dose IFN-α is the most active adjuvant therapy for high-risk melanoma. Treatment decisions for

TABLE
32-4 **ADJUVANT THERAPY OF PATIENTS WITH MELANOMA METASTATIC
TO REGIONAL LYMPH NODES AT HIGH RISK FOR TUMOR RECURRENCE**

Trial, Year of Publication	No. of Patients	Interferon	Control	Outcome	Ref.
WHO Melanoma 16, Cascinelli et al, 1994	424	IFN-α2a 3 MU SC 3 × per week for 3 years	Observation	No significant RFS or OS benefit	102
SWOG 8642, Meykens et al, 1995	127	IFN-γ 0.2 mg SC 3 × per week for 1 year	Observation	No significant RFS or OS benefit	93
NCCTG, Creagan et al, 1995	160	IFN-α2a 20 MU/m² IM 3 × per week for 3 months	Observation	No significant RFS or OS benefit	94
ECOG 1684, Kirkwood et al, 1996	249	IFN-α2b 20 MU/m²/day IV × 5 q 7 days for 4 weeks then 10 MU/m² SC 3 × per week for 11 months	Observation	IFN has significant RFS or OS benefit	95
ECOG 1690, Kirkwood et al, 2000	632	IFN-α2b 20 MU/m²/day IV × 5 q 7 days for for 4 weeks then 10 MU/m² SC 3 × per week × 11 months vs 3 MU SC 3 × per week for 2 years	Observation	No significant RFS or OS benefit	98
ECOG 1694, 2001	678	IFN-α2b 20 MU/m² day IV × 5 q 7 days for 4 weeks then 10 MU/m² SC 3 × per week for 11 months	G$_{M2}$ ganglioside vaccine	IFN has significant DFS and OS benefit	99
EORTC 18952, 2001	1300	IFN-α2b 10 MU/dx5 q 7 days × 4 weeks, 5 MUSC 3 × per week for 23 months vs. 10 MU/dx5 q 7 days for 4 weeks, 10 MU SC 3 × per week for 11 months	Observation	Significant RFS but no OS benefit with low-dose IFN vs. control	100
EORTC 18871, 2001	490	IFN-α2b 1 MU 3 × per week for 1 year	IFN-γ 0.2 mg SC 3 × per week for 1 year	No significant RFS or OS benefit	100
UKCCCR, Hancock et al, 2001	529	IFN-α2a 3 MU SC 3 × per week for 2 years	Observation	No significant RFS or OS benefit	101

OS = overall survival; RFS = relapse-free survival.

such patients should be individualized depending on the patient's desire for aggressive therapy and an acceptance of therapy-related toxicity for potential benefit.

New combinations involving IFN with either melanoma vaccine, interleukin-2 (IL-2), or the combination of IL-2 and chemotherapy are currently under evaluation in high-risk melanoma patients. The result of such a clinical trial with a combination of IFN-α2b and IL-2 was recently reported by Hauschild et al. (104). Two hundred twenty five patients with resected intermediate-high-risk primary melanoma without detectable node metastasis were randomized either to observation or to therapy with a combination of low-dose (3 MU/m² per day for 7 days and then twice weekly during weeks 3 to 6) and IFN-α2b with IL-2 (9 MU/m² per day for 4 days during the second week). There was no significant improvement in RFS or OS with biotherapy. A trial comparing the efficacy of high-dose IFN-α2b to IL-2–based biochemotherapy is currently under way nationally. In this SWOG study, stage III melanoma patients are prospectively randomized following surgery to receive either high-dose IFN administered for 1 year or three courses of biochemotherapy including cisplatin, vinblastine, DTIC, IFN, and IL-2 over a 9-week period. The effects of these treatments on RFS and OS will be compared. A similar study is currently ongoing at MD Anderson Cancer Center (MDACC).

■ MANAGEMENT OF METASTATIC DISEASE

It is estimated that between 2 and 5% of patients will present with metastatic disease. On the whole, survival time in patients with metastasis ranges from 6 to 9 months with long-term survival of less than 10%. In these patients, the site of metastasis is of prognostic value. Patients with skin, subcutaneous, and distant lymph node metastasis have a better prognosis than those with lung or liver and bone metastasis. The development of brain metastasis has a significant adverse impact on prognosis (survival of 3 to 4 months). The number of metastatic sites is also predictive of patient outcome. In those patients with a single metastatic focus to the brain, lungs, gastrointestinal tract, skin, or subcutaneous tissue following a long disease free interval after treatment of local/regional disease, surgical excision may render the patient disease-free. Such patients have respectable 2-year survival rates. Unfortunately, patients who are not candidates for surgical intervention are left with few medical treatment options. These options include single-agent chemotherapy, combination chemotherapy, biotherapy, biochemotherapy, radiation therapy, and vaccines (Table 32-5). Since metastatic melanomas of skin/mucosal primary in general respond to systemic chemotherapy and immunotherapy better than metastatic melanomas of choriodal origin, their management is described separately.

METASTATIC SKIN/MUCOSAL MELANOMA

Single-Agent Chemotherapy

Dacarbazine (DTIC) remains the most active single agent in malignant melanoma and is the only cytotoxic drug approved by the FDA for the treatment of metastatic disease. DTIC has a response rate (RR) of about 20%; however, complete responses (CRs) are rare and the response duration is short (4 to 6 months) (105–107). Side effects include nausea and mild marrow suppression; rare cases of hepatic venoocclusive disease have also been reported (108).

Temozolomide (TMZ), a DTIC analog, has several properties that are advantageous compared to DTIC. TMZ has high oral bioavailability, does not require metabolic conversion to an active metabolite, and readily crosses the blood-brain barrier. This last is a feature that makes the use of TMZ especially appealing for the management of brain metastasis. Clinical studies to determine the efficacy of TMZ in this subgroup of patients are currently ongoing. A recent phase III European study comparing DTIC to TMZ reported similar RRs, time to progression (TTP), overall survival (OS), and disease-free survival (DFS) between the two treatment arms (109). However, quality of life was significantly improved in the TMZ arm. Patients with brain metastasis were excluded from the study.

Cisplatin has been shown to have modest activity in melanoma, with an RR of approximately 15% (110). Higher doses of cisplatin have resulted in RRs as high a 53%, but at the cost of increased toxicity even when used in combination with amifostine (85). Substitution of carboplatin for cisplatin, as a single agent or in combination with other cytotoxic drugs, is currently being studied.

Nitrosoureas, which include carmustine and CCNU, have RRs that range from 13 to 18% (110). Several

TABLE 32-5 | BIOCHEMOTHERAPY TRIALS AT MD ANDERSON CANCER CENTER DURING THE PAST DECADE

Author/Year	Regimen	No. of Patients	% Overall Response	% CR	TTP (months)	Median Survival (months)	Ref.
Legha et al, 1997	Alternating BiochemoRx	39	33	3	5.8	11	126
Legha et al, 1997	Sequential BiochemoRx	61	59	21	7.5	11.8	126
Legha et al, 1998	Concurrent BiochemoRx	53	62	20	5.0	11.8	127
Buzaid et al, 1998	Neoadjuvant BiochemoRx	64	50	6.5	N/A	N/A	128
Eton et al, 2002	Sequential BiochemoRx vs. CVD	190	25% vs. 48%	2 vs. 7%	2.4 vs. 4.9 months $p = 0.008$	9.2 vs. 11.9 months $p = 0.06$	129

CVD = cisplatin, vinblastine, dacarbazine; CR = complete remission; TTP = time to progression.

phase II studies have shown the nitrosourea fotemustine to have superior single-agent RRs ranging from 12 to 47% (112–115). In these trials the average RR was 20% (116). Furthermore, the median response duration was 18 to 26 weeks, significantly longer than that seen with other active single agents. Fotemustine also demonstrated significant efficacy in brain metastasis (average RR 21%) (116).

Other agents with single-agent efficacy in melanoma include the *vinca alkaloids* (vindesine and vinblastine), RR 16 to 17% (110,117), and the *taxanes* (paclitaxel and docetaxel), with RRs similar to those of the vinca alkaloids (118,119). Other taxane derivatives, including BMS-184476 and epothilone, are currently being investigated in phase II clinical studies (116). Piritrexim isethionate, new lipid-soluble dihydrofolate reductase inhibitor, produced an RR of 23% (120).

Interferons exhibit antiviral, immunomodulatory, and growth-inhibitory properties. A low but consistent RR has been observed in patients with metastatic malignant melanoma treated with IFN. In 439 patients treated with IFN, an overall RR of 15% was observed (121). No clear dose-response relationship was seen. Despite the low RR, durable responses have been observed in patients with low-volume and soft-tissue disease.

Interleukin-2 (IL-2) is a cytokine with immunostimulatory effects including activation of natural killer cells and T cells. In addition, it induces production of IFN–α and tumor necrosis factor. IL-2 has been investigated for activity against metastatic melanoma in several dosages and schedules. The high-dose bolus IL-2 regimen has been approved by the FDA. In this regimen, IL-2 is administered intravenously over 15 min once every 8 h under the supervision of medical and nursing personnel. Rosenberg et al. (122) reported an RR of 16%, with a 6% rate of complete remission among 270 consecutive patients with metastatic melanoma. About half the patients who had complete remission remained relapse-free at 5 years. Patients with metastatic melanoma confined to the skin or subcutaneous sites had a higher RR to IL-2 than patients with metastasis to visceral organs in addition to these sites (50 vs. 16%) (123).

Combination Chemotherapy

The principle of combining drugs that have single-agent efficacy to achieve additive or synergistic effects has been extensively studied in metastatic melanoma.

The *CVD regimen* (cisplatin, vinblastine, and DTIC) was initially evaluated at MDACC and found to be effective against metastatic malignant melanoma with a complete remission rate of 10% and an overall RR of 50% (124). Further evaluation of this regimen produced RRs ranging from 30 to 40%.

The *Dartmouth regimen*—consisting of cisplatin, DTIC, carmustine, and tamoxifen—reported a RR of 46% among 141 treated patients (125). Unfortunately, this high RR was not confirmed in subsequent phase II clinical trails. Phase III randomized multi-institutional trials comparing DTIC alone to either CVD or the Dartmouth regimen showed no significant advantage of the combination regimens over DTIC, either in RRs or patient survival. Despite this, the CVD and Dartmouth regimens have remained the "standard of care" in the management of metastatic melanoma over the past decade.

Interleukin-2–Based Biochemotherapy

Based on clinical observations about lack of cross-resistance between chemotherapy and biotherapy with IL-2 and the possibility of synergy between these treatments, different combinations of chemotherapy with IL-2 and IFN have been investigated. The most common chemotherapy regimens used in these biochemotherapy trials were the CVD and Dartmouth regimens. Several phase II clinical trials at MDACC showed significant improvement with biochemotherapy in overall RR over CVD (Table 32-5). In these trials, the CVD regimen was administered together with biotherapy, including IFN and IL-2. The CVD regimen consisted of cisplatin, 20 mg/m^2 IV for 4 days; vinblastine, 1.6 mg/m^2 IV for 4 to 5 days; and DTIC, 800 mg/m^2 IV for 1 day. The biotherapy (BIO) consisted of IL-2, 9 MU/m^2 IV by C. I. over 24 h for 4 days; and IFN, 5 MU/m^2 SQ for 5 days, starting on the first day of IL-2. Courses were repeated every 3 weeks. In the first study (alternating biochemotherapy), patients received either two courses of CVD followed by three courses of BIO or the reverse sequence (126) (Fig. 32-14). In the sequential biochemotherapy, patients were randomized to receive either CVD/BIO followed by 6 days of rest, then BIO/CVD/BIO; the other group received BIO/CVD/BIO followed by rest, then BIO/CVD every 6 weeks (126). In the third and fourth studies, the BIO and chemotherapy were administered concurrently (127–128). In this study, the doses of CVD and BIO were the same as in the previous trial except for vinblastine, which was administered for 4 days instead of 5. In addition, after the administration of 5 days of biochemotherapy, IFN was administered, using an alternate-day schedule when possible. In the fifth (phase III) study, patients were randomly assigned to *either* the sequential CVD/BIO regimen as described above or to CVD alone (129).

The eligibility criteria for the patients in these studies were similar. Table 32-5 shows the outcome of these therapies. Compared with CVD, the sequential biochemotherapy and concurrent biochemotherapy showed better RRs and survival. Phase II clinical trials with concurrent biochemotherapy similar to one described above or using the Dartmouth regimen together with IL-2 and IFN were conducted over the past decade. The outcome of these studies was markedly inconsistent. RRs ranging from 20 to 65% were observed.

The superiority of IL-2 based biochemotherapy over combination therapy has not been established. To date only three prospectively randomized phase III studies comparing biochemotherapy with combination chemotherapy have been completed. The outcome of the MDACC trial is summarized in Table 32-5 (129). It showed superiority of sequential biochemotherapy over CVD regimen in RR, and survival. Rosenberg et al. reported on the result of a randomized trial comparing chemotherapy including cisplatin, DTIC, and tamoxifen with or without high-dose IL-2 and IFN (130). While the biochemotherapy arm gave a superior RR (44 vs. 27%; $p = 0.07$), the survival of the chemotherapy group was superior, with a median survival time of 15.8 vs. 10.7 months, respectively (130). ECOG conducted a phase III clinical trial to test the superiority of concurrent biochemotherapy including CVD plus IL-2/IFN-α2b over CVD alone in patients with no prior chemotherapy for stage IV melanoma. The trial was designed to detect a 33% improvement in survival. Interim analysis performed after 397 patients were registered showed no significant superiority of biochemotherapy over chemotherapy. The results as presented during the 2003 meeting of the American Society of Clinical Oncology showed no significant advantage for biochemotherapy in RR (17 vs. 11% progression-free survival (5.3 vs. 3.6 months) or OS (8.4 vs. 8.7 months) over chemotherapy alone (131). Compared to patients treated in the MDACC phase III trial, a larger proportion of patients in the ECOG trial were previously treated with adjuvant high-dose IFN.

METASTATIC CHOROIDAL MELANOMA

Only a handful of clinical trials have assessed the impact of systemic therapy on metastatic uveal melanoma. Besides, most of these reports lack the large number of patients needed to give meaningful information. Therefore a clear-cut conclusion about the efficacy of treatment regimens is difficult to draw from these pilot studies. Overall, metastatic choroidal melanoma is considered to be chemoresistant, and the outcome of therapy is dependent on the extent of spread of disease.

Disease Confined to the Liver

In selected cases of solitary metastasis, surgical excision was reported to yield long-lasting control of local disease. In view of the fact that in most patients with metastatic choroidal melanoma is multifocal even if the metastatic disease is confined to one organ, only a few patients are candidates for resection of metastatic disease. In patients with metastatic melanoma confined to the liver, several regional therapies have given responses in 40 to 60% of patients, with a median survival of about 11 to 14 months (57,132). These therapies include hepatic-arterial chemotherapy with fotemustine, hyperthermic hepatic isolation perfusion with melphalan and tumor necrosis factor, and chemoembolization of liver metastasis with cisplatin and starch particles. Radiofrequency thermal ablation for melanoma metastatic to the liver has been shown to be beneficial if the liver metastasis is limited to a segment of the liver and the treated lesion is between 1 and 6 cm in largest diameter.

Multiorgan Metastasis

Anticancer drugs such as DTIC, TMZ, cisplatin, paclitaxel, and biologicals such as IFN and IL-2 alone or together with combination chemotherapy have been shown to be ineffective. Regional biotherapy with IFN and IL-2 with or without LAK cells failed to induce partial responses in patients with choroidal melanoma confined to the liver. CVD, Dartmouth, or IL-2–based biochemotherapy has yielded responses in less than 10% of the patients. The most commonly used multidrug regimen, BOLD-IFN [bleomycin + oncovin + (lomustine CCNU) + DTIC + IFN], is of marginal efficacy, with an RR of about 20% (57). Participation of patients in phase II clinical trials with new anticancer agents should be encouraged in view of the poor outcomes of available therapies in patients with choroidal melanoma metastasized to multiple organs.

References

1. Jemal A, Murray T, Ward E, et al. Cancer statistics, 2005. *CA Cancer J Clin* 2005;55:10–30.
2. Brochez L, Naeyaert JM. Understanding the trends in melanoma incidence and mortality: Where do we stand? *Eur J Dermatol* 2000;10:71–75; quiz 76.
3. Jones WO, Harman CR, Ng AK, et al. Incidence of malignant melanoma in Auckland, New Zealand: Highest rates in the world. *World J Surg* 1999;23:732–735.
4. Dennis LK, White E, Lee JA. Recent cohort trends in malignant melanoma by anatomic site in the United States. *Cancer Causes Control* 1993;4:93–100.
5. Swerdlow AJ, English JS, Qiao Z. The risk of melanoma in patients with congenital nevi: A cohort study. *J Am Acad Dermatol* 1995;32:595–599.

6. Weiss J, Bertz J, Jung EG. Malignant melanoma in southern Germany: Different predictive value of risk factors for melanoma subtypes. *Dermatologica* 1991;183:109–113.

7. Greene MH, Clark WH Jr, Tucker MA, et al. High risk of malignant melanoma in melanoma-prone families with dysplastic nevi. *Ann Intern Med* 1985;102:458–465.

8. Tucker MA, Halpern A, Holly EA, et al. Clinically recognized dysplastic nevi. A central risk factor for cutaneous melanoma. *JAMA* 1997;277:1439–1444.

9. Sahin S, Levin L, Kopf AW, et al. Risk of melanoma in medium-sized congenital melanocytic nevi: A follow-up study. *J Am Acad Dermatol* 1998;39:428–433.

10. Valyi-Nagy IT, Hirka G, Jensen PJ, et al. Undifferentiated keratinocytes control growth, morphology, and antigen expression of normal melanocytes through cell-cell contact. *Lab Invest* 1993;69:152–159.

11. Shih IM, Elder DE, Hsu MY, et al. Regulation of Mel-CAM/MUC18 expression on melanocytes of different stages of tumor progression by normal keratinocytes. *Am J Pathol* 1994;145:837–845.

12. Koukoulis GK, Patriarca C, Gould VE. Adhesion molecules and tumor metastasis. *Hum Pathol* 1998;29:889–892.

13. Bani MR, Rak J, Adachi D, et al. Multiple features of advanced melanoma recapitulated in tumorigenic variants of early stage (radial growth phase) human melanoma cell lines: Evidence for a dominant phenotype. *Cancer Res* 1996;56:3075–3086.

14. Luca M, Hunt B, Bucana CD, et al. Direct correlation between MUC18 expression and metastatic potential of human melanoma cells. *Melanoma Res* 1993;3:35–41.

15. Shih LM, Hsu MY, Palazzo JP, et al. The cell-cell adhesion receptor Mel-CAM acts as a tumor suppressor in breast carcinoma. *Am J Pathol* 1997;151:745–751.

16. Shih IM, Elder DE, Speicher D, et al. Isolation and functional characterization of the A32 melanoma-associated antigen. *Cancer Res* 1994;54:2514–2520.

17. Johnson JP, Bar-Eli M, Jansen B, et al. Melanoma progression-associated glycoprotein MUC18/MCAM mediates homotypic cell adhesion through interaction with a heterophilic ligand. *Int J Cancer* 1997;73:769–774.

18. Mills L, Tellez C, Huang S, et al. Fully human antibodies to MCAM/MUC18 inhibit tumor growth and metastasis of human melanoma. *Cancer Res* 2002;62:5106–5114.

19. Hsu MY, Wheelock MJ, Johnson KR, et al. Shifts in cadherin profiles between human normal melanocytes and melanomas. *J Invest Dermatol Symp Proc* 1996;1:188–194.

20. Sanders DS, Blessing K, Hassan GA, et al. Alterations in cadherin and catenin expression during the biological progression of melanocytic tumors. *Mol Pathol* 1999;52:151–157.

21. Scott GA, Cassidy L. Rac1 mediates dendrite formation in response to melanocyte stimulating hormone and ultraviolet light in a murine melanoma model. *J Invest Dermatol* 1998;111:243–250.

22. Tang A, Eller MS, Hara M, et al. E-cadherin is the major mediator of human melanocyte adhesion to keratinocytes in vitro. *J Cell Sci* 1994;107(Pt 4):983–992.

23. Hsu M, Andl T, Li G, et al. Cadherin repertoire determines partner-specific gap junctional communication during melanoma progression. *J Cell Sci* 2000;113(Pt 9):1535–1542.

24. Li G, Schaider H, Satyamoorthy K, et al. Downregulation of E-cadherin and Desmoglein 1 by autocrine hepatocyte growth factor during melanoma development. *Oncogene* 2001;20:8125–8135.

25. Li G, Satyamoorthy K, Herlyn M. N-cadherin-mediated intercellular interactions promote survival and migration of melanoma cells. *Cancer Res* 2001;61:3819–3825.

26. Sandig M, Voura EB, Kalnins VI, et al. Role of cadherins in the transendothelial migration of melanoma cells in culture. *Cell Motil Cytoskel* 1997;38:351–364.

27. Voura EB, Sandig M, Siu CH. Cell-cell interactions during transendothelial migration of tumor cells. *Microsc Res Tech* 1998;43:265–275.

28. Gruss C, Herlyn M. Role of cadherins and matrixins in melanoma. *Curr Opin Oncol* 2001;13:117–123.

29. McGary EC, Lev DC, Bar-Eli M. Cellular adhesion pathways and metastatic potential of human melanoma. *Cancer Biol Ther* 2002;1:459–465.

30. Becker D, Lee PL, Rodeck U, et al. Inhibition of the fibroblast growth factor receptor 1 (FGFR-1) gene in human melanocytes and malignant melanomas leads to inhibition of proliferation and signs indicative of differentiation. *Oncogene* 1992;7:2303–2313.

31. Wang Y, Becker D. Antisense targeting of basic fibroblast growth factor and fibroblast growth factor receptor-1 in human melanomas blocks intratumoral angiogenesis and tumor growth. *Nat Med* 1997;3:887–893.

32. Natali PG, Nicotra MR, Winkler AB, et al. Progression of human cutaneous melanoma is associated with loss of expression of c-kit proto-oncogene receptor. *Int J Cancer* 1992;52:197–201.

33. Lassam N, Bickford S. Loss of c-kit expression in cultured melanoma cells. *Oncogene* 1992;7:51–56.

34. Zakut R, Perlis R, Eliyahu S, et al. KIT ligand (mast cell growth factor) inhibits the growth of KIT-expressing melanoma cells. *Oncogene* 1993;8:2221–2229.

35. Giebel LB, Spritz RA. Mutation of the KIT (mast/stem cell growth factor receptor) proto-oncogene in human piebaldism. *Proc Natl Acad Sci USA* 1991;88:8696–8699.

36. Carroll M, Ohno-Jones S, Tamura S, et al. CGP 57148, a tyrosine kinase inhibitor, inhibits the growth of cells expressing BCR-ABL, TEL-ABL, and TEL-PDGFR fusion proteins. *Blood* 1997;90:4947–4952.

37. Herlyn M, Satyamoorthy K. Activated ras. Yet another player in melanoma? *Am J Pathol* 1996;149:739–744.

38. Sherr CJ, Weber JD. The ARF/p53 pathway. *Curr Opin Genet Dev* 2000;10:94–99.

39. Satyamoorthy K, Herlyn M. Cellular and molecular biology of human melanoma. *Cancer Biol Ther* 2002;1:14–17.

40. Huang S, Jean D, Luca M, et al. Loss of AP-2 results in downregulation of c-KIT and enhancement of melanoma tumorigenicity and metastasis. *Embo J* 1998;17:4358–4369.

41. Jean D, Gershenwald JE, Huang S, et al. Loss of AP-2 results in up-regulation of MCAM/MUC18 and an increase in tumor growth and metastasis of human melanoma cells. *J Biol Chem* 1998;273:16501–16508.

42. Bar-Eli M. Gene regulation in melanoma progression by the AP-2 transcription factor. *Pigment Cell Res* 2001;14:78–85.

43. Jean D, Harbison M, McConkey DJ, et al. CREB and its associated proteins act as survival factors for human melanoma cells. *J Biol Chem* 1998;273:24884–24890.

44. Jean D, Bar-Eli M. Regulation of tumor growth and metastasis of human melanoma by the CREB transcription factor family. *Mol Cell Biochem* 2000;212:19–28.

45. Jean D, Tellez C, Huang S, et al. Inhibition of tumor growth and metastasis of human melanoma by intracellular anti-ATF-1 single chain Fv fragment. *Oncogene* 2000;19:2721–2730.

46. Jean D, Bar-Eli M. Targeting the ATF-1/CREB transcription factors by single chain Fv fragment in human melanoma: Potential modality for cancer therapy. *Crit Rev Immunol* 2001;21:275–286.

47. Xie S, Price JE, Luca M, et al. Dominant-negative CREB inhibits tumor growth and metastasis of human melanoma cells. *Oncogene* 1997;15:2069–2075.

48. Leiter U, Schmid RM, Kaskel P, et al. Anti-apoptotic bcl-2 and bcl-xL in advanced malignant melanoma. *Arch Dermatol Res* 2000;292:225–232.

49. Olie RA, Hafner C, Kuttel R, et al. Bcl-2 and bcl-xL antisense oligonucleotides induce apoptosis in melanoma cells of different clinical stages. *J Invest Dermatol* 2002;118:505–512.

50. Banerjee D. Genasense (Genta Inc). *Curr Opin Invest Drugs* 2001;2:574–580.

51. Langley RG, Sober AJ. Clinical recognition of melanoma and its precursors. *Hematol Oncol Clin North Am* 1998;12:699–715, v.

52. Weinstock MA, Sober AJ. The risk of progression of lentigo maligna to lentigo maligna melanoma. *Br J Dermatol* 1987;116:303–310.

53. Reintgen DS, McCarty KM Jr, Cox E, et al. Malignant melanoma in black American and white American populations. A comparative review. *JAMA* 1982;248:1856–1859.

54. Jain S, Allen PW. Desmoplastic malignant melanoma and its variants. A study of 45 cases. *Am J Surg Pathol* 1989;13:358–373.

55. Cooper PH, Mills SE, Allen MS Jr. Malignant melanoma of the anus: Report of 12 patients and analysis of 255 additional cases. *Dis Colon Rectum* 1982;25:693–703.

56. Hungerford J. Uveal melanoma. *Eur J Cancer* 1993;29A:1365–1368.

57. Bedikian AY, McIntyre S, Hodges C, et al. *Treatment of Metastatic Uveal and Conjunctival Melanoma. In press.*

58. Langley RG, Sober AJ. Clinical recognition of melanoma and its precursors. *Hematol Oncol Clin North Am* 1998;12:699–715, v.

59. Ross MI, Balch CM. Surgical treatment of primary melanoma. In Balch CM, Houghton AN, Sober AJ, Soong SJ (eds). *Cutaneous Melanoma*, 3d ed. St Louis: Quality Medical Publishing; 1998:141–153.

60. Zitelli JA, Brown C, Hanusa BH. Mohs micrographic surgery for the treatment of primary cutaneous melanoma. *J Am Acad Dermatol* 1997;37:236–245.

61. Zitelli JA, Brown CD, Hanusa BH. Surgical margins for excision of primary cutaneous melanoma. *J Am Acad Dermatol* 1997;37:422–429.

62. Coit DG, Rogatko A, Brennan MF. Prognostic factors in patients with melanoma metastatic to axillary or inguinal lymph nodes. A multivariate analysis. *Ann Surg* 1991;214:627–636.

63. Morton DL, Wanek L, Nizze JA, et al. Improved long-term survival after lymphadenectomy of melanoma metastatic to

64. Buzaid AC, Tinoco LA, Jendiroba D, et al. Prognostic value of size of lymph node metastases in patients with cutaneous melanoma. *J Clin Oncol* 1995;13:2361–2368.

regional nodes. Analysis of prognostic factors in 1134 patients from the John Wayne Cancer Clinic. *Ann Surg* 1991;214:491–499; discussion 499–501.

65. Drepper H, Kohler CO, Bastian B, et al. Benefit of elective lymph node dissection in subgroups of melanoma patients. Results of a multi-center study of 3616 patients. *Cancer* 1993;72:741–749.

66. Coates AS, Ingvar CI, Petersen-Schaefer K, et al. Elective lymph node dissection in patients with primary melanoma of the trunk and limbs treated at the Sydney Melanoma Unit from 1960 to 1991. *J Am Coll Surg* 1995;180:402–409.

67. Slingluff CL Jr, Stidham KR, Ricci WM, et al. Surgical management of regional lymph nodes in patients with melanoma. Experience with 4682 patients. *Ann Surg* 1994;219:120–130.

68. Veronesi U, Adamus J, Bandiera DC, et al. Delayed regional lymph node dissection in stage I melanoma of the skin of the lower extremities. *Cancer* 1982;49:2420–2430.

69. Morton DL, Wen DR, Wong JH, et al. Technical details of intraoperative lymphatic mapping for early stage melanoma. *Arch Surg* 1992;127:392–399.

70. Krag DN, Weaver DL, Alex JC, et al. Surgical resection and radiolocalization of the sentinel lymph node in breast cancer using a gamma probe. *Surg Oncol* 1993;2:335–339; discussion 340.

71. Albertini JJ, Cruse CW, Rapaport D, et al. Intraoperative radio-lympho-scintigraphy improves sentinel lymph node identification for patients with melanoma. *Ann Surg* 1996;223:217–224.

72. Kelley MC, Ollila DW, Morton DL. Lymphatic mapping and sentinel lymphadenectomy for melanoma. *Semin Surg Oncol* 1998;14:283–290.

73. Wang X, Heller R, VanVoorhis N, et al. Detection of submicroscopic lymph node metastases with polymerase chain reaction in patients with malignant melanoma. *Ann Surg* 1994;220:768–774.

74. Balch CM, Buzaid AC, Soong SJ, et al. Final version of the American Joint Committee on Cancer staging system for cutaneous melanoma. *J Clin Oncol* 2001;19:3635–3648.

75. Balch CM, Soong SJ, Gershenwald JE, et al. Prognostic factors analysis of 17,600 melanoma patients: Validation of the American Joint Committee on Cancer melanoma staging system. *J Clin Oncol* 2001;19:3622–3634.

76. Bedikian AY, Legha SS. Adjuvant chemotherapy for malignant melanoma. In: Kirkwood JM (ed). *Molecular Diagnosis and Treatment of Melanoma.* New York: Marcel Dekker; 1998:195–216.

77. Hill, II, GJ, Moss SE, Golomb FM, et al. DTIC and combination therapy for melanoma: III DTIC Surgical Adjuvant Study COG Protocol 7040. *Cancer* 1981;47:2556–2562.

78. Tranum BL, Dixon D, Quagliana J, et al. Lack of benefit of adjunctive chemotherapy in stage I malignant melanoma: A Southwest Oncology Group Study. *Cancer Treat Rep* 1998;71:643–644.

79. Morton DL, Eilber FR, Malmgren RA, et al. Immunologic factors which influence response to immunotherapy in malignant melanoma. *Surgery* 1970;68:158–164.

80. Cunningham TJ, Schoenfeld D, Nathanson L, et al. A controlled ECOG study of adjuvant therapy with BCG or BCG

plus DTIC in patients with stage I and II malignant melanoma. In: Terry WD, Rosenberg SA (eds). *Immunotherapy of Human Cancer.* New York: Excerpta Medica; 1982:271–277.

81. Terry WD, Hodges RJ, Rosenberg SA, et al. Treatment of stage I and II malignant melanoma with adjuvant immunotherapy or chemotherapy: Preliminary analysis of a prospective randomized trial. In: Terry W, Rosenberg SA (eds). *Immunotherapy of Human Cancer.* New York: Excerpta Medica; 1982:251–257.

82. Cunningham TJ, Schoenfeld DL, Nathanson L, et al. A controlled ECOG study of adjuvant therapy in patients with stage I & II malignant melanoma. In: Jones SE, Salmon SE (eds). *Adjuvant Therapy of Cancer IV.* New York: Grune & Stratton; 1984:507–277.

83. Veronesi U, Adamus J, Aubert C, et al. A randomized trial of adjuvant chemotherapy and immunotherapy in cutaneous melanoma. *N Engl J Med* 1982;307:913–916.

84. Misset JL, Mathe G, Cupissol D, et al. Eight year update of the Oncofrance Melanoma Adjuvant Trial. In: Jones SE, Salmon SE (eds). *Adjuvant Therapy of Cancer IV.* New York: Grune & Stratton; 1984:557–566.

85. Czarnetzki BM, Macher E, Behrendt H, et al. Current status of melanoma chemotherapy and immunotherapy. *Recent Results Cancer Res* 1982;80:264–268.

86. Spitler LE. A randomized trial of levamisole versus placebo as adjuvant therapy in malignant melanoma. *J Clin Oncol* 1991;9:736–740.

87. Quirt IC, Shelley WE, Pater JL, et al. Improved survival in patients with poor-prognosis malignant melanoma treated with adjuvant levamisole: A phase III study by the National Cancer Institute of Canada Clinical Trial Group. *J Clin Oncol* 1991;9:729–735.

88. Wallack MK, Sivanandham M, Balch CM, et al. A phase III randomized, double-blind multi-institutional trial of vaccinia melanoma oncolysate-active specific immunotherapy for patients with stage II melanoma. *Cancer* 1995;75:34–42.

89. Hersey P, Coates AS, McCarthy WH, et al. Adjuvant immunotherapy of patients with high-risk melanoma using vaccinia viral lysate of melanoma: Results of a randomized trial. *J Clin Oncol* 2002;20:4181–4190.

90. Sondak VK, Liu PY, Tuthill RJ, et al. Adjuvant immunotherapy of resected, intermediate-thickness, node-negative melanoma with an allogeneic tumor vaccine: Overall results of a randomized trial of the Southwest Oncology Group. *J Clin Oncol* 2002;20:2058–2066.

91. Livingston PO, Natoli EJ, Calves MJ, et al. Vaccines containing purified GM2 ganglioside elicit GM2 antibodies in melanoma patients. *Proc Natl Acad Sci USA* 1987;84:2911–2915.

92. Livingston PO, Wong GY, Adluri S, et al. Improved survival in stage III melanoma patients with GM2 antibodies: A randomized trial of adjuvant vaccination with GM2 ganglioside. *J Clin Oncol* 1994;12:1036–1044.

93. Meyskens FL Jr, Kopecky J, Taylor CW, et al. Randomized trial of adjuvant human interferon gamma versus observation in high-risk cutaneous melanoma: A Southwest Oncology Group Study. *J Natl Cancer Inst* 1995;87:1710–1713.

94. Creagan ET, Dalton RJ, Ahmann DL, et al. Randomized, surgical adjuvant clinical trial of recombinant interferon alpha-2a in selected patients with malignant melanoma. *J Clin Oncol* 1995;13:2776–2783.

95. Kirkwood JM, Strawderman MH, Ernstoff MS, et al. Interferon alpha-2b adjuvant therapy of high-risk resected cutaneous melanoma: The Eastern Cooperative Oncology Group Trial EST 1684. *J Clin Oncol* 1996;14:7–17.

96. Grob JJ, Dreno B, de la Salmoniere P, et al. for the French Cooperative Group on Melanoma. Randomized trial of interferon alpha-2a as adjuvant therapy in resected primary melanoma thicker than 1.5 mm without clinically detectable node metastases. French Cooperative Group on Melanoma. *Lancet* 1998;351:1905–1910.

97. Pehamberger H, Soyer HP, Steiner A, et al. Adjuvant interferon alpha-2a treatment in resected primary stage II cutaneous melanoma: Austrian Malignant Melanoma Cooperative Group. *J Clin Oncol* 1998;16:1425–1429.

98. Kirkwood JM, Ibrahim JG, Sondak VK, et al. High- and low-dose interferon alpha-2b in high-risk melanoma: First analysis of inter-group trial E1690/S9111/C9190. *J Clin Oncol* 2000;18:2444–2458.

99. Kirkwood JM, Ibrahim JG, Sosman JA, et al. High-dose interferon alpha-2b significantly prolongs relapse-free and overall survival compared with the GM2-KLH/QS-21 vaccine in patients with resected stage IIB-III melanoma: Results of intergroup trial E1694/S9512/C509801. *J Clin Oncol* 2001;19:2370–2380.

100. Kleeberg UR, Broker EB, Lejeune F, et al. Adjuvant trial in melanoma patients comparing rIFN-alpha to Iscador to a control group after curative resection of high risk primary (>3 mm) or regional lymph node metastasis (EORTC 18871). *Eur J Cancer* 1999;35(suppl 4):S82.

101. Hancock BW, Wheatley K, Harrison G. Aim high-adjuvant interferon in melanoma (high risk), a United Kingdom Coordinating Committee on Cancer Research (UKCCCR) randomized study of observation vs. adjuvant low-dose extended duration interferon alpha-2a in high-risk resected malignant melanoma. *Proc Am Soc Clin Oncol* 2001;20:349a.

102. Cascinelli N, Bufalino R, Morabito A, et al. Results of adjuvant interferon study in WHO melanoma programme. *Lancet* 1994;343:913–914.

103. Kirkwood JM, Manola J, Ibrahim J, et al. Pooled-analysis of four ECOG/Intergroup trials of high-dose interferon alpha-2b (HDI) in 1916 patients with high risk resected cutaneous melanoma. *Proc Am Soc Clin Oncol* 2001;20:350a.

104. Hauschild A, Weichenthal M, Balda B, et al. Prospective randomized trial of interferon alpha-2b and interleukin-2 adds adjuvant for treatment of resected intermediate- and high-risk primary melanoma without clinically detectable node metastasis. *J Clin Oncol* 2003;21:2883–2888.

105. Carbone PP, Costello W. Eastern Cooperative Oncology Group studies with DTIC (NSC-45388). *Cancer Treat Rep* 1976;60:193–198.

106. Costanza ME, Nathanson L, Schoenfeld D, et al. Results with methyl-CCNU and DTIC in metastatic melanoma. *Cancer* 1977;40:1010–1015.

107. Hill GJ II, Krementz ET, Hill HZ. Dimethyl triazeno imidazole carboxamide and combination therapy for melanoma. IV. Late results after complete response to chemotherapy (Central Oncology Group protocols 7130, 7131, and 7131A). *Cancer* 1984;53:1299–1305.

108. McClay E, Lusch CJ, Mastrangelo MJ. Allergy-induced hepatic toxicity associated with dacarbazine. *Cancer Treat Rep* 1987;71:219–220.

109. Middleton MR, Grob JJ, Aaronson N, et al. Randomized phase III study of temozolomide versus dacarbazine in the treatment of patients with advanced metastatic malignant melanoma. *J Clin Oncol* 2000;18:158–166.

110. Atkins MB. The treatment of metastatic melanoma with chemotherapy and biologics. *Curr Opin Oncol* 1997;9:205–213.

111. Glover D, Glick JH, Weiler C, et al. WR-2721 and high-dose cisplatin: An active combination in the treatment of metastatic melanoma. *J Clin Oncol* 1987;5:574–578.

112. Calabresi F, Aapro M, Becquart D, et al. Multicenter phase II trial of the single agent fotemustine in patients with advanced malignant melanoma. *Ann Oncol* 1991;2:377–378.

113. Jacquillat C, Khayat D, Banzet P, et al. Final report of the French multicenter phase II study of the nitrosourea fotemustine in 153 evaluable patients with disseminated malignant melanoma including patients with cerebral metastases. *Cancer* 1990;66:1873–1878.

114. Kleeberg UR, Engel E, Israels P, et al. Palliative therapy of melanoma patients with fotemustine. Inverse relationship between tumour load and treatment effectiveness. A multicentre phase II trial of the EORTC-Melanoma Cooperative Group (MCG). *Melanoma Res* 1995;5:195–200.

115. Schallreuter KU, Wenzel E, Brassow FW, et al. Positive phase II study in the treatment of advanced malignant melanoma with fotemustine. *Cancer Chemother Pharmacol* 1991; 29:85–87.

116. Bajetta E, Del Vecchio M, Bernard-Marty C, et al. Metastatic melanoma: Chemotherapy. *Semin Oncol* 2002;29:427–445.

117. Quagliana JM, Stephens RL, Baker LH, et al. Vindesine in patients with metastatic malignant melanoma: A Southwest Oncology Group study. *J Clin Oncol* 1984;2:316–319.

118. Bedikian AY, Weiss GR, Legha SS, et al. Phase II trial of docetaxel in patients with advanced cutaneous malignant melanoma previously untreated with chemotherapy. *J Clin Oncol* 1995;13:2895–2899.

119. Einzig AI, Hochster H, Wiernik PH, et al. A phase II study of taxol in patients with malignant melanoma. *Invest New Drugs* 1991;9:59–64.

120. Feun LG, Gonzalez R, Savaraj N, et al. Phase II trial of piritrexim in metastatic melanoma using intermittent, low-dose administration. *J Clin Oncol* 1991;9:464–467.

121. Legha SL. Current therapy for malignant melanoma. *Semin Oncol* 1989; (suppl 1):12–19.

122. Rosenberg SA, Yang JC, Topalian SL, et al. Treatment of 283 consecutive patients with metastatic melanoma or renal cell cancer using high-dose interleukin-2. *JAMA* 1994;271: 907–913.

123. Chang E, Rosenberg SA. Patients with melanoma metastases at cutaneous and subcutaneous sites are highly susceptible to interleukin-2-based therapy. *J Immunotherapy* 2001;24:88–90.

124. Legha SS, Ring S, Papadopoulos N, et al. A prospective evaluation of triple-drug regimen containing cisplatin, vinblastine, and dacarbazine (CVD) for metastatic melanoma. *Cancer* 1989;64:2024–2029.

125. McClay EF, Mastrangelo MJ, Berd D, et al. Effective combination chemo/hormonal therapy for malignant melanoma: Experience with three clinical trials. *Int J Cancer* 1992;50: 553–556.

126. Legha SS, Ring S, Eton O, et al. Development and results of biochemotherapy in metastatic melanoma. The University of Texas MD Anderson Cancer Center experience. *Cancer J Sci Am* 1997;3:S9–S15.

127. Legha SS, Ring S, Eton O, et al. Development of a biochemotherapy regimen with concurrent administration of cisplatin, vinblastine, DTIC, IFN-a and IL-2 for patients with metastatic melanoma. *J Clin Oncol* 1998;16:1752–1759.

128. Buzaid AC, Colome M, Bedikian A, et al. Phase II study of neoadjuvant concurrent biochemotherapy in melanoma patients with local regional metastases. *Melanoma Res* 1998;8: 549–556.

129. Eton O, Legha SS, Bedikian AY, et al. Sequential biochemotherapy versus chemotherapy for metastatic melanoma: Results from a phase III randomized trial. *J Clin Oncol* 2002; 20(8):2045–2052.

130. Rosenberg SA, Yang JC, Schwartzentruber DJ, et al. Prospective randomized trial of the treatment of patients with metastatic melanoma using chemotherapy with cisplatin, dacarbazine and tamoxifen alone or in combination with interleukin-2 and interferon alpha-2b. *J Clin Oncol* 1999;17: 968–975.

131. Atkins MB, Lee S, Flaherty LA, et al. A prospective randomized phase III trial of concurrent biochemotherapy (BCT) with cisplatin, vinblastine, dacarbazine (CVD), IL-2 and interferon alpha-2b (IFN) versus CVD alone in patients with metastatic melanoma (E3695): An ECOG-coordinated Intergroup trial. *Proc ASCO* 2003;22:708 (abstr 2847).

132. Alexander HR Jr, Libutti SK, Pingpank JF, et al. Hyperthermic isolated hepatic perfusion using melphalan for patients with ocular melanoma metastatic to liver. *Cancer Clin Res* 2003;9:6343–6349.

SOFT TISSUE AND BONE SARCOMAS

L. Johnetta Blakely
Jonathan C. Trent
Shreyaskumar Patel

Sarcomas are an extremely rare and heterogeneous group of tumors that arise from mesenchymal tissues. According to the estimates of the American Cancer Society, approximately 1.3 million people were diagnosed with cancer in the year 2004, with only 11,120 cases representing sarcomas (1). There are estimated to be 8680 new soft tissue sarcomas and 2440 bone sarcomas diagnosed in 2004, with 3660 and 1300 deaths, respectively, resulting from these tumors (1).

■ EPIDEMIOLOGY AND PATHOGENESIS

The etiology and pathogenesis of sarcomas, like those of most cancers, are not well understood. Multiple environmental factors have been associated with the development of soft tissue and bone sarcomas. Many studies have shown that patients who have received radiation therapy for prior cancers have an increased risk of developing soft tissue sarcomas near or within the field of radiation (2–7). In one series, patients developed sarcoma between 3 to 23 years after radiation therapy (5). The average time to development is between 10 to 13 years (2,4–6). Postirradiation sarcomas have been reported to occur most commonly in patients who received radiation for breast cancer, Hodgkin's and non-Hodgkin's lymphoma, and cervical cancer. These have also been reported in patients who received radiation for other benign and malignant conditions (2,3). Postirradiation sarcomas comprise a variety of histologic types, including malignant fibrous histiocytoma, osteosarcoma, fibrosarcoma, malignant peripheral nerve sheath tumor, and angiosarcoma (3,5,6). Most postirradiation sarcomas are associated with high-grade lesions, which are less responsive to chemotherapy than their de novo counterparts and are associated with a poorer prognosis (2–7).

Exposure to various chemicals and environmental toxins—such as asbestos, phenyl herbicides, chlorophenols (wood preservatives), dioxins (agent orange), and hexachlorobenzene (pesticide)—has been related to the development of sarcoma (8–15). Arsenic, vinyl chloride, and thorotrast have also been associated with the occurrence of sarcomas (15–18). Tamoxifen, which is used to treat and to prevent breast cancer, has been implicated in the etiology uterine sarcomas (19).

Trauma and foreign bodies have also been associated with sarcoma development. There are reports of sarcomas developing after recent trauma (20,21), although a causal relationship is unclear; it is likely that it is the trauma that is responsible for bringing the tumor to medical attention. Chronic inflammation has been associated with sarcoma development and may be a risk factor (15). Lymphangiosarcoma is associated with a type of chronic lymphoedema known as Stewart-Treves syndrome (22). Sarcoma has also been associated with viral infections; the best known are herpesvirus 8 (HHV-8), HIV-1, and AIDS, which is related to the development of Kaposi's sarcoma (15,16). Other viral infections have been suggested, but no epidemiologic data have been found to establish a true causal relationship (15).

Molecular and genetic alterations have been shown to be responsible for the development of sarcoma. While their occurrence is mostly sporadic in nature, some mutations are known to be inherited. One of the most notable of these is the Li-Fraumeni syndrome (23). First described in 1969 in four families with an autosomal dominant pattern of soft tissue sarcoma, breast cancer, and other cancers in children and young adults, subsequent studies found that the syndrome includes osteosarcoma, brain tumors, acute leukemia, adrenocortical carcinoma, and germ cell tumors (15,23). Li-Fraumeni syndrome is associated with a germline mutation of the *p53* tumor suppressor gene, which is located on chromosome 17p13 (24). Inherited retinoblastoma is also associated with the development of sarcomas, both osteosarcoma and soft tissue sarcoma (15). In retinoblastoma there is a germline mutation in the *rb-1* tumor suppressor gene, which is associated with the development of sarcoma (15,18). Neurofibromatosis-1 (von Recklinghausen disease) is a single-gene disorder inherited in an autosomal dominant pattern (25). The *nf-1* gene is located on chromosome 17 and codes for a protein called neurofibromin, which is involved in the regulation of Ras oncoproteins (18,25,26). Neurofibromatosis-1 is associated with an increased

risk of development of sarcoma, specifically, malignant nerve sheath tumors (18,25–27). Sarcomas have been associated with other cancer family syndromes including basal cell nevus syndrome, Werner's syndrome, familial adenomatous polyposis, and Gardner's syndrome (15,28).

Many sarcomas are known to have characteristic cytogenetic abnormalities (Table 33-1).

Because many of these are relatively tumor-specific, it has been postulated that molecular therapies could be developed for each of them (26,29). Imatininb (Gleevec) in the treatment of gastrointestinal stromal tumors is one example of a successful targeted therapy. Many of these specific abnormalities can also be useful in the diagnosis of certain histologies (26,30). Molecular testing of tumors is becoming more useful in the diagnosis and treatment of soft tissue sarcomas. For example the t(x; 18) translocation is a specific marker for synovial sarcomas. The transcript formed from this translocation (SYT-SSX) can be detected using polymerase chain reaction (PCR) testing. Coindre et al. evaluated over 200 cases of synovial sarcoma and classified these into three groups: (1) those in which the diagnosis of synovial sarcoma was certain; (2) those in which the diagnosis of synovial sarcoma was probable; and (3) those in which the diagnosis of synovial sarcoma was possible but where it was not the first on the list. After evaluation all the specimens underwent PCR examination for the SYT-SSX transcript. Tumors in the first category

TABLE 33-1 | CYTOGENETIC TRANSLOCATION AND OTHER ABNORMALITIES IN SARCOMA

Tumor	Cytogenetic Abnormality	Gene Product
Alveolar rhabdomyosarcoma	t(2;13)(q35;q14)	PAX3-FOXO1A
Alveolar soft tissue sarcoma	t(X;17)(p11.2;q25)	ASPL-TFE3
Clear cell sarcoma	t(12;22)(q13;q12)	EWSR1-ATF1
Congenital fibrosarcoma	t(12;15)(p13;q25)	ETV6-NTRK3
Dermatofibrosarcoma protuberans	t(17;22)(q22;q13)	COL1A1-PDGFB
Desmoplastic small round cell tumor	t(11;22)(p13;q12)	EWSR1-WR1
Endometrial stromal sarcoma	t(7,17)	
Ewing's sarcoma	t(11;22)(q24;q12)	EWSR1-FLI1
	t(21;22)(q22;q12)	EWSR1-ERG
	t(7;22)(p22;q12)	EWSR1-ETV1
	t(17;22)(q21;q12)	EWSR1-ETV4
	t(2;22)(q33;q12)	EWSR1-FEV
Lipoma	12q abnormalities	Amplified 12q
Myxoid chondrosarcoma	t(9,22)(q22-31;q11-12)	EWSR1-NR4A3
Myxoid liposarcoma	t(12;16)(q13;p11)	FUS-DDIT3
	t(12;22)(q13;q12)	EWSR1-DDIT3
Synovial sarcoma	T(X;18)(p11;q11)	SYT-SSX
Uterine leiomyosarcoma	t(12,14)(q7-)	

did not need molecular evaluation, as 84.5% of these tumors were positive for the transcript. In the second category, where the diagnosis of synovial sarcoma was probable, these tumors were found to have the SYT-SSX transcript 74.4% of the time. However, for the third category, where the diagnosis of synovial sarcoma was possible but not the first in the differential, 24.3% tumors were positive for the transcript, which aided in the diagnosis of synovial sarcoma (31). These data suggest that molecular genetics may also be useful in the diagnosis of some sarcomas.

■ SOFT TISSUE SARCOMA

Soft tissues are the nonepithelial extraskeletal tissues of the body that support, connect, and surround other discrete anatomic structures. These tissues include fibrous, adipose, and vascular structures as well as muscles and tendons; they represent more than 50% of body weight. Soft tissues are derived embryologically primarily from the mesoderm, making tumors from these tissues mesenchymal in origin. Soft tissue sarcomas represent approximately 0.6% of all adult cancers and tend to occur more frequently in men (1). These cancers are also more common in older adults, but this is somewhat dependent on tumor type as well (32).

Soft tissue sarcomas are an extremely heterogeneous group. Most sarcomas are classified by the tissue that they most closely resemble histopathologically. Unfortunately, because tumors have decreasing histologic differentiation, it becomes more and more difficult to classify these sarcomas. Sometimes it can be almost impossible to classify some spindle cell and round cell soft tissue tumors despite immunohistochemical techniques and electron microscopy. Each tumor type has a varying degree of aggressiveness and ability to metastasize, depending on the degree of differentiation or histologic grade.

CLINICAL PRESENTATION

Soft tissue sarcomas can occur in any anatomic region of the body because of the ubiquitous nature of connective tissue. The majority of soft tissue sarcomas arise from the extremities (60%), with mostly in the lower extremities. They can also develop in the trunk region (30%) and in the head and neck region (10%). Because the majority of these tumors develop in the extremities, the most common symptom reported is that of a soft tissue mass or swelling. Pain is reported by only about one-third of patients with soft tissue sarcoma at presen-

tation (33). Therefore, because of the lack of symptoms, there is often a delay in the diagnosis (34). Many times these tumors are mistaken for other benign tumors, such as hematomas or lipomas. In the case of retroperitoneal and intraabdominal sarcomas, delay in diagnosis is likely due the fact that tumors can grow extensively in this area without causing any symptoms.

EVALUATION

As with any suspected illness or disease, evaluation should start with a thorough history and physical examination. This can give some indication as to how long the symptoms have been present and can help guide further study, including imaging and biopsy.

The imaging modalities recommended for the evaluation of sarcomas depend on the site of disease. A plain film of the involved area, if possible, is a good initial imaging modality. For soft tissue tumors of the extremities as well as the head and neck, magnetic resonance imaging (MRI) is preferred (35,36). By using T1- and T2-weighted images, MRI studies can provide maximal contrast between tumor, fat, vessels, bone, and other surrounding structures (34,35). Soft tissue sarcomas of the pelvis may also be better visualized with MRI studies, which may thus enhance decision making. Soft tissue sarcomas found in the retroperitoneum and abdomen are generally best evaluated by computed tomography (CT) imaging. Arteriograms and other invasive studies are almost never required to evaluate soft tissue sarcomas.

A biopsy should be performed in any soft tissue mass if it is symptomatic, enlarging, is greater than 5 cm, and has persisted for more than 4 to 6 weeks. The method of biopsy chosen depends on the least invasive technique available to make a definitive diagnosis of both histology and grade of the tumor. Most often a core-needle biopsy is sufficient to provide enough tissue for definitive diagnosis; however open biopsy may still need to be performed in cases where more tissue is needed to evaluate the histology (37,38). If an open biopsy is performed, the biopsy site should be removed at the time of definitive surgical resection, as there are some reports of tumor recurrences within the needle tract after percutaneous biopsy (39). An excisional biopsy may be used for small or superficial lesions; however, careful examination of margins and planning of the orientation of the resection should always be performed. Fine-needle aspiration can also be a useful tool in diagnosis, assuming that an experienced sarcoma cytopathologist is available (40–42). When it is possible to obtain them, core biopsies are better for the diagnosis of sarcoma.

Once the diagnosis of sarcoma is established, screening for metastatic disease is also required. The most common site of metastatic disease in sarcoma is the lung; however in abdominal and retroperitoneal sarcomas, the liver is also a common site. Therefore staging workup should include chest x-ray but may also include chest CT, depending on the size, grade, and location of the primary tumor. Patients with low-grade or intermediate/high-grade tumors less than 5 cm in diameter need only a chest x-ray during staging; those with high-grade tumors greater than 5 cm in diameter need a chest CT at diagnosis for staging (43). Patients with abdominal or retroperitoneal soft tissue sarcomas should also undergo CT scanning of the abdomen and pelvis, with appropriate imaging of the liver and peritoneal space, to evaluate for metastatic disease.

PATHOLOGY

Malignancies are classified according to histologic grade, which is determined by assessment of several features: (1) degree of cellularity, (2) cellular pleomorphism or anaplasia, (3) mitotic activity, (4) degree of necrosis, and (5) expansive or infiltrative and invasive growth (44). Sarcomas are classified primarily according to their tissue appearance, histologic grade, and size. This can be quite difficult, as approximately 70 different histologic types of soft tissue sarcoma are recognized (Table 33-2).

Generally, sarcomas are classified into several major histologic categories according to the cell of origin. The clinical course of sarcomas depends in large part on the tissue they resemble histologically. The clinical course of saromas depends in large part on the aggressiveness of the original tumor; this can vary not only between the major histologic categories but also among individual lesions of the same type. Pathologists often separate sarcomas into three histologic grades based on tumor grade. Grade 1 (low-grade) describes tumors thath are well differentiated; grade 2 describes those tumors that have an intermediate differentiation, and grade 3 (high-grade) describes tumors that have a poorly differentiated histology. Biological aggressiveness can be predicted based on histologic grade, and this spectrum varies among the histologic subtypes of sarcoma (Fig. 33-1) (45,46).

STAGING AND PROGNOSIS

The staging system of the American Joint Committee on Cancer (AJCC) is one of the most often used such systems for soft tissue sarcomas (Table 33-3) (47).

TABLE 33-2	SOFT TISSUE SARCOMA— HISTOLOGIC DIAGNOSIS

Sarcomas of adipose tissue	Sarcomas of blood vessels and lymphatics
Liposarcoma	Epithelioid hemangioendothelioma
Atypical lipomatous tumor	Hemangiopericytoma
Myxoid liposarcoma	Angiosarcoma
Cellular myxoid liposarcoma	
Round cell liposarcoma	Sarcomas of skeletal muscle
Dedifferentiated liposarcoma	Embryonal rhabdomyosarcoma
Pleomorphic liposarcoma	Alveolar rhabdomyosarcoma
	Pleomorphic rhabdomyosarcoma
Sarcomas of peripheral nervous tissue	
Malignant peripheral nerve sheath tumor	Sarcomas of unknown origin
(Malignant schwannoma, neurofibrosarcoma,	Synovial sarcoma
neurogenic sarcoma)	Monophasic
	Biphasic
Sarcomas of smooth muscle	Alveolar soft tissue sarcoma
Leiomyosarcoma	Epithelioid sarcoma
	Unclassified sarcoma
	Extraskeletal osteosarcoma
Sarcomas of fibrous tissue	Extraskeletal chondrosarcoma
Desmoid fibromatosis	Extraskeletal Ewing's sarcoma (PNET)
Dermatofibrosarcoma protuberans	
Low-grade fibromyxoid sarcoma	
Fibrosarcoma	Soft tissue tumors of melanocytic tissue
Malignant fibrous histiocytoma (MFH)	Melanoma of soft tissue or clear cell sarcoma

PNET = primitive neuroectodermal tumor.

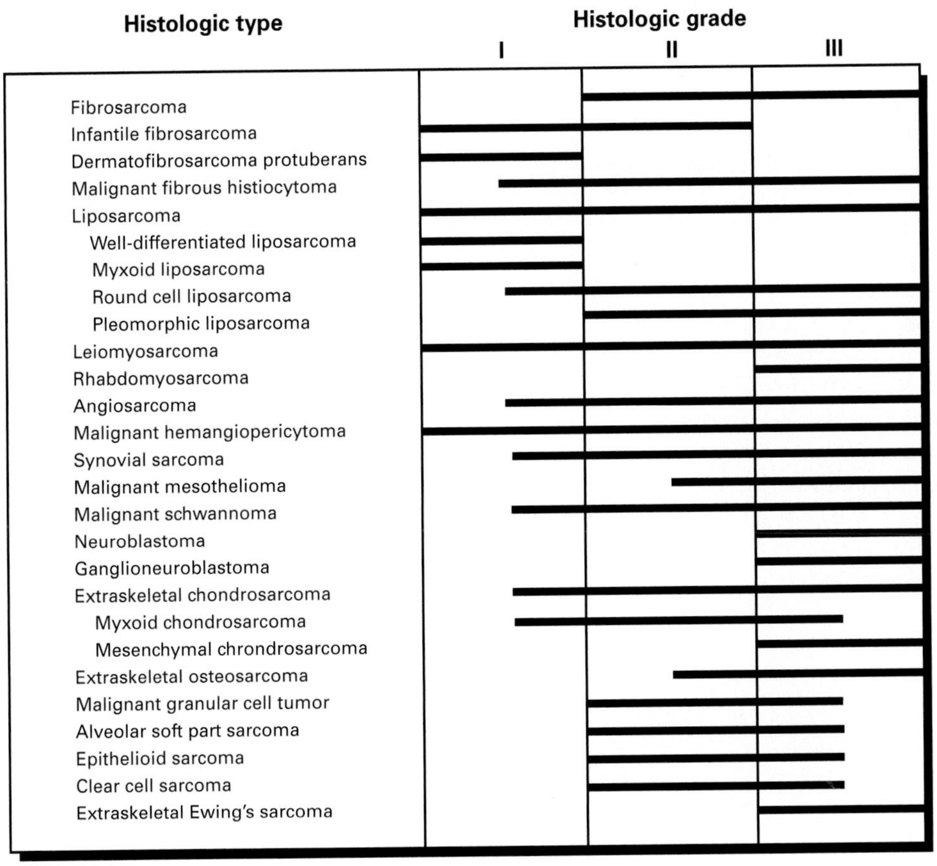

Histologic type

Histologic grade

I II III

Fibrosarcoma
Infantile fibrosarcoma
Dermatofibrosarcoma protuberans
Malignant fibrous histiocytoma
Liposarcoma
  Well-differentiated liposarcoma
  Myxoid liposarcoma
  Round cell liposarcoma
  Pleomorphic liposarcoma
Leiomyosarcoma
Rhabdomyosarcoma
Angiosarcoma
Malignant hemangiopericytoma
Synovial sarcoma
Malignant mesothelioma
Malignant schwannoma
Neuroblastoma
Ganglioneuroblastoma
Extraskeletal chondrosarcoma
  Myxoid chondrosarcoma
  Mesenchymal chrondrosarcoma
Extraskeletal osteosarcoma
Malignant granular cell tumor
Alveolar soft part sarcoma
Epithelioid sarcoma
Clear cell sarcoma
Extraskeletal Ewing's sarcoma

FIGURE 33-1 Spectrum of grades observed among histologic subtypes of soft tissue sarcoma. [*From Enzinger and Weiss (32). With permission.*]

All soft tissue sarcoma subtypes are included except Kaposi's sarcoma, dermatofibrosarcoma protuberans, infantile fibrosarcoma, and angiosarcoma.

This system is designed to classify tumors of the extremities, trunk, head and neck, and retroperitoneum, but it was not designed to be used to evaluate sarcomas of the gastrointestinal tract. This system is limited because anatomic site is not taken into account. This, however, is a very important factor, as anatomic location is known to influence outcome (48,49).

There are several clinicopathologic factors that are important in terms of prognosis and treatment planning. These are primarily tumor grade, size of the primary tumor, depth of invasion, and extent of disease (45,46,50). Patients at highest risk for local recurrence or distant metastases would be those with a high-grade lesion, a primary tumor >5 cm, and deep tumor location (45,46, 49,50). Whether local recurrence of soft tissue sarcomas affects overall survival is unclear (51). And in soft tissue sarcomas, the adverse prognostic factors for local recurrence differ from those that predict distant metastasis and tumor-related mortality (45).

TREATMENT

Evaluation for the treatment of sarcoma requires a multidisciplinary approach with experienced medical oncologists, surgical oncologists, pathologists, radiologists, and radiation oncologists working together to develop the best plan of action. The treatment depends on the tumor type, location, and extent of disease. The primary endpoint of any sarcoma therapy is to eradicate all gross and microscopic evidence of disease with aggressive multimodality treatment. In patients in whom this endpoint is achievable, the therapeutic intent is cure; where this is not achievable, the intent is palliation of existing or potential symptoms and perhaps extension of life.

Treatment of Local Disease

Surgery

For local disease, surgical resection has been the mainstay of therapy in most cases. Sarcomas tend to expand and compress tissue planes, which produces a pseudocapsule comprising normal tissue interlaced with tumor tissue. When surgical resection does not include the

TABLE 33-3	STAGING—FROM THE AMERICAN JOINT COMMITTEE ON CANCER

Primary tumor (T)

TX	Primary tumor cannot be assessed
T0	No evidence of primary tumor
T1	Tumor 5 cm or less in greatest dimension
	T1a Superficial tumor*
	T1b Deep tumor*
T2	Tumor more than 5 cm in greatest dimension
	T2a Superficial tumor
	T2b Deep tumor

Regional lymph nodes (N)

NX	Regional lymph nodes cannot be assessed
N0	No regional lymph node metastasis
N1	Regional lymph node metastasis

Distant metastasis (M)

MX	Distant metastasis cannot be assessed
M0	No distant metastasis
M1	Distant metastasis

Histologic grade (G)

GX	Grade cannot be assessed
G1	Well differentiated
G2	Moderately differentiated
G3	Poorly differentiated
G4	Poorly differentiated or undifferentiated (four-tiered systems only)

Stage grouping

Stage	T	N	M	G	G	
Stage I	T1a, 1b, 2a, 2b	N0	M0	G1–2	G1	Low
Stage II	T1a, 1b, 2a	N0	M0	G3–4	G2–3	High
Stage III	T2b	N0	M0	G3–4	G2–3	High
Stage IV	Any T	N1	M0	Any G	Any G	High or Low

* Superficial tumors are located exclusively above the superficial fascia without invasion of the fascia; deep tumors are located either exclusively beneath the superficial fascia, superficial to the fascia with invasion of or through the fascia, or both superficial yet beneath the fascia. Retroperitoneal, mediastinal, and pelvic sarcomas are classified as deep tumors.
SOURCE: The American Joint Committee on Cancer (47). With permission.

plane of tissue adjacent to the pseudocapsule, the local recurrence rates are between 33 and 66% (52–54). Wide local resection with a margin of normal tissue surrounding the tumor is associated with better results; that is, local recurrence rates of approximately 10 to 30% (55–57). Often wide local resection is used in conjunction with preoperative or postoperative radiation therapy; however, there are select situations when surgical resection alone is sufficient. Radiation and chemotherapy should be considered in treating patients in whom a wide negative margin of resection is not possible or in whom the risk for local recurrence or metastatic disease is high.

Adult sarcomas have a less than 4% prevalence of lymph node metastases (58,59). For this reason routine

regional lymph node dissection is often not required. However, patients with clear cell sarcoma, rhabdomyosarcoma, angiosarcoma, and epithelioid sarcoma have a higher incidence of lymph node metastases and should be evaluated closely for lymphadenopathy; if found, this should be treated appropriately (58,59).

Because of better surgical techniques and a multimodality approach to the care of patients, there has been a decrease in radical resection of extremity tumors, such as amputation or compartment resection. There has been a corresponding rise in limb-sparing procedures combining wide local resection with preoperative or postoperative chemotherapy and radiotherapy (60,61). Of patients with localized sarcomas of the extremities, approximately 90% can safely undergo limb-sparing procedures which maintain function and adequately maintain local control (61,62). There are times when a limb-sparing approach is contraindicated; specifically when a margin-free resection is impossible and/or when radiation therapy is risky. Also if major vessels and nerves are involved at the site where resection would critically compromise function, limb-sparing surgeries are not typically performed (63). A study conducted at the National Cancer Institute (NCI) showed that there was no survival advantage to amputation over limb-sparing surgery with postoperative radiation; thus, amputation should be used only as a last resort surgical option (64).

Isolated limb perfusion has been studied in patients with soft tissue sarcoma of the extremities and is still being investigated as a treatment modality (65–67). During this form of treatment, the artery and vein to an extremity are cannulated and all the blood flow for that extremity is passed through a cardiopulmonary bypass pump. The limb is perfused with a biological agent or chemotherapy—for example, high-dose tumor necrosis factor alpha (TNF-α), interferon-gamma (IFN-γ), or melphalan. The results of these studies have been promising, especially in patients with locally advanced, unresectable disease where occasionally limb-salvage therapies have been achieved after limb perfusion. This treatment modality continues to be investigated and should be performed at an experienced sarcoma center.

The same principles of surgical resection for soft tissue sarcomas of extremities are applied to soft tissue sarcomas in other parts of the body. However many times these lesions are located in areas that are not amenable to "radical" resection. This makes it even more important to incorporate radiation and/or chemotherapy in a sequence deemed appropriate by a multidisciplinary group with experience and expertise in these areas. Unfortunately, even with the multimodality approach, local recurrences are common in retroperitoneal sarcomas.

Radiation

Although radiation is not effective for the treatment of gross disease, it has been a useful adjunct to surgery in the treatment of microscopic local disease and for palliation of symptoms. In the past, soft tissue sarcomas were thought to be relatively resistant to radiation for several reasons. Tumors treated with radiation regress slowly, low-energy radiation beams initially used in treatment of these tumors were less effective than the beams currently available, and previous clinical experience demonstrating resistance was based in large part on studies where radiation was the sole therapy used (68). Now, however, both experimental and clinical studies have shown that radiation is an effective adjuvant treatment modality for soft tissue sarcomas (68,69). In patients with sarcomas arising from certain anatomic locations, there are limitations on the amount of radiation that may be delivered to the tumor or tumor bed due to the proximity to vital normal tissues. These locations include the abdomen, paraspinal region, head and neck, and mediastinum.

Radiation therapy is occasionally used as the sole treatment modality for palliation for some patients with soft tissue sarcomas. These patients are often those who have unresectable disease or who are not appropriate candidates for surgery and/or chemotherapy. There have been reports of 5-year survival rates ranging from 25 to 40% with radiation therapy alone, and of local control rates of approximately 30%, depending on the primary tumor's size (69–71).

Radiation therapy is commonly used in the preoperative or postoperative adjuvant setting. Studies comparing preoperative and postoperative radiation therapy found that wound complications were twice as common with preoperative as opposed to postoperative radiation; however, larger field sizes were required with postoperative radiation and grade 2 or greater fibrosis or edema was more common in patients receiving this treatment (72–74). Because there are pros and cons as to the timing of radiation therapy, this topic remains controversial; appropriate discussion between radiation oncologists, medical oncologists, and surgeons is required in planning the treatment of each patient (75,76).

Preoperative radiation has several advantages over postoperative radiation, including smaller radiation portals, easier surgical resection from vital structures, conversion to a limb-sparing procedure, reduction of the extent of the surgical procedure, and lower radiation doses, which can be utilized because there are theoretically fewer radio-resistant hypoxic cells within the tumor (72,77–79). However, preoperative radiotherapy may lead to difficulty in assessing pathologic responses to preoperative chemotherapy may also contribute to delayed wound healing. Several studies have shown improved local control rates with preoperative radiation, especially with larger tumors that were initially considered unresectable (56,64,80–82). A dose of 50 Gy or more is often required to obtain local control. At these dose levels, the entire circumference of the extremity must not be irradiated in order to avoid lymphedema (56,64,82). Adjuvant radiation should be considered in all patients with positive or close microscopic margins in whom reexcision is impossible or impractical.

Brachytherapy, sometimes called interstitial implant therapy, is also used in the treatment of soft tissue sarcomas and is an alternative approach to external-beam radiation therapy. Brachytherapy has been shown to be effective in the treatment of soft tissue sarcomas, with local control rates approaching 90% (55,83). Radiation is delivered to the area desired by implanting catheters in a parallel orientation along the operative bed at the time of surgical resection (Fig. 33-2).

On postoperative days 5 to 7, a radioactive source, usually iridium 192, is inserted into the catheters, where it remains for 3 to 5 days to deliver the prescribed dose of radiation. After delivery of the radiation, the wires and catheters are removed. This type of therapy is used in some centers as a radiation boost to the tumor bed following adjuvant external-beam radiation, or it can be used in lieu of traditional external-beam radiation. There are advantages to using brachytherapy: the total time required for therapy is usually <2 weeks, and it can be done during the required hospital stay for resection of the tumor. While delivering the same dose of radiation, it costs approximately $1000 less per patient for

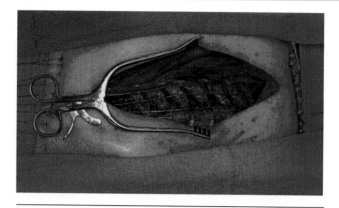

FIGURE 33-2 Brachytherapy wires used intraoperatively. (*Courtesy of Dr. Matthew Ballo, Department of Radiation Oncology, The University of Texas M.D. Anderson Cancer Center.*)

brachytherapy than external-beam radiation, and the irradiated volume is smaller, which may improve function of the radiated area (84).

Chemotherapy

The goals of chemotherapy in the local treatment of disease are to eradicate micrometastasis, decrease risk of local recurrence, and downsize tumors to facilitate either limb-sparing procedures for extremity tumors or resection for tumors initially deemed unresectable. For all patients with small cell sarcomas [e.g., rhabdomyosarcoma, Ewing's/primitive neuroectodermal tumor (PNET)] of any size, systemic chemotherapy is considered standard of care. Patients who have high-risk local primary tumors should be considered for preoperative or postoperative chemotherapy as well (Fig. 33-3).

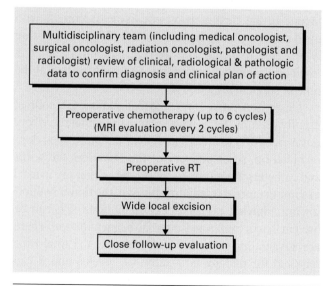

FIGURE 33-3 Treatment approach for patients with stage III soft-tissue sarcomas.

Some soft tissue sarcomas are more sensitive to chemotherapy than others. Small cell sarcomas, synovial sarcomas, angiosarcomas, uterine leiomyosarcomas, and myxoid liposarcomas are sensitive to conventional chemotherapy. Extraskeletal osteosarcomas, chondrosarcomas, and Ewing's sarcomas are treated in a similar fashion as soft tissue sarcomas. One study performed at the University of Texas M.D. Anderson Cancer Center (MDACC) showed that extraskeletal osteosarcomas were not as responsive to chemotherapy as osseous osteosarcomas (85). Gastrointestinal stromal tumors (GISTs, discussed further on), gastrointestinal leiomyosarcomas, alveolar soft part sarcomas, and clear cell sarcomas, on the other hand, are resistant to standard chemotherapy; therefore these tumors should not be treated with standard therapies, as the toxicities and risks clearly outweigh any benefit.

The two most active agents in the treatment of soft tissue sarcoma are doxorubicin and ifosfamide. Unfortunately very few other known active agents are currently available. Studies have shown that both doxorubicin and ifosfamide also exhibit a positive dose-response curve (Fig. 33-4) (86,87).

Doxorubicin is most active at doses of ≥ 75 mg/m^2, with single-agent response rates of approximately 20 to 35%; when given by a 48- to 96-h continuous infusion, it is less cardiotoxic (86). Ifosfamide has been shown to produce single-agent response rates similar to those of single-agent doxorubicin when used at doses of 10 g/m^2 or higher (87). Ifosfamide has also been shown to have greater efficacy when administered as a 2- to 3-h infusion as opposed to a 24-h infusion (87–90). Dacarbazine (DTIC) has activity as a single agent, with response rates of 10 to 15%. The three-drug regimen MAID [mesna, Adriamycin (doxorubicin), ifosfamide, dacarbazine] has been studied and has shown response rates varying from 25 to 47% (91,92). When the MAID regimen was studied at MDACC, significant toxicities related to the addition of DTIC were seen (93). The combination of doxorubicin (75 or 90 mg/m^2) and ifosfamide at 10 g/m^2 without DTIC was then evaluated in two pilot studies at MDACC in patients with soft tissue sarcomas; objective response rates of 66% [95% confidence interval (CI): 46 to 82%] were seen. This regimen is most often used in the clinic at MDACC in patients who are otherwise healthy, ≤ 65 years of age, and with high-risk tumors (94). Because of these encouraging results, this regimen was further studied, and thrombopoietin was added for platelet support. The results showed a 75% response rate [95 CI: 59 to 71%; complete response (CR) 12%] in patients with primary tumors of the extremities and a 68% response rate (95%

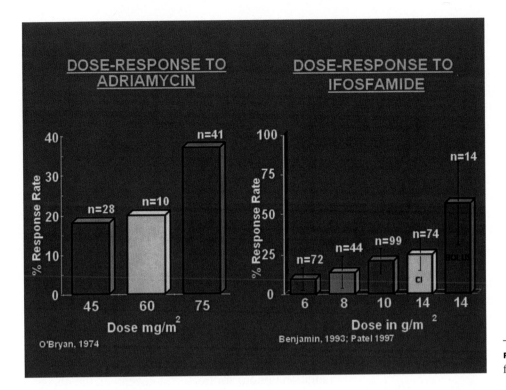

FIGURE 33-4 Doxorubicin and ifosfamide dose-response curves.

CI: 56 to 80%; CR 12%) for patients with primary disease at any site (95). The breakdown of response rates according to histology from this study was as follows: malignant fibrous histiocytoma (MFH) 69%, synovial sarcoma 88%, unclassified sarcomas 60%, non-GI–leiomyosarcomas 50%, liposarcomas 56%, angiosarcomas 83%, neurogenic sarcomas 40%, other miscellaneous histologies demonstrated objective response rates of 45% (95). These data show that sensitivity to chemotherapy depends on the histologic type of sarcoma and points to the importance of proper histologic diagnosis in determining prognosis.

Other agents have been studied in soft tissue sarcomas. Often these are used after failure of doxorubicin and ifosfamide. Response rates in patients whose disease failed doxorubicin-based therapy and then received high-dose ifosfamide as a single agent was 29% for soft tissue sarcomas (87). The response rate (RR) was higher (30 to 40%) for the bolus schedule; therefore, high-dose ifosfamide as a single agent with doses of 14 g/m^2 is often used as a salvage regimen at MDACC.

Gemcitabine alone or in combination with docetaxel is frequently used for the treatment of advanced, recurrent, or metastatic disease once patients fail doxorubicin- and ifosfamide-based therapy or in patients who may not tolerate intensive chemotherapy. A two-arm phase II study using gemcitabine as a single agent was performed using doses of 1g/m^2 on a weekly schedule.

A response rate of 18% (95% CI: 7 to 29%) was seen even though many patients had received prior chemotherapies (96). The median duration of response was 3.5 months, ranging from 2 to 13 months (96). Four patients with leiomyosarcomas of nongastrointestinal origin achieved a partial response, which suggests that there may be selective activity in this subset of patients (96). Studies performed by the GI medical oncology group at MDACC have shown a benefit with prolonged infusions of gemcitabine at 10 mg/m^2/min, or a "fixed dose rate" (97,98). Another study evaluated gemcitabine given at 900 mg/m^2 on days 1 and 8 and docetaxel 100 mg/m^2 on day 8, after gemcitabine, repeated every 21 days in patients with unresectable leiomyosarcomas of gynecologic origin. The results showed that 3 of 34 patients achieved CR and 15 achieved a partial response, for an overall response rate of 53% (95% CI: 35 to 70%) (99). The data from these two trials show that gemcitabine is an active agent for the treatment of soft tissue sarcoma. The contribution of docetaxel is currently being investigated in a randomized trial, given the fact that docetaxel as a single agent has been shown to have very little activity (100,101).

Other agents under investigation include ecteinascidin (ET-743), temozolomide, irinotecan, 9-nitrocamptothecin, and several angiogenesis inhibitors (102–108). Many of these agents have shown moderate efficacy. Most of them remain investigational, and the number of patients studied is small. Thus, any treatment of soft tissue sarcomas with these agents should be done in the context of a clinical trial.

Targeted therapy is also becoming useful in the treatment of soft tissue sarcomas. Imatinib mesylate (Gleevec, or STI-571) is effective in the treatment of metastatic GIST. GISTs express the tyrosine kinase KIT (CD-117), the molecular target of imatinib. Imatinib has also been used in dermatofibrosarcoma protuberans, where it may have therapeutic effect (109). Tamoxifen, raloxifene, and toremifene have been used as targeted agents in the treatment of desmoid tumors with some success (110–113). Targretin and rosiglitazone have been used as targeted agents in the treatment of liposarcoma (114,115).

Preoperative chemotherapy is often used for patients with large, high-grade tumors and also for tumors whose location or size prohibit primary surgical excision. At MDACC, preoperative chemotherapy is preferred in patients with high-risk (>5 cm or high-grade) tumors.

Postoperative chemotherapy and its benefits have been debated over the last couple of decades. The majority of randomized trials conducted, mainly in the 1970s and '80s, were very small (understandable, given the rarity of this disease); they were therefore underpowered to evaluate significant improvements in disease-free and overall survival. Many of these studies also used suboptimal doses of chemotherapy and included patients with a variety of tumor histologies and grades, making evaluation of these studies difficult in terms of the current knowledge of chemotherapy dose and prognostic factors. The Sarcoma Meta-Analysis Collaboration undertook a quantitative intention-to-treat metaanalysis of all 14 randomized trials of adjuvant chemotherapy from the 1970s and '80s to answer some of the questions regarding benefit of doxorubicin-based chemotherapy in patients with localized, resectable soft tissue sarcomas. This metaanalysis showed a significant improvement for local and distant recurrence-free survival and for overall survival in patients with extremity sarcomas; however, the survival advantage for the entire group failed to achieve statistical significance (116). The Italian Sarcoma Group conducted a randomized trial enrolling the true high-risk patients with high-grade, $\geq$5 cm primary or locally recurrent extremity soft tissue sarcomas. The 104 patients were randomized to receive five cycles of adjuvant chemotherapy of epirubicin (a doxorubicin analog) at 60 mg/m^2 on days 1 and 2 and ifosfamide 9 g/m^2 over 5 days versus observation following appropriate local therapy (either surgery or radiation) (117). Results showed that with a median follow-up of 59 months, there was significant improvement in disease-free survival in patients who received chemotherapy (48 versus 16 months, p = 0.04); there was also significant improvement in overall survival (75 versus 46 months, p = 0.03) (117). The absolute benefit in overall survival for the chemotherapy arm was 13% at 2 years and 19% at 4 years, which was also statistically significant (p = 0.04) (117).

Recurrent Disease

Even with a multimodality approach to patients with soft tissue sarcoma, locally recurrent disease occurs up to 50% of the time. Once local recurrence has been identified, these patients are treated much like patients initially diagnosed with soft tissue sarcomas. During the evaluation of the patient with locally recurrent disease, an attempt is made to determine possible reasons for treatment failure and whether this is truly recurrent disease versus a new primary tumor. Workup is conducted to evaluate the primary tumor as well to look for metastatic disease. Surgical, chemotherapeutic, and radiation options for treatment depend on the management of the initial tumor and are sometimes limited; however, patients with local recurrence can be cured of their disease. Surgery, radiation, and chemotherapy should be considered as outlined above.

Metastatic Disease

Patients with obvious metastatic disease to multiple organ systems are generally incurable and considered appropriate for palliative systemic therapy. The subset of patients with lung-only metastatic disease, especially with a greater than 12-month disease-free interval, have a favorable biology and prognosis and should be considered for resection if feasible. This approach results in 3- to 5-year survival of up to 20%. Chemotherapy is the mainstay of therapy for patients with metastatic disease; although surgical resection of residual disease to render patients free of gross disease is often pursued. The sequencing of chemotherapy is similar to that of isolated local disease. In a study done at MDACC, patients with metastatic disease showed a 57% response rate to doxorubicin (75 to 90 mg/m^2) and ifosfamide (10 g/m^2) (118). If patients fail this regimen, high-dose ifosfamide as described above is a salvage therapy. Because every patient is different, there will be times when the clinical picture dictates that such intensive chemotherapy is not possible. For these situations, gemcitabine alone or in combination with docetaxel is a possibility. Most other therapies would be best utilized in the context of a clinical trial. There are times when surgery and/or radiation may also be used for palliation of symptoms. These cases are very select and should be discussed in a multimodality planning conference, as the risks and benefits of such therapies must be weighed carefully. Radiotherapy to the pelvis may limit the ability to deliver systemic chemotherapy, since the pelvis is a major site of bone marrow production.

GASTROINTESTINAL STROMAL TUMORS

GISTs are the most common mesenchymal tumors of the gastrointestinal tract (119). Until recently, they were often designated smooth muscle tumors of the GI tract—specifically, GI leiomyosarcoma, leiomyoblastoma, leiomyosarcoma, and leiomyomas. Recently investigators have found that GISTs express the KIT (CD-117) receptor tyrosine kinase. These tumors are thought to originate from the interstitial cell of Cajal, the intestinal pacemaker cell responsible for peristalsis (120). These tumors most commonly arise in the stomach (60 to 70%), small intestine (20 to 30%), colon and rectum (5%), and esophagus (<5%), although they can arise anywhere in the GI tract or omentum/peritoneum (extra-GI GIST). The liver, peritoneum, and abdominal wall are the most common sites of metastatic disease; however, there are reports of associated central nervous system (CNS), lymph node, lung, and bone metastasis (121). The incidence of GIST tumors is equal in men and women; it generally peaks between the fourth and

sixth decades of life, and patients are more commonly Caucasian. Presenting symptoms often represent the site of tumor origin, but they may be vague, including abdominal pain, anorexia, weight loss, and dyspepsia.

Traditional chemotherapy or radiotherapy has historically not been effective in the treatment of GIST. As early as 1975, Gottlieb at MDACC observed that leiomyosarcomas arising from the GI tract did not respond to doxorubicin-based chemotherapy, as leiomyosarcomas that arose from other organ systems did (122). Other agents have been studied in GISTs, also with disappointing results. A phase II study of gemcitabine in patients with metastatic GI leiomyosarcoma found no objective responses in 17 patients treated (96). Prior to the availability of imatinib, we published a phase II trial of temozolamide in patients with GIST in which there were no objective responses (123). The standard treatment for localized/primary GISTs continues to be complete surgical resection with negative margins. We are currently investigating the use of imatinib in the neoadjuvant and adjuvant settings.

Imatinib mesylate selectively inhibits ABL, BCR-ABL, ARG, KIT, and PDGFR tyrosine kinase and therefore inhibits growth of tumor cells that express high levels of these kinases (Fig. 33-5) (124,125).

The first study reported described a patient with widely metastatic, chemotherapy-resistant GIST who, within a few weeks of starting therapy with imatinib

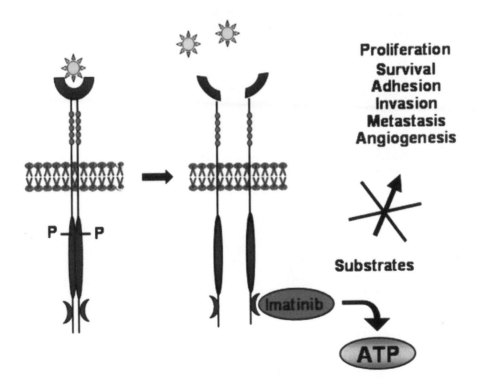

FIGURE 33-5 Imatinib mesylate is thought to displace ATP from the ATP binding site of the Kit kinase domain. This results in abrogation of downstream signaling and reversal of the tumor phenotype.

mesylate, was found to have a major objective clinical response, which was maintained for more than 18 months (126). Recent clinical trials with imatinib mesylate have indicated that the majority of patients with malignant GIST show some benefit with treatment, with response rates ranging from 33 to 69% (127–130). There have been reports of patients with GISTs who respond to imatinib mesylate and whose tumors have very low or no expression of c-KIT, perhaps mediated by expression of the PDGFRα (Platelet Derived Growth Factor Recipient Alpha) (131). As with many treatments in oncology, there are patients who ultimately fail imatinib therapy and/or develop resistance; an effective method of managing these patients is not currently known. There are clinical trials in development to evaluate imatinib in combination with other agents and to evaluate the mechanisms of tumor resistance to imatinib.

Recommended radiographic imaging of GISTs is in evolution. The imaging technique most often used is CT. This modality tends to be useful because of the intraabdominal nature of these tumors. Unlike other soft tissue sarcomas, GISTs metastasize to the lungs approximately 2% of the time. Thus, if the initial CT of the chest does not show evidence of disease, a subsequent chest x-ray is sufficient. The standard measurement of response by CT scan, such as RECIST (Response Evaluation Criteria In Solid Tumors) criteria, may underestimate early tumor response seen in GIST. Patients who respond to imatinib clinically may show a decrease in tumor size or a decrease in tumor radiodensity by CT radiography (Fig. 33-6).

We have also seen tumors enlarge after 2 months of therapy with Gleevec, only to regress later on.

Positron emission tomography (PET) may be a useful imaging modality in GISTs. We have found that patients treated with imatinib mesylate have responses by PET scanning earlier than with conventional CT radiography. We have observed complete responses by PET criteria as early as 5 days after the start of imatinib therapy. This has laid the groundwork for additional clinical trials designed to determine whether the rapid assessment and prediction of clinical response is possible with PET scans performed in the first few days of therapy. Van den Abbeele et al. reported that patients with advanced GIST who had a PET response (79%, SUV [Standardized Uptake Value] < 2.0) as early as day 1 maintained a long-term response. However, patients who had no PET response or only a temporary one (21%, SUV > 2.0) were found to have a poor response or progression. PET scanning often predicted response prior to a decrease in tumor size (132). At MDACC, we have developed a novel clinical trial designed to study the

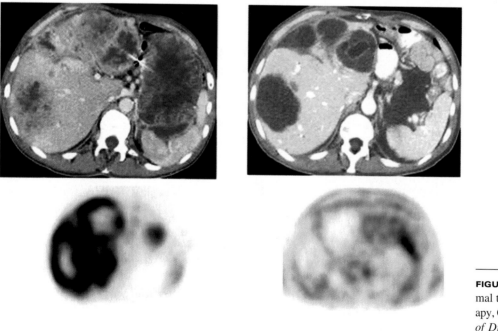

Pretreatment   **8 Weeks Posttreatment**

FIGURE 33-6 Gastrointestinal stromal tumor response to Gleevec therapy, CT, and PET imaging. (*Courtesy of Dr. Haesun Choi, Department of Diagnostic Radiology, The University of Texas M.D. Anderson Cancer Center.*)

early biological effects of preoperative imatinib in patients with resectable GISTs who show early responses on PET imaging. It is hoped that this will provide insight into the direct molecular and radiographic effects of imatinib in GIST. The Radiation Therapy Oncology Group (RTOG) in conjunction with the American College of Radiology Imaging Network is also evaluating the utility of early PET scanning (1 to 7 days after initiation of therapy with imatinib mesylate) in patients with operable malignant GIST who receive preoperative imatinib. It is our experience that decisions to discontinue therapy should not be based solely on CT radiography or PET imaging but instead should take into consideration the patient's overall clinical condition.

FOLLOW-UP MANAGEMENT

The major goals of follow-up surveillance and management should be early identification of potentially curable recurrences, identification of treatment-related complications, and patient reassurance. Much of the surveillance of patients treated for soft tissue sarcomas is based on known prognostic factors, outcomes in individual subsets of patients, and patterns of tumor recurrence. These patterns vary depending on the anatomic site of the primary tumor; it is also important to realize that lymph node metastases occur extremely rarely in soft tissue sarcomas (<5%). Patients with extremity and superficial trunk primaries often have distant lung metastasis rather than local or regional recurrences, whereas patients whose primary is located in the retroperitoneum, head and neck, or visceral organs tend to have higher incidences of local rather than distant metastasis.

For patients with low-risk T1 primaries of the extremities (or other sites) who have undergone treatment with curative intent and are free of any gross evidence of disease, follow-up should include a history and physical, cross-sectional imaging to encompass the tumor bed to evaluate for local recurrence, and routine chest x-rays for surveillance of metastatic disease (43). Imaging of the primary tumor site should be done with the modality best for that particular site. For tumors of the head and neck and extremities, MRI imaging is appropriate; for tumors of the chest cavity, abdomen, and retroperitoneum, CT scans are appropriate (43). Ultrasound technology can be a useful tool in imaging primary tumor sites of the extremity and superficial trunk when in the hands of an experienced ultrasonographer, but this is extremely operator-dependent and requires expertise, experience, and consistency (43). The routine use of chest CT for evaluation of metastatic disease in soft tissue sarcomas has been studied and found not to be cost-effective; further, when it was used, the group that underwent both CT and chest x-ray was found to have a lower (65%) 5-year metastases-free survival than the group followed with chest x-ray alone (90%) (133). The interval and length of time to follow these patients depends on the clinician to some degree. The National Comprehensive Cancer Network recommends follow-up with annual scanning of the primary site for at least 5 years; however, often these patients are seen every 3 to 4 months in the immediate postoperative period for the first 2 years, then every 4 to 6 months for the next 2 years, and yearly thereafter (43,134).

Patients with high-risk T2 (>5 cm) soft tissue sarcomas are at a greater risk for distant lung metastases than those with low-risk tumors. In patients with high-risk tumors who have undergone treatment with curative intent and are free of any gross evidence of disease, follow-up should include a history and physical, cross-sectional imaging to encompass the tumor bed to evaluate for local recurrence, routine chest x-rays, and CT for surveillance of metastatic disease (43). These patients are followed in the same manner as low-risk patients, with follow-up visits with the above studies every 3 months for the first 1 to 2 years, then visits every 4 months for the next 1 to 2 years, followed by visits every 6 months for 1 to 2 years, and yearly visits thereafter (43). As for local recurrence surveillance, the cross-sectional imaging is omitted after 5 years, as most local recurrences appear within 5 years of initial treatment (43). There is a fair amount of variability in the frequency of visits based on the clinician's suspicion for the possibility of metastatic or locally recurrent disease, as well as patient preference.

■ BONE SARCOMA

Bone sarcomas are very rare tumors. In 2004 it was estimated that 2440 new cases of bone sarcoma would be diagnosed in the United States and that 1300 deaths would be due to such tumors (1). Bone tumors account for approximately 9% of all childhood cancers and comprise approximately 15% of all cancer deaths in patients below 20 years of age (1). The most common malignant tumor of bone is osteosarcoma, which accounts for approximately 20 to 45% of all bone tumors. Chondrosarcoma is the second most common, accounting for approximately 20%, and the Ewing's/PNET family of tumors accounts for approximately 11% of malignant bone tumors. The incidence of osteosarcoma is slightly higher in men than in women and that of chondrosarcoma is roughly equal. The Ewing's/PNET family of tumors also has a slightly greater predilection for men (135, 136). Tumors of this family of tumors tend to occur more frequently in children and adolescents (135,136), whereas osteosarcoma has a biphasic pattern of incidence that peaks in adolescents, with the growth of long bones, and in the elderly, with tumors arising in association with Paget's disease or previously radiated tissues (137,138). Chondrosarcomas are usually seen in patients after the fifth decade of life, but they can also occur in younger patients, where the tumors tend to be of a higher-grade malignancy.

CLINICAL PRESENTATION

The clinical presentation of any bone tumor depends on its location. Virtually any bone in the body may be affected by a sarcoma (Table 33-4).

Most osteosarcomas tend to occur in the metaphyseal region of long bones, specifically the distal femur, proximal tibia, and proximal humerus. Approximately 55% of osteosarcomas occur around the knee joint. Chondrosarcomas can also arise in any bone in the body; however, they have been noted to occur in the pelvis and other flat bones. Ewing's/PNET tumors tend to occur in the diaphyseal portions of the long bones, although they can also occur anywhere in bone. These lesions are also known to arise in the flat bones of the body—e.g., the pelvis and scapula.

The most common presenting symptom is pain and swelling or a mass. This pain is often described as initially insidious and transient, gradually becoming progressively more severe and unremitting. Swelling can also occur; it is usually localized and can be associated with warmth and erythema. Patients can have decreased range of motion and increased pain with movement or weight bearing in the affected extremity. Patients who have pelvic tumors may have neurologic impairment and severe pain, typically because these tumors are often not recognized until late in the disease course.

EVALUATION

As with all patients, evaluation of those with sarcoma should begin with a careful history, physical examination, and routine laboratory tests, followed by imaging tailored to the given complaint. The imaging of any bone tumor should begin with a plain film of the involved area. Such an x-ray image is often helpful in the diagnosis of bone sarcomas; for example, osteosarcoma often has a "sunburst" appearance of calcification on x-ray imaging, which is virtually diagnostic (Fig. 33-7).

The amount of calcification associated with osteosarcoma depends on the histologic subtype, e.g., osteoblastic osteosarcoma usually has very dense calcification, whereas telangietatic osteosarcoma is usually primarily lytic with little or no calcification. Chondrosarcoma also has a distinct appearance on x-ray imaging, with destruction of the bone and endosteal scalloping of the bony cortex and a chondroid matrix, which appears lobulated (see Fig. 33-7). Ewing's sarcoma has a typical "onion-skin" appearance on x-ray imaging (see Fig. 33-7). Other initial imaging should include a CT scan and/or MRI of the primary lesion to further evaluate involvement of the neurovascular structures, surrounding soft tissues, and adjacent joints and to better evaluate any associated soft tissue mass. MRI may be useful to evaluate soft tissue masses associated with extremity and pelvic tumors; CT tends to be more useful in defining the cortical/bony details of involvement. These scans are often used together in the workup of bone sarcomas as complementary tests. Plain x-rays and CT scans are usually adequate for the evaluation of tumors arising from the thoracic skeleton.

TABLE 33-4	FEATURES OF COMMON BONE TUMORS					
Type	*Frequency*	*Age Distribution*	*Gender*	*Common Sites*	*Radiologic Features*	*Pathologic Features*
Osteosarcoma	45%	10–20 years	M > F	Metaphysis	Sunburst calcifications	Spindle cells, osteoid matrix
MFH	8%	20–80 years	M > F	Long bones	Radiolucent with ill-defined margins	Pleomorphic spindle cells, NO osteoid
Chondrosarcoma	22%	20–80 years	M > F	Pelvis/shoulder girdles	Lobulated appearance	Lobules, chondroid matrix
Ewing's/PNET	15%	10–20 years	F > M	Diaphyses	Lytic with soft tissue component	Small round blue cells

MFH = malignant fibrous histiocytoma; PNET = primitive neuroectodermal tumor.

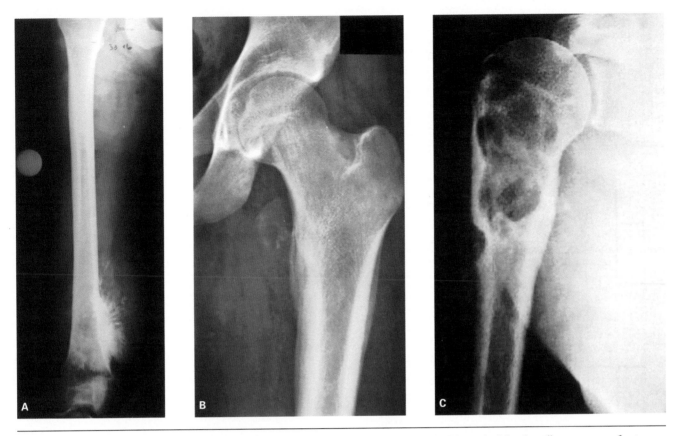

FIGURE 33-7   X-ray imaging of osteosarcoma, Ewing's sarcoma, and chondrosarcoma. **A.** The typical "sunburst" appearance of osteosarcoma. **B.** The "onionskin" appearance often seen in Ewing's sarcoma. **C.** The lobulated appearance of chondrosarcoma.

As with soft tissue sarcomas, biopsy of bone sarcomas is critical to the diagnosis, and careful planning is essential. When patients are diagnosed with bone sarcoma or the diagnosis is suspected, it is important to have a multidisciplinary team approach with physicians who are experienced in the treatment of bone sarcomas. The biopsy method chosen should be the least invasive required to make the diagnosis; most often, however, a core-needle biopsy is performed, as this tends to suffice. A open biopsy should be performed only when core-needle biopsy does not provide enough material for a conclusive diagnosis (139). When surgery is ultimately performed, care should be taken that the biopsy site is also completely resected. The pathologist should be provided not only with the specimen but also with the patient's x-ray images, as these can help make the diagnosis (140).

Once the diagnosis of sarcoma has been made, a chest x-ray, CT scan of the chest, and bone scan should also be performed to evaluate for metastatic disease. As with many sarcomas, the most common site of metastasis from bone sarcoma is the lungs; therefore a thorough examination to screen for pulmonary metastasis is warranted. A bone scan should be included in the workup for metastatic disease in patients with bone sarcoma to evaluate for distant bone metastases or "skip" metastases. For patients with Ewing's sarcoma, an MRI of the spine should be done in the metastatic or staging workup, as there is a risk of bone marrow metastases in these patients. The usefulness of positron emission tomography (PET) and dynamic MRI scans for the workup of bone sarcomas remains to be defined. These scans can be helpful in evaluating viable tumor after or during therapy, especially when patients have a baseline scan with which to compare.

PATHOLOGY

As with soft tissue sarcomas, there are many histologic subsets of bone sarcoma. Osteosarcoma can be broken down into two major categories: conventional osteosarcoma and variant osteosarcoma (Fig. 33-8).

Conventional osteosarcoma comprises approximately 60 to 75% of all osteosarcomas, while the variants comprise the other 35 to 40% (141). Conventional osteosarcoma includes osteoblastic osteosarcoma, chondroblastic osteosarcoma, and fibroblastic osteosarcoma. These classifications are made based on the histologic features

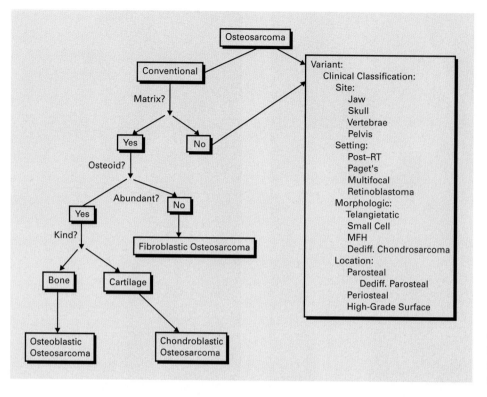

FIGURE 33-8 Flowchart of osteosarcoma: pathologic diagnosis rationale.

of the tumor, such as the amount of matrix present within the tumor and whether bone or cartilage is predominant. The classification of the osteosarcoma variants relies more on the clinical correlation, such as the site of disease (i.e., jaw, skull, or pelvis), the setting in which the disease presents (i.e., postradiation, Paget's disease, multifocal and retinoblastoma), and the morphology, such as telangiectatic, small cell, malignant fibrous histiocytoma of bone (MFH), dedifferentiated chondrosarcoma, and surface lesions such as parosteal, periosteal, and high-grade surface osteosarcoma.

MFH of bone is similar to MFH of soft tissue histologically and often appears to constitute the high-grade component of dedifferentiated chondrosarcoma. MFH is also sometimes seen as a component of fibroblastic osteosarcomas, the only difference between the two being the presence or absence of osteoid. MFH is thought to be part of a spectrum of osteosarcoma where the spindle cells do not produce osteoid visible by light microscopy; however, it may become possible to visualize these at some time in the future.

Chondrosarcoma is a malignant tumor of bone characterized by malignant cartilaginous proliferation. These tumors produce chondroid, a primitive form of cartilage, and can arise from benign processes such as enchondroma. Chondrosarcoma is characterized by the permeation of cartilage into the bone marrow. This process

is virtually pathognomonic for chondrosarcoma when other possibilities, such as chondroblastic osteosarcoma and fracture callus formation, have been excluded. It should be noted that chondroblastic osteosarcoma and chondrosarcoma are two completely separate entities with different prognoses and treatments. Dedifferentiated chondrosarcoma is a unique subset of chondrosarcomas, where the overriding component of MFH or osteosarcoma dictates therapeutic strategy, as opposed to the low-grade chondrosarcoma.

Ewing's sarcoma is a completely separate histology and is grouped with the primitive neuroectodermal tumors owing to their similarities in histology, immunohistochemistical staining, molecular genetics, and tissue culture. This family of tumors includes Ewing's tumors of bone, extraosseus Ewing's, primitive neuroectodermal tumors (PNETs), and Askin's tumors (PNET of the chest wall). These tumors are often referred to as "small round blue cell tumors" because, under the microscope, the cells contain scanty cytoplasm and round to oval nuclei with fine chromatin that are tightly packed together.

An important part of the pathologic review of bone tumors is the grading of the tumors by the pathologist. Bone sarcomas are classified as either high- or low-grade lesions, similar to the three-tier grading system of soft tissue sarcomas. Grading is an important factor that helps to determine the overall "stage" and prognosis.

STAGING AND PROGNOSIS

The staging of bone sarcomas is an area of debate. There are two widely accepted staging systems, that of the American Joint Committee on Cancer and that of the Musculoskeletal Tumor Society (142,143). In a comparison of these systems, there was no significant difference between them and neither had any notable advantage (144). At MDACC, instead of routinely using a staging system, we prefer to emphasize prognostic factors—e.g., size of the primary, location and extent of bone involvement, soft tissue involvement, histologic grade, and presence or absence of distant metastases. The prognosis of patients with bone sarcomas largely depends on the specific histology, grade, location, and presence of metastatic disease. A major predictive factor relating to prognosis and survival of patients with bone sarcoma is the percent of tumor necrosis achieved with preoperative chemotherapy.

TREATMENT

The treatment of bone sarcomas is best accomplished by a multidisciplinary team comprising medical oncologists, surgical oncologists, pathologists, and radiation oncologists working together to provide comprehensive care. The treatment required depends on the tumor type, location, and extent of disease. As with soft tissue sarcomas, the primary endpoint of therapy is to eradicate all gross and microscopic evidence of disease with multimodality treatment whenever possible.

▒ Osteosarcoma

Osteosarcoma is the prototype of most other bone sarcomas. Chemotherapy is the mainstay of treatment for osteosarcoma which is a systemic disease, because most patients have micrometastatic disease at presentation. That is why there is a <20% long-term survival in patients who are treated with surgery alone (145). Patients who receive surgery alone as treatment for localized osteosarcoma tend to have pulmonary metastasis within months of surgery. Aggressive combination chemotherapy with adjuvant surgery for local control can offer "cure" rates of close to 70% in patients with localized, conventional osteosarcoma of an extremity (145). With the use of preoperative chemotherapy, the majority of patients can undergo limb-sparing procedures, which offer increased function and a better quality of life.

At MDACC, patients with conventional high-grade osteosarcoma of an extremity receive treatment consisting of preoperative chemotherapy followed by limb-sparing surgery, followed by postoperative chemotherapy (Fig. 33-9).

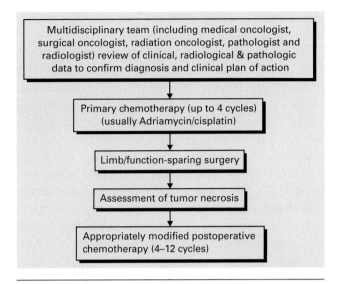

FIGURE 33-9 Treatment approach for patients with osteosarcoma/malignant fibrous histocytoma/dedifferentiated chondrosarcoma.

The postoperative therapy chosen is based on the knowledge of the percent necrosis found in the pathologic specimen after surgery. The most active agents for the treatment of osteosarcoma are cisplatin, doxorubicin (Adriamycin), ifosfamide, and high-dose methotrexate (87,88,146–149). Intraarterial administration of cisplatin (120 mg/m^2) in combination with doxorubicin (90 mg/m^2 continuous infusion over 96 h) given preoperatively has been studied by investigators at MDACC (145). This regimen is given every 3 to 4 weeks for a total of four cycles prior to surgery. Tumor is continually reassessed prior to each two cycles of therapy. The correct assessment of response to this therapy is judged by the percentage of tumor necrosis, as this was found to be the single most important predictor of long-term disease-free and overall survival (150). Generally, patients who had ≥90% tumor necrosis after preoperative chemotherapy were shown to have a 5-year continuous disease-free survival of approximately 80% (145). The 5-year continuous disease-free survival of patients with <90% tumor necrosis after preoperative chemotherapy with doxorubicin and cisplatin depended on their postoperative chemotherapy. If the same doxorubicin-based regimen was continued, it was 13%, compared to 34% with the addition of high-dose methotrexate and 67% with the addition of high-dose methotrexate and ifosfamide (145). For patients who achieved ≥90% tumor necrosis with four cycles of doxorubicin and cisplatin preoperatively, we recommend four additional cycles of doxorubicin (75 mg/m^2) combined with ifosfamide (10 g/m^2). For those who have <90% tumor necrosis after preoperative doxorubicin and cisplatin, we favor six cycles of high-dose ifosfamide and six cycles of high-dose methotrexate given sequentially.

Memorial Sloan Kettering Cancer Center randomized patients to receive the T10 regimen (high-dose methotrexate, bleomycin, cyclophosphamide, dactinomycin) preoperatively, followed by doxorubicin and cisplatin postoperatively, or patients received a more intense regimen of two cycles of doxorubicin or cisplatin in addition to the T10 chemotherapy (T12 protocol) followed by doxorubicin or cisplatin postoperatively (151). The 5-year event-free survival was similar in both groups, at 78 and 73%, respectively. Researchers in Italy performed a series of studies in which they used high-dose methotrexate with one of three combinations (cisplatin and ifosfamide, cisplatin and doxorubicin, or doxorubicin and ifosfamide) (152). Each of the four chemotherapeutic agents was used as a single agent in the postoperative setting. A total of 121 patients with primary osteosarcoma of an extremity were evaluated; the resulting data showed that the limb-salvage rate was 97% and that 32% of patients achieved total tumor necrosis. With a median follow-up of 36 months, 76% of patients remained without recurrence. The projected 3-year continuous disease-free survival was 75%, and the overall survival was 91%. Several other studies using similar combinations have continued to support the use of doxorubicin, cisplatin, ifosfamide, and high-dose methotrexate in the pre- and postoperative treatment of osteosarcoma (153–156).

Patients with high-grade osteosarcomas of other sites are treated in a similar fashion; however, their overall outcome appears to be poorer than that of patients with extremity tumors. This may be due in part to poor sensitivity to the chemotherapy agents and also to difficulties in achieving a negative surgical margin of resection owing to anatomic constraints. Patients with low-grade and variant osteosarcomas—such as well-differentiated intramedullary osteosarcoma or parosteal osteosarcoma and jaw osteosarcoma, typically arising in the mandible, which have a lower tendency to produce distant metastases—are treated with surgical resection with negative margins alone without routine use of adjuvant chemotherapy. If surgical resection with negative margins cannot be achieved in osteosarcoma of the jaw, preoperative chemotherapy should be considered. Patients with intermediate-grade periosteal osteosarcoma should also receive preoperative chemotherapy.

MFH of bone is treated according to the same basic principles as conventional osteosarcoma. Patients are given preoperative chemotherapy, followed by surgical resection, followed by postoperative chemotherapy, which is based on the knowledge of the response to

preoperative chemotherapy or percent tumor necrosis. Studies performed at MDACC showed that with preoperative chemotherapy with doxorubicin and cisplatin, approximately 50% of the patients with localized MFH of bone had percent tumor necrosis of ≥90% (157). The median survival was 23 months for all patients who received this preoperative regimen, with the patients who achieved ≥90% having a median survival of 66 months and patients with <90% necrosis a median survival of 20 months. The European Osteosarcoma Intergroup had similar results in studies using doxorubicin and cisplatin preoperatively and postoperatively, with 5-year progression-free survival and overall survival of 56 and 59%, respectively (158).

With regard to rare histologic variants of osteosarcoma—such as small cell osteosarcoma, unclassified sarcoma, or dedifferentiated osteosarcoma—it should be noted that while these are treated in the same fashion as described, they have a worse prognosis than the histologies discussed above. Patients with these tumors are better treated on investigational protocols that evaluate more intensive regimens or standard regimens in combination with biological agents to improve efficacy.

Metastatic and Recurrent Disease

Most often osteosarcoma metastasizes to the lung; however, osteosarcoma can also metastasize to almost any bone in the body. Rarely are lymph node metastases seen; when they are, it is usually later in the disease process, after or in conjunction with other metastasis. Patients who have resectable pulmonary metastases are treated with curative intent with primary chemotherapy, as described above, followed by surgical resection of all lesions either at the same time or in staged operations. These patients have a 15 to 30% chance of long-term disease-free survival and potential cure, depending on the biology of the disease. Patients with bony metastasis have a poorer prognosis, with therapy usually directed at palliation and prolongation of life as the primary outcomes.

Patients with metastasis or recurrence later are approached in a similar way as those with metastasis at the time of diagnosis; however, options for chemotherapy may be somewhat limited. There are ongoing studies using gemcitabine with or without taxotere as a salvage regimen, as these agents have had some activity in sarcomas (see "Soft Tissue Sarcoma," above).

Chondrosarcoma

Chondrosarcoma is refractory to most of the chemotherapeutic agents used for the treatment of bone sarcomas. Most patients with chondrosarcoma are treated primarily with surgical resection regardless of the grade of the tumor. The exceptions to this rule are mesenchymal chondrosarcoma and dedifferentiated chondrosarcoma. Dedifferentiated chondrosarcoma is associated with low-grade chondrosarcoma, with foci of high-grade sarcoma that resemble osteosarcoma of MFH of bone and are often thought of as variants of osteosarcoma. These tumors can respond to chemotherapy and are treated in the same manner as conventional osteosarcomas (159). Mesenchymal chondrosarcoma is a very rare variant that presents in the jaw, spinal column, and ribs with lytic lesions on x-ray. The histology shows benign to low-grade cartilaginous components with poorly differentiated small cell components. Mesenchymal chondrosarcomas do respond to chemotherapy; they are treated in a similar fashion as Ewing's sarcoma, discussed below.

Ewing's Sarcoma

Like osteosarcoma, Ewing's sarcoma and the PNET family of tumors are treated primarily with chemotherapy prior to surgery, because patients with localized disease most likely have occult metastasis at the time of diagnosis. These tumors are extremely responsive to the following chemotherapeutic agents: doxorubicin, actinomycin D, ifosfamide, cyclophosphamide, vincristine, and VP-16. The most commonly used combinations are vincristine, Adriamycin (doxorubicin) and cyclophosphamide (VAC); ifosfamide and etoposide (IE); and vincristine, Adriamycin, and ifosfamide (VAI). Multiple trials have shown that with these combinations of chemotherapy, survival rates greater than 50% can be achieved (160–163). At MDACC, we usually give vincristine (up to 2 mg) with doxorubicin (75 to 90 mg/m^2) and ifosfamide (10 g/m^2) as our preoperative chemotherapy regimen. This is followed by surgical resection, if possible, or radiation therapy. Ewing's sarcoma is very radiosensitive; often, when surgical resection is not an option or positive margins remain, consolidative radiation therapy is used. There are studies that show good survival results in patients who have consolidative radiation therapy when needed (164). After definitive resection, tumor necrosis is assessed and postoperative therapy modified as needed (Fig. 33-10).

Metastatic/Recurrent Disease

Metastatic or recurrent Ewing's sarcoma is treated in a similar manner as metastatic or recurrent disease in osteosarcoma. Patients who have metastatic disease in their lungs at the time of presentation are treated as out-

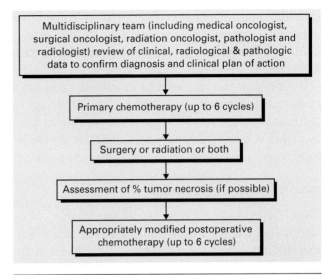

FIGURE 33-10 Treatment approach for patients with Ewing's sarcoma/primitive neuroectodermal tumor and mesenchymal chondrosarcoma.

lined above, with curative intent. Those patients with recurrent or metastatic disease after primary therapy are treated on the basis of their disease-free interval. If there is a long interval (>12 months), a retrial of previous chemotherapeutic regimens preferably at higher dose intensity (e.g., high-dose ifosfamide) is reasonable. For patients with a shorter interval between therapy and recurrence or metastasis, investigational therapies are appropriate. Patients who have bone or bone marrow metastasis are more difficult, as they have a poor prognosis.

FOLLOW-UP MANAGEMENT

Similar to other treatable and potentially curable malignancies, long-term follow up is essential. It is important to follow patients frequently with good-quality chest x-rays to evaluate for pulmonary metastasis and plain films of the primary tumor area to evaluate for local recurrence and to determine the condition of any prosthesis that may be in place. Patients are followed at MDACC with x-rays and physical examination every 3 months for the first 2 years, every 4 months for the next 2 years, every 6 months for the next 2 years, and then yearly thereafter. There are also occasional side effects from chemotherapy that are seen later after treatment. Cardiomyopathy due to doxorubicin is rare, the incidence varying with the cumulative dose and the duration of infusion. Nephrotoxicity due to ifosfamide can be present within weeks to months after chemotherapy, especially when patients are simultaneously taking nonsteroidal anti-inflammatory drugs (NSAIDs) or other nephrotoxic agents. Sensory neuropathy due to cisplatin is often seen in patients who receive more than a 300 mg/m^2 cumulative dose; while this tends to be self-limited, it can take several months to years after chemotherapy before it resolves. The incidence of secondary malignancies such as leukemia is low; however, this is a real possibility and clinicians should be aware of it.

RARE BONE TUMORS

Some mention should be made of tumors that, while rare, are occasionally seen. Chordoma is a "benign" tumor that arises from the remnants of the primitive notochord. While biologically indolent, it can be locally aggressive, with a tendency to occur at either end of the spinal canal. These tumors rarely metastasize. Chordomas occur more frequently in men; they affect younger adults and patients present with symptoms relating to their location. Treatment of these tumors is primarily surgical when feasible. Unresectable chordomas are treated with radiation therapy, as chemotherapy is of little value for chordoma unless dedifferentiation is seen.

Another rare tumor is giant cell tumor of the bone. This is characterized by osteoclast-like giant cells that tend to occur more frequently in young adult women. The tumor tends to involve the epiphyses of long bones and presenting symptoms are usually pain, swelling, and decreased range of motion. Giant cell tumors appear as lytic, eccentrically located lesions in the epiphyses of a long bone on x-ray imaging. While this is also a "benign" tumor histologically, it has been known to recur and to metastasize, primarily to the lungs. Giant cell tumors are treated initially with surgical resection, consisting of intralesional curettage and cementation. If they recur or metastasize and surgical resection becomes prohibitive, they can be treated with systemic therapy. The rationale for systemic therapy is that they are vascular tumors and antiangiogenic therapy might be beneficial. At MDACC, we treat patients with interferon therapy with either 3 million units subcutaneously every day for 6 to 12 months or 10 million units subcutaneously every Monday, Wednesday, and Friday for 6 to 12 months (165). Clinicians must be aware that these tumors respond gradually and can even grow initially on treatment. Often responses are not fully appreciated until after interferon therapy has been completed.

References

1. Jemal A, Tiwari RC, Murray T, et al. Cancer statistics, 2004. *CA Cancer J Clin* 2004;54:8–29.
2. Mark RJ, Poen J, Tran LM, et al. Postirradiation sarcomas. A single-institution study and review of the literature. *Cancer* 1994;73:2653–2662.
3. Brady MS, Gaynor JJ, Brennan MF. Radiation-associated sarcoma of bone and soft tissue. *Arch Surg* 1992;127:1379–1385.
4. Pitcher ME, Davidson TI, Fisher C, et al. Post irradiation sarcoma of soft tissue and bone. *Eur J Surg Oncol* 1994;20:53–56.
5. Wiklund TA, Blomqvist CP, Raty J, et al. Postirradiation sarcoma. Analysis of a nationwide cancer registry material. *Cancer* 1991;68:524–531.
6. Laskin WB, Silverman TA, Enzinger FM. Postradiation soft tissue sarcomas. An analysis of 53 cases. *Cancer* 1988;62:2330–2340.
7. Robinson E, Neugut AI, Wylie P. Clinical aspects of postirradiation sarcomas. *J Natl Cancer Inst* 1988;80:233–240.
8. Kogevinas M, Kauppinen T, Winkelmann R, et al. Soft tissue sarcoma and non-Hodgkin's lymphoma in workers exposed to phenoxy herbicides, chlorophenols, and dioxins: Two nested case-control studies. *Epidemiology* 1995;6:396–402.
9. Grimalt JO, Sunyer J, Moreno V, et al. Risk excess of soft-tissue sarcoma and thyroid cancer in a community exposed to airborne organochlorinated compound mixtures with a high hexachlorobenzene content. *Int J Cancer* 1994;56:200–203.
10. Smith JG, Christophers AJ. Phenoxy herbicides and chlorophenols: A case control study on soft tissue sarcoma and malignant lymphoma. *Br J Cancer* 1992;65:442–448.
11. Johnson CC, Feingold M, Tilley B. A meta-analysis of exposure to phenoxy acid herbicides and chlorophenols in relation to risk of soft tissue sarcoma. *Int Arch Occup Environ Health* 1990;62:513–520.
12. Wingren G, Fredrikson M, Brage HN, et al. Soft tissue sarcoma and occupational exposures. *Cancer* 1990;66:806–811.
13. Eriksson M, Hardell L, Adami HO. Exposure to dioxins as a risk factor for soft tissue sarcoma: A population-based case-control study. *J Natl Cancer Inst* 1990;82:486–490.
14. Hardell L, Eriksson M. The association between soft tissue sarcomas and exposure to phenoxyacetic acids. A new case-referent study. *Cancer* 1988;62:652–656.
15. Zahm SH, Fraumeni JF Jr. The epidemiology of soft tissue sarcoma. *Semin Oncol* 1997;24:504–514.
16. Froehner M, Wirth MP. Etiologic factors in soft tissue sarcomas. *Onkologie* 2001;24:139–142.
17. Marion MJ, Boivin-Angele S. Vinyl chloride-specific mutations in humans and animals. *IARC Sci Publ* 1999:315–324.
18. Helman LJ, Meltzer P. Mechanisms of sarcoma development. *Nat Rev Cancer* 2003;3:685–694.
19. Wickerham DL, Fisher B, Wolmark N, et al. Association of tamoxifen and uterine sarcoma. *J Clin Oncol* 2002;20:2758–2760.
20. Raney RB Jr. Localized sarcoma of the chest wall. *Med Pediatr Oncol* 1984;12:116–118.
21. Joss R, Ganz R, Ryssel HJ, et al. [Posttraumatic soft tissue sarcoma: A case study of a malignant fibrous histiocytoma of the elbow joint which appeared six and a half years after a severe injury]. *J Suisse Med* 1980;110:2021–2024.
22. Stewart FW, Treves N. Classics in oncology: Lymphangiosarcoma in postmastectomy lymphedema: A report of six cases in elephantiasis chirurgica. *CA Cancer J Clin* 1981;31:284–299.

23. Li FP, Fraumeni JF Jr. Soft-tissue sarcomas, breast cancer, and other neoplasms. A familial syndrome? *Ann Intern Med* 1969;71:747–752.

24. Malkin D, Li FP, Strong LC, et al. Germ line p53 mutations in a familial syndrome of breast cancer, sarcomas, and other neoplasms. *Science* 1990;250:1233–1238.

25. Goldberg Y, Dibbern K, Klein J, et al. Neurofibromatosis type 1—An update and review for the primary pediatrician. *Clin Pediatr (Phila)* 1996;35:545–561.

26. Tuveson DA, Fletcher JA. Signal transduction pathways in sarcoma as targets for therapeutic intervention. *Curr Opin Oncol* 2001;13:249–255.

27. Neville H, Corpron C, Blakely ML, et al. Pediatric neurofibrosarcoma. *J Pediatr Surg* 2003;38:343–346; discussion 343–346.

28. Lynch HT, Deters CA, Hogg D, et al. Familial sarcoma: Challenging pedigrees. *Cancer* 2003;98:1947–1957.

29. Mackall CL, Meltzer PS, Helman LJ. Focus on sarcomas. *Cancer Cell* 2000;2:175–178.

30. Sandberg AA, Bridge JA. Updates on the cytogenetics and molecular genetics of bone and soft tissue tumors: Osteosarcoma and related tumors. *Cancer Genet Cytogenet* 2003;145: 1–30.

31. Coindre JM, Pelmus M, Hostein I, et al. Should molecular testing be required for diagnosing synovial sarcoma? A prospective study of 204 cases. *Cancer* 2003;98:2700–2707.

32. Weiss SW, Goldblum JR. *Enzinger and Weiss's Soft Tissue Tumors,* 4th ed. St. Louis: Mosby; 2001.

33. Mann GB, Lewis JJ, Brennan MF. Adult soft tissue sarcoma. *Aust N Z J Surg* 1999;69(5):336–343.

34. Lawrence W Jr, Donegan WL, Natarajan N, et al. Adult soft tissue sarcomas. A pattern of care survey of the American College of Surgeons. *Ann Surg* 1987;205:349–359.

35. Hanna SL, Fletcher BD. MR imaging of malignant soft-tissue tumors. *Magn Reson Imaging Clin North Am* 1995;3:629–650.

36. Chang AE, Matory YL, Dwyer AJ, et al. Magnetic resonance imaging versus computed tomography in the evaluation of soft tissue tumors of the extremities. *Ann Surg* 1987;205: 340–348.

37. Skrzynski MC, Biermann JS, Montag A, et al. Diagnostic accuracy and charge-savings of outpatient core needle biopsy compared with open biopsy of musculoskeletal tumors. *J Bone Joint Surg Am* 1996;78:644–649.

38. Heslin MJ, Lewis JJ, Woodruff JM, et al. Core needle biopsy for diagnosis of extremity soft tissue sarcoma. *Ann Surg Oncol* 1997;4:425–431.

39. Schwartz HS, Spengler DM. Needle tract recurrences after closed biopsy for sarcoma: Three cases and review of the literature. *Ann Surg Oncol* 1997;4:228–236.

40. Kilpatrick SE, Cappellari JO, Bos GD, et al. Is fine-needle aspiration biopsy a practical alternative to open biopsy for the primary diagnosis of sarcoma? Experience with 140 patients. *Am J Clin Pathol* 2001;115:59–68.

41. Ward WG, Savage P, Boles CA, et al. Fine-needle aspiration biopsy of sarcomas and related tumors. *Cancer Control* 2001;8:232–238.

42. Palmer HE, Mukunyadzi P, Culbreth W, et al. Subgrouping and grading of soft-tissue sarcomas by fine-needle aspiration cytology: A histopathologic correlation study. *Diagn Cytopathol* 2001;24:307–316.

43. Patel SR, Zagars GK, Pisters PW. The follow-up of adult soft-tissue sarcomas. *Semin Oncol* 2003;30:413–416.

44. Broders AC, Hargrave R, Meyerding HW. Pathologic features of soft tissue fibrosarcoma with special reference to the grading of its malignancy. *Surg Gynecol Obstet* 1939;69.

45. Pisters PW, Leung DH, Woodruff J, et al. Analysis of prognostic factors in 1,041 patients with localized soft tissue sarcomas of the extremities. *J Clin Oncol* 1996;14:1679–1689.

46. Coindre JM, Terrier P, Bui NB, et al. Prognostic factors in adult patients with locally controlled soft tissue sarcoma. A study of 546 patients from the French Federation of Cancer Centers Sarcoma Group. *J Clin Oncol* 1996;14:869–877.

47. Soft tissue sarcoma. In: Green FL, Page DL, Fleming ID, et al (eds): *AJCC Cancer Staging Handbook, From the AJCC Cancer Staging Manual,* 6th ed. Philadelphia: Lippincott-Raven; 2002:221–228.

48. Kattan MW, Leung DH, Brennan MF. Postoperative nomogram for 12-year sarcoma-specific death. *J Clin Oncol* 2002; 20:791–796.

49. Stojadinovic A, Yeh A, Brennan MF. Completely resected recurrent soft tissue sarcoma: Primary anatomic site governs outcomes. *J Am Coll Surg* 2002;194:436–447.

50. Gaynor JJ, Tan CC, Casper ES, et al. Refinement of clinicopathologic staging for localized soft tissue sarcoma of the extremity: A study of 423 adults. *J Clin Oncol* 1992;10: 1317–1329.

51. Lewis JJ, Leung D, Heslin M, et al. Association of local recurrence with subsequent survival in extremity soft tissue sarcoma. *J Clin Oncol* 1997;15:646–652.

52. Bowden L, Booher RJ. The principles and technique of resection of soft parts for sarcoma. *Surgery* 1958;44:963–977.

53. Cantin J, McNeer GP, Chu FC, et al. The problem of local recurrence after treatment of soft tissue sarcoma. *Ann Surg* 1968;168:47–53.

54. Gerner RE, Moore GE, Pickren JW. Soft tissue sarcomas. *Ann Surg* 1975;181:803–808.

55. Pisters PW, Harrison LB, Leung DH, et al. Long-term results of a prospective randomized trial of adjuvant brachytherapy in soft tissue sarcoma. *J Clin Oncol* 1996;14:859–868.

56. Yang JC, Chang AE, Baker AR, et al. Randomized prospective study of the benefit of adjuvant radiation therapy in the treatment of soft tissue sarcomas of the extremity. *J Clin Oncol* 1998;16:197–203.

57. Karakousis CP, Proimakis C, Walsh DL. Primary soft tissue sarcoma of the extremities in adults. *Br J Surg* 1995;82: 1208–1212.

58. Fong Y, Coit DG, Woodruff JM, et al. Lymph node metastasis from soft tissue sarcoma in adults. Analysis of data from a prospective database of 1772 sarcoma patients. *Ann Surg* 1993;217:72–77.

59. Weingrad DN, Rosenberg SA. Early lymphatic spread of osteogenic and soft-tissue sarcomas. *Surgery* 1978;84:231–240.

60. Rosenberg SA, Tepper J, Glatstein E, et al. Prospective randomized evaluation of adjuvant chemotherapy in adults with soft tissue sarcomas of the extremities. *Cancer* 1983;52: 424–434.

61. Williard WC, Collin C, Casper ES, et al. The changing role of amputation for soft tissue sarcoma of the extremity in adults. *Surg Gynecol Obstet* 1992;175:389–396.

62. Johnstone PA, Wexler LH, Venzon DJ, et al. Sarcomas of the hand and foot: Analysis of local control and functional result

with combined modality therapy in extremity preservation. *Int J Radiat Oncol Biol Phys* 1994;29:735–745.

63. Yang JC, Rosenberg SA. Surgery for adult patients with soft tissue sarcomas. *Semin Oncol* 1989;16:289–296.

64. Rosenberg SA, Tepper J, Glatstein E, et al. The treatment of soft-tissue sarcomas of the extremities: Prospective randomized evaluations of (1) limb-sparing surgery plus radiation therapy compared with amputation and (2) the role of adjuvant chemotherapy. *Ann Surg* 1982;196:305–315.

65. Eggermont AM, Schraffordt Koops H, Lienard D, et al. Isolated limb perfusion with high-dose tumor necrosis factor-alpha in combination with interferon-gamma and melphalan for nonresectable extremity soft tissue sarcomas: A multicenter trial. *J Clin Oncol* 1996;14:2653–2665.

66. Yang JC, Fraker DL, Thom AK, et al. Isolation perfusion with tumor necrosis factor-alpha, interferon-gamma, and hyperthermia in the treatment of localized and metastatic cancer. *Recent Results Cancer Res* 1995;138:161–166.

67. Lienard D, Ewalenko P, Delmotte JJ, et al. High-dose recombinant tumor necrosis factor alpha in combination with interferon gamma and melphalan in isolation perfusion of the limbs for melanoma and sarcoma. *J Clin Oncol* 1992;10:52–60.

68. Suit H, Spiro I. Radiation as a therapeutic modality in sarcomas of the soft tissue. *Hematol Oncol Clin North Am* 1995;9:733–746.

69. Tepper JE, Suit HD. Radiation therapy alone for sarcoma of soft tissue. *Cancer* 1985;56:475–479.

70. Pickering DG, Stewart JS, Rampling R, et al. Fast neutron therapy for soft tissue sarcoma. *Int J Radiat Oncol Biol Phys* 1987;13:1489–1495.

71. Slater JD, McNeese MD, Peters LJ. Radiation therapy for unresectable soft tissue sarcomas. *Int J Radiat Oncol Biol Phys* 1986;12:1729–1734.

72. O'Sullivan B, Davis AM, Turcotte R, et al. Preoperative versus postoperative radiotherapy in soft-tissue sarcoma of the limbs: A randomised trial. *Lancet* 2002;359:2235–2241.

73. O'Sullivan B, Davis A. A randomized phase III trial of preoperative compared to postoperative radiotherapy in extremity soft tissue sarcoma. *Proc ASTRO* 2001;151.

74. Wayne JD, Langstein H, Pollack A, et al. Preoperative radiotherapy for extremity soft tissue sarcoma (STS): Site-specific wound complication rates and the impact of reconstructive surgery. New Orleans, LA. *Proc Am Soc Clin Oncol* 2000:558a.

75. Robinson MH, Keus RB, Shasha D, et al. Is pre-operative radiotherapy superior to postoperative radiotherapy in the treatment of soft tissue sarcoma? *Eur J Cancer* 1998;34:1309–1316.

76. Zagars GK, Ballo MT, Pisters PW, et al. Preoperative vs postoperative radiation therapy for soft tissue sarcoma: A retrospective comparative evaluation of disease outcome. *Int J Radiat Oncol Biol Phys* 2003;56:482–488.

77. Suit HD, Mankin HJ, Wood WC, et al. Preoperative, intraoperative, and postoperative radiation in the treatment of primary soft tissue sarcoma. *Cancer* 1985;55:2659–2667.

78. Nielsen OS, Cummings B, O'Sullivan B, et al. Preoperative and postoperative irradiation of soft tissue sarcomas: Effect of radiation field size. *Int J Radiat Oncol Biol Phys* 1991;21:1595–1599.

79. Stinson SF, DeLaney TF, Greenberg J, et al. Acute and long-term effects on limb function of combined modality limb

sparing therapy for extremity soft tissue sarcoma. *Int J Radiat Oncol Biol Phys* 1991;21:1493–1499.

80. Pollack A, Zagars GK, Goswitz MS, et al. Preoperative vs postoperative radiotherapy in the treatment of soft tissue sarcomas: A matter of presentation. *Int J Radiat Oncol Biol Phys* 1998;42:563–572.

81. Suit HD, Mankin HJ, Wood WC, et al. Treatment of the patient with stage M0 soft tissue sarcoma. *J Clin Oncol* 1988;6:854–862.

82. Fein DA, Lee WR, Lanciano RM, et al. Management of extremity soft tissue sarcomas with limb-sparing surgery and postoperative irradiation: Do total dose, overall treatment time, and the surgery-radiotherapy interval impact on local control? *Int J Radiat Oncol Biol Phys* 1995;32:969–976.

83. Brennan MF, Hilaris B, Shiu MH, et al. Local recurrence in adult soft-tissue sarcoma. A randomized trial of brachytherapy. *Arch Surg* 1987;122:1289–1293.

84. Janjan NA, Yasko AW, Reece GP, et al. Comparison of charges related to radiotherapy for soft-tissue sarcomas treated by preoperative external-beam irradiation versus interstitial implantation. *Ann Surg Oncol* 1994;1:415–422.

85. Ahmad SA, Patel SR, Ballo MT, et al. Extraosseous osteosarcoma: Response to treatment and long-term outcome. *J Clin Oncol* 2002;20:521–527.

86. O'Bryan RM, Baker LH, Gottlieb JE, et al. Dose response evaluation of Adriamycin in human neoplasia. *Cancer* 1977;39:1940–1948.

87. Patel S, Vadhan-Raj S, Papadopoulos N, et al. High-dose ifosfamide in bone and soft-tissue sarcomas: Results of phase II and pilot studies—Dose response and schedule dependence. *J Clin Oncol* 1997;15:2378–2384.

88. Patel SR, Benjamin RS. Ifosfamide in sarcomas: Is it a schedule-dependent drug? *Cancer Invest* 1996;14:290–291.

89. Benjamin RS, Legha SS, Patel SR, et al. Single-agent ifosfamide studies in sarcomas of soft tissue and bone: The MD Anderson experience. *Cancer Chemother Pharmacol* 1993;31(suppl 2):S174–S179.

90. Antman KH, Ryan L, Elias A, et al. Response to ifosfamide and mesna: 124 previously treated patients with metastatic or unresectable sarcoma. *J Clin Oncol* 1989;7:126–131.

91. Bramwell V, Quirt I, Warr D, et al. Combination chemotherapy with doxorubicin, dacarbazine, and ifosfamide in advanced adult soft tissue sarcoma. Canadian Sarcoma Group—National Cancer Institute of Canada Clinical Trials Group. *J Natl Cancer Inst* 1989;81:1496–1499.

92. Elias A, Ryan L, Sulkes A, et al. Response to mesna, doxorubicin, ifosfamide, and dacarbazine in 108 patients with metastatic or unresectable sarcoma and no prior chemotherapy. *J Clin Oncol* 1989;7:1208–1216.

93. Vadhan-Raj S, Patel S, Burgess MA, et al. Phase II trial of Adriamycin (A), ifosfamide (I), mesna (M), uroprotection, darcarbazine (D) (MAID) with PIXY321 (GM-CSF/IL-3 fusion protein) of G-CSF in patients (PTS) with soft tissue sarcoma (STS). *Proc Am Soc Clin Oncol* 1996:525.

94. Patel S, Vadhan-Raj S, Burgess M, et al. Results of two consecutive trials of dose-intensive chemotherapy with doxorubicin and ifosfamide in patients with sarcomas. *Am J Clin Oncol* 1998;21:317–321.

95. Patel SR. *Dose Intensive Chemotherapy for Soft Tissue Sarcoma.* American Society of Clinical Oncology Educational

Booklet. Alexandria, VA: Lippincott Williams & Wilkins; 2000:453–457.

96. Patel SR, Gandhi V, Jenkins J, et al. Phase II clinical investigation of gemcitabine in advanced soft tissue sarcomas and window evaluation of dose rate on gemcitabine triphosphate accumulation. *J Clin Oncol* 2001;19:3483–3489.

97. Touroutoglou N, Gravel D, Raber MN, et al. Clinical results of a pharmacodynamically-based strategy for higher dosing of gemcitabine in patients with solid tumors. *Ann Oncol* 1998;9:1003–1008.

98. Tempero M, Plunkett W, Ruiz van Haperen V, et al. Randomized phase II comparison of dose-intense gemcitabine: Thirty-minute infusion and fixed dose rate infusion in patients with pancreatic adenocarcinoma. *J Clin Oncol* 2003; 21:3402–3408.

99. Hensley ML, Maki R, Venkatraman E, et al. Gemcitabine and docetaxel in patients with unresectable leiomyosarcoma: Results of a phase II trial. *J Clin Oncol* 2002;20:2824–2831.

100. Edmonson JH, Ebbert LP, Nascimento AG, et al. Phase II study of docetaxel in advanced soft tissue sarcomas. *Am J Clin Oncol* 1996;19:574–576.

101. van Hoesel QG, Verweij J, Catimel G, et al. Phase II study with docetaxel (Taxotere) in advanced soft tissue sarcomas of the adult. EORTC Soft Tissue and Bone Sarcoma Group. *Ann Oncol* 1994;5:539–542.

102. Delaloge S, Yovine A, Taamma A, et al. Ecteinascidin-743: A marine-derived compound in advanced, pretreated sarcoma patients—Preliminary evidence of activity. *J Clin Oncol* 2001;19:1248–1255.

103. Demetri GD. ET-743: The US experience in sarcomas of soft tissues. *Anticancer Drugs* 13(suppl 1):S7–S9.

104. Talbot SM, Keohan ML, Hesdorffer M, et al. A phase II trial of temozolomide in patients with unresectable or metastatic soft tissue sarcoma. *Cancer* 2003;98:1942–1946.

105. Woll PJ, Judson I, Lee SM, et al. Temozolomide in adult patients with advanced soft tissue sarcoma: A phase II study of the EORTC Soft Tissue and Bone Sarcoma Group. *Eur J Cancer* 1999;35:410–412.

106. Cosetti M, Wexler LH, Calleja E, et al. Irinotecan for pediatric solid tumors: The Memorial Sloan-Kettering experience. *J Pediatr Hematol Oncol* 2002;24:101–105.

107. Patel SR, Beach J, Papadopoulos N, et al. Results of a 2-arm phase II study of 9-nitrocamptothecin in patients with advanced soft-tissue sarcomas. *Cancer* 2003;97:2848–2852.

108. Patel SR, Jenkins J, Papadopolous N, et al. Pilot study of vitaxin—An angiogenesis inhibitor-in patients with advanced leiomyosarcomas. *Cancer* 2001;92:1347–1348.

109. Sirvent N, Maire G, Pedeutour F. Genetics of dermatofibrosarcoma protuberans family of tumors: From ring chromosomes to tyrosine kinase inhibitor treatment. *Genes Chromosomes Cancer* 2003;37:1–19.

110. Clark SK. Sulindac and tamoxifen in the treatment of desmoid tumours in patients with familial adenomatous polyposis. *Colorectal Dis* 2002;4:68.

111. Hansmann A, Adolph C, Vogel T, et al. High-dose tamoxifen and sulindac as first-line treatment for desmoid tumors. *Cancer* 2004;100:612–620.

112. Tonelli F, Ficari F, Valanzano R, et al. Treatment of desmoids and mesenteric fibromatosis in familial adenomatous polyposis with raloxifene. *Tumori* 2003;89:391–396.

113. Heidemann J, Ogawa H, Otterson MF, et al. Antiangiogenic treatment of mesenteric desmoid tumors with toremifene and interferon alpha-2b: Report of two cases. *Dis Colon Rectum* 2004;47:118–122.

114. Debrock G, Vanhentenrijk V, Sciot R, et al. A phase II trial with rosiglitazone in liposarcoma patients. *Br J Cancer* 2003;89:1409–1412.

115. Agarwal VR, Bischoff ED, Hermann T, et al. Induction of adipocyte-specific gene expression is correlated with mammary tumor regression by the retinoid X receptor-ligand LGD1069 (Targretin). *Cancer Res* 2000;60:6033–6038.

116. Adjuvant chemotherapy for localised resectable soft-tissue sarcoma of adults: meta-analysis of individual data. Sarcoma Meta-analysis Collaboration. *Lancet* 1997;350:1647–1654.

117. Frustaci S, Gherlinzoni F, De Paoli A, et al. Adjuvant chemotherapy for adult soft tissue sarcomas of the extremities and girdles: Results of the Italian randomized cooperative trial. *J Clin Oncol* 2001;19:1238–1247.

118. Patel SR. *Dose-Intensive Chemotherapy for Soft Tissue Sarcomas.* American Society of Clinical Oncology;2000:453–457.

119. Fletcher CD, Berman JJ, Corless C, et al. Diagnosis of gastrointestinal stromal tumors: A consensus approach. *Hum Pathol* 2002;33:459–465.

120. Kindblom LG, Remotti HE, Aldenborg F, et al. Gastrointestinal pacemaker cell tumor (GIPACT): Gastrointestinal stromal tumors show phenotypic characteristics of the interstitial cells of Cajal [see comments]. *Am J Pathol* 1998;152:1259–1269.

121. DeMatteo RP, Lewis JJ, Leung D, et al. Two hundred gastrointestinal stromal tumors: Recurrence patterns and prognostic factors for survival. *Ann Surg* 2000;231:51–58.

122. Gottlieb J, Baker L, O'Bryan R, et al. Adriamycin (NSC-123-127) used alone and in combination for soft tissue and bony sarcomas. *Cancer Chemother Rep* 1974;6:271–282.

123. Trent JC, Beach J, Burgess MA, et al. A two-arm phase II study of temozolomide in patients with advanced gastrointestinal stromal tumors and other soft tissue sarcomas. *Cancer* 2003;98:2693–2699.

124. Buchdunger E, Cioffi CL, Law N, et al. Abl protein-tyrosine kinase inhibitor STI571 inhibits in vitro signal transduction mediated by c-Kit and platelet-derived growth factor receptors [In Process Citation]. *J Pharmacol Exp Ther* 2000;295:139–145.

125. Savage DG, Antman KH. Imatinib mesylate—A new oral targeted therapy. *N Engl J Med* 2002;346:683–693.

126. Joensuu H, Roberts P, Sarlomo-Rikala M, et al. Effect of the tyrosine kinase inhibitor STI571 in a patient with a metastatic gastrointestinal stromal tumor. *N Engl J Med* 2001; 344:1052–1056.

127. van Oosterom AT, Judson IR, Verweij J, et al. Update of phase I study of imatinib (STI571) in advanced soft tissue sarcomas and gastrointestinal stromal tumors: A report of the EORTC Soft Tissue and Bone Sarcoma Group. *Eur J Cancer* 2002;38(suppl 5):S83–S87.

128. Verweij J, van Oosterom A, Blay JY, et al. Imatinib mesylate (STI-571 Glivec, Gleevec) is an active agent for gastrointestinal stromal tumours, but does not yield responses in other soft-tissue sarcomas that are unselected for a molecular target. Results from an EORTC Soft Tissue and Bone Sarcoma Group phase II study. *Eur J Cancer* 2003;39:2006–2011.

129. Van Oosterom A, Judson I, Verweij J. STI57, an active drug in metastatic gastrointestinal stromal tumors (GIST), an EORTC phase I study. *Proc Am Soc Clin Oncol* 2001;(abstr 2).

130. Demetri GD, von Mehren M, Blanke CD, et al. Efficacy and safety of imatinib mesylate in advanced gastrointestinal stromal tumors. *N Engl J Med* 2002;347:472–480.

131. Bauer S, Corless CL, Heinrich MC, et al. Response to imatinib mesylate of a gastrointestinal stromal tumor with very low expression of KIT. *Cancer Chemother Pharmacol* 2003; 51:261–265.

132. Van den Abbeele A, Badawi R, Cliche J-P, et al. 18F-FDG PET predicts response to imatinib mesylate (Gleevec) in patients with advanced gastrointestinal stromal tumors (GIST). *Proc Am Soc Clin Oncol* 2002;(abstr 1610).

133. Fleming JB, Cantor SB, Varma DG, et al. Utility of chest computed tomography for staging in patients with T1 extremity soft tissue sarcomas. *Cancer* 2001;92:863–868.

134. Demetri GD, Delaney T. NCCN: Sarcoma. *Cancer Control* 2001;8:94–101.

135. Paulussen M, Ahrens S, Craft AW, et al. Ewing's tumors with primary lung metastases: Survival analysis of 114 (European Intergroup) Cooperative Ewing's Sarcoma Studies patients. *J Clin Oncol* 1998;16:3044–3052.

136. Cotterill SJ, Ahrens S, Paulussen M, et al. Prognostic factors in Ewing's tumor of bone: Analysis of 975 patients from the European Intergroup Cooperative Ewing's Sarcoma Study Group. *J Clin Oncol* 2000;18:3108–3114.

137. Dahlin DC, Coventry MB. Osteogenic sarcoma. A study of six hundred cases. *J Bone Joint Surg Am* 1967;49:101–110.

138. Wick MR, Siegal GP, Unni KK, et al. Sarcomas of bone complicating osteitis deformans (Paget's disease): Fifty years' experience. *Am J Surg Pathol* 1981;5:47–59.

139. Ayala AG, Raymond AK, Ro JY, et al. Needle biopsy of primary bone lesions. MD Anderson experience. *Pathol Annu* 1989;24(pt 1):219–251.

140. Raymond AK, Simms W, Ayala AG. Osteosarcoma. Specimen management following primary chemotherapy. *Hematol Oncol Clin North Am* 1995;9:841–867.

141. Raymond AK. Basic Pathology of Osteosarcoma. In: Blakely LJ (ed): Houston, TX: 2004.

142. Enneking WF, Spanier SS, Goodman MA. A system for the surgical staging of musculoskeletal sarcoma. *Clin Orthop* 1980;106–120.

143. Bone, in Green FL, Page DL, Fleming ID, et al (eds): *AJCC Cancer Staging Handbook*, 6th ed. New York: Springer-Verlag; 2002:213–319.

144. Heck RK Jr, Stacy GS, Flaherty MJ, et al. A comparison study of staging systems for bone sarcomas. *Clin Orthop* 2003:64–71.

145. Jaffe N, Patel SR, Benjamin RS. Chemotherapy in osteosarcoma. Basis for application and antagonism to implementation: Early controversies surrounding its implementation. *Hematol Oncol Clin North Am* 1995;9:825–840.

146. Petrilli S, Penna V, Lopes A, et al. IIB osteosarcoma. Current management, local control, and survival statistics—São Paulo, Brazil. *Clin Orthop* 1991;60–66.

147. Cortes EP, Holland JF, Glidewell O. Osteogenic sarcoma studies by the Cancer and Leukemia Group B. *Natl Cancer Inst Monogr* 1981;207–209.

148. Antman KH, Montella D, Rosenbaum C, et al. Phase II trial of ifosfamide with mesna in previously treated metastatic sarcoma. *Cancer Treat Rep* 1985;69:499–504.

149. Jaffe N. Recent advances in the chemotherapy of metastatic osteogenic sarcoma. *Cancer* 1972;30:1627–1631.

150. Raymond AK, Chawla SP, Carrasco CH, et al. Osteosarcoma chemotherapy effect: A prognostic factor. *Semin Diagn Pathol* 1987;4:212–236.

151. Meyers P, Heller G, Healey J. Chemotherapy for nonmetastatic osteogenic sarcoma: The Memorial Sloan-Kettering experience. *J Clin Oncol* 1992;10:5–15.

152. Bacci G, Ferrari S, Mercuri M, et al. Neoadjuvant chemotherapy for extremity osteosarcoma: Preliminary results of the Rizzoli's 4th study. *Acta Oncol* 1998;37:41–48.

153. Goorin AM, Schwartzentruber DJ, Devidas M, et al. Presurgical chemotherapy compared with immediate surgery and adjuvant chemotherapy for nonmetastatic osteosarcoma: Pediatric Oncology Group Study POG-8651. *J Clin Oncol* 2003;21:1574–1580.

154. Souhami RL, Craft AW, Van der Eijken JW, et al. Randomised trial of two regimens of chemotherapy in operable osteosarcoma: A study of the European Osteosarcoma Intergroup. *Lancet* 1997;350:911–917.

155. Benjamin RS, Patel SR, Armen T, et al. The value of ifosfamide in the postoperative neoadjuvant chemotherapy of osteosarcoma. *Proc Am Soc Clin Oncol* 1995;516.

156. Link M, Goorin A, Miser A. The effect of adjuvant chemotherapy on relapse-free survival in patients with osteosarcoma of the extremity. *N Engl J Med* 1986;314:1600–1606.

157. Patel SR, Armen T, Carrasco CH, et al. Primary chemotherapy in malignant fribrous histiocytoma of bone. In: Banzet P, Holland J, Khayat D, et al (eds): *U.T.M.D. Anderson Cancer Center Experience. Cancer Treatment—An Update.* Houston, TX: MDACC; 1994:577–580.

158. Bramwell VH, Steward WP, Nooij M, et al. Neoadjuvant chemotherapy with doxorubicin and cisplatin in malignant fibrous histiocytoma of bone: A European Osteosarcoma Intergroup study. *J Clin Oncol* 1999;17:3260–3269.

159. Benjamin RS, Chu P, Patel SR, et al. *De-differentiated Chondrosarcoma: A Treatable Disease.* American Association of Cancer Research; 1995.

160. Paulussen M, Ahrens S, Dunst J, et al. Localized Ewing tumor of bone: Final results of the cooperative Ewing's Sarcoma Study CESS 86. *J Clin Oncol* 2001;19:1818–1829.

161. Burgert EO Jr, Nesbit ME, Garnsey LA, et al. Multimodal therapy for the management of nonpelvic, localized Ewing's sarcoma of bone: Intergroup study IESS-II. *J Clin Oncol* 1990;8:1514–1524.

162. Rosito P, Mancini AF, Rondelli R, et al. Italian Cooperative Study for the treatment of children and young adults with localized Ewing sarcoma of bone: A preliminary report of 6 years of experience. *Cancer* 1999;86:421–428.

163. Craft A, Cotterill S, Malcolm A, et al. Ifosfamide-containing chemotherapy in Ewing's sarcoma: The Second United Kingdom Children's Cancer Study Group and the Medical Research Council Ewing's Tumor Study. *J Clin Oncol* 1998; 16:3628–3633.

164. Dunst J, Schuck A. Role of radiotherapy in Ewing tumors. *Pediatr Blood Cancer* 2004;42:465–470.

165. Benjamin RS, Patel SR, Gutterman JU, et al. Interferon alpha-2b as anti-angiogenesis therapy of giant cell tumor of bone: Implications for the study of newer angiogenesis-inhibitors. *Proc Am Soc Clin Oncol* 1999:548a.

CHAPTER
34

AIDS-RELATED MALIGNANCIES

Maricer P. Escalón
Fredrick B. Hagemeister

First described in 1983, HIV is now recognized worldwide as a cause of the acquired immunodeficiency syndrome (AIDS). Since the onset of the AIDS epidemic, advances in therapy have prolonged the median life expectancy of patients with HIV infection to more than 12 years (1). However, a consequence of this improved survival rate is a rising incidence of HIV-related malignancies. Levine has predicted that up to 40% of persons with AIDS will develop cancer (2). Therapy for these malignancies will thus pose a significant challenge to physicians caring for these patients in the future.

HIV induces immune dysfunction in a variety of ways. Immune abnormalities observed in HIV infection include depletion and dysfunction of CD4-positive T cells, polyclonal activation of B cells (often associated with hypergammaglobulinemia and autoimmune phenomena), and diminished function of monocytes, macrophages, and natural killer cells (3). Patients also exhibit impaired B-cell response to T-cell–dependent antigens, dysfunction of cell-mediated immunity, poor delayed-type hypersensitivity, and abnormal cytokine expression. Collectively, these defects of the immune system provide multiple opportunities for malignant transformation on the molecular level and, once this is established, the maintenance of malignant cell growth (3–5).

By the time the HIV epidemic was under way, investigators had already realized that transplant recipients develop atypical lymphomas involving extranodal sites or the central nervous system (CNS) at 25 to 50 times the rate expected among nontransplant populations, anogenital cancer at 100 times, Kaposi's sarcoma at 400 to 500 times, and squamous-cell cancers of the skin at 3 to 20 times the expected rate (6–8). These patients present with malignancy within 2 to 8 years of the onset of immunosuppressive therapy and often exhibit particularly virulent tumors (8). Similarly, HIV-infected patients present with malignancy at a higher than expected rate, at younger ages, and with more virulent courses than the general population.

Malignancy in patients with impaired immunity is the result of multiple factors. Immunosuppression itself can impair immune surveillance, which controls virally mediated cancers. Immunosuppressed patients often demonstrate chronic antigenic stimulation induced by an allograft or by repetitive acquired infections, which may increase the opportunity for random transforming mutations. Finally, dysregulation of the immune system, with a lack of the proper suppressor mechanisms, may result in malignant transformation (7).

Although many malignancies have been reported in association with HIV infection, only three are conclusively associated with HIV infection and are considered AIDS-defining conditions. These include Kaposi's sarcoma (KS), intermediate or high-grade non-Hodgkin's B-cell lymphomas (including primary CNS lymphoma), and cervical carcinoma (9–12). Other malignancies (e.g., Hodgkin's lymphoma, anorectal carcinoma, pediatric smooth muscle tumors, noncervical gynecologic cancers, and nonmelanoma skin cancers) may be associated with AIDS, as their incidence is higher in patients with HIV-positive serology. This chapter focuses on those malignancies that define AIDS.

■ KAPOSI'S SARCOMA

Prior to the AIDS epidemic, KS appeared mostly as an indolent, pigmented lesion involving the lower extremities in older men of Jewish, eastern European, or Mediterranean descent (13,14). The disease rarely involved lymph nodes, mucous membranes, or visceral organs. However, up to one-third of these patients demonstrated a second primary malignancy, most frequently non-Hodgkin's lymphoma (13,14).

Aggressive KS has been reported as the most prevalent cancer among HIV-1–infected patients (Fig. 34-1) (15,16), and may appear at any stage of HIV disease. Immune impairment is usually present: less than one-sixth of HIV-infected patients have CD4-positive T-cell counts of more than 500/μL; most cases develop when the CD4-positive cell count is more than 200/μL (6,14,17). The incidence and severity of the disease has

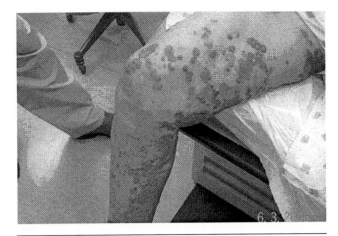

FIGURE 34-1 An example of Kaposi's sarcoma.

especially declined in the era of effective HIV treatment, especially highly active antiretroviral therapy (HAART).

The prevalence of KS varies among different categories of AIDS patients by the route of HIV infection and by geographic location (5,14). KS is six times more common in male homosexuals than in other risk groups, and 95% of AIDS-related KS cases in the United States and Europe are diagnosed in homosexual males (13). For this reason, a sexually transmitted agent was thought to be responsible for the pathogenesis of the disease even before the discovery of KS-associated herpesvirus/human herpesvirus 8 (KSHV/HHV-8) in 1994 (18).

PATHOLOGY

All forms of KS are characterized by a proliferation of spindle cells in a background network of reticular and collagen fibers, vascular and lymphatic proliferation, and the presence of mononuclear cells, including macrophages, lymphocytes, and plasma cells. Tumors are highly vascular, accounting for their purplish hue. Lesions may involve only the reticular dermis (patch stage) or the full thickness of the dermis (plaque or nodular stage). As lesions evolve to the plaque and nodular stages, the number of interstitial cells increases. The abundance of cells is thought to reflect a cytokine-rich environment (2,6,14,19).

The cell of origin of KS lesions is unknown. Investigators have observed endothelial (factor VIIIa) and spindle cell markers and expression of the gene for smooth muscle alpha-actin in vitro, implicating a vascular or lymphatic endothelial cell or vascular smooth muscle cell as the cell of origin (6,10,14,19,20). KS cells also coexpress macrophage markers such as PAM-1, CD68, and CD14 (21). Therefore the lesions have

been thought to originate from a pluripotent mesenchymal precursor cell. However, investigators have recently proposed that KS spindle cells belong to the endothelial lineage that differentiates into lymphatic cells (22).

PATHOGENESIS

The discovery of KS-associated herpesvirus/human herpesvirus 8 (KSHV/HHV-8) in cells isolated from a KS lesion 9 years ago was rapidly followed by molecular and hematologic data confirming an etiologic link between the virus and development of KS lesions (22). KSHV, a novel human γ-herpesvirus, is present in KS spindle cells and in flat endothelial cells lining vascular spaces of KS lesions (23). KSHV chemokines and cytokines, such as IL-6, have been shown to stimulate spindle cells and promote angiogenesis, which may contribute to the pathogenesis of KS (24,25).

KS is believed to be caused by KSHV, but the tumor's microenvironment also plays an important role in the pathogenesis of the disease (22). KS cells maintained in culture can induce angiogenesis, but they also produce cytokines that promote their own growth and the growth of normal endothelial cells, fibroblasts, and other mesenchymal cells (19). Angiogenic cytokines include interleukin (IL)-1 beta, basic fibroblast growth factor, acidic fibroblast growth factor, endothelial cell growth factor, and vascular endothelial growth factor receptor 3 (15,19,22). Other cytokines include IL-6, granulocyte-macrophage colony-stimulating factor (GM-CSF), transforming growth factor beta (TGF-β), and platelet-derived growth factor alpha (PDGF-α). KS cells also respond to exogenously produced cytokines originating from HIV-infected T cells, including IL-1, fibroblast growth factor, IL-6, and oncostatin M (2,6,14, 15,19,20). Oncostatin M acts directly to stimulate KS cells and induces KS cells to produce IL-6, which acts to sustain growth in an autocrine fashion.

The HIV virus itself may be responsible for the transformation of nonmalignant to malignant KS cells. When Vogel et al. transfected fertilized eggs from mice with a recombinant HIV transactivating (TAT) gene with a long terminal repeat sequence, they observed the development of lesions resembling KS in 15% of male offspring (26). Investigators have also demonstrated that the TAT gene product can promote the growth of AIDS-associated KS cells (2), possibly by stimulating KSHV replication (24). The process of oncologic transformation may be associated with the expression of certain receptors such as IL-6 and oncostatin M, distinguishing KS cells from their normal counterparts.

CLINICAL FEATURES

Typical lesions range from violaceous to brown and may be flat or raised and ulcerated. They are usually multicentric and symmetric and may be in various stages of development. The lesions do not blanch and are usually not tender. A biopsy must be obtained to exclude bacillary angiomatosis or pyogenic granuloma, which may have a similar presentation in AIDS patients (2,14). The tumor is often widespread, involving the skin, mucous membranes, gastrointestinal tract, lymph nodes, genitalia, oral cavity, conjunctiva, and/or lungs and airways.

Oral KS is a marker of more advanced HIV infection. Patients exhibit CD4 cell counts of less than 200/μL and associated involvement of the gastrointestinal tract in 50% of cases. Gastrointestinal KS may be manifest by bleeding, diarrhea, or weight loss. Because barium enema studies may fail to demonstrate flat lesions, these patients should instead undergo endoscopy. Patients with pulmonary KS can present with shortness of breath, fever, cough, hemoptysis, or chest pain or be asymptomatic. The radiographic appearance of the disease is nonspecific and may demonstrate infiltrates, poorly defined nodules, or effusions. Effusions are exudative and often bloody (2,27). Involvement of either the gastrointestinal (GI) tract or lung causes death in 10 to 20% of patients (14). Patients may also present with disease limited to nodes, in which case lymph node biopsy is required to establish the diagnosis. Significant lymphedema may occur and is cytokine mediated (2,13).

STAGING AND PROGNOSTIC FACTORS

The development of a universally accepted staging system for KS is complicated by the fact that the usual indicators of tumor burden in other metastatic cancers do not have the same prognostic significance in KS. However, Chachoua et al. reported three adverse prognostic factors for survival in a cohort of epidemic KS patients: prior or coexistent opportunistic infection (OI), the presence of B symptoms (weight loss, fever, and night sweats), and an absolute CD4-positive T-cell count of less than 300/μL (28). The most important of these, OI, was associated with a median survival of only 7 months, versus

20 months for those without prior OI. Other features, including the ratio of helper to suppressor cells and extent of disease, were not independent predictors of survival in this study.

Based on these findings, the AIDS Clinical Trials Group Oncology Committee of the National Institute for Allergy and Infectious Diseases proposed and revised a KS staging system incorporating extent of disease, severity of immune dysfunction, and the presence of systemic B symptoms (Table 34-1).

They also recommended the following staging methods for these patients: complete physical examination (including rectal and oral examination), biopsy of skin lesions and/or lymph nodes, chest x-ray, gastroscopy and colonoscopy (bronchoscopy in patients with abnormal chest x-ray), computed tomography (CT) scan of the abdomen, and laboratory studies (complete blood count, common serum chemistries, HIV serology, T4-T8 lymphocyte counts) (29,30).

TREATMENT

Highly Active Antiretroviral Therapy

The widespread use of HAART has dramatically decreased the incidence of KS and altered its natural history (31). KS lesions have been found to regress after initiation of HAART therapy (32–35). Since the dawn of HAART, treatment goals have shifted from palliation to long-term remission. HAART therapy consists of one protease inhibitor combined with two nucleoside

TABLE 34-1	TIS STAGING SYSTEM FOR AIDS-RELATED KAPOSI'S SARCOMA AND RISK STATUS	
	GOOD RISK (0)	**POOR RISK (1)**
Characteristics	*All of the following:*	*Any of the following:*
Tumor (T)	Tumor confined to skin and lymph nodes and/or minimal oral disease*	Tumor-associated edema or ulceration; extensive oral KS; gastrointestinal KS; KS in other nonnodal viscera
Immune system (I)	CD4 cells ≥150/mm³	CD4 cells <150/mm³
Systemic illness (S)	No history of opportunistic infection or thrush; no B symptoms;† performance status ≥70 (Karnofsky)	History of opportunistic infection and/or thrush; B symptoms; performance status <70 (Karnofsky); other HIV-related illness (e.g., neurologic disease, lymphoma)

KS = Kaposi's sarcoma.

* Minimal oral disease defined as nonnodular KS confined to the palate.

† B symptoms: fever, drenching night sweats, and/or >10% involuntary weight loss.

SOURCE: Levine and Tulpule (31). With permission.

reverse transcriptase inhibitors (NRTI). An available alternative is the combination of two NRTIs with one non-NRTI. There is an ongoing search for new drugs and better drug combinations for the treatment of HIV. All KS patients with positive HIV serology should receive HAART; this initial treatment is usually sufficient for asymptomatic disease. In one large study, HAART, with or without protease inhibitors, prolonged time to progression by more than 1 year (31). For symptomatic visceral disease, cytotoxic therapy should be combined with HAART. For symptomatic lesions, with pain or extensive ulceration, local treatment may be added.

LOCAL THERAPY

Local therapy for KS patients is palliative and directed toward improving symptoms and overall quality of life, since local therapy will not control disease outside the treatment area. Also, most patients with AIDS-associated KS die of opportunistic infections rather than KS (1,14). Indications for treatment include cosmetic control, bulky oral lesions, lesions resulting in pain or significant edema, extensive cutaneous disease, or the presence of symptoms referable to viscera, such as bleeding or obstruction (36,37).

Cryotherapy

Treatment of KS lesions with liquid nitrogen may result in a complete or partial resolution of disease in more than 85% of cases regardless of anatomic location or activity of underlying HIV infection (38), although persistent KS can often be demonstrated in the deep reticular dermis by biopsy, and therapy will permanently destroy melanocytes, particularly in dark-skinned patients. Patients considered candidates for cryotherapy include those with indolent KS and macular or papular lesions less than 1 cm in diameter. Advantages of cryotherapy are the short duration of treatment, minimal pain, ease of administration and repeated treatments, and potential combination with other modalities of treatment.

Laser and Surgical Therapies

Laser photocoagulation therapy, which can be performed in the outpatient setting, can completely shrink smaller lesions, partially resolve larger lesions, lessen bleeding and pain, improve cosmetic appearance, and allow minimal wound care. However, like cryotherapy, it offers limited tissue penetration and is unlikely to resolve large, deep, or exophytic lesions.

Surgery has traditionally been reserved for lesions that cause visceral morbidity (bowel obstruction or bleeding) and for skin lesions that are large, are ulcer-ated, infiltrate underlying tissues or bone, or occur in areas that can cause morbidity, such as the face. Furthermore, the potential for HIV infection of the surgeon or laser operator remains a concern, and these modalities should be reserved for selected patients only.

Radiation Therapy

Studies have shown that radiation therapy may benefit patients with KS lesions. Tappero et al. reported that more than two-thirds of patients attained at least a partial response (PR) to radiation of KS lesions (14). More recently, Berson et al. achieved response rates of more than 80% with appropriate patient selection (39). Current indications for radiotherapy include bleeding, pain, mass effect (large intraoral lesions, localized painful lymphadenopathy, localized lymphedema of extremities or genitalia), or cosmetically disfiguring lesions at selected sites (facial, ocular, or periorbital lesions or lesions of the feet) that fail to respond to intralesional or cryotherapy (40).

Toxicities of radiotherapy include residual purple pigmentation, hyperpigmentation, desquamation, or ulceration in treated skin lesions; mucositis of the oral cavity, pharynx, and larynx (often ameliorated by prophylactic systemic antifungal and antiherpetic medication); and dry mouth or altered taste during treatment of oral lesions (41–43). It has been suggested that patients with oral lesions or lesions of the feet are especially sensitive to conventional doses of radiotherapy with enhanced toxicities; this may limit the effectiveness of such therapy for these lesions (42,43). Observed responses to radiotherapy vary by site of disease and the overall condition of the patient. Lesions treated to palliate pain or visceral symptoms are less likely to demonstrate objective responses and are more likely to recur locally than are lesions treated for cosmetic reasons (40,42). When present, lymphedema is also less likely to resolve: studies have shown only PR in 40% of fields treated (39).

Alitretinoin Topical Gel (Panretin Gel)

This topical gel has been associated with response rates of 35 to 50% (31). It is applied twice daily, and responses can be expected at 2 to 14 weeks following initiation of therapy. Adverse effects include local inflammation, lightening of the skin, and inadequate cosmesis (44).

Intralesional Therapy

Intralesional injections of vinblastine, vincristine, or bleomycin reportedly result in objective response rates of 60 to 88% with minimal or no systemic effects. As with cryotherapy, cosmetic response is often better than histologic response, with residual disease by biopsy. Median duration of response varies from 4 to 6 months, with 40% of patients experiencing recurrent disease (14).

Reported concentrations of intralesional vinblastine vary from 0.1 to 0.6 mg/mL, with larger doses recommended for oral lesions or larger papulonodular lesions. Total doses administered at a treatment session are limited to 1 to 3 mg (14,45–47). Patients are allowed a recovery time of 3 to 4 weeks before retreatment. Lesions may require two to three injections for maximal response. Pain at the injection site is the most common side effect, but investigators have also reported hyper- or hypopigmentation, edema, blistering and ulceration, alopecia, and transient mononeuropathy.

THERAPY FOR SYSTEMIC DISEASE

Patients with widely disseminated, progressive, or symptomatic disease are candidates for systemic therapy, including biological-agent therapies, antiretroviral therapies, or single- or multiagent chemotherapies (Fig. 34-2). However, systemic therapies may be limited by severe toxicities or the intercurrent development of opportunistic infections.

Immunomodulators

Interferon alpha (IFN-α) was the first agent approved for AIDS-associated KS. Its testing was prompted by its antiviral, antiproliferative, antiangiogenic, and immunoregulatory activities. Like other biological-therapy agents, interferon offers the advantages of less myelosuppres-

sion and fewer systemic toxicities. Responses have been reported to differ depending on extent of disease, prior treatment with chemotherapy, prior or coexistent OI, and CD4-positive T-cell count.

A number of trials have confirmed the activity of single-agent interferon in AIDS-associated KS. Initial studies were designed to determine the optimal dose and schedule and whether a dose-response relationship exists for interferon (48). In general, higher doses resulted in an improved response rate, responses of 20 to 40% being reported with doses of more than 20 million units (MU)/m^2 (48,49). Responders demonstrated improved survival rates compared to nonresponders. The most prominent toxicities included malaise, flu-like syndrome, and depression. Studies of combined interferon and cytotoxic chemotherapy demonstrated increased toxicity but not synergistic or additive activity (48,49).

Factors predicting a poor response to interferon include extensive disease, constitutional symptoms, a CD4-positive cell count of less than 200/μL at initiation of therapy, anemia, and current or prior OI (49,50). Subsequent studies excluding patients with the worst prognostic indicators have resulted in improved response rates approaching 50%. Patients with CD4-positive cell counts of more than 200/μL are almost four times as likely to respond as patients with CD4 cell counts below 200/μL.

Investigators have suggested that IFN-α acts against HIV by suppressing the translation of its mRNA into protein, thus blocking the assembly of viral proteins into intact virions. Zidovudine (Retrovir), although not directly antiviral, acts by blocking the infection of previ-

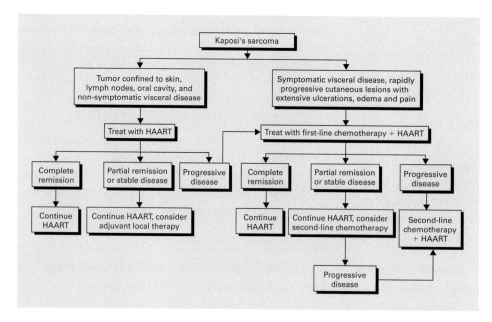

FIGURE 34-2 Algorithm for the management of AIDS-related Kaposi's sarcoma. *Monthly evaluation of Kaposi's sarcoma clinical response and estimation of CD4+ cell count and HIV-RNA levels. **HAART regimen should be changed in the case of immunovirologic failure. HAART, highly active antiretroviral therapy. [*From Catellan et al. (79). With permission.*]

ously uninfected cells (50). When used in combination, these agents have demonstrated synergistic activity both in vitro and in vivo.

Trials combining interferon and zidovudine have been primarily phase I studies. In one, Krown et al. reported a maximum tolerated interferon dose of 18 MU with 100 mg zidovudine every 4 h (an alternative schedule of 4.5 MU of interferon with 200 mg of zidovudine was also tolerated) (51). However, the excessive toxicity of lymphoblastoid interferon (IFN-α-N 1) and zidovudine resulted in early closure of the third study arm.

Dose-limiting toxicities included neutropenia (defined as a cell count of 500 to 750/μL, accounting for 10 of 17 dose reductions) as well as severe fatigue, malaise, and elevated transaminase levels. A decrease in hemoglobin concentration to 10 g/dL or lower occurred in all patients treated for 2 or more weeks. Although the interferon/zidovudine study reported by Krown et al. was not designed specifically to evaluate response, they observed a response rate of 46%. Similar results were noted by Fischl et al. (52) and Kovacs et al. (53). Studies examining the combination of interferon and HAART are under way.

Chemotherapy

Vincristine-, vinblastine-, and bleomycin-containing regimens were the first combinations to be studied as treatment for disseminated KS. Etoposide (Vepesid)- and doxorubicin-containing regimens were generally used as second-line therapy. Subsequently, studies demonstrated the combination of Adriamycin (doxorubicin), bleomycin, and vinca alkaloids (ABV) was effective, with response rates of approximately 85%. Although active, this regimen was limited by myelosuppression, especially neutropenia, and concomitant development of opportunistic infections (OIs).

Other investigators have studied doxorubicin-containing therapies. Gill et al. compared the combination of ABV versus doxorubicin alone in 61 patients with mucocutaneous KS (54). The overall response rate for ABV was 88 versus 48% for doxorubicin alone; however, the median survival was the same (9 months) in both groups. A higher dose version of ABV was also studied by Laubenstein et al. In that study, the response rate was 84%, but 61% of patients developed OIs and 44% required dose reductions to minimize hematologic toxicity (55).

This situation has improved since the discovery of liposomal anthracyclines and paclitaxel (31). Liposomal preparations alter pharmacodynamics and prolong the half-life of medications, and investigators have de-

scribed increased accumulation of these drugs in KS lesions when compared to normal cells (31). Liposomal daunorubicin (DaunoXome) and doxorubicin (Doxil) have been extensively studied. In a phase III clinical trial of liposomal doxorubicin versus ABV conducted by Northfelt et al. at the University of California, San Francisco, the overall response rate of liposomal doxorubicin was found to be superior to ABV, 45.9 versus 24.8% ($p < 0.001$) (56). The lower reported response rate of ABV in these later studies are due to higher doses of doxorubicin, which also increased toxicity. In the same study, the toxicity profile also strongly favored liposomal doxorubicin, with decreased cardiac toxicity and hair loss. Other studies have reported similar results with liposomal doxorubicin or daunorubicin (57–59). These results have led these preparations to become the first-line chemotherapy treatment of KS.

Another active agent is paclitaxel. In a pilot study of 20 patients reported by Saville et al., the response rate was 65% (60). Later studies confirmed the efficacy of paclitaxel in severely immunocompromised and heavily pretreated patients (61,62). In a recently published multicenter trial of patients with advanced KS who had failed to respond to prior chemotherapy, the response rate was 56% (62). In this study, many patients also safely received a protease inhibitor during paclitaxel treatment. The most significant toxicities reported were myelosuppression, especially neutropenia, and hair loss. This agent is commonly used as second-line therapy.

FUTURE THERAPIES

Because KS is a highly vascular tumor, angiogenesis inhibitors such as thalidomide have been investigated as KS treatment. In a phase II study of thalidomide in 20 KS patients with positive HIV serology, the overall response rate, based on an intention-to-treat model, was 40%, with a median response duration of 7 months in assessable patients (63). Most of these patients were on HAART therapy; however, study entry criteria required disease progression in the preceding 2 months, and only 4 had previously received cytotoxic chemotherapy. Toxicities of therapy included somnolence, neutropenia, and depression (63).

Fumagillin analogs (64,65) and sulfated polysaccharide peptidoglycan compounds produced by bacteria (66,67) are potent inhibitors of angiogenesis and are currently being investigated for activity in AIDS-associated KS. AGM 1470 (TNP 470) is a semisynthetic fumagillin analog that inhibits spindle cell proliferation in vitro. In a phase I study of TNP 470 in 38 patients, the drug was well tolerated overall (68). In this preliminary study the partial and overall response rate was 18% and the median duration of response was short, only 11 weeks (68). Tecogalan sodium is a polysaccharide that has been shown to inhibit KS-derived spindle cell growth in vitro (66), but results in phase I clinical trials have been discouraging, with response rates close to 0% (69,70). This drug may show improved activity in combination with other agents.

Another antiangiogenic compound under study is glufanide disodium (IM-862), a dipeptide identified from soluble fractions of the thymus (31). Results of a randomized phase II study using IM-862 nasal solution are promising: the overall response rate was 36%, with 5 complete responses and 11 PRs (71). The median response duration was more than 33 weeks. The majority of the patients on this study were concurrently treated with HAART. How much of the response can be attributable to the antiretroviral therapy is unclear. A phase III study is under way.

An interesting epidemiologic aspect of KS is its male predominance, more than can be explained by the patterns of KSHV infection. For this reason hormonal approaches are being studied. Initial in vitro studies conducted by Gill et al. demonstrated inhibitory effects of β-hCG (72). However, more recently, these effects were shown to be mediated through a yet undefined hCG-associated factor. Work is currently being conducted to identify this protein (73).

The discovery of KSHV promoted interest in antiviral approaches to KS. Anecdotally, responses to foscarnet and gancyclovir, but not acyclovir, have been cited (74–76). The large multicenter AIDS cohort study in 1996 found a reduction of relative risk of developing KS in patients taking ganciclovir (48%) and foscarnet (60%) (77). Mocroft et al. reported a reduction of 60% in KS occurrence in patients treated with either ganciclovir or foscarnet (76).

Optimum therapy for patients with multiple KS relapses and HAART resistance is yet undefined. To address this concern, targeted therapies are being developed. Pentosan polysulfate, an inhibitor of basic fibroblast growth factor (bFBF), is being investigated (78). In a phase II study of 16 males, the response rate was 6%, with a favorable toxicity profile (77). Newer antiangiogenic compounds directed against bFGF, such as matrix metalloproteinase inhibitors (MMPs) and oligonucleotides, are promising (79). In a recently reported phase I study of the MMP COL-3, the overall response rate in a total of 18 treated patients was 44%, including one complete response (80). The median response duration was greater than 25 weeks. Grade 3 to 4 toxicity was experienced by one-third (6) of the pa-

tients. These toxicities included photosensitivity, rash, and headache (80).

In conclusion, the epidemiology and natural history of KS have been markedly affected by HAART. HAART has decreased the incidence of the disease and allowed for control of early disease. Although there are several effective therapies for KS, the activity of novel agents is encouraging, and the search for new and targeted therapies continues.

■ NON-HODGKIN'S LYMPHOMA

EPIDEMIOLOGY

The Surveillance, Epidemiology, and End Results (SEER) program of the National Cancer Institute has demonstrated a more than 50% increase in non-Hodgkin's lymphoma (NHL) cases from 1973 to 1987 (81). The overall incidence of NHL (HIV- and non-HIV–related) continues to rise. Although the factors contributing to this increase are not fully understood, the increased incidence of NHL in HIV-infected individuals has contributed in some part to this figure. However, AIDS-associated NHL is not entirely responsible for the increased incidence, as the increase predates the AIDS epidemic.

High- or intermediate-grade B-cell HIV-related lymphoma (HRL) first became an AIDS-defining illness in 1985 (82). With the addition of cervical cancer, recurrent bacterial infection, tuberculosis, and others to the list of AIDS-defining illnesses, the peak of the AIDS epidemic occurred in 1993 (83). The incidence began to drop in 1995 due to the widespread use of HAART (83). Although the incidence of AIDS, opportunistic infections, and KS has declined since the advent of HAART, the impact of HAART itself on the incidence of HIV-related lymphoma is not well established (83).

Initially, investigators thought that HAART had no impact on the incidence of HRL; however, recent data have demonstrated a decreased incidence of HRL since the advent of HAART. Because HAART has had such a significant effect in reducing the incidence of KS and OIs and a relatively smaller effect on the incidence of HRL, the proportion of AIDS cases defined by HRL has increased from 4% in 1994 to 16% in 1998 (83,84). The risk of developing NHL is approximately 60 to 100 times higher in the HIV-positive population (84,85); after HAART, the incidence of HRL is about 1.6% per year (86).

As the AIDS epidemic has evolved, it has become apparent that all HIV risk groups are susceptible to the development of NHL. Prior to the HAART era, the

World Health Organization European Region measured the frequency of NHL in all groups (87). They noted a higher frequency of NHL in homosexual and bisexual men and hemophiliacs than in abusers of intravenous drugs, who exhibited a downward trend in NHL. This same pattern was recorded in a U.S. study of AIDS-associated NHL (88). Also pre-HAART, Northfelt et al. examined the degree of immunodeficiency in terms of CD4-positive cell counts at the time of diagnosis of non-CNS AIDS-associated NHL (89). The median CD4 cell count at diagnosis was 110/μL. The authors concluded that the degree of immunodeficiency at diagnosis as measured by CD4 cells varies over a wide range and that no specific CD4 cell count is a useful marker for the development of non-CNS AIDS-associated NHL. These data contrast with those from a study by Pluda et al., which suggested that NHL is a late manifestation

of HIV infection (90). However, others have also suggested that lymphoma is a late manifestation of HIV infection, since the incubation period between infection and the development of lymphoma in transfusion recipients is approximately 50 months, similar to that for the development of opportunistic infections (91).

The demographics of HRL patients have changed in the last decade. In a retrospective study including 369 patients published by Levine et al. in 2000 (Table 34-2), the differences observed in 1995–1998 (post-HAART) versus 1987–1990 (pre-HAART) include a higher prevalence in women (7 versus 2%,), in Hispanics (55% versus 33%), and in those who acquired HIV through heterosexual contact (18 versus 5%) (92).

The median age of HRL was unchanged. Also, the median CD4-positive cell count at diagnosis of AIDS-related lymphoma was reduced from 113 to 53/μL. The

TABLE 34-2 | **DEMOGRAPHIC PROFILE OF 369 PATIENTS WITH AIDS-RELATED LYMPHOMA OVER DIFFERENT TIME INTERVALS**

	1982–1986 (%)	1987–1990 (%)	1991–1994 (%)	1995–1998 (%)	Total (%)	p value
No. of patients	44	88	132	105	369	
Median age (years)	40	36	38	39	38	0.18
Sex						0.25
Female	0 (0)	2 (2)	6 (5)	7 (7)	15 (4)	
Male	44 (100)	86 (98)	126 (95)	98 (93)	354 (96)	
Race						0.001
Caucasian	33 (75)	50 (57)	64 (48)	42 (40)	189 (51)	*
Hispanic	7 (16)	26 (33)	51 (39)	58 (55)	145 (39)	†
Black	4 (9)	4 (5)	17 (13)	5 (5)	30 (8)	
Asian	0 (0)	5 (6)	0 (0)	0 (0)	5 (1)	
Risk						0.039
MSM	37 (84)	67 (76)	105 (80)	69 (66)	278 (75)	‡
IDU ± MSM	3 (7)	7 (8)	4 (3)	3 (3)	17 (5)	
Hetero	2 (5)	4 (5)	13 (10)	19 (18)	38 (10)	#
Transfusion	0	3 (3)	1 (0.5)	4 (4)	8 (2)	
Unknown	2 (5)	7 (8)	9 (7)	10 (10)	28 (8)	
KPS						0.0008
>80%	14 (32)	28 (32)	75 (57)	45 (43)	162 (44)	
<80%	30 (68)	60 (68)	57 (43)	60 (57)	207 (56)	
Prior OI§	14 (32)	40 (45)	58 (44)	53 (50)	165 (45)	0.22
Prior KS§	2 (5)	13 (15)	11 (8)	14 (13)	40 (11)	0.20
Median CD4¶	177	113	54	53	66	0.0006
Range	0–1703	2–1927	0–710	0–700	0–1927	

MSM = men who have sex with men; IDU = injection drug use; Hetero = heterosexual risk factor for HIV; KPS = Karnofsky performance status; OI = opportunistic infection; KS = Kaposi's sarcoma.
* p value = 0.0007, comparing Caucasian versus all other races.
† p value = <0.0001, comparing Hispanics versus all other races.
‡ p value = 0.045, comparing MSM with all other HIV risk groups.
# p value = 0.011, comparing heterosexual transmission with all other HIV risk groups.
§ Patients without a diagnosis of OI or KS prior to development of lymphoma presented with lymphoma as the first AIDS-defining condition.
¶ CD4 cell count at time of diagnosis of AIDS-related lymphoma.
SOURCE: Levine et al. (92). With permission.

difference in overall survival in patients with systemic NHL did not reach statistical significance, but was prolonged in later years (5.7 versus 8.2 months). Similar results were obtained in a study conducted in the United Kingdom involving 7840 patients in whom the 2-year overall survival in the pre-HAART versus the post-HAART era was improved in the latter (29 versus 41%), but again this was not statistically significant (93). However, a French study published in 2001 demonstrated a significantly decreased incidence and increased overall survival (6 versus 20 months) of HRL over time (94). They also found that the CD4-positive cell count at diagnosis had increased from 63 to 191/µL. Many researchers believe that further studies will demonstrate a trend toward a decreased incidence and improved overall survival of HRL patients.

PATHOGENESIS

Although the precise mechanisms of lymphoma development in AIDS have not been determined, host factors are predominantly responsible for such lymphomas. The HIV virus itself is not directly involved in malignant B-cell transformation. HIV sequences are not uniformly detected in lymphoma tissue or in the reactive B-cell hyperplasia of persistent generalized lymphadenopathy that precedes the development of lymphoma in 30% of cases (95). Polymerase chain reaction (PCR) analysis reveals HIV to be present only in infiltrating T cells. Therefore, HIV infection does not appear to be an absolute prerequisite for the development of these lymphomas; in fact, more important than HIV infection itself is the immune dysregulation it causes (95).

HIV-infected cells produce multiple cytokines, some of which serve as stimuli for B-cell proliferation and differentiation. These include IL-1, 2, 4, 6, 7, 10, IFN-γ, tumor-necrosis factor, lymphotoxin, and B-cell growth factor. In particular, IL-6 is an autocrine growth factor for B-cell malignancies, including multiple myeloma and chronic lymphocytic leukemia. HIV may also directly stimulate IL-6 from monocytes and macrophages, and elevated levels of IL-6 may predict the development of lymphoma in HIV infection (95). Also, Epstein-Barr virus (EBV)–positive B-cell lines from patients with AIDS-associated Burkitt's lymphoma express large amounts of IL-10, suggesting a role for this cytokine in B-cell growth and immortalization. In addition, HIV itself is capable of direct polyclonal activation of B cells.

Ongoing B-cell proliferation and differentiation may result in an increased incidence of random mutations, which may in turn result in transformation (96). The normally occurring DNA rearrangements involving the immunoglobulin heavy- and light-chain genes may provide vulnerable sites for mutations or translocations (97). Molecular events may occur stepwise, with several molecular events required to induce transformation. Patients with reactive lymphadenopathy demonstrate multiple clonal rearrangements of immunoglobulin genes (98). These lesions may be early precursor lesions, with additional molecular events required for transformation of a single malignant clone. The classic translocations of Burkitt's lymphoma, t(8;14), t(8;22), and t(2;8), are all demonstrated in AIDS-associated Burkitt's lymphomas, and rearrangements involving the c-myc oncogene have been observed in AIDS-associated lymphomas (96). Such rearrangements of c-myc imply a molecular mechanism similar to that in sporadic Burkitt's lymphomas. In addition, HIV infection of already immortalized B-cell lines can lead to upregulation of c-myc transcripts. C-myc activation, in turn, may result in altered phenotypic features that allow cells to escape immune surveillance by cytotoxic T cells, including absence or low expression of class I major histocompatibilty complex antigens, insufficient expression of adhesion molecules required for effector–target cell interactions, and downregulation of EBV-coded antigens (96). However, no consistent c-myc rearrangements occur in AIDS-associated lymphoma tissue, suggesting the presence of other operative mechanisms (95).

Investigators have studied the role of EBV in the development of AIDS-associated lymphoma. Collectively, data suggest that the virus is responsible for at least a portion of cases of AIDS-associated lymphomas and is likely involved in all cases of primary CNS lymphoma in patients with AIDS. A proportion (less than 50%) of systemic AIDS-associated lymphomas show signs of latent EBV infection and may also express combinations of EBV antigens not previously observed in B-cell lymphomas (99).

Lymphomas that are both EBV- and HIV-positive demonstrate evidence of clonal EBV infection, indicating that EBV integration occurs before clonal B-cell expansion and that EBV may play a role in lymphomagenesis (100). Studies attempting to identify EBV-positive persistent generalized lympadenopathy (lymphadenopathy syndrome) as a precursor of EBV-positive HIV lymphoma have had differing results. In a study conducted by Shibata et al., approximately one-third of patients with lymphadenopathy syndrome demonstrated EBV DNA, and the presence of EBV DNA correlated with development of lymphoma at a later time (101). However, a subsequent study by Dolcetti et al. concluded that EBV-positive lymphadenopathy syndrome did not correlate with the subsequent development of EBV-positive lymphomas (102).

Mutation or allelic loss of tumor suppressor genes has also been investigated in AIDS-associated NHL. For example, some smaller studies indicate that *p53* mutations occur as often as 37% in NHL, especially in association with c-*myc* overexpression. One study using a more sensitive assay detected *p53* mutations in 55% of Burkitt's/Burkitt's-like HRL and 25% of DLCL (103). *Ras* mutations and *BCL-6* rearrangements have also been described in a minority of HRLs (104). In contrast, there is no evidence of *BCL-1* and *BCL-2* rearrangements or retinoblastoma gene inactivation in AIDS-associated NHL (104,105). The defect in tumor suppression and the deregulation of oncogene-induced growth may be central to the pathogenesis of these lymphomas. Also, viral proteins may bind to and inactivate *p53,* leading to dysregulation of cell growth (97). In summary, B-cell proliferation induced by HIV or EBV may foster mutations in critical oncogenes, or tumor suppressor genes may occur along with abnormal DNA rearrangements, leading to c-*myc* activation, clonal selection, and the development of a monoclonal B-cell lymphoma.

HISTOPATHOLOGY

Most systemic AIDS-associated lymphomas (>90%) are aggressive B-cell neoplasms, including diffuse large cell, immunoblastic, or small noncleaved cell lymphomas, including Burkitt's and Burkitt's-like lymphoma (85). The small noncleaved cell type usually occurs at higher CD4 cell counts than the other variants (150 versus 50/μL) (85). Under the Revised European-American Classification of Lymphoid Neoplasms/World Health Organization Classification of Lymphoid Neoplasms (REAL/WHO), these histologic subtypes are categorized as mature (peripheral) B-cell neoplasms.

A rare subtype under the same REAL/WHO classification that is increased in incidence in HIV-seropositive individuals is primary effusion lymphoma (PEL). PEL has been associated with KSHV/HHV-8, the same virus linked to the pathogenesis of KS (86). These tumors are difficult to treat and the outcome is generally poor (86).

Other B-cell malignancies, including low-grade small cleaved cell lymphoma, chronic lymphocytic leukemia (106), and myeloma (107), are not considered AIDS-defining illnesses but have been reported in HIV patients. A case series of 10 HIV patients with indolent lymphoma was recently reported by Levine et al (108). When compared to HIV patients with aggressive lymphoma, these patients had a higher incidence of bone marrow involvement (50 versus 17%), and had higher median CD4 cell counts (531 versus 90/μL). The median survival in this small group was 66.8 months, comparable to that seen in non-HIV indolent lymphoma.

T-cell lymphoma is also not an AIDS-defining illness; however, T-cell neoplasms—including cutaneous T-cell lymphoma (109,110), precursor T-cell lymphoma (111), lymphoblastic lymphoma (112), HTLV-I-associated T-cell leukemia (113), peripheral T-cell lymphoma (114), and anaplastic large cell lymphoma (115)—have been described in HIV-infected individuals. Although the incidence of T-cell lymphoma is increased in HIV, this increase is much smaller than that seen with B-cell lymphomas.

CLINICAL PRESENTATION

Patients often seek medical attention for B symptoms (fever, night sweats, and weight loss of more than 10% of body weight) or for a rapidly growing mass lesion. Although these symptoms occur in approximately 75% of patients with AIDS-associated lymphomas, it is important to exclude other etiologies, such as occult opportunistic infections.

Most patients with AIDS-associated NHL have advanced-stage disease at presentation and frequent involvement of extranodal sites, features confirmed in multiple series. Between 64 and 83% of patients present with stage III or IV disease and between 65 and 91% with extranodal disease (116,117). The most common extranodal sites in all reported series are bone marrow (25%), CNS parenchyma or meninges (32%), liver (12 to 48%), and gastrointestinal tract (26%) (118,119). Other reported sites include lung (120), pleura (121), rectum (119), testis (122,123), kidney (124), spleen (121), heart (125), and rarely common bile duct (85), muscle (85), and placenta and products of conception (85).

STAGING AND PROGNOSTIC FEATURES

Besides routine chest x-ray, blood studies, and computed tomography (CT) of the chest, abdomen, and pelvis, patients with AIDS-associated NHL should undergo bone marrow biopsy and lumbar puncture. CT or magnetic resonance imaging (MRI) of the brain or spinal cord, bone scans, and GI contrast studies should be done as needed if symptoms suggest disease. Gallium and/or 18F-fluorodeoxyglucose (FDG)-positron emission tomography (PET) scans can be performed at the discretion of the clinician. Disease should be staged according to the Ann Arbor system (Table 34-3).

Although patients with AIDS-associated NHL are a

TABLE 34-3	ANN ARBOR STAGING CLASSIFICATION FOR HODGKIN'S LYMPHOMA[227]
Stage	**Characteristics**
I	Involvement of a single lymph node region (I) or a single extralymphatic organ or site (IE).
II	Involvement of two or more lymph node regions on the same side of the diaphragm (II) or localized involvement of an extralymphatic organ or site (IIE).
III	Involvement of lymph node regions on both sides of diaphragm (III) or localized involvement of an extralymphatic organ or site (IIIE) or spleen (IIIS) or both (IIISE).
IV	Diffuse or disseminated involvement of one or more extralymphatic organs with or without associated lymph node involvement. The organ(s) involved should be identified by a symbol: A, asymptomatic; B, fever, sweats, weight loss >10% of body weight.

SOURCE: De Vita et al. With permission.

diverse group, several common factors predicting short survival have been identified. Gisselbrecht et al. treated non-CNS AIDS-associated lymphomas with a modified NHL (126) regimen consisting of three cycles of induction therapy with doxorubicin, cyclophosphamide, vindesine, bleomycin, and prednisone (127). Patients who achieved a complete response (CR) received consolidation therapy containing high-dose methotrexate, ifosfamide, etoposide, asparaginase, and cytarabine. All patients received CNS prophylaxis. Sixty-five percent achieved complete remission after induction therapy, 22% had a partial remission or failed, and 15% died during induction therapy. The median survival was 9 months. The authors performed a concurrent prospective analysis of prognostic determinants and confirmed that a performance status more than 1, localized disease (stage I or II), absence of bone marrow involvement, nonimmunoblastic histology, absence of B symptoms, no previous AIDS-defining diagnosis, and a CD4 cell count of more than 100/μL were predictors of improved survival. They also found that 50% of patients having CD4 cell counts of more than 100/μL, no B symptoms, a performance status of less than 2, and nonimmunoblastic histology were alive at 2 years, suggesting that factors that reflect the patient's underlying immunodeficiency are at least as important and perhaps more important determinants of survival than are factors intrinsic to the lymphoma itself. Levine et al. retrospectively studied a group of 49 patients treated for systemic AIDS-associated lymphoma (128). A Karnofsky performance status of less than 70%, history of AIDS before the diagnosis of lymphoma, and bone marrow involvement were independently associated with poor prognosis. In the absence of all three risk factors, median survival was 11.3 months; for the remaining patients, it was only 4 months. A complete response to therapy was associated with prolonged survival in the good-prognosis group (17.8 versus 5 months in patients without a complete response) but not in the poor-prognosis group. Patients in either group who attained a CR to antilymphoma therapy remained at risk for dying of AIDS during lymphoma remission. Thus, attempts at prolonging survival must address both the neoplasm and the underlying HIV infection. In a larger study, Straus and colleagues, using the Cox proportional hazards model, were able to identify four factors associated with shorter survival: age greater than 35 years, intravenous drug use, stages III/IV, and CD4 cell counts less than 100/μL (129). The median overall survival for patients with none or one of the adverse factors was 46 weeks; with two adverse factors, it was 44 weeks; and with three or four such factors, was 18 weeks. The International Prognostic Index for aggressive lymphoma has also been validated for patients with HRL (130,131).

THERAPY FOR AIDS-RELATED NON-HODGKIN'S LYMPHOMA

Difficulties in Managing NHL in Patients with HIV Infection

The major factor limiting the use of chemotherapy in AIDS-related NHL either alone or with antiretroviral therapy is hematologic toxicity and poor bone marrow reserve at initiation of therapy. Infection with the HIV virus often results in bone marrow dysplasia, anemia, thrombocytopenia, and leukopenia, and both ineffective hematopoiesis and peripheral destruction of blood cells are responsible for cytopenias. Decreased survival of blood cells may be related to autoimmune phenomena as well as increased turnover driven by multiple infections (132). A positive Coombs test is observed in 20% of HIV-infected patients with hypergammaglobulinemia. Hemolytic anemia, however, is rarely observed. Nonspecific attachment of other antibodies to red cells is also frequently observed and is usually clinically silent (132).

Between 70 and 95% of AIDS patients are anemic at presentation, with mean hemoglobin levels ranging between 9.1 and 11.7 g/dL (132,133). Less ill patients with HIV exhibit anemia in 5 to 16% of cases (132).

However, the incidence of anemia and other cytopenias increases with the degree of immunologic dysfunction and with progression from HIV seropositivity to frank AIDS.

Anemia in HIV disease is normochromic and normocytic, although 70% of patients receiving zidovudine demonstrate macrocytosis, with a mean corpuscular volume (MCV) of more than 100 after 2 weeks of therapy. Anemic HIV patients demonstrate an inappropriately low reticulocyte count, suggesting a hypoproliferative anemia or ineffective hematopoiesis. Iron studies demonstrate patterns consistent with chronic disease marked by an increased serum ferritin and decreased serum iron and total iron binding capacity. Serum ferritin levels parallel disease activity and are higher in AIDS than in HIV seropositivity. Serum ferritin levels may also be elevated owing to the protein's role as an acute-phase reactant (132).

The incidence of thrombocytopenia also increases with increasing severity of immune dysregulation, ranging from 5 to 12% in HIV-seropositive patients and reaching as high as 30% in patients with AIDS (132). Patients can exhibit classic immune thrombocytopenic purpura (with increased numbers of megakaryocytes in the bone marrow) or may develop thrombocytopenia as a result of impaired thrombopoiesis, the toxic effect of medications, or a thrombotic thrombocytopenic purpura (TTP)-hemolytic uremia syndrome (132). Furthermore, therapies in these patients vary in their effectiveness. Therapy with prednisone offers a durable response in only 10 to 20% of patients and may further worsen immune status. The most effective therapy seems to be intravenous gamma globulin (IVIG), which has a response rate of 88% but a median response duration of only 3 weeks (132).

Leukopenia, encompassing both granulocytopenia and lymphocytopenia, is also observed in up to 75% of AIDS patients. Atypical lymphocytes, hyposegmented granulocytes, and vacuolated monocytes can be seen on peripheral smears. Phagocytosed pathogens may be observed in neutrophils or monocytes (132,133). Antibodies to granulocytes are also frequent in HIV disease, and, although they do not necessarily correlate with the degree of neutropenia, they do correlate with progression to AIDS (132).

Anemia, leukopenia, and pancytopenia are well-documented effects of treating HIV infection with zidovudine (134). Such treatment is also associated with lower mean hemoglobin levels and an increased need for red cell transfusions (132). Up to 20% of patients may develop severe neutropenia (cell numbers below 500/μL).

However, because zidovudine's toxicity is dose-dependent, reducing the dose often ameliorates cytopenias.

In addition, zidovudine-related myelosuppression and synergistic effects may occur when zidovudine is combined with other drugs commonly administered to treat infections, including ganciclovir, pentamidine, trimethoprim-sulfamethoxazole, pyrimethamine, sulfadiazine, dapsone, and amphotericin B. Other retroviral drugs such as suramin, ribavirin, ddC, ddI, and interferon also produce hematologic toxicity. In particular, the combination of interferon and zidovudine in therapy of KS causes significant hematologic toxicity.

CHEMOTHERAPY: TRIALS FOR PATIENTS WITH HIV-RELATED LYMPHOMAS

Although some experts advise universal CNS prophylaxis in HIV-related lymphoma (HRL), most believe it should be restricted to patients with Burkitt's or Burkitt's-like lymphoma or those with bone marrow involvement (85). The results of trials of therapeutic regimens for AIDS-associated NHL are summarized in Table 34-4.

Comparison of these regimens is limited, however, by the fact that various histologies are often grouped together, inclusion criteria vary among the studies, and few prospective trials have been completed. However, investigators have drawn several conclusions from their experience in treating AIDS-associated NHL.

Dose-Intensive Regimens

The favorable results of dose escalation in non-AIDS–associated high-grade lymphomas are not easily demonstrated in the treatment of patients with AIDS-associated lymphomas. Gill et al. (135) analyzed results of two sequential phase II trials: in the first of these, patients received m-BACOD (methotrexate, leucovorin, bleomycin, doxorubicin, cyclophosphamide, vincristine, dexamethasone); in the second trial, they received a regimen containing high doses of cytarabine and methotrexate and standard doses of cyclophosphamide, vincristine, prednisone, bleomycin, and L-asparaginase. The second regimen was designed to expose patients to high-dose cytarabine and high-dose methotrexate early in the course of therapy to prevent the high CNS relapse rate observed in two-thirds of the patients who received m-BACOD. Complete remission was achieved in 54% of the m-BACOD group but in only 33% of the high-dose group, with significantly greater numbers of patients with OIs and hematologic toxicity appearing in the group

| TABLE 34-4 | SUMMARY OF SELECTED HRL TRIALS |

Chemo Regimen	N	Median CD4 Cell Count at Enrollment (per microliter)	CR (%)	ORR (%)	HAART	OI (%)	OS	Year (ref.)
Modifed m-BACOD vs	98	100	41	69	NR	22	35 weeks	1997 (137)
m-BACOD+G-CSF	94	107	52	78	NR	23	31 weeks	
MTX/LV	29	132	46	77	AZT	NR	12 months	1999 (139)
CHOP-HAART vs	24	190	50	NR	Yes	18	62% at 8.5 months	2001 (154)
CHOP	80	146	36	NR	No	52	7 months	
G-CSF+CHOP-R vs	95	133 total	58	NR	NR	NR	Median F/U	2003 (155)
G-CSF+CHOP	47		50	NR	NR	NR	26 weeks	
Infusional CDE	62	NR	48	74	NR	NR	2.7 years	2002 (148)
G-CSF+CDE-R	30	132	86	90	Yes	7	80% at 2 years	2002 (151)
EPOCH	39	198	74	87	Held during chemotherapy	*	60% at 53 months	2003 (149)

AZT = azidothymidine; CR = complete response; HAART = highly active antiretroviral therapy; NR = not reported; OI = opportunistic infection; OS = overall survival; ORR = overall response rate.
* 0% during chemotherapy, 9% after.

receiving high-dose therapy. The median survival in the m-BACOD group was 11 months, compared with only 6 months in the high-dose group, and the trial was terminated early because of the high rates of OI and hematologic toxicity.

In a trial by Kaplan et al. (117), a new intensive chemotherapy regimen, COMET-A, consisting of cyclophosphamide, vincristine, methotrexate, etoposide, and cytarabine with CNS prophylaxis, was compared with standard therapies including CHOP, m-BACOD, Pro-MACE-MOPP, COMLA, CVP, COMP, and radiation therapy alone. Although the complete remission rate for COMET-A was 58%, 28% of patients developed OI and the median survival was only 5.2 months. The investigators concluded that patients receiving "dose-intensive" regimens, defined as regimens containing a cyclophosphamide dose of more than 1 g/m^2, had significantly shorter survival times (median 4.6 months) than did patients receiving less intensive regimens (median 12.2 months).

Low-Dose Regimens

Levine et al. (136) have reported results for a regimen of low-dose m-BACOD (50% reduction in cyclophosphamide and doxorubicin doses) with early CNS prophylaxis and the initiation of zidovudine at completion of chemotherapy. A complete remission rate of 46% was reported, with long-term lymphoma-free survival in 75% of complete responders suggesting that low-

dose therapy may be effective. No patient had an isolated CNS relapse; however, despite prophylaxis, OI developed in 20% of patients.

Kaplan et al. and the AIDS clinical trials group compared the low-dose m-BACOD and standard-dose m-BACOD regimen combined with growth factors (GM-CSF) (137). In this study, overall and disease-free survival were similar in both arms. However, grade 3 toxicity was more frequent in the patients who received standard-dose m-BACOD and growth factors (70 versus 51%). In addition, the recurrence rate in the patients treated with low-dose chemotherapy was lower than that seen in the patients who received standard doses, and there were no differences in the incidence of OIs or deaths from HIV progression.

Remick et al. reported results of therapy employing a lower-dose, orally administered combination chemotherapy regimen for HRL consisting of lomustine (CCNU) 100 mg/m^2 on day 1, etoposide 200 mg/m^2 on days 1 through 3, cyclophosphamide 100 mg/m^2 on days 22 through 31, and procarbazine 100 mg/m^2 on days 22 through 31 at 6-week intervals (138). The overall response rate was 61%, with 39% complete remissions. The treatment-related mortality was 11%, and median overall survival was 7 months.

Tosi and colleagues evaluated the combination of oral zidovudine (administered to each patient at 2, 4, and 6 mg/m^2) and moderate-dose intravenous methotrexate and leukovorin rescue (139). The overall response rate was 77%, with 46% complete responses. There was one treatment-related death (3%) from septic shock. Grades III to IV neutropenia was observed in 52%. Median survival was 12 months.

Supportive Care

Despite the development of lower-dose regimens designed to minimize toxicity, significant hematologic toxicities were often still observed and resulted in delays in therapy, dose reductions, or termination of therapy. It has been suggested that HAART therapy may have reduced the incidence of toxicity and prolonged survival (84). In addition, the use of growth factors has been shown to ameliorate these toxicities and allow improved dose intensity (Table 34-5).

Walsh et al. and the AIDS Clinical Trials Group (ACTG) conducted a phase I study of m-BACOD with GM-CSF (140). Three different doses of m-BACOD were used along with fixed doses of GM-CSF (140). Eight of 16 patients could be treated at the highest dose level, and none of these patients experienced dose-limiting hematologic toxicity. However, OI developed in one patient on dose level 1 and in one patient on dose level 2, and the level of p24 antigenemia increased in some patients given GM-CSF.

Kaplan et al. also studied the use of GM-CSF with the CHOP regimen (141). Patients receiving GM-CSF all had higher mean nadirs of absolute neutrophil count, fewer chemotherapy cycles complicated by neutropenia and fever, fewer days hospitalized for fever and neutropenia, fewer reductions in chemotherapy doses, and less frequent delays in chemotherapy administration. However, these patients had a significant increase in p24 antigenemia (243%) baseline by week 3 after initiation of chemotherapy, suggesting stimulation of HIV

| TABLE 34-5 | SUGGESTED SUPPORTIVE CARE FOR THE PATIENT WITH HIV INFECTION AND LYMPHOMA OR OTHER MALIGNANCIES |

Indication	*Drug(s)*
Primary infection prophylaxis	
Pneumocystis carinii, Toxoplasma	Trimethoprim-sulfamethoxazole 1 DS qd
Oral and/or oesophageal candidiasis	Fluconazole 100 mg qd
MA1 complex (CD4 <50/μL)	Azithromycin 1200 mg weekly
Secondary infection prophylaxis	
Herpes simplex infections	Acylovir 400 mg bid or 200 mg tid
Cytomegalovirus infection	Ganciclovir 1 g tid
Mycobacterium–avium complex	Clarithromycin 500 mg bid plus ethambutol 15 mg/kg qd, with or without rifabutin 300 mg qd
Toxoplasma gondii	Sulphadiazine 1–1.5 gm q6h pyrimethamine 25–75 mg QD, Leucovorin 10–25 mg qd–qid
Cryptococcus neoformans	Fluconazole 200 mg qd
Salmonella bacteremia	Ciprofloxacin 500 mg bid
Hematopoietic growth factors	
For selected patients in whom the risk of febrile neutropenia ≥40%	G-CSF μg/kg or GM-CSF 250 μg/m² SC daily beginning after completion of chemotherapy and continuing until neutrophil recovery
Antiretroviral agents	
Selecting patients for therapy	Follow NIH guidelines (http://www.hivatis.org)
Role of therapy in controlling malignancy	
Kaposi's sarcoma	Essential
Lymphoma	Unknown
Other tumors	Unknown
May be used with myelosuppressive drugs	Didanosine, zalcitabine
Avoid with myelosuppressive drugs/regimens	Zidovudine
Avoid with neurotoxic drugs/regimens	Didanosine, zalcitabine, stavudine
May alter the metabolism of cytotoxic drugs metabolized by cytochrome P-450 enzymes	All protease inhibitors and nonnucleoside RTIs

bid = two times daily; G-CSF = granulocyte colony-stimulating factor; GM-CSF = granulocyte-macrophage colony-stimulating factor; NIH = National Institute of Health; qd = daily; qid = four times daily; RTIs = reverse transcriptase inhibitors; SC = subcutaneous; tid = three times daily.
SOURCE: Sparano (85). With permission.

activity. On the other hand, other trials have demonstrated an increase in CD4 cell count and a reduced viral burden with administration of GM-CSF (142,143). The use of growth factors is generally recommended when the expected incidence of febrile neutropenia exceeds 40% for the chemotherapy regimen selected (85).

Infusional Chemotherapy

Infusional cyclophosphamide, doxorubicin, and etoposide (CDE) given over 4 days was developed and evaluated by Sparano et al. (144–148) and found to be superior to bolus administration. The combination was found to be safe and effective when combined with growth factors and antiretroviral agents (146,147). A large phase II ECOG trial of infusional CDE plus filgastim in 62 chemotherapy-naïve patients yielded an overall response rate of 74%, with 48% complete responses and a median overall survival of 2.7 years (148). However, when these data was compared to controls matched according to the International Prognostic Factors Index, there were no significant differences in failure-free or overall survival rates. In addition, toxicity, especially myelosuppression and infection, was higher than that associated with EPOCH, another infusional regimen under study at the time. This regimen—containing infusional doxorubicin, etoposide, and vincristine (over 4 days) and bolus cyclophosphamide, oral prednisone, and granulocyte colony-stimulating factor (G-CSF)—was investigated by Little et al. (Table 34-6) (149).

In their study of 39 newly diagnosed patients with HRL, Little et al. reported a CR rate of 74% and an overall survival rate of 60% at a median follow-up of 53 months. Antiretroviral therapy was withheld during treatment and restarted shortly thereafter. This manipulation did not have a negative impact with respect to complications associated with AIDS, for several possible reasons. Compliance with HAART becomes challenging during chemotherapy administration, and HIV mutations may occur during periods of poor compliance. Pharmacokinetic interactions between HAART and chemotherapy can be avoided by withholding drugs during treatment for NHL, with no apparent added risk of increased opportunistic infections. Finally, HAART may inhibit lymphocyte apoptosis, thereby reducing the effects of chemotherapy (149).

In this study, molecular and immunohistochemical analysis revealed that HRLs had a higher proliferative rate, higher rate of mutated *p53,* and a lower rate of *bcl-2* expression than non-HIV related aggressive lymphomas. This higher proliferative rate was thought to explain the sensitivity of the HRL to an infusional schedule of chemotherapy. Interestingly, *p53* overexpression did not correlate with a poor prognosis in this population, implying a difference in pathogenesis from lymphomas in patients without HIV seropositivity. A lower *bcl-2* expression rate also suggested a better

TABLE 34-6	DOSE-ADJUSTED EPOCH		
Drug	*Dose*	*Route*	*Treatment Days*
Infused agents*			
Etoposide	50 mg/m^2/day	CIV	1,2,3,4 (96 h)
Doxorubicin	10 mg/m^2/day	CIV	1,2,3,4 (96 h)
Vincristine[†]	0.4 mg/m^2/day	CIV	1,2,3,4 (96 h)
Bolus agents			
Cyclophosphamide (cycle 1)			
CD4$^+$ cells ≥100/mm^3	375 mg/m^2/day	IV	5
CD4$^+$ cells <100/mm^3	187 mg/m^2/day	IV	5
Cyclophosphamide dose-adjustment (after cycle 1)[‡]			
nadir ANC >500/µL	↑187 mg above previous cycle	NA	NA
nadir ANC <500/µL or platelets <25000/µL	↓187 mg below previous cycle	NA	NA
Prednisone	60 mg/m^2/day	PO	1,2,3,4,5
Filgrastim	5 µg/kg/day	SC	6→ANC >5000/µL (past nadir)
Next cycle[#]		Day 21	

ANC = absolute neutrophil count; NA = not applicable.

* Etoposide, doxorubicin, and vincristine can be admixed in the same solution. Etoposide, doxorubicin, and vincristine are never dose-adjusted for hematologic toxicity.

[†] Vincristine dose should never be routinely capped.

[‡] Dose based on previous cycle absolute neutrophil count (ANC) nadir (CBC BIW); maximum cyclophosphamide dose 750 mg/m^2.

[#] Begin day 21 if ANC ≥1000/µL and platelets ≥50 000/µL.

[¶] Data are for cycle 1 except where noted in "Cyclophosphamide dose-adjustment."

SOURCE: From Little et al. (149). With permission.

prognosis in this population. These results led the authors to conclude that tumor biology at presentation, and not immune function during treatment, determined the prognosis of HRL. A multicenter trial of this regimen is under way through the U.S. AIDS Malignancy Consortium (150).

Tirelli and colleagues evaluated the addition of rituximab to CDE/G-CSF/HAART (151). Although the study consisted of only 29 patients and the median follow-up was only 9 months, the initial efficacy data were promising, with a CR rate of 89%. However, toxicity rates were also high, with 79% of patients experiencing grade 3 to 4 neutropenia and a 41% infection rate.

CHOP chemotherapy has been used to treat lymphoma in patients with and without HIV seropositivity. However, there have been relatively few studies in HRL published in the literature. Investigators of one Danish retrospective study reported, in abstract form, a CR rate of 52% with a median survival of 6.8 months (152). A study by Ratner et al. evaluated the combination of HAART therapy with either modified-dose CHOP (mCHOP) or standard-dose CHOP (sCHOP) and G-CSF (153). The CR rates seen in the patients treated with mCHOP and sCHOP were 30 and 48%, respectively. Overall response rates in both groups were similar, 60% and 57%. Both combinations were equally well tolerated, with the most common toxicity observed being transaminase elevation. Vaccher et al. retrospectively compared a group of 24 patients treated with CHOP and HAART to 80 patients treated with CHOP alone (154). The group treated with CHOP-HAART had a superior CR rate (50 versus 36%) and overall survival (62% were alive at a median follow-up of 8.5 months versus a median overall survival of 7 months) and significantly fewer OIs (18 versus 52%). However, the patients treated with CHOP-HAART had a better overall performance status than those treated with CHOP alone, and the great majority of those treated with CHOP alone never received HAART therapy before or after chemotherapy.

Kaplan and Scadden reported the results of a phase III trial comparing CHOP to CHOP plus rituximab (CHOP-R) (155). The CR rate was similar in the two arms of this study, 50 versus 58%. However, complications and mortality were increased in the patients who received CHOP-R. For this reason CHOP-R is not currently recommended for treatment of HRL.

Burkitt's Lymphoma

AIDS-associated Burkitt's lymphoma is particularly difficult to treat and is associated with a poor prognosis.

Hyperfractionated cyclophosphamide, vincristine, Adriamycin (doxorubicin), and dexamethasone (Hyper-CVAD) in addition to HAART therapy was found to be tolerable and effective, with a CR rate of 92% and a median survival of 12 months (156).

Relapsed and Refractory Disease

Effective salvage therapy for relapsed or refractory HRL has yet to be defined. In a small retrospective analysis conducted by Bi and colleagues, ESHAP (etoposide, methylprednisolone, cytosine arabinoside, platinol) was found to be superior to DHAP (dexamethasone, cytosine arabinoside, platinol) in this setting, with CR rates of 31 versus 0%, ORR 54 versus 7%, and median survival rates of 7.1 months versus 3 months (157). Sixty-three percent of patients receiving ESHAP experienced neutropenic fever. Studies are being conducted to evaluate the role of autologous transplantation in this patient population, and preliminary data indicate that this may be a feasible approach (158,159).

HIV-Related Lymphoma: The Challenge

HRL is a complex condition with rapidly evolving therapeutic options. Infusional chemotherapy may be superior to bolus administration, although the optimal combination of drugs is still unknown. Although antiviral therapy is essential to HIV management, a temporary discontinuation of these medications during HRL treatment does not appear to have a negative effect on AIDS or HRL treatment (149). Rituximab, although widely used to treat HIV-negative patients with NHL, seems to add toxicity without improving efficacy in HRL and is therefore not currently recommended for treatment (155). Higher-dose chemotherapy also seems to add toxicity without improving efficacy. Growth factors and OI prophylaxis are generally recommended for the duration of chemotherapy. Unresolved issues in the therapy for AIDS-associated NHL include the significance and influence on prognosis of pathologic subtype, the selection of therapy based on prognostic indicators, and the contribution of antiretroviral therapy to overall survival.

■ PRIMARY CNS LYMPHOMA

EPIDEMIOLOGY

Prior to the AIDS epidemic, primary central nervous system (PCNS) lymphoma was a rare disorder, accounting for 1 to 2% of all cases of NHL and fewer than 5% of all cases of primary intracranial neoplasm (160).

Increasing numbers of cases of PCNS lymphoma were reported in the 1970s, paralleling an increase in the number of patients with congenital and iatrogenic immunosuppression. The incidence of PCNS lymphoma rose significantly in the 1980s with the onset of the AIDS epidemic and was designated an AIDS-defining disease early in the epidemic. As many as 6% of AIDS patients may develop PCNS lymphoma during their illness (161,162). Interestingly, there has simultaneously been a threefold rise in the incidence of PCNS lymphoma in patients who are immunocompetent. The reasons for this are unknown.

To learn more about PCNS lymphoma, Fine and Mayer retrospectively analyzed PCNS lymphomas in 792 immunocompetent patients and 315 patients with AIDS (160). The mean age of patients with AIDS was significantly less than that of those without AIDS (30.8 versus 55.2 years), and the ratio of men to women with disease was different in AIDS lymphomas, with men representing a greater proportion of AIDS/PCNS lymphoma patients. Eighty percent of the AIDS patients had a history of OI, and 20% had PCNS lymphoma as their AIDS-defining illness (161).

CLINICAL PRESENTATION AND DIAGNOSIS

Clinically, patients with PCNS lymphoma present with a wide variety of symptoms and physical findings, including headache, new-onset seizures, hemiparesis, signs of increased intracranial pressure such as nausea and vomiting, mental status changes, or subtle cognitive or personality changes (160). The differential diagnosis of neurologic abnormalities in AIDS is long (163), and diligent evaluation may be necessary to obtain the correct diagnosis. However, PCNS lymphoma can often be confused with cerebral toxoplasmosis, the most common cause of focal cerebral masses in patients with AIDS. With the use of HAART and toxoplasmosis prophylaxis, the number of patients with PCNS may surpass that of those with toxoplasmosis in the near future. CT imaging reveals lymphomas to involve the cerebrum, brainstem, and cerebellum in decreasing order of frequency (160,164); such lesions are often periventricular in location and necrotizing. Extension to the ventricles or subarachnoid space may allow cytologic diagnosis through the cerebrospinal fluid (163).

Immunophenotyping reveals almost all lymphomas to be of B-cell origin with intermediate- to high-grade histology. Sixty percent of AIDS patients exhibit high-grade histologies of small noncleaved cells or immunoblasts, compared with only 22% of non-AIDS patients

(160,164). Lymphoma lesions may appear as single or multifocal masses that are isodense, hyperdense, or hypodense and thus difficult to distinguish from other mass lesions such as those due to toxoplasmosis (Fig. 34-3).

However, lymphomas tend to exhibit larger and fewer (more than 3 cm) lesions than toxoplasmosis (119). Ten percent of lesions may be radiographically occult (160). In contrast to non-AIDS–associated lymphomas, which almost never exhibit ring enhancement, AIDS-associated lymphomas are twice as frequently multifocal and have ring (50% of cases) or solid enhancement, which may be due to central tumor necrosis (162).

PCNS lymphomas usually appear hypointense on T1-weighted MRI images and isointense or hyperintense on T2-weighted images (160). Although the diagnosis can be suggested by CT or MRI, a definitive diagnosis by cerebrospinal fluid (CSF) cytology, EBV-DNA PCR, or brain biopsy is recommended, especially in patients with negative toxoplasmosis titers and whose condition worsens on empiric antitoxoplasmosis therapy (85,119,164). CSF may be analyzed for markers of clonality such as B-cell gene rearrangement or kappa or lambda light-chain analysis (160,164). De Luca et al. conducted a prospective study on 19 patients with HIV-positive serology and focal brain lesions (FBL) and 21 patients with HIV-positive serology with or without

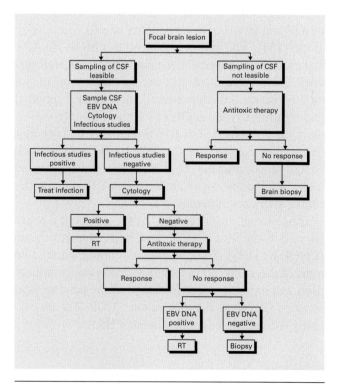

FIGURE 34-3 Evaluation of brain lesions in patients with HIV disease. CSF, cerebrospinal fluid; EBV, Epstein-Barr virus; RT = radiotherapy. [*From Sparano (85). With permission.*]

other neurologic disorders (165). Seven of eight patients with biopsy-proven PCNS were positive for EBV-DNA by PCR. The eighth patient had EBV-negative PCNS lymphoma tissue. Nevertheless, the sensitivity of the test was deemed to be 87.5%. The other 11 patients with FBL of other etiologies all tested negative for EBV-DNA by PCR. The remaining 21 control patients with other neurologic disorders also tested negative for EBV-DNA by PCR. Therefore the specificity of the test was 100% (165). Investigators of a small study performed FDG-PET scans on patients with the diagnosis of PCNS lymphoma or toxoplasmosis and found that such scans can accurately differentiate these disorders by the differences in standardized uptake values (range 1.7 to 3.1 versus 0.3 to 0.7, $p < 0.05$) (166). These results should be validated in a larger prospective study. Other investigators have reported that thallium-20 SPECT scans can be useful in diagnosing PCNS lymphoma and, by measuring a value called the retention index, can accurately distinguish between toxoplasmosis and neoplasm (167). These methods should be tested by others to establish the value of the test, and randomized comparisons among available imaging modalities should be performed.

PATHOGENESIS

The detection of EBV in nearly all cases of AIDS-associated PCNS lymphomas and the fact that these tumors are often polyclonal suggests a primary role for this virus in the pathogenesis of PCNS lymphomas. This is in contrast to the case in lymphomas in immunocompetent individuals and systemic lymphomas in patients with AIDS, where EBV expression is variable and occurs in less than 50% of cases. It is theorized that EBV infection causes a clonal expansion of B cells that goes unchecked by the abnormal immunoregulatory mechanisms of a dysfunctional immune system. Oncogene activation (c-myc is implicated) may result in transformation of one clone and a selective growth advantage. In addition, these effects may be enhanced by the decreased immune surveillance normally found in the CNS (160). Although HHV-8 has been implicated in the pathogenesis of PCNS lymphoma, this has recently been disproven (168).

STAGING

Upon confirmation of a diagnosis of PCNS lymphoma, a full neurologic evaluation for staging should be performed, including lumbar puncture, MRI of the spinal axis, and slit-lamp examination of the eye (7 to 18% of patients have ocular involvement at presentation) (161).

The extent of systemic staging required is controversial. However, if physical examination, chest x-ray, and routine laboratory results are unremarkable, further imaging is rarely useful (160). Other studies that may be done include bone marrow examination, abdomino-pelvic CT, chest CT, and gallium or FDG-PET (169) scanning (161). Thallium scans may also be helpful in diagnosis (167).

PROGNOSTIC FACTORS AND SURVIVAL

The median overall survival for patients with AIDS who have PCNS lymphomas is 2 to 3 months, compared with 12 to 20 months for similar patients without AIDS (160,161,170). The reasons for this difference are unclear, but several theories exist. It is possible that the tumors are biologically distinct and thus differ in their inherent responsiveness to chemoradiotherapy. Also, as Fine observed, trials have tended to use lower doses of radiotherapy in AIDS patients: 56% of patients with AIDS received less than 3500 cGy, compared with only 12% of patients without AIDS (160).

As with patients who have HRL, most patients with AIDS and PCNS lymphoma die of sequelae of advanced HIV disease rather than PCNS lymphoma (160,170). CNS lymphoma is a late manifestation of HIV disease, with most patients having CD4 cell counts less than 50/μL and a well-established AIDS diagnosis manifest by prior or concurrent opportunistic infections. Some 25 to 100% of autopsied patients with AIDS and CNS lymphoma have coexisting CNS infections, including HIV encephalitis, toxoplasmosis, cryptococcal meningitis, or cytomegalovirus encephalitis (161). However, patients who present with PCNS lymphoma as their AIDS-defining disease live longer than those with a prior history of opportunistic infections; they represent the few cases in the literature with long-term survival (160). Nevertheless, long-term remission in several patients was reported by Raez et al. in a retrospective study using treatments with intravenous zidovudine, ganciclovir, and low-dose IL-2 (85,171). According to a retrospective analysis, patients treated with HAART therapy also have improved survival over untreated patients (172).

THERAPY

With symptomatic therapy alone, the median survival is 2 to 3 months (173). Tumor resection is contraindicated due to the infiltrative nature of PCNS lymphoma; standard therapy consists of whole-brain radiation (160, 170). The optimal dose and fractionation schedule are undefined, but complete responses have been achieved at doses of 40 to 60 Gy; this is generally given in 1.8- to 2.0-Gy daily fractions (85,160,162,170,174). Survival in most analyses has been 12 to 42 months with treatment (175). Radiation therapy can substantially improve quality of life even if survival is not prolonged. Steroids are commonly used to decrease the edema surrounding the FBL or reduce mass effect, and tumor shrinkage with steroids alone has been reported.

Although there are minimal data regarding the use of chemotherapy, investigators have reported response and survival rates similar to those reported with radiotherapy (161). DeAngelis et al. reported a median survival time of 44 months with a regimen consisting of systemic methotrexate, steroids, whole-brain radiation, systemic cytarabine, and intraventricular methotrexate (176). This regimen was labeled "the DeAngelis protocol" and widely adopted until a follow-up report revealed its severe neurotoxic effects, especially in patients over 60 years of age (162). Other studies of systemic methotrexate in conjunction with whole-brain radiation have revealed good response and survival-rate data but compromised cognitive function (162). More intensive preradiation chemotherapy regimens are poorly tolerated (162).

The impact of HAART on PCNS lymphoma is largely unknown, although survival seems to be prolonged in treated patients (12). Anecdotal spontaneous regression of PCNS lymphoma with HAART therapy alone has been reported (177,178). Further study of chemotherapy and radiation combinations used in tandem or concurrently in the era of HAART is needed.

■ HODGKIN'S LYMPHOMA

Although several studies suggest an eightfold increase in the incidence of Hodgkin's lymphoma (HL) in patients with HIV (179,180), it is still not considered an AIDS-defining malignancy (181). However, HL is the most common type of non-AIDS-defining malignancy in the HIV population (179). There is evidence that concurrent HIV infection alters the natural history of HL (182). Many investigators recommend that all patients diagnosed with HL be tested for HIV infection, since those found to be HIV-positive may require modified treatment.

Investigators have reported that HIV-positive patients with HL have been younger (median age of 32) (86); they have a high frequency of stage III and IV disease, with atypical patterns of disease spread, extranodal presentations, and a high frequency of B symp-

toms at presentation (179,181,183). In most series, about two-thirds of patients have extranodal disease; of these, roughly half will have bone marrow involvement at diagnosis (179,184,185).

Patients with HIV disease have a higher incidence of mixed cellularity and lymphocyte-depleted histologies, subtypes considered to carry a poor prognosis (179,183, 186,187). The survival of patients with concurrent HIV and HL is also much shorter than for those with HL alone but better than for those with AIDS-associated non-Hodgkin's lymphomas (188). Median overall survival in HIV patients with HL is approximately 1.5 years in most studies (181,189–192). Patient deaths occur as a consequence of progressive HIV or OIs, but in contrast to HIV-associated NHL, they are also commonly a result of progressive HL.

Epstein-Barr virus (EBV) is strongly linked to the pathogenesis of HIV-associated HL, with rates of EBV positivity between 80 and 100% (193). This is much higher than the 40% rate observed in the non-HIV HL population (193). Reed-Sternberg cells, the malignant cells of HL, almost always express EBV-encoded latent membrane protein-1 (LMP-1). LMP-1 has demonstrated oncogenic properties and has been implicated in the pathogenesis of EBV-associated malignancies (193). Further studies are required to determine its role in HIV-associated malignancies, specifically HL.

Optimal therapy for HL in the HIV setting has yet to be defined. Standard therapies are usually employed but are often limited by severe cytopenias, exacerbated by involvement of bone marrow by HL when present. The AIDS Clinical Trial Group evaluated the efficacy of ABVD [Adriamycin (doxorubicin) bleomycin, vinblastine, and dacarbazine] with G-CSF in 21 HIV-seropositive patients (184). Although antiretrovirals were not used, these patients had an overall response rate of 62%, with 43% CR and 19% PR. The median survival in this cohort was 1.5 years. Almost half the patients experienced grade 4 neutropenia, and 29% of patients developed OIs. Although these results are far from optimal, no combination has yet to be proven to be more effective than this regimen (179,185). The role of HAART therapy during treatment is unknown.

■ CERVICAL NEOPLASM

EPIDEMIOLOGY

In 1993, the Centers for Disease Control (CDC) designated cervical cancer as an AIDS-defining illness (194). An association between cervical cancer and AIDS was anticipated on the basis of common sexual risk factors.

Also, immunosuppressed women such as transplant recipients have long been known to be at increased risk for lower genital tract neoplasia (195). Furthermore, both transplant patients and AIDS patients are at increased risk for human papillomavirus (HPV) infection, long known to be involved in the pathogenesis of cervical cancer (195). HPV infection is the most important risk factor for the development of cervical cancer (Table 34-7) (196,197). For HIV-infected women, the greatest risk factors for HPV infection may be a CD4 count less than 200/μL and elevated HIV viral load >10,000 HIV-RNA copies (198).

The association between HPV infection and cervical dysplasia and carcinoma is well established; in fact, HPV subtypes are identified by their ability to cause genital tract neoplasia. The risk of genital tract neoplasia is low for subtypes 6 and 11, which cause condyloma accumulata, and high for subtypes 16 and 18 (195). Sixty-four percent of HPV strains isolated in cervical cancer specimens are subtypes 16 and 18 (199). HPV's oncogenic properties are mediated through E6 and E7, viral encoded transforming proteins (200). These proteins inactivate the products of host tumor suppressor genes *p53* and *Retinoblastoma* (200). Once contracted, the infection is lifelong and places the patient at continued risk of cervical dysplasia. Immunosuppression induced by HIV infection can result in reactivation of HPV infection.

The incidence of high-risk HPV strains in HIV-seropositive women is 1.5 to 3 times that in their HIV-negative counterparts (201). The risk is even higher for persistent infection. The New York Cervical Disease Study, a prospective study of 328 HIV-seropositive women and 325 uninfected women, found that the ratio of HIV-positive and HIV-negative patients who tested positive for HPV was almost 2:1 (202,203). Almost all (95%) of patients with CD4 count of less than 500/μL tested positive for HPV-DNA. In addition, persistent infection was demonstrated in 20% of seropositive women and 3% of seronegative women (202). In a study by Maiman et al., 97% of HIV-positive patients versus

only 50% of HIV-negative patients had evidence of HPV infection (204). Other studies have confirmed these results (205).

CERVICAL CYTOLOGY AND SCREENING

HIV-infected women demonstrate a wide range of cytologic abnormalities, including inflammatory changes, hyperkeratosis, parakeratosis, trichomoniasis, herpetic changes, HPV-related changes, and varying degrees of cervical neoplasia. HIV-positive women show cytologic abnormalities in 30 to 60% of Pap smears and cervical dysplasia in 15 to 40% of smears (195,206,207). The prevalence of these abnormalities increases as the immunodeficiency becomes more severe (208), with patients with cervical dysplasia demonstrating lower absolute CD4 counts and CD4:CD8 ratios.

A disturbing feature of cervical dysplasia in HIV-infected women is the inconsistent resporting of the accuracy of cytologic examination (Pap smear) in predicting dysplasia on biopsy (206,208). Wright et al. (207) reported a 19% false-negative rate for Pap tests in HIV-seropositive patients, yet, even though this rate fell within the range for such tests in the general population (10 to 40%), the authors still recommended repeat Pap screening to reduce the risk of missing dysplasia on Pap smears. Other studies have also demonstrated the Pap smear's comparable accuracy in HIV positive and negative women (199). The "ThinPrep" technique may be preferable if available (199). Current U.S. Public Health Service (USPHS) and Infectious Diseases Society of America (IDSA) guidelines recommend Pap smears every 6 months during the first year after HIV diagnosis; if both are normal, annual screening is suggested (209). Some authorities advocate more aggressive screening, with either more frequent Pap smears or colposcopic examinations. Compliance and morbidity, however, are of concern in incorporating these programs.

Higher rates of concomitant vaginal infections in seropositive women may obscure smears. Minimally abnormal Pap smear results, such as inflammation, must be viewed as suspicious in the seropositive population as their likelihood of underlying high-grade dysplasia exceeds 10% (199). Colposcopy, or at least repeat Pap smear within a prudent time increment, is recommended. All HIV seropositive women with atypical squamous cells of undetermined significance (ASCUS), Pap smears read as "atypical squamous cells cannot exclude high grade squamous intraepithelial lesion" (HGSIL), atypical glandular cells of undetermined significance, low-grade squamous intraepithelial lesion (LGSIL), HGSIL, adenocarcinoma, and squamous

TABLE 34-7	TRADITIONAL FACTORS FOR CERVICAL CANCER RISK

History of more than six sexual partners
Cigarette smoking
Early age of first intercourse
History of sexually transmitted disease
Immunosuppression
Human papillomavirus

SOURCE: Data from Stier (199). With permission.

carcinoma must be evaluated with colposcopic examination (Fig. 34-4) (199).

Given the increased rates of HPV infection in HIV seropositive women and their increased risk for persistent infection, the higher incidence of cervical cancer seen in these patients is not surprising. Studies have demonstrated an increase in cervical cancer by five- to ninefold (199). HIV-positive patients with invasive cer-

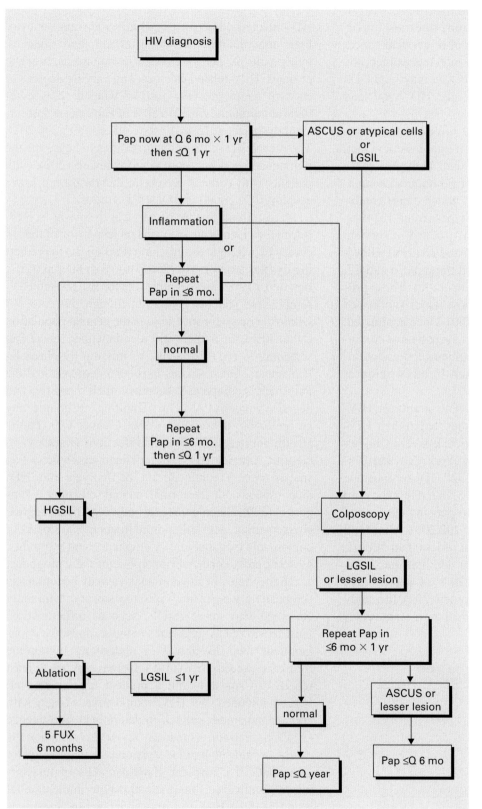

FIGURE 34-4 Screening/treatment algorithm for cervical cancer.

vical cancer also more frequently present with higher-stage disease.

THERAPY

Treatment is indicated for HGSIL or LGSIL that persists for 1 to 2 years (LGSIL may regress on its own) (199). For seropositive women treated with ablation or excision, overall results have been disappointing, with recurrence rates of 40 to 60% (195,199,206). Recurrence has been directly linked to the extent of immune deficiency: rates of more than 50% occur in patients with CD4 cell counts of less than 500/μL. Although the actual rate of progression of these lesions to invasive cancer is unknown, it is known that untreated lesions are more likely to progress in HIV-positive women (206). The AIDS Clinical Trials Group investigated topical fluorouracil (5-FU) plus ablative therapy as prophylaxis against recurrent dysplasia (210). In that study, patients were randomized to receive ablative therapy alone versus ablative therapy plus 2 g of 5% fluorouracil cream vaginally every 2 weeks for 6 months. The patients treated with 5-FU had fewer recurrences (28 versus 46%), longer time to recurrence, and lower-grade recurrences. The 5-FU was well tolerated. Patients with cervical dysplasia often require repetitive treatments and close surveillance to avoid progression of lesions.

INVASIVE CERVICAL CARCINOMA

Management of HIV-positive patients with invasive cervical cancer is complicated by the fact that patients are younger, present with more advanced stages of disease, present with metastatic disease at uncommon sites, and demonstrate a significantly poorer prognosis. Unlike patients with other AIDS-related malignancies, most patients die from advanced cervical carcinoma rather than from HIV disease (206). Patients with CD4 cell counts of more than 500/μL fare better than patients with lower counts.

Therapies for invasive cervical carcinoma are the same as in HIV seronegative individuals. (See "Tumors of the Uterine Cervix," Chap. 24.) These therapies include surgery, radiation, and concomitant chemoradiation and chemotherapy (211). The usual indications for surgery are early disease with curative intent or complications of advanced disease such as bowel obstruction. Concurrent chemoradiation with curative intent is commonly employed following hysterectomy in patients with extracervical disease (199). Cisplatin is the most commonly used agent in this setting. Chemotherapy

alone is reserved for palliation, and is complicated by a high rate of hematologic toxicity.

FUTURE DIRECTIONS

Extensive research to find an HPV vaccine is ongoing. A prophylactic vaccine would optimally be administered prior to initiating sexual activity. Therapeutic vaccine trials are also under way; however, it is unclear whether this strategy would be useful in the HIV population.

The impact of HAART on cervical dysplasia is unclear. As HAART improves immune function, HPV infection may be better controlled and dysplastic lesions may regress. Several studies have demonstrated such an effect (212–215). The effect of HAART on the incidence and prognosis of cervical cancer is also unclear, with studies showing no statistically significant change in incidence or survival (216–218). However, these studies were small and had short-term follow-up. Even if only for the other positive effects of HAART therapy, it should be administered to patients with cervical dysplasia and cancer.

■ ANORECTAL CARCINOMA

EPIDEMIOLOGY

Studies confirm an increasing incidence of anal cancer in both men and women that predates the AIDS epidemic (219) and that has doubled in recent decades (220). Suspected reasons for this increase include changing sexual habits and, more probably, increased exposure to HPV. Men with a history of homosexual activity are at highest risk. This is supported by a study of single, never-married men aged 20 to 49 in San Francisco between 1973 and 1989 (219), which showed a sevenfold increase in cases of squamous cell carcinoma of the anus in that group. Risk factors have been well defined (Table 34-8).

PATHOGENESIS

The subtypes of HPV associated with cervical cancer are also implicated in malignant transformation in anal cancer (219). However, other factors probably contribute as well to cervical and anal cancer, as not all cancers are HPV-positive. Many HPV-negative anal and cervical cancers contain *p53* mutations, and it is known that HPV E6 protein transforms epithelial cells by inactivating *p53*. It is likely that *p53* mutation or inactivation represents the final common pathway of malignant transformation for these epithelial cells. In addition, c-*myc*

TABLE 34-8	RISK FACTORS FOR AIDS-ASSOCIATED ANAL CARCINOMA
HIV seropositivity	
Low CD4 cell count	
Persistent HPV infection	
High-risk HPV genotypes	
Multiple HPV genotypes	
History of anal intercourse	
Cigarette smoking	
Immunosuppression	

HPV = Human papillomavirus.
SOURCE: Martin and Bowers (227). With permission.

activation occurs in approximately 30% of HPV-16–associated anal cancers and in premalignant anal lesions (219).

DISEASE FEATURES

Like HIV-infected cervical cancer patients, HIV-infected anorectal cancer patients demonstrate a higher incidence of precancerous lesions, a higher incidence of high-grade lesions, lower CD4 cell counts, and a higher overall incidence of HPV infection, often with multiple subtypes present simultaneously. Patients with lower CD4 cell counts (and frank AIDS) demonstrate more severe disease than do those with asymptomatic HIV infection (211,219,221). Futhermore, the natural history is one of rapid progression to invasive and morbid lesions.

SCREENING

Although screening for anal preinvasive neoplasia or anal cancer is available, it has not yet been widely utilized. Screening involves routine Pap smears and anoscopy, with biopsy of any suspicious lesions. Anal Pap smears have a reported sensitivity of approximately 70% (equivalent to that of cervical smears) and, as in cervical cancer, tend to underestimate the grade and incidence of neoplasia (211). There are currently no standard recommendations regarding the optimal type and frequency of screening tests for anal cancer (211). In any case, vigilant screening should be performed in patients who complain of abnormal discharge, bleeding, pruritus, bowel irregularity, or rectal or pelvic pain and in those with previous preinvasive lesions or abnormal Pap smears. Other patients who should be considered for screening include HIV-negative men with a history of anal-receptive intercourse, HIV-positive men, women with CD4 cell counts below 500/μL, and HIV-positive

or HIV-negative women with a history of high-grade cervical intraepithelial neoplasia (Fig. 34-5) (219).

THERAPY

Intraepithelial neoplasia II and III (AIN II and III), also referred to as high-grade squamous intraepithelial lesions (HGSILs), should be considered for therapy (Fig. 34-6) (211).

Therapeutic options depend on the size and location of the lesion; they include podophyllotoxin, 80% trichloroacetic acid, imiquimod, liquid nitrogen, and laser surgery (220,222). Patients with LGSIL or AIN can usually be evaluated every 6 months, as these lesions may spontaneously regress or progress slowly enough to allow detection before invasive cancer develops (211,219). If the lesion is small and morbidity of treatment is low, these lesions may be treated earlier (Fig. 34-7) (222).

Studies of HAART in AIN are limited but have not yet demonstrated an effect on the incidence or mortality of AIN (222).

Invasive lesions are treated, as in the general population (see "Anal Cancer," Chap. 17), with concurrent chemoradiation. Anecdotal experience suggests that HIV-infected patients have a decreased tolerance to full pelvic radiotherapy, with increased myelotoxicity and mucositis, thus limiting the size of treatment fields (223). It has been suggested that the addition of HAART may improve tolerance to therapy (220).

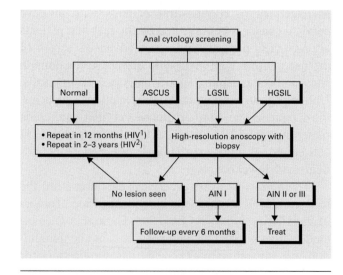

FIGURE 34-5 Protocol for screening anal intraepithelial neoplasia (AIN). ASCUS, atypical squamous cells of indeterminate significance; HGSIL, high-grade squamous intraepithelial lesion; LGSIL, low-grade squamous intraepithelial lesion. [*From Chin-Hong and Palevsky (222). With permission.*]

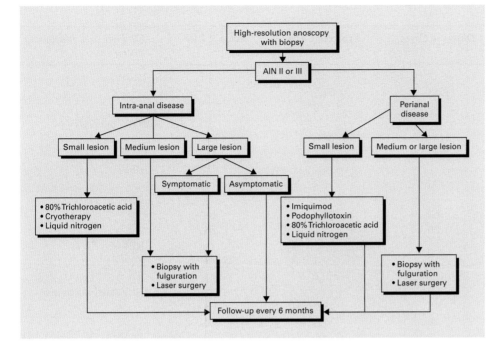

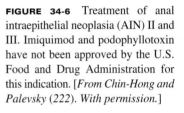

FIGURE 34-6 Treatment of anal intraepithelial neoplasia (AIN) II and III. Imiquimod and podophyllotoxin have not been approved by the U.S. Food and Drug Administration for this indication. [*From Chin-Hong and Palevsky (222). With permission.*]

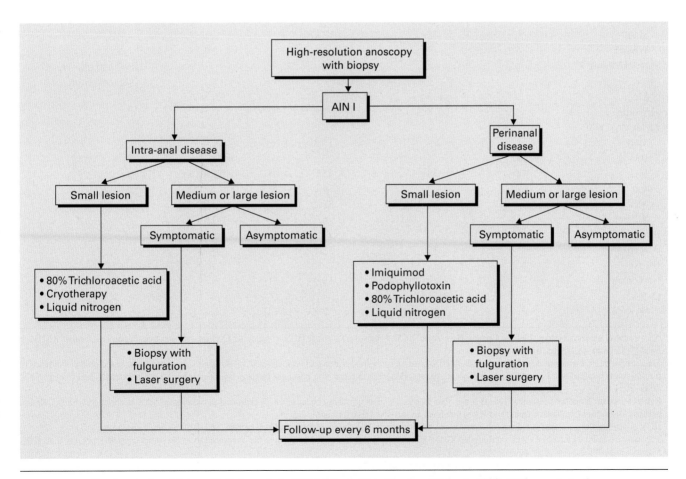

FIGURE 34-7 Treatment of anal intraepithelial neoplasia (AIN). [*From Chin-Hong and Palevsky (222). With permission.*]

TABLE 34-9	AIDS-ASSOCIATED CANCERS*			

Cancer Type	Observed Cases	Expected Cases	Relative Risk	Etiologic or Contributing Factors
Kaposi's sarcoma				KSHV
Men	5583	57.3	97.5[†]	
Women	200	1.0	202.7[†]	
Non-Hodgkin's lymphoma				EBV and KSHV
Men	2434	65	37.4	
Women	342	6.3	54.6	
Cervical, invasive				HPV
Women	133	14.7	9.1	
Hodgkin's disease				EBV
Men	160	20	8	
Women	20	3.1	6.4	
Tongue				HPV and EBV
Men	17	9.3	1.8	
Women	5	0.7	7.1	
Rectal, rectosigmoidal and anal				HPV (anal carcinoma)
Men	75	22.7	3.3	
Women	9	3.0	3.0	
Liver (primary only)				HCV,[‡] HBV, alcohol
Men	36	7.1	5.1	
Tracheal, bronchial and lung				Smoking[#]
Men	217	66.1	3.3	
Women	50	6.7	7.5	
Brain and CNS				EBV for CNS lymphoma
Men	42	13.4	3.1	
Women	7	2.0	3.4	
Skin, excluding KS				HPV[§] and ultraviolet-light exposure
Men	133	6.4	20.8	
Women	8	1.1	7.5	
Melanoma, skin				
Men	24	17.3	1.4	
Testicular				
Men	38	25.6	1.5	
Colon				
Men	32	38.2	0.8	
Women	5	6.3	0.8	
Prostate				
Men	37	53.7	0.7	
Breast				
Women	47	59.9	0.8	
Ovarian				
Women	6	7.8	0.8	

CNS = central nervous system; EBV = Epstein-Barr virus; HBV = hepatitis B virus; HCV = hepatitis C virus; HPV = human papillomavirus; KSHV = Kaposis's sarcoma–associated herpesvirus.

* Data are based on the observed number of cases in HIV-positive individuals (men and women aged 15–69 years), expected cases based on the incidence in a nonimmunocompromised population in New York State (NYS), relative risk and etiologic factors. Data from the AIDS/Cancer Matched Cohort NYS, 1981–1991.

[†] Relative risk for Kaposis's sarcoma (KS) is lower than in other studies, probably because the background population in NYS is enriched with population groups (for example, Italians, Greeks, and Jews) that have an increased risk for classic KS.

[‡] HCV contributes to increased incidence of liver cancer, particularly in HIV-infected men with hemophilia, and in intravenous drug users.

[#] The increase in lung cancer might be confounded by the fact that HIV-infected individuals have been reported to smoke more cigarettes per day than HIV-negative individuals.

[§] In Africa, HPV and ultraviolet-light exposure have been implicated in the high incidence of conjunctival squamous carcinoma, and HPV is also implicated as the cause of skin cancers seen after an organ transplant. Misdiagnosis of KS might also contribute to increased risk of skin cancer.

SOURCE: Reproduced with permission from *Nature Reviews Cancer.* Boshoff C, Weiss R. AIDS-related malignancies. *Nature* 2002;2:373–382. MacMillan Magazines Ltd.

■ OTHER HIV-ASSOCIATED MALIGNANCIES

Many other solid tumors reportedly occur in conjunction with HIV infection, including head and neck malignancies, skin cancers, lung cancers, GI malignancies, testicular germ cell tumors, breast cancers, melanomas, thymomas, gliomas, and leiomyosarcomas (Table 34-9) (224,225). However, information about such tumors is found only in small series or case reports, and not enough epidemiologic evidence exists to demonstrate conclusively the increased incidence of these tumors. Collectively, however, these tumors do have some traits in common: often atypical and aggressive presentations, onset at an earlier than expected age, and absence of commonly defined risk factors.

References

1. Cremer KJ, Spring SB, Gruber J. Role of human immunodeficiency virus type 1 and other viruses in malignancies associated with acquired immunodeficiency disease syndrome. *J Natl Cancer Inst* 1990;82:1016–1024.
2. Levine AM. AIDS-related malignancies: The emerging epidemic. *J Natl Cancer Inst* 1993;85:1382–1397.
3. Zunich KM, Lane HC. Immunologic abnormalities in HIV infection. *Hematol Oncol Clin North Am* 1991;5:215–228.
4. Lazo PA, Tsichlis PN. Biology and pathogenesis of retroviruses. *Semin Oncol* 1990;17:269–294.
5. Valentine FT. Pathogenesis of the immunological deficiencies caused by infection with the human immunodeficiency virus. *Semin Oncol* 1990;17:321–334.
6. Weiss RA. Retroviruses and human cancer. *Semin Cancer Biol* 1992;3:321–328.
7. Appelbaum JW. The role of the immune system in the pathogenesis of cancer. *Semin Oncol Nurs* 1992;8:51–62.
8. Levine AM. Cancer in AIDS: Editorial overview. *Curr Opin Oncol* 1989;1:55–56.
9. Gallo RC, Nerurkar LS. Human retroviruses: Their role in neoplasia and immunodeficiency. *Ann NY Acad Sci* 1987;567:82–94.
10. Safai B, Diaz B, Schwartz J. Malignant neoplasms associated with human immunodeficiency virus infection. *CA Cancer J Clin* 1992;42:74–95.
11. Bernstein L, Hamilton AS. The epidemiology of AIDS-related malignancies. *Curr Opin Oncol* 1993;5:822–830.
12. Centers for Disease Control and Prevention. Surveillance for AIDS-defining opportunistic illnesses, 1992–1997. *MMWR* 1999; :SS2.
13. Krigel RL, Friedman-Kien AE. Epidemic Kaposi's sarcoma. *Semin Oncol* 1990;17:350–360.
14. Tappero JW, Conant MA, Wolfe SF. Kaposi's sarcoma. *J Am Acad Dermatol* 1993;28:371–395.
15. Kaplan MH. Human retroviruses and neoplastic disease. *Clin Infect Dis* 1993; 17(suppl 2):S400–S406.
16. Biggar RJ, Rabkin CS. The epidemiology of AIDS-related neoplasms. *Hematol Oncol Clin North Am* 1996;10:997–1010.
17. Biggar RJ, Rosenberg PS, Cote T. Kaposis's sarcoma and non-Hodgkin's lymphoma following the diagnosis of AIDS. Multistate AIDS/Cancer Match Study Group. *Int J Cancer* 1996;68:754–758.
18. Beral V, Peterman TA, Berkelman RL, Jaffe HW. Kaposi's sarcoma among persons with AIDS: A sexually transmitted infection? *Lancet* 1990;335:123–128.
19. Ensoli B, Barillari G, Gallo R. Pathogenesis of AIDS-associated Kaposi's sarcoma. *Hematol Oncol Clin North Am* 1991;5:281–295.
20. Miles SA. Pathogenesis of human immunodeficiency virus-related Kaposi's sarcoma. *Curr Opin Oncol* 1992;14:875–882.
21. Uccini S, Ruco LP, Monardo F, et al. Co-expression of endothelial cell and macrophage antigens in Kaposi's sarcoma cells. *J Pathol* 1994;173:23–31.
22. Boshoff C, Weiss R. AIDS-related malignancies. *Nature* 2002;2:373–382.
23. Boshoff C, Schulz TF, Kennedy MM, et al. Kaposi's sarcoma-associated herpesvirus infects endothelial and spindle cells. *Nat Med* 1995;1:1274.
24. Sarid R, Klepfish A, Schattner A. Virology, pathogenic mechanisms, and associated diseases of Kaposi sarcoma-associated herpesvirus (human herpesvirus 8). *Mayo Clin Proc* 2002;77:941–949.
25. Boshoff C, Endo Y, Collins PD, et al. Angiogenic and HIV-inhibitory functions of KSHV-encoded chemokines. *Science* 1997;278:290–294.
26. Vogel J, Hinrichs SH, Reynolds RK, et al. The HIV tat gene induces dermal lesions resembling Kaposi's sarcoma in transgenic mice. *Nature* 1998;335:606–611.
27. Judson MA, Sahn SA. Endobronchial lesions in HIV-infected individuals. *Chest* 1994;105:1314–1323.
28. Chachoua A, Krigel R, Lafleur F, et al. Prognostic factors and staging classification of patients with epidemic Kaposi's sarcoma. *J Clin Oncol* 1989;7:774–780.
29. Errante D, Vaccher E, Tirelli U, et al. Management of AIDS and its neoplastic complications. *Eur J Cancer* 1991;27:380–389.
30. Krown SE, Testa MA, Huang J. AIDS-related Kaposi's sarcoma: Prospective validation of the AIDS Clinical Trials Group Oncology Committee. *J Clin Oncol* 1997;15:3085–3092.
31. Levine AM, Tulpule A: Clinical aspects and management of AIDS-related Kaposi's sarcoma. *Eur J Cancer* 2001;37:1288–1295.
32. Dupont C, Vasseur E, Beauchet A, et al. Long-term efficacy on Kaposi's sarcoma of highly active antiretroviral therapy in a cohort of HIV-positive patients. *AIDS* 2000;14:987–993.
33. Cattelan AM, Calabro ML, Gasperini P, et al. Acquired immunodeficiency syndrome-related Kaposi's sarcoma regression after highly active antiretroviral therapy: Biologic correlates of clinical outcome. *J Natl Cancer Inst Monogr* 2000;28:44–49.
34. Cattelan AM, Calabro ML, Averso SML, et al. Regression of AIDS-related Kaposi's sarcoma following antiretroviral therapy with protease inhibitors: Biological correlates of clinical outcome. *Eur J Cancer* 1999;35:1809–1815.
35. Dupin N, Rubin de Cervantes V, Gorin I, et al. The influence of highly active antiretroviral therapy on AIDS-associated Kaposi's sarcoma. *Br J Dermatol* 1999;140:875–881.

36. Krown SE, Myskowski PL, Paredes J. Kaposi's sarcoma. *Med Clin North Am* 1992;76:235–252.

37. Pluda JM, Broder S, Yarchoan R. Therapy of AIDS and AIDS-related tumors. *Cancer Chemother Biol Response Modif* 1991;12:395–429.

38. Tappero JW, Berger TG, Kaplan LD, et al. Cryotherapy for cutaneous Kaposi's sarcoma (KS) associated with acquired immune deficiency syndrome (AIDS): A phase II trial. *J AIDS* 1991;4:839–846.

39. Berson AM, Quivey JM, Harris JW, et al. Radiation therapy for AIDS-related Kaposi's sarcoma. *Int J Radiat Oncol Biol Phys* 1990;19:569–575.

40. Cooper JS, Steinfeld AD, Lerch I. Intentions and outcomes in the radiotherapeutic management of epidemic Kaposi's sarcoma. *Int J Radiat Oncol Biol Phys* 1991;20:419–421.

41. deWit R, Smit WGJM, Veenhof KHN, et al. Palliative radiation therapy for AIDS-associated Kaposi's sarcoma by using a single fraction of 800 cGy. *Radiother Oncol* 1990;19:131–136.

42. Chak LY, Gill PS, Levine AM, et al. Radiation therapy for acquired immunodeficiency syndrome-related Kaposi's sarcoma. *J Clin Oncol* 1988;6:863–867.

43. Cooper JS, Fried PR. Toxicity of oral radiotherapy in patients with acquired immunodeficiency syndrome. *Arch Otolaryngol Head Neck Surg* 1987;113:327–328.

44. Walmsley S, Northfelt DW, Melosky B, et al. Treatment of AIDS related cutaneous Kaposi's sarcoma with topical alitretinoin (9-cis retinoic) gel. *J Acquir Immune Defic Syndr* 1999;22:235–246.

45. Serfling U, Hood AF. Local therapies for cutaneous Kaposi's sarcoma in patients with acquired immunodeficiency syndrome. *Arch Dermatol* 1991;127:1479–1481.

46. Newman SB. Treatment of epidemic Kaposi's sarcoma (KS) with intralesional vinblastine injection (IL-VLB) (abstr). *Proc Am Soc Clin Oncol* 1988;7:5.

47. Brambilla L, Boneschi V, Beretta G, et al. Intralesional chemotherapy for Kaposi's sarcoma. *Dermatologica* 1984;169:150–155.

48. Abrams DI, Volberding PA. Alpha interferon therapy of AIDS-associated Kaposi's sarcoma. *Semin Oncol* 1987;14:43–47.

49. deWit R. AIDS-associated Kaposi's sarcoma and the mechanisms of interferon alpha's activity: A riddle within a puzzle. *J Intern Med* 1992;231:321–325.

50. Safai B, Bason M, Friedman-Birnbaum R, et al. Interferon in the treatment of AIDS-associated Kaposi's sarcoma: The American experience. *J Invest Dermatol* 1990;95:166–169.

51. Krown SE, Gold JWM, Niedzwiecki D, et al. Interferon-alpha with zidovudine: Safety, tolerance, and clinical and virologic effects in patients with Kaposi sarcoma associated with the acquired immunodeficiency syndrome (AIDS). *Ann Intern Med* 1990;112:812–821.

52. Fischl MA, Uttamchandani RB, Resnick L, et al. A phase I study of recombinant human interferon-alpha 2A or human lymphoblastoid interferon-alpha Nl and concomitant zidovudine in patients with AIDS-related Kaposi's sarcoma. *J AIDS* 1991;4:1–10.

53. Kovacs JA, Deyton L, Davey R, et al. Combined zidovudine and interferon-alpha therapy in patients with Kaposi's sarcoma and the acquired immunodeficiency syndrome (AIDS). *Ann Intern Med* 1989;111:280–287.

54. Gill PS, Rarick M, McCutchan JA, et al. Systemic treatment of AIDS-related Kaposi's sarcoma: Results of a randomized trial. *Am J Med* 1991;90:427–433.

55. Laubenstein LJ, Krigel RL, Odajnyk CM, et al. Treatment of epidemic Kaposi's sarcoma with etoposide or a combination of doxorubicin, bleomycin, and vinblastine. *J Clin Oncol* 1984;12:1115–1120.

56. Northfelt DW, Dezube BJ, Thommes JA, et al. Pegylated-liposomal doxorubicin versus doxorubicin, bleomycin, and vincristine in the treatment of AIDS related Kaposi's sarcoma: Results of a randomized phase III clinical trial. *J Clin Oncol* 1998;16:2445–2451.

57. Stewart S, Jablonowski H, Goebel FD, et al. Randomized comparative trial of pagylated liposomal doxorubicin versus bleomycin and vincristine in the treatment of AIDS-related Kaposi's sarcoma. International Pegylated Liposomal Doxorubicin Study Group. *J Clin Oncol* 1998;16:683–691.

58. Gill PS, Wernz J, Scadden DT, et al. Randomized phase III trial of liposomal daunorubicin versus doxorubicin, bleomycin, and vincristine in AIDs-related Kaposi's sarcoma. *J Clin Oncol* 1996;14:2233–2364.

59. Rosenthal E, Poizot-Martin I, Saint-Marc T, et al. Phase IV study of liposomal daunorubicin (DaunoXome) in AIDS-related Kaposi's sarcoma. *Am J Clin Oncol* 2002;25:57–59.

60. Saville MW, Lietzau J, Pluda JM, et al. Treatment of HIV-associated Kaposi's sarcoma with paclitaxel. *Lancet* 1995;346:26–28.

61. Welles L, Savelle MW, Lietzau J, et al. Phase II trial with dose titration of paclitaxel for the therapy of human immunodeficiency virus-associated Kaposi's sarcoma. *J Clin Oncol* 1998;16:1112–1121.

62. Tulpule A, Groopman J, Saville MW, et al. Multicenter trial of low-dose paclitaxel in patients with advanced AIDS-related Kaposi ssarcoma. *Cancer* 2002;95:147–154.

63. Little RF, Wyvill KM, Pluda JM, et al. Activity of thalidomide in AIDS-related Kaposi's sarcoma. *J Clin Oncol* 2000;18:2593–2602.

64. Ingber D, Fukita T, Kishimoto S, et al. Synthetic analogues of fumagillin that inhibit angiogenesis and suppress tumour growth. *Nature* 1990;348:555–557.

65. Pluda JM, Wyvill K, Figg WD, et al. A phase I study of an angiogenesis inhibitor, TNP-470 (AGM-1470), administered to patients (PTS) with HIV-associated Kaposi's sarcoma (KS) (abstr). *Proc Am Soc Clin Oncol* 1994;13:51.

66. Nakamura S, Sakurada S, Salahuddin SZ, et al. Inhibition of development of Kaposi's sarcoma-related lesions by a bacterial cell wall complex. *Science* 1992;255:1437–1440.

67. Eckhardt SG, Burris HA, Eckardt JR, et al. Phase I assessment of the novel angiogenesis inhibitor DS4152 (tecogalan sodium) (abstr). *Proc Am Soc Clin Oncol* 1994;13:55.

68. Dezube BJ, Von Roenn JH, Holden-Wiltse J, et al. Fumagillin analog in the treatment of Kaposi's sarcoma: A phase I AIDS Clinical Trial Group study. *J Clin Oncol* 1998;14(4):1444–1449.

69. Tulpule A, Snyder JC, Espina BM, et al. A phase I study of tecogalan, a novel angiogenesis inhibitor in the treatment of AIDS-related Kaposi's sarcoma and solid tumor (abstr). *Blood* 1994;84(suppl 1):248a.

70. Eckhardt SG, Burris HA, Eckardt JR, et al. A phase I clinical and pharmacokinetic study of the angiogenesis inhibitor, tecogalan sodium. *Ann Oncol* 1996;7:491–496.

71. Tulpule A, Scadden DT, Espina BM, et al. Results of a randomized study of IM862 nasal solution in the treatment of AIDS-related Kaposi's sarcoma. *J Clin Oncol* 2000;18(4):716–723.

72. Gill PS, Lunardi-Iskandar Y, Louie S, et al. Human chorionic gonadotropin has antitumor activity in AIDS-related Kaposi's sarcoma. *N Engl J Med* 1996;335:261–269.

73. Lunardi-Iskandar Y, Bryant JL, Blattner WA, et al. Effects of a urinary factor from women in early pregnancy on HIV-1, SIV and associated disease. *Nat Med* 1998;4:428–434.

74. Morfeldt L, Torssander J. Long-term remission of Kaposi's sarcoma following foscarnet treatment in HIV-infected patients. *Scand J Infect* Dis 1994;26:749–752.

75. Humphrey RW, Davis DA, Newcomb FM, et al. Human herpesvirus 8 (HHV-8) in the pathogenesis of Kaposis's sarcoma and other diseases. *Leuk Lymph* 1998;28:255–264.

76. Mocroft A, Youle M, Gazzard B, et al. Anti-herpesvirus treatment and the risk of Kaposi's sarcoma in HIV infection: Royal Free/Chelsea and Westminster Hospitals Collaborative Group. *J Clin Invest* 1997;99:2082–2086.

77. Gelsby MJ, Hoover DR, Weng S, et al. Use of antiherpes drugs and the risk of Kaposi's sarcoma: Data from the Multicenter AIDS Cohort Study. *AIDS* 1996;10:1101–1105.

78. Schwartsmann G, Sander E, Prolla G, et al. Phase II trial of pentosan polysulfate (PPS) in patients (PTS) with AIDS-related Kaposi's sarcoma (KS) (abstr). *Proc Am Soc Clin Oncol* 1993;12:54.

79. Cattelan AM, Trevenzoli M, Aversa SML, et al. Recent advances in the treatment of AIDS-related Kaposi's sarcoma. *Am J Clin Dermatol* 2002;3(7):451–462.

80. Cianfrocca M, Cooley TP, Lee JY, et al. Matrix metalloproteinase inhibitor COL-3 in the treatment of AIDS-related Kaposi's sarcoma: A phase I AIDS malignancy consortium study. *J Clin Oncol* 2002; 20(1):153–159.

81. Biggar RJ, Rabkin CS. The epidemiology of acquired immunodeficiency syndrome-related lymphomas. *Curr Opin Oncol* 1992;4(5):883–893.

82. Centers for Disease Control. Revision of the case definition of acquired immunodeficiency syndrome for national reporting-United States. *Ann Intern Med* 1985;103:402–403.

83. Levine AM, Scadden DT, Zaia JA, et al. Hematologic aspects of HIV/AIDS. (Am Soc Hematol Educ Program). *Hematology* 2001:463–478.

84. Tirelli U, Bernardi D. Impact of HAART on the clinical management of AIDS-related cancers. *Eur J Cancer* 2001;37(10):1320–1324.

85. Sparano JA. Clinical aspects and management of AIDS-related lymphoma. *Eur J Cancer* 2001;37(10):1296–1305.

86. Ng VL, McGrath MS. Pathogenesis of HIV-associated NHL. HIV InSite Knowledge Base Chapter. Published November 2002. http://hivinsite.ucsf.edu

87. Serraino D, Salamina G, Franceschi S, et al. The epidemiology of AIDS-associated non-Hodgkin's lymphoma in the World Health Organization European region. *Br J Cancer* 1992;66:912–916.

88. Northfelt DW, Kaplan LD. Clinical aspects of AIDS-related non-Hodgkin's lymphoma. *Curr Opin Oncol* 1991;3:872–880.

89. Northfelt DW, Volberding PA, Kaplan LD. Degree of immunodeficiency at diagnosis of AIDS-associated non-Hodgkin's lymphoma (abstr). *Proc Am Soc Clin Oncol* 1992;11:45.

90. Pluda JM, Yarchoan R, Jaffe ES, et al. Development of non-Hodgkin lymphoma in a cohort of patients with severe human immunodeficiency virus (HIV) infection on long-term antiretroviral therapy. *Ann Intern Med* 1990;113:276–282.

91. Beral V, Peterman T, Berkelman R, Jaffe H. AIDS-associated non-Hodgkin lymphoma. *Lancet* 1991;337:805–809.

92. Levine AM, Seneviratne L, Espina BM, et al. Evolving characteristics of AIDS-related lymphoma. *Blood* 2000;96(13):4084–4090.

93. Matthews GV, Bower M, Mandalia S, et al. Changes in AIDS-related lymphoma. *Blood* 2000;96:2730–2734.

94. Besson C, Goubar A, Gabarre J, et al. Changes in AIDS related lymphomas since the era of highly active anti-retroviral therapy. *Blood* 2001;98:2339–2344.

95. Levine AM. Acquired immunodeficiency-syndrome related lymphoma. *Blood* 1992;80:8–20.

96. Pluda JM, Yarchoan R, Broder S. The occurrence of opportunistic non-Hodgkin's lymphomas in the setting of infection with the human immunodeficiency virus. *Ann Oncol* 1991; 2(suppl 2):191–200.

97. Karp JE, Broder S. The pathogenesis of AIDS lymphomas: A foundation for addressing the challenges of therapy and prevention. *Leuk Lymph* 1992;8:167–188.

98. Pelicci P, Knowles DM, Arlin ZA, et al. Multiple monoclonal B cell expansions and c-myc oncogene rearrangements in acquired immune deficiency syndrome-related lymphoproliferative disorders. *J Exp Med* 1986;164:2049–2076.

99. Shibata D, Weiss LM, Hernandez AM, et al. Epstein-Barr virus-associated non-Hodgkin's lymphoma in patients infected with the human immunodeficiency virus. *Blood* 1983; 81:2102–2109.

100. Neri A, Barriga F, Inghirami G, et al. Epstein-Barr virus infection precedes clonal expansion in Burkitt's and acquired immunodeficiency syndrome-associated lymphoma. *Blood* 1991;77:1092–1095.

101. Shibata D, Weiss LM, Nathwani BN, et al. Epstein-Barr virus in benign lymph node biopsies from individuals infected with the human immunodeficiency virus is associated with concurrent or subsequent development of non-Hodgkin's lymphoma. *Blood* 1991;77:1527–1533.

102. Dolcetti R, Gloghini A, De Vita S, et al. Characteristics of EBV-infected cells in HIV-related lymphadenopathy: Implications for the pathogenesis of EBV-associated and EBV-unrelated lymphomas of HIV-seropositive individuals. *Int J Cancer* 1995;63:652–659.

103. Martin A, Flaman JM, Frebourg T, et al. Functional analysis of the p53 protein in AIDS-related non-Hodgkin's lymphomas and polymorphic lymphoproliferations. *Br J Haematol* 1998;101(2):311–317.

104. Nador RG, Horenstein MG, Chadburn A, et al. Molecular analysis of 70 AIDS-related systemic non-Hodgkin's lymphomas from the east and west coasts of the United States of America (USA). *Ann Oncol* 1996;7(suppl. 3):16.

105. DM. Biologic aspects of AIDS-associated non-Hodgkin's lymphoma. *Curr Opin Oncol* 1993;15:845–851.

106. Knowles DM, Chamulak GA, Subar M, et al. Lymphoid neoplasia associated with the acquired immunodeficiency syndrome (AIDS). *Ann Intern Med* 1988;108:744–753.

107. Voelkerding KV, Sandhaus LM, Kim HC, et al. Plasma cell malignancy in the acquired immune deficiency syndrome. *Am J Clin Pathol* 92:222–228, 1989.

108. Levine AM, Sadeghi S, Espina B, et al. Characteristics of indolent non-Hodgkin lymphoma in patients with type 1 human immunodeficiency virus infection. *Cancer* 2002 Mar 1;94(5):1500–1506.

109. Janier M, Katlama C, Flageul B, et al. The pseudo-Sezary syndrome with CD8 phenotype in a patient with the acquired immunodeficiency syndrome (AIDS). *Ann Intern Med* 1989; 110:738–740.

110. Goldstein J, Becker N, Del Rowe J et al. Cutaneous T-cell lymphoma in a patient infected with human immunodeficiency virus type 1. Use of radiation therapy. *Cancer* 1990; 66:1130–1132.

111. Ruff P, Bagg A, Papadopoulos K: Precursor T-cell lymphoma associated with human immunodeficiency virus type 1 (HIV-1) infection. *Cancer* 1989;64:39–42.

112. Ciobanu N, Andreeff M, Safai B, et al. Lymphoblastic neoplasia in a homosexual patient with Kaposi's sarcoma. *Ann Intern Med* 1983;98:151–155.

113. Shibata D, Byrnes RK, Rabinowitz A, et al. Human T-cell lymphotropic virus type I (HTLV-I)-associated adult T-cell leukemia-lymphoma in a patient infected with human immunodeficiency virus 1 (HIV-1). *Ann Intern Med* 1989;111: 871–875.

114. Sternlieb J, Mintzer D, Kwa D, et al. Peripheral T-cell lymphoma in a patient with the acquired innumodeficiency syndrome. *Am J Med* 1988;85:445.

115. Gonzales-Clemente JM, Ribera JM, Campo E, et al. Ki-1 plus anaplastic large-cell lymphoma of T-cell origin in an HIV-infected patient. *AIDS* 1991;5:751–755.

116. Ziegler JL, Beckstead JA, Volberding PA, et al. Non-Hodgkin's lymphoma in 90 homosexual men. Relation to generalized lymphadenopathy and the acquired immunodeficiency syndrome. *N Engl J Med* 1984;311:565–570.

117. Kaplan LD, Abrams DI, Feigal E, et al. AIDS-associated non-Hodgkin's lymphoma in San Francisco. *JAMA* 1989; 261:719–724.

118. Freter CE. Acquired immunodeficiency syndrome-associated lymphomas. *J Natl Cancer Inst* 1990;10:45–54.

119. Levine AM. Epidemiology, clinical characteristics, and management of AIDS-relatd lymphoma. *Hematol Oncol Clin North Am* 1991;5:331–342.

120. Heitzman ER. Pulmonary neoplastic and lymphoproliferative disease in AIDS: A review. *Radiology* 1990;177:347–351.

121. Dodd GD III, Greenler DP, Confer SR. Thoracic and abdominal manifestations of lymphoma occurring in the immunocompromised patient. *Radiol Clin North Am* 1992;30:597–610.

122. Sokovich RS, Bormes TD, McKiel CF. Acquired immunodeficiency syndrome presenting as testicular lymphoma. *J Urol* 1992;147:1110–1111.

123. Green ST, Nathwani D, Goldberg DJ, et al. Urological manifestations of HIV-related disease. A case of AIDS-associated testicular seminoma, Kaposi's sarcoma, and possible intracranial lymphoma. *Br J Urol* 1991;167:188–190.

124. Tsang K, Kneafsey P, Gill MJ. Primary lymphoma of the kidney in the acquired immunodeficiency syndrome. *Arch Pathol Lab Med* 1993;117:541–543.

125. Holladay AO, Siegel RJ, Schwartz DA. Cardiac malignant lymphoma in acquired immune deficiency syndrome. *Cancer* 1992;70:2203–2207.

126. Levine AM. AIDS-associated malignant lymphoma. *Med Clin North Am* 1992;76:253–268.

127. Gisselbrecht C, Oksenjendler E, Tirelli U, et al. Non-Hodgkin's lymphoma associated with human immunodeficiency virus: Treatment with LNH 84 regimen in a selected group of patients. *Leukemia* 1992;6(suppl 3):10–IIS.

128. Levine AM, Sullivan-Halley J, Pike MC, et al. Human immunodeficiency virus-related lymphoma. Prognostic factors predictive of survival. *Cancer* 1991;68:2466–2472.

129. Straus DJ, Huang J, Testa MA, et al. Prognostic factors in the treatment of human immunodeficiency virus-associated non-Hodgkin's lymphoma: Analysis of AIDS Clinical Trials Group protocol 142-low-dose versus standard-dose m-BACOD plus granulocyte-macrophage colony-stimulating factor. National Institute of Allergy and Infectious Diseases. *J Clin Oncol* 1998;16:3601–3606.

130. Navarro JT, Ribera JM, Oriol A, et al. International prognostic index is the best prognostic factor for survival in patients with AIDS-related non-Hodgkin's lymphoma treated with CHOP. A multivariate study of 46 patients. *Haematologica* 1998;83:508–513.

131. Rossi G, Donisi A, Casari S, et al. The International Prognostic Index can be used as a guide to treatment decisions regarding patients with human immunodeficiency virus-related systemic non-Hodgkin's lymphoma. *Cancer* 1999;86:2391–2397.

132. Aboulafia DM, Mitsuyasu RT. Hematologic abnormalities in AIDS. *Hematol Oncol Clin North Am* 1991;5:195–214.

133. Calenda V, Chermann JC. The effects of HIV on hematopoiesis. *Eur J Hematol* 1992;148:181–186.

134. Pluda JM, Mitsuya H, Yarchoan R. Hematologic effects of AIDS therapies. *Hematol Oncol Clin North Am* 1991;5:229–248.

135. Gill PS, Levine AM, Krailo M, et al. AIDS-related malignant lymphoma: Results of prospective treatment trials. *J Clin Oncol* 1987;5:1322–1328.

136. Levine AM, Wemz JC, Kaplan L, et al. Low-dose chemotherapy with central nervous system prophylaxis and zidovudine maintenance in AIDS-related lymphoma. *JAMA* 1991; 266:84–88.

137. Kaplan LD, Straus DJ, Testa MA, et al. Low-dose compared with standard-dose m-BACOD chemotherapy for non-Hodgkin's lymphoma associated with human immunodeficiency virus infection. National Institute of Allergy and Infectious Diseases AIDS Clinical Trials Group. *N Engl J Med* 1997;336:1641–1648.

138. Remick SC, McSharry JJ, Wolf BC, et al. Novel oral combination chemotherapy in the treatment of intermediate-grade and high-grade AIDS-related non-Hodgkin's lymphoma. *J Clin Oncol* 1993;11:1691–1702.

139. Tosi P, Gherlinzoni F, Mazza P, et al. 3'-Azido 3'-deoxythymidine + methotrexate as a novel antineoplastic combination in the treatment of human immunodeficiency virus-related non-Hodgkin's lymphomas. *Blood* 1997;89:419–425.

140. Walsh C, Wernz JC, Levine A, et al. Phase I trial of m-BACOD and granulocyte macrophage colony stimulating factor in HIV-associated non-Hodgkin's lymphoma. *J AIDS* 1993;6: 265–271.

141. Kaplan LD, Kahn JO, Crowe S, et al. Clinical and virologic effects of recombinant human granulocyte-macrophage colony-stimulating factor in patients receiving chemotherapy for human immunodeficiency virus-associated non-Hodgkin's lymphoma: Results of a randomized trial. *J Clin Oncol* 1991; 9:929–940.

142. Perrella O, Finelli E, Perrella A, et al. Combined therapy with zidovudine, recombinant granulocyte colony stimulating factors and erythropoietin in asymptomatic HIV patients. *J Chemother* 1996;8:63–66.

143. Skowron G, Stein D, Drusano G, et al. Safety and anti-HIV effect of GM-CSF in patients on highly active antiretroviral therapy. 5th Conference on Retroviruses and Opportunistic Infections, 1998 (abstr 615).

144. Sparano JA, Wiernik PH, Strack M, et al. Infusional cyclophosphamide, doxorubicin, and etoposide in human immunodeficiency virus- and human T-cell leukemia virus type I-related non-Hodgkin's lymphoma: A highly active regimen. *Blood* 1993;81(10):2810–2815.

145. Sparano JA, Wiernik PH, Leaf A, Dutcher JP. Infusional cyclophosphamide, doxorubicin, and etoposide in relapsed and resistant non-Hodgkin's lymphoma: Evidence for a schedule-dependent effect favoring infusional administration of chemotherapy. *J Clin Oncol* 1993;11(6):1071–1079.

146. Sparano JA, Wiernik PH, Hu X, et al. Pilot trial of infusional cyclophosphamide, doxorubicin, and etoposide plus didanosine and filgrastim in patients with human immunodeficiency virus-associated non-Hodgkin's lymphoma. *J Clin Oncol* 1996; 14(11):3026–3035.

147. Sparano JA, Wiernik PH, Hu X, et al. Saquinavir enhances the mucosal toxicity of infusional cyclophosphamide, doxorubicin, and etoposide in patients with HIV-associated non-Hodgkin's lymphoma. *Med Oncol* 1998;15(1):50–57.

148. Sparano JA, Weller E, Nazeer T, et al. Phase 2 trial of infusional cyclophosphamide, doxorubicin, and etoposide in patients with poor-prognosis, intermediate-grade non-Hodgkin lymphoma: An Eastern Cooperative Oncology Group trial (E3493). *Blood* 2002;100(5):1634–1640.

149. Little RF, Pittaluga S, Grant N, et al. Highly effective treatment of acquired immunodeficiency syndrome-related lymphoma with dose-adjusted EPOCH: Impact of antiretroviral therapy suspension and tumor biology. *Blood* 2003;101(12): 4653–4659.

150. Scadden DT. AIDS lymphomas: Beginning of an EPOCH? *Blood* 2003;101:4647.

151. Tirelli U, Spina M, Jaeger U, et al. Infusional CDE with rituximab for the treatment of human immunodeficiency virus-associated non-Hodgkin's lymphoma: Preliminary results of a phase I/II study. *Recent Results Cancer Res* 2002;159:149–153.

152. Gronemann UT, Helweg-Larsen J, Jensen-Fangel S, et al. HIV-associated NHLs in Denmark post-HAART—A retrospective analysis of 61 consecutive cases. *Blood* 2002; (abstr 3652).

153. Ratner L, Lee J, Tang S, et al. Chemotherapy for human immunodeficiency virus-associated non-Hodgkin's lymphoma in combination with highly active antiretroviral therapy. *J Clin Oncol* 2001;19(8):2171–2178.

154. Vaccher E, Spina M, di Gennaro G, et al. Concomitant cyclophosphamide, doxorubicin, vincristine, and prednisone chemotherapy plus highly active antiretroviral therapy in patients with human immunodeficiency virus-related, non-Hodgkin lymphoma. *Cancer* 2001;91(1):155–163.

155. Kaplan LD, Scadden DT. No benefit from rituximab in a randomized phase III trial of CHOP with or without rituximab for patients with HIV-associated non-Hodgkin's lymphoma: AIDS malignancies consortium study 010. *Proc Am Soc Clin Oncol* 2003; (abstr 2268).

156. Cortes J, Thomas D, Rios A, et al. Hyperfractionated cyclophosphamide, vincristine, doxorubicin, and dexamethasone and highly active antiretroviral therapy for patients with acquired immunodeficiency syndrome-related Burkitt lymphoma/leukemia. *Cancer* 2002;94:1492–1499.

157. Bi J, Espina BM, Tulpule A, et al. High-dose cytosine-arabinoside and cisplatin regimens as salvage therapy for refractory or relapsed AIDS-related non-Hodgkin's lymphoma. *J AIDS* 2001;28:416–421.

158. Ellent DP, Rowley D, Godberg L, et al. Autologous hematopoietic stem cell transplantation (HSCT) for the treatment of HIV-infected patients on HAART with non-Hodgkin's lymphoma. *Proc Am Soc Oncol* 2003; (abstr 2413).

159. Krishnan A, Molina A, Zaia J, et al. Autologous stem cell transplantation for HIV-associated NHL. *Blood* 2001;98: 3857–3859.

160. Fine HA, Mayer RJ. Primary central nervous system lymphoma. *Ann Intern Med* 1993;119:1093–1104.

161. Deangelis LM. Current management of primary central nervous system lymphoma. *Oncology* 1995;9:63–71.

162. Schlegel U, Schmidt-Wolf IG, Deckert M. Primary CNS lymphoma: Clinical presentation, pathological classification, molecular pathogenesis and treatment. *J Neurol Sci* 2000; 181(1–2):1–12.

163. Davenport C, Dillon WP, Sze G. Neuroradiology of the immunosuppressed state. *Radiol Clin North Am* 1992;30:611–637.

164. Xerri L, Gambarelli D, Horschowski N, et al. What's new in primary central nervous system lymphomas? *Pathol Res Pract* 1990;186:809–816.

165. De Luca A, Antinori A, Cingolani A, et al. Evaluation of cerebrospinal fluid EBV-DNA and IL-10 as markers for in vivo diagnosis of AIDS-related primary central nervous system lymphoma. *Br J Haematol* 1995;90(4):844–849.

166. Villringer K, Jager H, Dichgans M, et al. Differential diagnosis of CNS lesions in AIDS patients by FDG-PET. *J Comput Assist Tomogr* 1995;19(4):532–536.

167. Lorberboym M, Wallach F, Estok L, et al. Thallium-201 retention in focal intracranial lesions for differential diagnosis of primary lymphoma and nonmalignant lesions in AIDS patients. *J Nucl Med* 1998;39(8):1366–1369.

168. Antinori A, Larocca LM, Fassone L, et al. HHV-8/KSHV is not associated with AIDS-related primary central nervous system lymphoma. *Brain Pathol* 1999;9(2):199–208.

169. Roelcke U, Leenders KL. Positron emission tomography in patients with primary CNS lymphomas. *J Neurooncol* 1999; 43(3):231–236.

170. Goldstein JD, Dickson DW, Moser FG, et al. Primary central nervous system lymphoma in acquired immune deficiency syndrome. A clinical and pathologic study with results of treatment with radiation. *Cancer* 1991;67:2756–2765.

171. Raez LE, Patel P, Feun L, Restrepo A, et al. Natural history and prognostic factors for survival in patients with acquired immune deficiency syndrome (AIDS)-related primary central nervous system lymphoma (PCNSL). *Crit Rev Oncol* 1998; 9(3–4):199–208.

172. Skiest DJ, Crosby C. Survival is prolonged by highly active antiretroviral therapy in AIDS patients with primary central nervous system lymphoma. *AIDS* 2003;17(12):1787–1793.

173. Jellinger K, Radaskiewicz TH, Slowik F. Primary malignant lymphomas of the central nervous system in man. *Acta Neuropathol Suppl (Berl)* 1975;(suppl 6):95–102.

174. Formenti SC, Gill PS, Lean E, et al. Primary central nervous system lymphoma in AIDS. Results of radiation therapy. *Cancer* 1989;63:1101–1107.

175. Nelson DF. Radiotherapy in the treatment of primary central nervous system lymphoma (PCNSL). *J Neurooncol.* 1999; 43(3):241–247.

176. DeAngelis LM, Yahalom J, Thaler HT, et al. Combined modality therapy for primary CNS lymphoma. *J Clin Oncol* 1992;10(4):635–643.

177. McGowan JP, Shah S. Long-term remission of AIDS-related primary central nervous system lymphoma associated with highly active antiretroviral therapy. *AIDS* 1998;12(8):952–954.

178. Terriff BA, Harrison P, Holden JK. Apparent spontaneous regression of AIDS-related primary CNS lymphoma mimicking resolving toxoplasmosis. *J AIDS* 1992;5(9):953–954.

179. Vaccher E, Spina M, Tirelli U. Clinical aspects and management of Hodgkin's disease and other tumours in HIV-infected individuals. *Eur J Cancer* 2001;37(10):1306–1315.

180. Hessol NA, Katz MH, Liu JU, et al. Increased incidence of Hodgkin's disease in homosexual men with HIV infection. *Ann Intern Med* 1992;117:309–311.

181. Ames ED, Conjalka MS, Goldberg AF, et al. Hodgkin's disease and AIDS. Twenty-three new cases and a review of the literature. *Hematol Oncol Clin North Am* 1991;5:343–356.

182. Gold JE, Altarac D, Ree HJ, et al. HIV-associated Hodgkin's disease: A clinical study of 18 cases and review of the literature. *Am J Hematol* 1991;36:93–99.

183. Pelstring RJ, Zellmer RB, Sulak LE, et al. Hodgkin's disease in association with human immunodeficiency virus infection. Pathologic and immunologic features. *Cancer* 1991;67:1865–1873.

184. Levine AM, Li P, Cheung T, et al. Chemotherapy consisting of doxorubicin, bleomycin, vinblastine, and dacarbazine with granulocyte-colony-stimulating factor in HIV-infected patients with newly diagnosed Hodgkin's disease: A prospective, multi-institutional AIDS clinical trials group study (ACTG 149). *J AIDS* 2000;15(5):444–450.

185. Errante D, Gabarre J, Ridolfo AL, et al. Hodgkin's disease in 35 patients with HIV infection: An experience with epirubicin, bleomycin, vinblastine and prednisone chemotherapy in combination with antiretroviral therapy and primary use of G-CSF. *Ann Oncol* 1999;10(2):189–195.

186. Serraino D, Carbone A, Franceschi S, et al. Increased frequency of lymphocyte depletion and mixed cellularity subtypes of Hodgkin's disease in HIV-infected patients. *Eur J Cancer* 1993;29A:1948–1950.

187. Tirelli U, Vaccher E, Rezza G, et al. Hodgkin's disease in association with acquired immunodeficiency syndrome (AIDS). A report on 36 patients. *Acta Oncol* 1989;28:637–639.

188. Newcom S, Ward M, Napoli V, et al. Treatment of HIV-associated Hodgkin's disease (HIV-HD): Is there a clue regarding the etiology of Hodgkin's disease (abstr)? *Proc Am Soc Clin Oncol* 1992;11:44.

189. Tirelli U, Errante D, Dolcetti R, et al. Hodgkin's disease and human immunodeficiency virus infection: Clinicopathologic and virologic features of 114 patients from the Italian Cooperative Group on AIDS and tumors. *J Clin Oncol* 1995:13: 1758–1767.

190. Rubio R. Hodgkin's disease associated with human immunodeficiency virus infection. A clinical study of 46 cases. *Cancer* 1994;73:2400–2407.

191. Andrieu JM, Roithmann S, Tourani JM, et al. Hodgkin's disease during HIV-1 infection: The French registry experience. *Ann Oncol* 1993;4:635–641.

192. Ree HJ, Strauchen JA, Khan AA, et al. Human immunodeficiency virus-associated Hodgkin's disease. Clinicopathologic studies of 24 cases and preponderance of mixed cellularity type characterized by the occurrence of fibrohistiocytoid stromal cells. *Cancer* 1991;67:1614–1621.

193. Dolcetti R, Boiocchi M, Gloghini A, et al. Pathogenetic and histiogenetic features of HIV-associated Hodgkin's disease. *Eur J Cancer* 2001;37:1276–1287.

194. Centers for Disease Control. 1993 revised classification system for HIV infection and expanded case surveillance definition for AIDS among adolescents and adults. *JAMA* 1993; 269:729–730.

195. Stratton P, Ciacco K. Cervical neoplasia in the patient with HIV infection. *Curr Opin Obstet Gynecol* 11994;6:86–91.

196. Nobbenhuis MA, Walboomers JM, Helmerhorst TJ, et al. Relation of human papillomavirus status to cervical lesions and consequences for cervical-cancer screening: A prospective study. *Lancet* 1999;354:20–25.

197. Ho GY, Bierman R, Beardsley L, et al. Natural history of cervicovaginal papillomavirus infection in young women. *N Engl J Med* 1998;338:423–428.

198. Jamieson DJ, Duerr A, Burk R, et al. Characterization of genital human papillomavirus infection in women who have or who are at risk of having HIV infection. *Am J Obstet Gynecol* 2002;186:21–27.

199. Stier E. Cervical neoplasia and the HIV-infected patient. *Hematol Oncol Clin North Am* 2003;17:873–887.

200. Robinson W. Invasive and preinvasive cervical neoplasia in human immunodeficiency virus-infected women. *Semin Onol* 2000; 27:463–470.

201. Knowles DM, Pirog EC. Pathology of AIDS-related lymphomas and other AIDS-defining neoplasms. *Eur J Cancer* 2001;37:1236–1250.

202. Sun XW, Kuhn L, Ellerbrock TV, et al. Human papillomavirus infection in women infected with the human immunodeficiency virus. *N Engl J Med* 1997;337:1343–1349.

203. Ellerbrock TV, Chiasson MA, Bush TJ, et al. Incidence of cervical squamous intraepithelial lesions in HIV-infected women. *JAMA* 2000;282:1031–1037.

204. Maiman M, Fruchter RG, Serur E, et al. Human immunodeficiency virus infection and cervical neoplasia. *Gynecol Oncol* 1990;38:377–382.

205. Vermund SH, Kelley KF, Klein RS, et al. High risk of human papillomavirus infection and cervical squamous intraepithelial lesions among women with symptomatic human immunodeficiency virus infection. *Am J Obstet Gynecol* 1991;165: 392–400.

206. Maiman M. Cervical neoplasia in women with HIV infection. *Oncology* 1994;8:83–94.

207. Wright TC, Ellerbrock TV, Chiasson MA, et al. Cervical intraepithelial neoplasia in women infected with human immunodeficiency virus: Prevalence, risk factors, and validity of Papanicolaou smears. *Obstet Gynecol* 1994;84:591–597.

208. US Public Health Service (USPHS) and Infectious Diseases Society of America (IDSA0.2001 USPHA_IDSA guidelines for the prevention of opportunistic infections in persons infected with human immunodeficiency virus. Available at: http://www.guideline.gov/VIEWS/summary.asp?guideline=

=2306&summary_type=brief_summary&aSearch_string=. Accessed May 1, 2003.

209. Maiman M, Tarricone N, Vieira J, et al. Colposcopic evaluation of human immunodeficiency virus-seropositive women. *Obstet Gynecol* 1991;78:84–88.

210. Maiman M, Watts H, Andersen J. Vaginal 5-fluorouracil for high grade cervical dysplasia in HIV-infected women: A randomized trial. *Obstet Gynecol* 1999;94:954–961.

211. Northfelt DW. Cervical and anal neoplasia and HPV infection in persons with HIV infection. *Oncology* 1994;8:33–40.

212. Heard I, Tassie JM, Kazatchkine MD, et al. Highly active antiretroviral therapy enhances regression of cervical intraepithelial neoplasia in HIV-seropositive women. *AIDS* 2002;16:1799–1802.

213. Minkoff H, Ahdieh L, Massad LS, et al. The effect of highly active antiretroviral therapy on cervical cytologic changes associated with oncogenic HPV among HIV-infected women. *AIDS* 2001 15:2157–2164.

214. Robinson WR, Hamilton CA, Michaels SH, et al. Effect of excisional therapy and highly active antiretroviral therapy on cervical intraepithelial neoplasia in women infected with human immunodeficiency virus. *Am J Obstet Gynecol* 2001;184:538–543.

215. Lillo FB, Ferrari D, Veglia F, et al. Human papillomavirus infection and associated cervical disease in HIV-infected women: Effect of highly active antiretroviral therapy. *J Infec Dis* 2001;184:547–551.

216. International Collaboration on HIV and Cancer. Highly active antiretroviral therapy and incidence of cancer in human immunodeficiency virus-infected adults. *J Natl Cancer Inst* 2000;92:1823–1830.

217. Conti S, Masocco M, Pezzotti P, et al. Differential impact of combined antiretroviral therapy on the survival of Italian patients with specific AIDS-defining illnesses. *J AIDS* 2000;25:451–458.

218. Robinson W, Lee P, and Clark R. The effect of improved therapy for HIV on the outcome of cervical cancer in HIV-infected women. Proceedings of the 29th annual meeting of the western association of gynecologic oncologists. *Gynecol Oncol* 2000;79:135 (abstr 8).

219. Palefsky JM. Anal human papillomavirus infection and anal cancer in HIV-positive individuals: An emerging problem. *AIDS* 1994;8:283–295.

220. Klencke BJ, Palefsky JM. Anal cancer: An HIV-associated cancer. *Hematol Oncol Clin North Am* 2003;17:859–872.

221. Lipsey LR, Northfelt DW. Anogenital neoplasia in patients with HIV infection. *Curr Opin Oncol* 1993;5:861–866.

222. Chin-Hong PV, Palefsky JM. Natural history and clinical management of anal human papillomavirus disease in men and women infected with human immunodeficiency virus. *HIV/AIDS* 2002;35:1127–1134.

223. Holland JM, Swift PS. Tolerance of patients with human immunodeficiency virus and anal carcinoma to treatment with combined chemotherapy and radiation therapy. *Radiology* 1994;193:251–254.

224. Cooley TP. Non-AIDS-defining cancer in HIV-infected people. *Hematol Oncol Clin North Am* 2003;17:889–899.

225. Cohen P. Miscellaneous cancers associated with AIDS. *Curr Opin Oncol* 1989;1:68–71.

226. Martin F, Bowers M. Anal intraepithelial neoplasia in HIV-positive people. *Sex Transm Inf* 2001;77:327–331.

227. Carbone PP, Kaplan HS, Mushoff K, et al. Report of the Committee on Hodgkin's Disease Staging. *Cancer Res* 1971;31:1860–1861.

UNKNOWN PRIMARY CARCINOMAS

Alberto J. Montero
Gauri R. Varadhachary
James L. Abbruzzese

Unknown primary carcinomas, with their heterogeneous presentations, pose a major problem for oncologists; depending on the extent of evaluation, they comprise 3 to 10% of all tumors diagnosed (1–3). A working definition for unknown primary carcinoma (UPC) is biopsy-proven metastatic cancer with no identifiable primary source by history, physical examination, chest radiography, complete blood count, chemistry, computed tomography (CT) of the abdomen/pelvis, prostate-specific antigen (PSA) in men, and mammography in women. The natural history of disease for UPC is diverse and is dependent on multiple variables such as, age, number of metastatic sites, dominant area of disease, and histology (2,4,5). It is this considerable heterogeneity that has

presented a challenge to the systematic study of UPC. Depending on histologic features and sites of disease, a small but significant minority of patients will be long-term survivors (4,6).

This chapter discusses the evaluation of patients with UPC and optimal therapeutic strategies. The differing natural histories in UPC, depending on both the sites of disease and histology, are also discussed. Studies show that in this population, a search for the primary tumor is unrewarding in approximately 75% of cases, even after the most thorough evaluation (2,3,7). This fact has caused much consternation for both patients and physicians. The treatment of malignancy is traditionally based on the identification of the origin of the tumor, and treatment is chosen and initiated on the basis of the natural history and most specific therapies available for a certain type of tumor. Without knowledge of the primary site, the oncologist is often hesitant to recommend therapy. Furthermore, the physician may believe that not being able to identify a primary malignancy implies that he or she has somehow failed to serve the patient adequately. To complicate matters further, the oncologist is presented with an assortment of disparate clinical trials, which often exclusively stress the overall poor prognosis for these patients. In the past, this has contributed to a nihilistic outlook among oncologists treating patients with UPC. Although most patients with metastatic UPC have tumors that respond poorly to current treatments and will consequently have a poor prognosis, it has become evident over the last two decades that subsets of patients with UPC have a favorable prognosis and respond to chemotherapy; some of these can be successfully treated with regional therapy alone.

■ EPIDEMIOLOGY

The incidence of UPC is difficult to determine because many patients are given other diagnoses, and UPC is therefore underreported (6). In 2005, it was estimated that 28,590 new cases of "other and unspecified primary sites" will be diagnosed in the United States, or 2% of all cancers (8). The true incidence is thought to be much higher, closer to 6% of all new cancers (9). From the available data, UPCs seem to affect men and women equally. The median age at presentation in recent large series ranges between 59 and 66 years (1,5,10).

A minority of patients (10%) with UPCs have a history of an antecedent cancer (11). In autopsies performed before the advent of CT, the occult primary tumor was identified in 60 to 80% of cases. In one autopsy series, the two most commonly identified primary sites were the pancreas (20%) and lung (18%) (12). The poor prognosis for patients with these malignancies reflects the overall poor prognosis for those with UPCs as a group. Although breast and prostate cancers represent the most common cancers in women and men, these usually account for only 4 and 2%, respectively, of the primary sites found (13).

■ BIOLOGY AND CHROMOSOMAL ABERRATIONS

UPCs, despite their heterogeneity, are a clinically unique oncologic entity; as such, they share many common features that set them apart from other malignancies. The central unifying clinical feature of UPC is the absence of a detectable primary tumor. Even after autopsy, the primary site will not be identified in 20 to 40% of cases (14). At present, it is unknown why primary carcinomas exhibit this unique biological behavior. A current hypothesis is that the acquisition of a "metastatic phenotype" is an early event in UPCs, soon after oncogenesis, thus enabling cells to metastasize early, before the development of a clinically detectable tumor (15–17). It has also been hypothesized that the primary tumors may regress or involute before the metastases become clinically evident, attributed to a host immunologic response. A third hypothesis is that the primary tumor is exposed to antiangiogenic factors locally, whereas the metastases acquire the angiogenic phenotype after a period of dormancy (18).

Several studies have demonstrated a specific nonrandom pattern of chromosomal aberrations that seems to be unique to UPCs. These data suggest that some of these genetic changes may be the underlying cause of the metastatic phenotype. UPC is characterized by greater genetic instability, with massive genomic alterations, when compared with other distant metastases. In a recent study by Pantou and colleagues (19), cytogenetic profiling of tumors from 20 patients with UPC was performed, revealing an average of 11 chromosomal changes per case. Of the three histologic subtypes in this study, adenocarcinomas not only had the highest number of cytogenetic changes (16 versus 3) but also had involvement of distinct sites (4q31, 6q15, 10q25, and 13q22) when compared with carcinomas or undifferentiated malignancies. The latter group was distinguished by the involvement of changes at 11q22. Overall, the most commonly rearranged chromosomal regions were 1q21, 3p13, 6q21-23, 7q22, 11p15-12, and 11q14-24. The number of cytogenetic alterations was found to be prognostically relevant. Median survival was significantly greater for patients with 5 or fewer cytogenetic changes compared with those with more than 5 changes (3 versus 18 months, $P = 0.003$) (19). An older study of 12 UPC cell lines also demonstrated a preponderance of chromosome 1 abnormalities. These changes were observed on both the long arm (e.g., 1p deletion, isochromosome 1p, and translocations with a 1p breakpoint) and on the short arm (1q21), suggesting the importance of chromosome 1 in the biology of UPCs (16). Chromosome 1p aberrations are also commonly associated with advanced malignancies (20).

Chromosome 12 abnormalities have also been shown to be frequent in UPC. This is of particular interest because one of the observed alterations, isochromosome

12p (i12p), is present in as many as 80% of germ cell tumors. Motzer and colleagues (21,22) reported that 30% of patient tumors in their series had either i12p or 12q deletions. The presence of either of these two cytogenetic abnormalities was found to be predictive of a complete response to cisplatin-based chemotherapy (75 versus 17%, $P = 0.002$) (21,22).

The tumor suppressor gene *p53* is commonly mutated in human cancers, especially in advanced malignancies. Paradoxically, this does not seem to be true in UPC. Bar-Eli (15) found *p53* mutations to be less frequent than expected (26%) in UPC after evaluating 15 biopsy specimens and 8 cell lines (15). Immunohistochemical studies of *p53* in UPC, though, have found this protein to be highly expressed in 70% of the tumors examined, conflicting with the findings of Bar-Eli, because *p53* mutations typically lead to protein overexpression (23,24). Nevertheless, *p53* expression has not been found to have prognostic relevance. Molecular studies have also demonstrated the overexpression of other oncogenes, such as c-*myc, ras, bcl-2,* and *Her2/neu,* in UPCs, but none have been found to have any correlation with either survival or response to chemotherapy (23,25).

■ NATURAL HISTORY AND CLINICAL PRESENTATION

The clinical course of patients with UPC varies widely. Consequently, median survival in large retrospective studies has ranged from 11 weeks to 11 months (1,5,42). In the University of Texas M.D. Anderson Cancer Center database, the 5-year overall survival (OS) rate was only 11%. Although survival is poor as a whole, there are certain prognostic variables that correlate with longer survival, such as disease limited to one organ site, involvement of lymph nodes only, and histologic diagnoses of squamous or neuroendocrine carcinoma. Variables suggestive of a poor prognosis include male sex, histologic diagnosis of adenocarcinoma, and metastatic involvement of the liver, lung, bone, pleura, or brain (Table 35-1) (5,10).

By performing multivariate analyses on a consecutive series of 1000 patients with UPC with a different method, classification and regression tree (CART) analysis, Hess and colleagues (5) were able to more closely study the interactions between different clinical variables and how this influenced survival (Fig. 35-1).

As a result, some novel prognostic clinical factors in UPC were identified that had not been previously recognized. The initial tree constructed with CART analy-

TABLE 35-1	FAVORABLE-VERSUS POOR-PROGNOSIS UNKNOWN PRIMARY CARCINOMA	
Favorable	*Poor Prognosis*
Extragonadal germ cell syndrome	Liver metastases (non-neuroendocrine)
Isolated single small metastasis	Pleural and/or lung metastases
Papillary peritoneal adeno-carcinoma (women)	Adrenal metastases
Isolated axillary adenocarcinoma (women)	Multiple brain metastases
Cervical adenopathy (squamous cell)	
Isolated inguinal adenopathy	
Neuroendocrine histology	

sis had an initial split on the presence or absence of liver metastases, with 10 subgroups. The other variables that determined these terminal subgroups included specific sites of disease (bone, adrenal, lymph node, and pleura), histology, age, and number of metastatic sites. In this analysis, a group of 127 patients with no liver, bone, or adrenal metastases, two or fewer sites of disease, and nonadenocarcinoma histology had the longest median overall survival (OS) (40 months). The group with the shortest median OS (5 months) consisted of 150 patients who had liver metastases of nonneuroendocrine histology and were 61.5 years or older. A second alternate tree was constructed with the initial split on lymph node involvement. In this analysis, patients with lymph node involvement, two or fewer metastases, and nonadenocarcinoma histology had the best median survival (45 months). Interestingly, each CART analysis identified a small subset of patients with adrenal metastases who had a median survival of only 5 months. Additionally, the initial tree also identified a subset of patients with pleural-based metastases who also had a poorer than average survival of 9 months. These two clinical subsets had not been previously recognized as clinical features indicative of poor prognosis in UPC.

Patients with UPC present with symptoms and signs similar to those of patients with advanced malignancies of known origin. In one review, the most common symptoms at presentation of UPC were: general deterioration (73%), digestive symptoms (58%), liver enlargement (58%), abdominal pain (56%), respiratory symptoms (45%), ascites (26%), and node enlargement (16%) (40). Most patients with UPC present with multiple metastases, with three or more organs involved (10). Moreover, UPCs are also distinguished from other solid

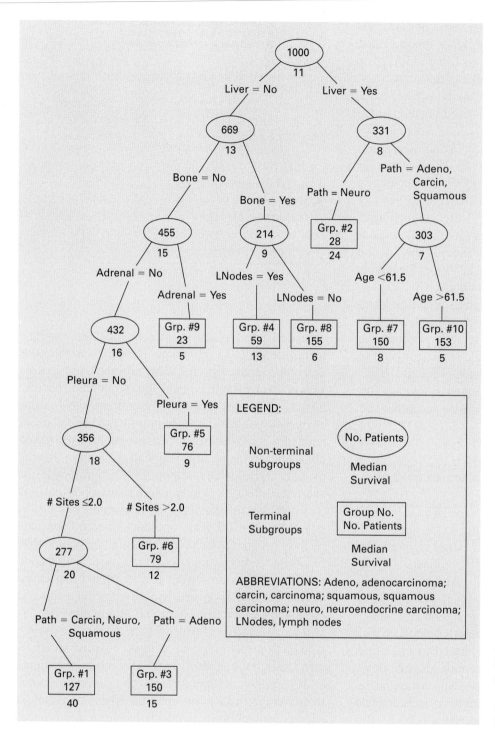

FIGURE 35-1 Classification and regression tree (CART) analysis of 1000 consecutive patients with UPC (default tree). [*From Hess KR et al. (5). With permission.*]

tumors by an unusual metastatic pattern, with a relatively high number of metastases found in the skin, kidneys, heart, and adrenal gland (12,41). In patients with a dominant (or sole) site of metastasis, the most common reported sites were liver (25%), bone (22%), lung (20%), lymph nodes (15%), pleural space (10%), and brain (5%) (10).

■ DIAGNOSTIC EVALUATION

Much has been written about the proper approach to the diagnostic evaluation of UPCs. In the past, minimalist diagnostic strategies had been advocated, limiting the scope of initial evaluations to differentiate only between treatable and untreatable disease (43). Others have supported a more aggressive approach, wherein a complete assessment of the extent of the disease and detection of the primary tumor site are attempted. In our experience, a more pragmatic approach is better. Extensive evaluation of all patients presenting with metastases of UPC is an expensive and wasteful extreme that does not benefit patients. In one study, the average cost of evaluating a patient with UPC was $17,973 (44). In that study, mean survival was 8.1 months, representative of the natural history of UPCs, with only 18% of patients surviving 1 year. However, a strictly minimalist approach may result in the oversight of treatable (and potentially curable) neoplasms.

An important determinant of the appropriate extent of evaluation for a given patient with an unknown primary is whether the data obtained by a diagnostic test will influence treatment decisions. If a treatable or potentially curable cancer is strongly suspected (e.g., a germ cell tumor or lymphoma), further investigation should proceed until a precise clinical diagnosis can be made provided that therapy is not unreasonably delayed. Clinical data support the observation that patients who have UPCs that are later proved to have originated from a particular site have an overall prognosis similar to that of patients who present with a known primary tumor (45). The recommended general approach is thus one of a directed evaluation based upon clinical presentation and initial pathologic findings.

PHYSICAL EXAMINATION AND LABORATORY TESTS INCLUDING SERUM TUMOR MARKERS

In each case, a thorough medical history should be obtained and a physical examination, including a digital prostate exam in men and a pelvic exam in women, should be performed. Determination of the patient's performance status, nutrition, and the presence or absence of concomitant medical illnesses and malignancy-related complications (e.g., paraneoplastic syndromes, painful metastases, or spinal cord compression) that may affect patient care is required.

Laboratory tests should include routine biochemical and hematologic surveys. The role of tumor markers in the evaluation of patients with UPCs is unclear. Most tumor markers are nonspecific and are not useful for identifying a primary site or for prognostic purposes. Adenocarcinoma markers [e.g., carcinoembryonic antigen (CEA), cancer antigen 125 (CA 125), CA 15-3, and CA 19-9] are often elevated in patients with UPCs and cannot be reliably used to identify a specific primary site or to predict either overall survival (OS) or the exact burden

of metastatic disease (37). Serum tumor markers may play an important role in helping to evaluate patients for responses to therapy, although levels are not always predictive of response to chemotherapy (38). Their selective use in a directed approach is more helpful than ordering a large battery of tumor markers on all patients who present with UPCs (39). Men who present with metastatic adenocarcinoma should have prostate-specific antigen (PSA) and prostatic acid phosphatase levels measured, even in the absence of bony metastases. In all men with undifferentiated carcinoma, beta-human chorionic gonadotropin and alpha-fetoprotein levels should be measured, especially if the clinical presentation suggests an extragonadal germ cell tumor (39). In patients with hepatic tumors, alpha-fetoprotein levels should also be measured to assist in the diagnosis of primary hepatocellular carcinoma.

DIAGNOSTIC IMAGING AND INVASIVE STUDIES

Initial radiographic studies should include chest radiography and CT of the abdomen. Pelvic CT or sonogram is routinely indicated in women, but in men it should be obtained only if relevant symptoms or physical findings exist (13). The benefit of CT scanning of the abdomen or pelvis in UPC is well established; detection of the primary site in 30 to 35% of these patients has been reported (46,47). Not surprisingly, the tumors most often identified on CT scans are those that arise from the pancreas, kidney, hepatobiliary tract, and ovary. CT scans of the chest should be performed for patients who have abnormalities evident on chest radiograph and/or immunohistochemical features on the biopsy that favor a primary lung cancer [e.g., thyroid transcription factor 1 (TTF-1)–positive]. Imaging or endoscopy of the upper and lower gastrointestinal (GI) tract is indicated for patients with abdominal complaints, ascites, liver metastases, or other findings in the initial workup that are suggestive of a possible GI primary tumor.

All women with UPC should undergo mammography and a careful pelvic examination. In cases of suspicious findings on a breast examination and negative mammography findings, patients should have breast sonography and a biopsy as indicated. As both the sensitivity (23% to 29%) and specificity (71% to 73%) of mammography in detecting an occult carcinoma are low, breast magnetic resonance imaging (MRI) has been evaluated as an alternative. In the setting of isolated axillary adenopathy, MRI is very sensitive in detecting occult primary breast cancers (>75%) and should be performed in women with isolated axillary adenopathy and negative mammography findings (48–51). Women with adenocarcinoma presenting with metastatic sites other than cervical or axillary adenopathy that are compatible with breast cancer (i.e., bone, liver, or lung) may also undergo breast MRI if the mammography findings are negative (52).

Patients with upper or midcervical adenopathy should undergo a thorough head and neck evaluation, including panendoscopy (i.e., laryngoscopy, bronchoscopy, and esophagoscopy) with random biopsies and an ipsilateral or bilateral tonsillectomy as part of the staging process. CT of the head and neck region is routinely done as part of the initial workup. Lower cervical or supraclavicular adenopathy suggests a primary tumor arising from below the clavicle. Patients with a pathologic diagnosis of adenocarcinoma or papillary carcinoma in the neck or chest region should be evaluated for thyroid carcinoma. Patients with inguinal lymphadenopathy may have a detectable primary site in the perineal or anorectal area, and anoscopy and colposcopy should be performed (2,59). Evaluation by an urologist may reveal a primary carcinoma of the distal urinary tract.

Recent studies have also further investigated the role of 18-fluorodeoxyglucose (FDG)-positron emission tomography (PET) in UPC. Even after PET and CT, the primary site remains undetermined in a small percentage of patients (53–56). In one retrospective study by Alberini and colleagues, the primary site remained unknown after complete imaging in 20% of patients (57).

There are a substantial number of studies that have evaluated the utility of PET scan in patients with occult primary head and neck cancers. In these small studies, a primary tumor was identified by PET in about 21 to 30% of patients. PET is of interest in this patient group since it may help to guide the biopsy, establish the extent of disease, and determine the appropriate treatment. Studies involving the cost-effectiveness of PET scans in this patient population are warranted. Finally, another nuclear imaging technology, ^{111}In-pentetreotide scanning, may also prove to be of use in helping to identify the primary site (58).

HISTOPATHOLOGIC EVALUATION INCLUDING IMMUNOHISTOCHEMICAL STUDIES AND ROLE OF CYTOGENETICS

All pathologic material obtained at biopsy from a patient with UPC should be evaluated by an experienced pathologist who is familiar with the special diagnostic problems of UPCs. The pathologist should also be informed of the patient's pertinent history and clinical findings so that he or she can recommend further analysis on the basis of this information. Adenocarcinoma is

the most common histologic diagnosis by light microscopy (approximately 55%). Another 30% of patients will have either undifferentiated or poorly differentiated carcinoma (PDC) or adenocarcinoma (PDAC). The remainder will have one of a variety of carcinomas that include squamous cell carcinomas (6%), neuroendocrine tumors (4%), and malignancies that upon more detailed study will be found to be sarcomas, lymphomas, germ cell tumors, melanomas, or unclassifiable undifferentiated malignant neoplasms (Table 35-2) (3,5).

Adequacy of tissue is essential, especially in cases where the pathologist has to make a diagnosis on deep fine-needle aspirations and there is insufficient tissue for immunohistochemical staining. The diagnosis of a poorly differentiated neoplasm implies that the pathologist is unable to classify it into any of the general neoplastic categories (carcinoma, lymphoma, melanoma, or sarcoma). Subsequent evaluation of this group of poorly differentiated lesions by means of special immunohistochemical techniques is warranted, because some of these patients will have tumors that are potentially curable and very responsive to treatment. Many immunohistochemical reagents are at the disposal of the pathologist, making the histologic classification of the tumor easier (Table 35-3).

Especially useful are the antibodies to common leukocyte antigens present in lymphoma and the antibodies to PSA present in most prostate cancers (26,27). Other useful immunohistochemical markers include cytokeratin (CK) 7 and 20 and TTF-1.

TTF-1 is a nuclear transcription factor that is normally expressed in lung and thyroid tissues and in their neoplasms. Staining for TTF-1 is frequently positive in lung cancer, especially in adenocarcinomas (60% to 75%) and small cell lung cancers (66% to 87%); however, it is inconsistently expressed in squamous cell carcinoma (31–38). Among the various monoclonal antibodies against various cytokeratins, CK7 and CK20 can help differentiate between different solid tumors. For instance, CK7 is more commonly associated with pul-

TABLE 35-2	MAJOR HISTOLOGIES IN UNKNOWN PRIMARY CARCINOMA
Histology	**Proportion (%)**
Well to moderately differentiated adenocarcinoma	55
Poorly differentiated adenocarcinoma, Poorly differentiated carcinoma	30
Squamous	6
Neuroendocrine	4
Undifferentiated malignancy	5

TABLE 35-3	COMMONLY UTILIZED IMMUNO-PEROXIDASE STAINS TO ASSIST IN THE DIFFERENTIAL DIAGNOSIS OF POORLY DIFFERENTIATED NEOPLASMS

Stain	*Likely Primary Site*
Estrogen/progesterone receptor, gross cystic disease fluid protein-15 (GCDFP-15), low molecular-weight cytokeratin (CK)	Breast cancer
Thyroid transcription factor (TTF-1), CK7, CK20, surfactant protein A precursor (SP-A1)	Lung cancer
Prostate-specific antigen (PSA), epithelial membrane antigen (EMA), alpha-methylacyl CoA racemase/P504S (AMACR/P504S)	Prostate cancer
Leukocyte common antigen (LCA), CD3, CD4, CD5, CD20, CD45	Lymphoma
Vimentin, desmin[†], factor VIII[‡]	Sarcoma
Chromogrannin/synaptophysin, neuron-specific enolase, cytokeratin	Neuroendocrine tumor
EMA, β-hCG, αFP, placental alkaline phosphatase (PLAP)	Germ cell tumor
CK7, CK20*, uroplakin III	Urothelial malignancies
S100, vimentin, HMB-45, neuron-specific enolase	Melanoma
CK7, CK20*, CDX-2, carcino-embryonic antigen (CEA)	Colorectal cancer

* Whereas a CK7+/CK20− staining pattern is typical of lung neoplasms, CK7−/CK20+ is suggestive of a colorectal primary. Dual CK7+/CK20+, however, is suggestive of urothelial primary.

[†] Positive in desmoid tumors, rhabdomyosarcomas, and leiomyosarcomas.

[‡] Positive in angiosarcomas.

monary or gynecologic malignancies, whereas CK20 is frequently seen in gastrointestinal adenocarcinomas. The CK7+/CK20− immunophenotype, in conjunction with TTF-1 staining, is suggestive of a lung primary and is a highly sensitive and specific method for differentiating primary pulmonary adenocarcinomas from metastatic extrapulmonary adenocarcinomas (Fig. 35-2) (32–34). By contrast, the CK7−/CK20+ immunophenotype is suggestive of a colorectal primary site. CK7+ and CK20+ dual staining suggest a malignancy of urothelial origin (35). Hep par 1 is an antigen whose expression is confined to benign and malignant hepatocytes and aids in the diagnosis of hepatocellular carcinoma in patients with UPC presenting with liver lesions. In women, depending on the pathology and pattern of metastasis, estrogen receptor (ER) and progesterone receptor (PR) staining is done to look for a breast primary. Another marker, for a breast primary is gross

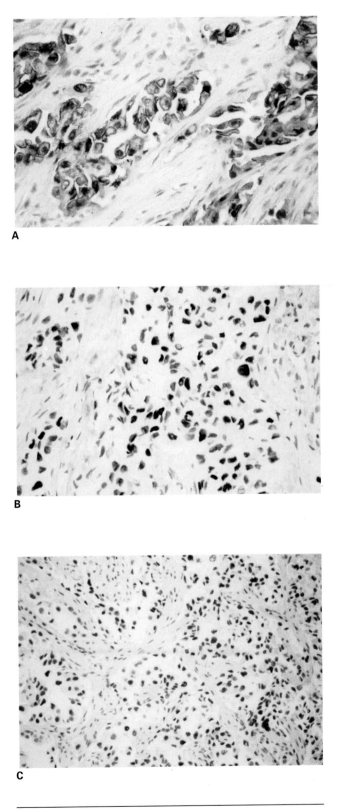

A

B

C

FIGURE 35-2 Immunohistochemical stains performed on the biopsy specimen from a patient with primary metastatic adenocarcinoma to a supraclavicular lymph node. Immunoperoxidase stains were positive for CK-7 (**A**) and TTF-1 (**B**) but negative for CK-20 (**C**), thus suggestive of metastatic non–small cell lung cancer. (*Courtesy of Dr Nelson Ordoñez, Department of Pathology MDACC.*)

cystic disease fluid protein 15 (GCDFP-15), which is pres-ent in 62 to 72% of breast cancers.

Dennis and colleagues (36) have identified other novel molecular markers using a bioinformatics approach. All publicly available gene expression data from various adenocarcinomas were pooled together and four novel proteins not previously recognized as tumor markers were found to be significantly upregulated. This was confirmed by reverse transcription–polymerase chain reaction. One example was lipophilin B, which was found to be restricted to breast, ovarian, and prostate cancers.

The use of cytogenetic analysis in the diagnosis of UPCs is limited. Specific chromosomal abnormalities have been identified in several types of lymphoma (8; 14 translocation in small non-cleaved-cell non-Hodgkin's lymphoma), germ cell tumors (i12p), and Ewing's sarcoma (t11; 22 or t21; 22). In the cytogenetic study by Pantou (19), lymphoma was diagnosed in 4 patients with UPC on the basis of the presence of IgH/Alk-1 rearrangement, which was identified by fluorescence in situ hybridization. Additionally, 1 patient was diagnosed with Ewing's sarcoma due to detection of characteristic rearrangement of chromosomes 11 and 22. Because the treatment of these malignancies is different, a correct diagnosis of the tumor is preferable to empiric treatment of all patients with cisplatin-based chemotherapy.

In the last update of our series of 1380 patients with suspected UPC, primary tumors were found in 27.5% by using the diagnostic approach outlined above. In this series, the most common sites of origin for epithelial histologies were lung (15%), pancreas (13%), colon/rectum (6%), kidney (5%), and breast (4%). Melanomas, sarcomas, and lymphomas each made up 6 to 8% of the total. The remaining cases were primary tumors of the stomach (4%), ovary (3%), liver (3%), esophagus (3%), mesothelial tissue (2%), prostate (2%), and a variety of other histologies (19%) (13).

■ MANAGEMENT OF SPECIFIC CLINICOPATHOLOGIC SUBGROUPS

UPC PRESENTING AS BRAIN METASTASES (WITHOUT ANY EXTRACRANIAL DISEASE)

It is estimated that brain metastases occur in 20 to 40% of patients with cancer. In as many as 15% of these, the primary site remains unknown (60). The important factor in treating patients with brain lesions is to distinguish patients with metastatic disease from those with primary brain tumors. Once this distinction has been made, patients with single metastatic lesions should be considered for surgery and those with multiple lesions should receive radiotherapy. In a recent small prospective study, patients with UPC who had single brain metastases treated with gross total resection and subsequent whole-brain radiotherapy (WBRT) had a median survival of 13 months. Patients with UPC who had multiple brain metastases and who underwent either WBRT alone or gross resection of symptomatic lesions followed by adjuvant WBRT had a median survival of only 6 to 8 months (61). After treatment, patients should be monitored for recurrence or the appearance of the primary site, which in most cases is the lung (61,62).

UPC PRESENTING AS METASTATIC CERVICAL ADENOPATHY

In this subgroup, patients present with high to midcervical or supraclavicular adenopathy; on histopathology, these tumors are squamous cell or PDCs. For squamous cell carcinoma, the primary site is eventually identified during follow-up in approximately 20% of patients, with the tonsil being the most common site, followed by the pyriform sinus and base of the tongue (63–65).

Adenocarcinoma is much less common and is generally from either metastatic nonpapillary thyroid carcinoma or advanced malignant disease from a distant site (gastrointestinal, lung, or breast carcinoma presenting as a metastatic supraclavicular node). Of all malignancies of the head and neck, only 5 to 10% are classified as unknown primary after imaging and panendoscopy (64). The prognosis for patients with cervical UPC overall is better than that for other UPC clinical subgroups; but even within this group, significant heterogeneity exists. Yalin et al. (66), in a retrospective study of 107 patients with cervical UPC (62% PDC, 24% squamous carcinoma, and 14% adenocarcinoma), reported a 5-year OS rate of 35.5% (66). In a recent retrospective study by Issing (63), 5- and 10-year OS rates were 42.7 and 30.6%, respectively. The prognosis is significantly worse in the presence of any of the following: adenocarcinoma, level III/IV lymphadenopathy, multiple lymph nodes, and bulky disease.

Patients with supraclavicular adenopathy have a far worse prognosis than those with adenopathy in other lymph node–bearing areas. Carcinoma affecting supraclavicular lymph nodes on the right most commonly arises from occult primary tumors of the lung and breast. When disease affects the lymph nodes on the left side, spread from intraabdominal malignancies by way of the thoracic duct (Virchow's node) is an additional possibility.

The management of patients with cervical UPC has become increasingly controversial, primarily because of the question of postoperative radiation therapy. The notion of adjuvant irradiation of all potential mucosal sites has been questioned because of the absence of any demonstrated survival benefit in randomized studies. To date, postoperative radiation therapy in cervical UPC significantly improves locoregional control, but this does not translate into improved OS (67). This being said, combined-modality therapy (surgery and radiation therapy) is better than either modality alone (67,68). Most patients with only cervical or supraclavicular involvement should have regional therapy consisting of surgery, postoperative radiation therapy, and close follow-up. Patients who undergo an excisional biopsy for diagnosis usually do not need additional surgery if: no gross disease is left behind, only a single lymph node measuring less than 6 cm is involved, and no extracapsular extension is noted on pathologic review. If any of these features are present, a neck dissection is indicated. Additionally, for patients with squamous cell carcinoma, unilateral tonsillectomy ipsilateral to the presenting neck mass is commonly advocated as part of the surgical treatment, because occult tonsillar carcinomas are usually found in 18 to 39% of patients who undergo tonsillectomy (64,65). Identification of the primary site would thereby reduce morbidity by limiting the field of radiation and would improve surveillance.

In patients with N1 or N2a disease (squamous cell), it is unclear whether postoperative radiation improves local control, because studies have been contradictory (2, 69). In this case, close surveillance would also be an acceptable option after surgery. All other patients should receive postoperative radiation to the bilateral neck covering all potential occult primary sites (i.e., nasopharynx, oropharynx, and hypopharynx). The 3-year survival rate after radical neck dissection and/or radical neck irradiation ranges from 35 to 60%. Within this group, patients with N1 disease have a better prognosis; patients with N3 disease, regardless of the local treatment modality used (surgery, radiotherapy, or both), fail to achieve complete remission in 65% of cases.

Although the role of chemotherapy in patients with cervical UPC remains poorly defined, extrapolation of phase II/III data in head and neck cancer indicates a role in patients with advanced nodal disease (N3). A recent large metaanalysis of more than 10,000 patients in 63 trials with head and neck squamous cell carcinoma demonstrated a small but significant absolute survival benefit of 4% at 5 years for chemotherapy (70). Intensive concurrent chemoradiotherapy in unresectable squamous cell head and neck cancers with cisplatin/

5-fluorouracil–based regimens has resulted in improved complete response rates, locoregional control, and preservation of organ function, albeit at the cost of significant toxicities. Taxanes have also been shown to be efficacious in this setting, either as single agents or in combination with cisplatin. In patients with N3 cervical UPC, there is a role for both chemotherapy and radiation therapy. Currently, insufficient data exist to know whether concurrent chemoradiation is superior to sequential chemotherapy followed by radiation in this group of patients with unresectable tumors (71).

WOMEN WITH UPC AND ISOLATED AXILLARY ADENOPATHY

Women who present with adenocarcinoma in the axillary lymph nodes compose another subset with a more favorable prognosis. Because the most likely primary is breast cancer, these patients are best managed as women with stage II breast cancer. This is an uncommon presentation of breast cancer, accounting for only 1 to 3 of every 1000 diagnosed breast cancers. In all women with isolated axillary adenopathy, mammography should be performed, and biopsies should be performed on any identified lesions. If mammography findings are normal, additional imaging of the breast with MRI is indicated because of its greater ability to detect primary breast tumors (70 to 95% sensitivity) (48–51). MRI has a very low false-negative rate. Of approximately 40 women reported in the literature with isolated axillary adenocarcinoma and negative breast MRI findings, only 4 were found to have breast cancer at surgery or during follow-up (50,72).

Modified radical mastectomy has been traditionally recommended in women with isolated axillary adenocarcinoma, even when physical examination and mammography studies fail to identify a primary breast cancer. A report by Ellerbroek et al. (73) documented actuarial disease-free survival rates of 71% at 5 years and 65% at 10 years (73). Survival rates were higher in patients who received systemic chemotherapy plus radiation therapy. Local control was also enhanced by irradiating the affected breast and axilla. Similar results were also reported by Foroudi and colleagues (74) in a small retrospective study of 20 women with axillary metastases who had received local therapy to the axilla (excisional biopsy, axillary dissection, or radiation). Recurrence-free survival was significantly longer for patients who had local therapy to the breast (either radiotherapy or mastectomy) than for those who did not (182 versus 7 months; $P = 0.003$). Interestingly, this was true despite the fact that a greater proportion of patients in the latter group received systemic therapy with tamoxifen and/or chemotherapy (74).

The present recommended management of women with UPC of the axilla includes axillary dissection, axillary radiotherapy for those at high risk of local recurrence (e.g., extracapsular invasion or more than four positive lymph nodes), and appropriate systemic therapy for breast cancer, depending on age and menopausal status. In cases where breast MRI findings are negative, neither mastectomy nor breast irradiation is recommended (75). If the breast MRI is positive or suspicious, radiation to the breast is usually recommended. The prognosis is not as favorable in men who present with axillary adenopathy only (76).

UPC PRESENTING AS ISOLATED INGUINAL ADENOPATHY

A few patients with UPC present with inguinal adenopathy. Undifferentiated (anaplastic) carcinoma is identified in at least half of these cases (6). Some of these anaplastic "carcinomas" appear to be melanomas with no obvious primary skin lesion. The remaining patients have squamous cell carcinomas arising from the skin, genitourinary tract, anus, or pelvis. A detailed investigation for primary lesions in these areas is important, because curative therapy is available for carcinomas of the anus, vulva, vagina, and cervix even with spread to regional lymph nodes. In patients with carcinomas and PDCs confined to the groin nodes, where no primary site was identified, a superficial groin dissection should be performed with or without radiation therapy (11). Chemotherapy, before definitive therapy and in the context of a clinical trial, may be offered in the face of systemic disease.

UPC WITH PULMONARY METASTASES AND PLEURAL EFFUSIONS

People with multiple pulmonary metastases constitute a large group of patients with UPCs, and lung cancer is the most frequent primary diagnosis made in this group. The diagnosis is commonly made on the basis of the results of chest radiography, CT scans, and either sputum cytology or bronchoscopy. It is very unusual for patients with pulmonary metastases to be candidates for surgical resection; these patients most often receive systemic chemotherapy. With the exception of some young patients whose tumors fit the criteria of germ cell equivalents, these patients usually do very poorly. Malignant pleural effusions are relatively common, affecting about 10% of patients with UPCs. Most of these patients have adenocarcinomas, which may be difficult to differentiate from mesotheliomas. Newer immunohistochemical

markers (e.g., calretinin, CK 5/6, and WT1) that are more sensitive in differentiating epithelioid malignant mesothelioma from pulmonary adenocarcinoma can assist in the diagnosis (77). Therapy for this group of patients is conservative. After initial diagnostic thoracentesis, patients are monitored for fluid reaccumulation. If the effusion reaccumulates quickly, pleurodesis may be attempted to slow the rate of fluid reaccumulation. If the effusion reaccumulates over a longer period or if new sites of disease develop, systemic chemotherapy should be administered.

UPC PRESENTING AS MALIGNANT ASCITES

Patients with malignant ascites usually belong to one of two subsets, each with a very different natural history of disease. The first group consists of patients with mucin-producing adenocarcinoma, who may present with ascitic fluid that contains signet ring cells. These patients often have multiple peritoneal implants with the primary site most likely being the GI tract (i.e., stomach, small bowel, appendix, or colon). This group has a poor prognosis and responds poorly to currently available treatment regimens. The second subset is composed of patients with primary peritoneal carcinomatosis. Typically, women are affected, with papillary adenocarcinoma in the peritoneal fluid. This disease is often also associated with pelvic adenopathy or masses. These patients may have elevated CA 125 levels but do not have detectable ovarian cancer. Some investigators consider these patients to have true unknown primary ovarian tumors or primary serous carcinomas of the peritoneum (78,79). Disease management should be the same as for women with ovarian carcinoma. A prolonged median survival of 13 months, with 25% of patients having a progression-free survival lasting more than 2 years, was reported for paclitaxel/carboplatin–based chemotherapy in patients with peritoneal carcinomatosis. In this study, a high overall response rate (ORR) and number of complete responses were reported for this subgroup of patients with UPC (68.4% and 20%, respectively) (80).

UPC PRESENTING AS ISOLATED BONY METASTASES

When bone metastases are detected, men should be evaluated for prostate cancer and women for breast cancer. Exclusion of these diagnoses leaves a group of patients with both a poor prognosis and a potentially painful condition. Patients with a single bony metastasis should be given local treatment with surgery and/or radiation and then monitored. Patients with multiple-site disease and good performance status and whose tumors progress after radiation therapy should be offered a trial of chemotherapy. Many experimental agents are currently available in ongoing clinical trials. Therapy with bone-seeking radioisotopes (e.g., strontium 89) may be useful in the treatment of disseminated painful bone metastases (81). Bisphosphonates are routinely used as in other malignancies, such as multiple myeloma, breast cancer, and prostate cancer (75).

UPC PRESENTING AS HEPATIC METASTASES

Patients with hepatic metastases constitute 20 to 30% of people with UPCs; they compose a clinical subgroup with a relatively poor prognosis, with reported median OS between 49 days and 7 months (82,83). The most important diagnostic considerations in this class are to distinguish primary liver and biliary tumors (hepatocellular carcinoma and cholangiocarcinoma) from cancers that have metastasized to the liver and to identify patients with neoplasms of a more indolent nature (e.g., neuroendocrine tumors). A careful pathologic review of liver biopsy specimens is therefore essential. The two most common histologies in primary UPC of the liver are adenocarcinoma (55%) and undifferentiated carcinoma (30%). The recommended initial therapy for unresectable disease is systemic chemotherapy. In one large retrospective study, the benefit of chemotherapy was most pronounced in patients with adenocarcinoma, significantly prolonging survival by 5 months compared with no chemotherapy ($P < 0.0001$) (83). Hepatic intra-arterial therapy is also an option for some patients, and surgery may be considered an option for those with resectable disease.

NEUROENDOCRINE TUMORS OF UNKNOWN PRIMARY SITE

Neuroendocrine tumors compose about 4% of all UPCs and commonly present with diffuse liver or bone metastases. Histologically, neuroendocrine tumors can be well differentiated or low grade, with features that are typical of carcinoid or islet cell tumors exhibiting a more indolent behavior. Management of these tumors should be similar to established guidelines for metastatic carcinoid tumors from a known primary site. In patients with limited disease, surgical resection or chemoembolization may be appropriate. If not amenable to local therapy, then a trial of chemotherapy may be considered. Cisplatin-based chemotherapy in well-differentiated neuroendocrine tumors has typically yielded low response rates (6).

A second group involves neuroendocrine tumors that are poorly differentiated by light microscopy but have neuroendocrine features revealed by immunohistochemistry (i.e., neuron-specific enolase, chromogranin A, and synaptophysin-positive) or electron microscopy (neurosecretory granules) (69). These high-grade neuroendocrine tumors act aggressively and are treated like small cell lung carcinoma with cisplatin/etoposide or carboplatin, with high reported response rates (84,85). A combination of paclitaxel, carboplatin, and oral etoposide has also been reported as an active regimen for patients with high-grade neuroendocrine tumors of unknown primary site (6,86).

UPC AND EXTRAGONADAL GERM CELL SYNDROME

As a group, patients who have undifferentiated carcinoma or PDC are less than 50 years old and present with rapidly growing midline tumors involving the lymph nodes, mediastinum, or retroperitoneum; their tumors have been found to be very responsive to chemotherapy, particularly to platinum-containing regimens. It is believed that these patients have poorly differentiated extragonadal germ cell tumors. They have response rates to chemotherapy of 35 to 50%, and those who achieve a complete response often enjoy a durable remission. In a prospective study by Hainsworth and colleagues (85) of 220 patients with PDC or PDAC treated between 1978 and 1989 with cisplatin-based chemotherapy regimens, approximately half of the patients had a predominant tumor location in the mediastinum, retroperitoneum, or peripheral lymph nodes. The ORR was 63%, with 26% complete responses and an actuarial 10-year disease-free survival rate of 16%.

However, this was not found to be true by Lenzi and colleagues (4), who retrospectively reviewed the clinical outcomes of 337 patients with PDC/PDAC. No prolonged survival was observed in this cohort of patients, and no significant survival advantage resulted from cisplatin-based chemotherapy. Moreover, elevated serum levels of alpha-fetoprotein or beta–human chorionic gonadotropin, contrary to other reports in the literature, were not found to be predictive of an improved median OS. This discrepancy may have resulted from several confounding factors.

First, older studies of extragonadal germ cell syndrome included patients with PDCs who in actuality did not have UPC but had other highly treatable malignancies (4). In a study by Hainsworth (85), of the 36 long-term survivors, 20% were subsequently found to have either lymphoma (5), testicular cancer (1), or leiomyosarcoma (1). Conversely, in the study by Lenzi, patients in whom the primary site was identified were excluded from the analysis. Most of these patients were found to have highly treatable malignancies, such as lymphoma (6%), breast cancer (8%), ovarian cancer (3%), germ cell tumors (2%), and prostate cancer (1%). Exclusion of these patients would significantly reduce response and median survival rates.

Second, even among patients with PDC/PDAC of unknown primary, significant heterogeneity exists. In the study by Lenzi, CART analysis on 337 patients revealed different groups with widely discrepant survival times. The group with the longest median OS (40 months) included patients with PDC, lymph node involvement, and only one or two metastatic sites. By contrast, patients with non–lymph node metastases had a very poor prognosis, with a median OS of only 7 months (4).

UPC AND SINGLE SITES DISCOVERED INCIDENTALLY ON RESECTION

UPCs are notorious for unusual, isolated presentations. Such lesions may appear on the skin, in single isolated lymph nodes removed during surgery for benign conditions, and at other, even more unusual sites. Patients should be examined for primary tumors and other sites of metastasis, as described earlier. If no primary tumor and no additional sites of metastasis are found, complete removal of the lesion must be ensured; this often requires additional excision with wider margins. The patient should then be monitored without therapy, regardless of the tumor histology involved. Many such patients may enjoy prolonged survival. Patients with isolated skin lesions may have an undifferentiated primary integumentary tumor with a potential for cure after adequate local surgical treatment.

UPC AND DISSEMINATED VISCERAL DISEASE

Developing a strategy to care for patients with UPC and disseminated visceral metastases has proven exceedingly difficult. As noted previously, some subsets of patients in this category have disease that is responsive to therapy (e.g., those with features of germ cell tumors and their equivalents, women with papillary abdominal carcinomatosis, and patients with neuroendocrine tumors). Such patients should be treated aggressively with platinum-based chemotherapy regimens and may have ORRs as high as 50% and complete response rates ranging from 20 to 35% (87,88).

■ CHEMOTHERAPEUTIC STRATEGIES FOR UPC

Data from chemotherapy trials enrolling patients with UPCs have historically been difficult to interpret. Many early studies were done before the era of controlled clinical trials, and the methods used in interpreting the results of these studies have been questioned. Additionally, combination regimens using newer chemotherapeutic agents have consistently demonstrated greater benefit than did older single-agent therapies. Several difficulties arise when survival and response rates reported in different chemotherapy trials are compared. For example, histologic criteria for patient selection often varied from study to study. Moreover, in older studies, immunohistochemical methods were not used to evaluate pathologic specimens. Despite these difficulties, no study has firmly established any chemotherapy regimen as the "gold standard" in UPC. The median survival in most studies, regardless of regimen, has ranged between 5 and 13 months, with response rates of less than 30% and without a significant improvement in survival (Table 35-4).

Nevertheless, patients with certain clinical subtypes (e.g., peritoneal carcinomatosis and lymph node–predominant disease) do benefit from chemotherapy. Historically, cisplatin-based combination chemotherapy regimens were frequently used to treat patients with UPC. Response rates in the literature range from 12 to 26% and median survival from 5 to 7 months. Combining paclitaxel with carboplatin has modestly improved both survival and response rates. In patients with widespread metastases and poor performance status however, systemic chemotherapy is unlikely to be beneficial, and only supportive therapy is usually indicated. Whenever possible, patients with UPC who do not belong in the previously defined subgroup should be treated within the context of a clinical trial.

In a phase II study by Hainsworth and colleagues (86), patients with UPC ($n = 55$) received paclitaxel (200 mg/m^2 day 1); carboplatin (AUC = 6 day 1); and oral etoposide (50 mg alternating with 100 mg days 1 to 10) every 21 days. Most were previously untreated, with only 4 having received prior chemotherapy. Most patients had moderately to well differentiated adenocarcinoma (55%) or PDC/PDAC (38%), with squamous (2%) and neuroendocrine (5%) histologies being less prevalent. The dominant sites of disease were: lymph nodes (25%), liver (16%), and lung (16%). Approximately 24% of patients in the study had multiple sites of disease, with 42% of patients having more than two metastatic sites. Response

TABLE 35-4 | SELECTED PHASE II STUDIES IN UNKNOWN PRIMARY CARCINOMA

Reference	N	Chemotherapy Regimen	Two or More Metastatic Sites (%)	ORR (%)	Median TTP (months)	OVERALL SURVIVAL Median (months)	1 year (%)	2 year (%)
Assersohn (94)	45	5-FU vs.	44	11.6	4.1	6.6	28	NR
	43	5-FU+ Mi		20	3.6	4.7	21	NR
Culine (95)	82	AC→EP, alt q 14 d + GCSF	68	39	NR	10		
McDonald (96)	31	Mi/P/CI 5-FU	52	27	3.4	7.7	28	
Greco (97)	120	Gem/Cb/Pac	65	25	NR	9	42	23
Saghatchian (98)	33	PDC/PDAC: EP×2→BI	57	40	8.1	9.4	NR	28
	18	Adeno: P/CI-5FU/IFN-α	44	44	8.6	16.1	NR	39
Hainsworth (93)	39	Gem	NR	33	5	NR		
Dowell (99)	17	Pac+ 5FU/leucovorin vs.	59	19	NR	8.4		
	17	CbE	65	19		6.5		
Briasoulis (80)	77	Cb+Pac	22% with 3 or more	38.7	6	13		
Greco (89)	23	DP vs.	73	26	NR	8	42	
	40	DCb	68	22		8	29	
Culine (90)	20	HDCT+Auto SCT vs.	80	42	NR	11		
	40	AC alt with EP	75	39		8		
Falkson (100)	43	Mi/Epi/P vs.	53	50	4.5*	9.4*		
	41	Mi	44	17	2.0	5.4		
Warner (101)	33	Cb+ E (PO)	91	23	NR	5.6	NR	
Hainsworth (86)	55	Pac/Cb/E (PO)	67	47	NR	13.4	58	NR
Hainsworth (85)	220	BEvP+/−Doxo; after 1985: BEP	74	63	NR			10-year survival: 16%
Van der Gaast (102)	34	BEP×4→EP×2	53	53	NR	NR		
Eagen, Robert (103)	28	MiA→CAM vs.	NR	14	NR	5.5	19	8
	27	MiAP→CAM		26		4.6	12	0

A = doxorubicin; Adeno = adenocarcinoma; alt = alternating; Auto SCT = autologous stem cell transplant; B = bleomycin; C = cyclophosphamide; Cb = carboplatin; CI = continuous infusion; D = docetaxel; Doxo = doxorubicin; E = etoposide; Epi = epirubicin; Gem = gemcitabine; HDCT = high-dose chemotherapy; I = ifosfamide; IFN = interferon; M = methotrexate; Mi = mitomycin; Neuro = neuroendocrine; NR = not reported; P = cisplatin; Pac = paclitaxel; PDC/PDAC = poorly differentiated carcinoma/adenocarcinoma; Undif = undifferentiated malignancy; v = vinblastine.
* Statistically significant difference $p = 0.05$.

rates were equivalent in all histologic subgroups, with a reported ORR of 47% and a median OS of 13.4 months. This regimen was well tolerated, with myelosuppression being the most common grade 3/4 toxicity. No treatment-related deaths were reported.

Briasoulis and colleagues (80) found equivalent response rates and median OS in UPC with carboplatin (AUC = 6) and paclitaxel (200 mg/m^2) without oral etoposide. In this phase II trial, patients ($n = 77$) were given a maximum of eight cycles of chemotherapy.

Additionally, granulocyte colony-stimulating factor was administered on days 5 to 12. The proportions of differing histologic subtypes were comparable to those in the Hainsworth study: adenocarcinoma (61%), undifferentiated (35%), and squamous (4%). Three distinct clinical subsets were present in this study: peritoneal carcinomatosis (25%, mostly women); visceral and/or bony metastases (43%); and predominant nodal and/or pleural disease (30%). The reported ORR, median response duration, and median OS were 38.7%, 6 months, and 13 months, respectively. Although response rates were equivalent for adenocarcinoma and undifferentiated carcinoma, significant differences were seen among the three clinical subsets: liver/bone or disseminated metastases (ORR, 15.1%; median OS, 10 months); nodal/pleural disease (ORR, 47.8%; median OS, 13 months); and peritoneal [ORR, 68.4% (75% for women); median OS, 15 months], $p = 0.01$. Three patients with nodal-predominant disease had durable responses lasting more than 2 years. Grade 3/4 neutropenia was only 4%, with two reported septic deaths.

The results of docetaxel in combination with carboplatin in one small phase II study appear to be inferior to that of paclitaxel/carboplatin in the above-mentioned trials. The ORR was 22%, the median OS was 8 months, and the 1-year OS rate was 29%. Differences in sites of disease and histology among these three studies may account for the discrepancy. Severe grade 3/4 myelosuppression was more frequent with docetaxel (50%) than with paclitaxel, with two reported septic deaths (89).

High-dose chemotherapy followed by autologous stem cell transplant has not been found to play any role in UPC. In a phase II study, patients ($n = 60$) were randomized to receive either high-dose chemotherapy followed by autologous stem cell rescue or conventional chemotherapy with doxorubicin at 50 mg/m^2 and cyclophosphamide at 1000 mg/m^2 alternating with etoposide at 300 mg/m^2 and cisplatin at 100 mg/m^2 on the basis of clinical features. Patients in the high-dose arm ($n = 12$) were less than 61 years of age, with good performance status, PDAC or PDC, and no evidence of brain or bone marrow involvement. ORRs (42% versus 39%) and median OS (11 versus 8 months) in the two arms were equivalent (90).

Patients with extragonadal germ cell syndrome or germ cell equivalent should be treated with a cisplatin-based regimen. Patients with undifferentiated or PDCs not fitting into the extragonadal germ cell or neuroendocrine clinical subgroups have traditionally been given a trial of a cisplatin-based regimen (59). Patients with squamous cell carcinomas who require chemotherapy are also often treated effectively using a cisplatin-based regimen. Investigators have discussed the merits of a combination of 5-fluorouracil and cisplatin in squamous cell carcinomas of the head and neck in addition to taxane-based chemotherapy (91,92).

The role of salvage chemotherapy in UPC is poorly defined. Gemcitabine is the only agent that has been shown to have modest activity as second-line therapy in patients with previously treated UPC. In a phase II study by Hainsworth and colleagues (93), gemcitabine was administered weekly at 1000 mg/m^2 (on days 1, 8, and 15 of a 28-day cycle). All patients ($n = 39$) received two cycles and were then evaluated for response. Chemotherapy was continued for a maximum of six cycles for either an objective response or stable disease. Approximately 90% of patients had failed a prior regimen containing platinum and a taxane. Most patients had either adenocarcinoma (59%) or PDC/PDAC (31%). Median time to progression was 5 months. Gemcitabine was well tolerated, with 92% of patients receiving two or more cycles. The most common grade 3 to 4 toxicities were fatigue/weakness and mucositis/esophagitis.

SUMMARY AND FUTURE TRENDS

It is unwise to consider all patients with UPCs to have an untreatable disease and a poor prognosis. Significant benefits may be achieved by administering regional or specific systemic therapies, and some patients can expect prolonged survival. All patients should undergo a directed diagnostic evaluation for the primary tumor. Some subsets of patients defined by clinical criteria (e.g., axillary nodes with adenocarcinoma in women or peritoneal carcinomatosis with a papillary or serous histology), histologic criteria (e.g., neuroendocrine, small cell, or germ cell tumor), or a combination of clinical and histologic criteria (e.g., undifferentiated tumors with a midline presentation in patients younger than 50 years) may benefit significantly from aggressive treatment with platinum-containing regimens.

For most patients who present with advanced UPCs, however, the prognosis remains poor, and no treatment of established efficacy is available. For those patients, enrollment into a clinical trial is appropriate. The role of DNA microarrays is evolving and the biggest challenge lies in their role as a diagnostic modality. The availability of targeted therapies and other novel agents promises an exciting future for better understanding the underlying biology of UPC and improving its management.

■ ACKNOWLEDGMENT

The authors thank David Galloway for critical review of the manuscript.

References

1. van de Wouw AJ, Janssen-Heijnen ML, Coebergh JW, et al. Epidemiology of unknown primary tumours; incidence and population-based survival of 1285 patients in Southeast Netherlands, 1984–1992. *Eur J Cancer* 2002;38(3):409–413.

2. Hainsworth JD, Greco FA. Treatment of patients with cancer of an unknown primary site. *N Engl J Med* 1993;329(4):257–263.

3. Greco FA, Burris HA, III, Erland JB, et al. Carcinoma of unknown primary site. *Cancer* 2000;89(12):2655–2660.

4. Lenzi R, Hess KR, Abbruzzese MC, et al. Poorly differentiated carcinoma and poorly differentiated adenocarcinoma of unknown origin: Favorable subsets of patients with unknown-primary carcinoma? *J Clin Oncol* 1997;15(5):2056–2066.

5. Hess KR, Abbruzzese MC, Lenzi R, et al. Classification and regression tree analysis of 1000 consecutive patients with unknown primary carcinoma. *Clin Cancer Res* 1999;5(11):3403–3410.

6. Greco FA, Hainsworth JD. Cancer of unknown primary site. In: DeVita VT (ed). *Cancer: Principles and Practice of Oncology.* Philadelphia: Lippincott, Williams & Wilkins; 2001:2537–2560.

7. Raber MN, Abbruzzese JL, Frost P. Unknown primary tumors. *Curr Opin Oncol* 1992;4(1):3–9.

8. Jemal A, Murray T, Ward E, et al. Cancer statistics, 2003. *CA Cancer J Clin* 2005;55:10–30.

9. Saad ED, Abbruzzese JL. Prognostic stratification in UPC: A role for assessing the value of conventional-dose and high-dose chemotherapy for unknown primary carcinoma. *Crit Rev Oncol Hematol* 2002;41(2):205–211.

10. Abbruzzese JL, Abbruzzese MC, Hess KR, et al. Unknown primary carcinoma: Natural history and prognostic factors in 657 consecutive patients. *J Clin Oncol* 1994;12(6):1272–1280.

11. Casciato DA, Tabbarah HJ. Metastases of unknown origin. In: Haskell CM (ed). *Cancer Treatment.* Philadelphia: Saunders; 1990:1128.

12. Nystrom JS, Weiner JM, Heffelfinger-Juttner J, et al. Metastatic and histologic presentations in unknown primary cancer. *Semin Oncol* 1977;4(1):53–58.

13. Abbruzzese JL, Abbruzzese MC, Lenzi R, et al. Analysis of a diagnostic strategy for patients with suspected tumors of unknown origin. *J Clin Oncol* 1995;13(8):2094–2103.

14. Daugaard G. Unknown primary tumours. *Cancer Treat Rev* 1994;20(2):119–147.

15. Bar-Eli M, Abbruzzese JL, Lee-Jackson D, et al. *p53* gene mutation spectrum in human unknown primary tumors. *Anticancer Res* 1993;13(5A):1619–1623.

16. Bell CW, Pathak S, Frost P. Unknown primary tumors: Establishment of cell lines, identification of chromosomal abnormalities, and implications for a second type of tumor progression. *Cancer Res* 1989;49(15):4311–4315.

17. van de Wouw AJ, Jansen RL, Speel EJ, et al. The unknown biology of the unknown primary tumour: A literature review. *Ann Oncol* 2003;14(2):191–196.

18. Naresh KN. Do metastatic tumours from an unknown primary reflect angiogenic incompetence of the tumour at the primary site? A hypothesis. *Med Hypoth* 2002;59(3):357–360.

19. Pantou D, Tsarouha H, Papadopoulou A, et al. Cytogenetic profile of unknown primary tumors: Clues for their pathogenesis and clinical management. *Neoplasia* 2003;5(1):23–31.

20. Atkin NB. Chromosome 1 aberrations in cancer. *Cancer Genet Cytogenet* 1986;21(4):279–285.

21. Motzer RJ, Rodriguez E, Reuter VE, et al. Molecular and cytogenetic studies in the diagnosis of patients with poorly differentiated carcinomas of unknown primary site. *J Clin Oncol* 1995;13(1):274–282.

22. Motzer RJ, Rodriguez E, Reuter VE, et al. Genetic analysis as an aid in diagnosis for patients with midline carcinomas of uncertain histologies. *J Natl Cancer Inst* 1991;83(5):341–346. B

23. Pavlidis N, Briassoulis E, Bai M, et al. The expression of *c-myc, ras,* and c-erbB-2 in patients with carcinoma of unknown primary. *Proc Am Soc Clin Oncol* 1994;13:(abst 1374).

24. Soong R, Robbins PD, Dix BR, et al. Concordance between p53 protein overexpression and gene mutation in a large series of common human carcinomas. *Hum Pathol* 1996;27(10):1050–1055.

25. Hainsworth JD, Lennington WJ, Greco FA. Overexpression of Her-2 in patients with poorly differentiated carcinoma or poorly differentiated adenocarcinoma of unknown primary site. *J Clin Oncol* 2000;18(3):632–635.

26. Warnke RA, Gatter KC, Falini B, et al. Diagnosis of human lymphoma with monoclonal antileukocyte antibodies. *N Engl J Med* 1983;309(21):1275–1281.

27. Allhoff EP, Proppe KH, Chapman CM, et al. Evaluation of prostate specific acid phosphatase and prostate specific antigen in identification of prostatic cancer. *J Urol* 1983;129(2):315–318.

28. Tan D, Li Q, Deeb G, et al. Thyroid transcription factor-1 expression prevalence and its clinical implications in non-small cell lung cancer: A high-throughput tissue microarray and immunohistochemistry study. *Hum Pathol* 2003;34(6):597–604.

29. Kaufmann O, Dietel M. Thyroid transcription factor-1 is the superior immunohistochemical marker for pulmonary adenocarcinomas and large cell carcinomas compared to surfactant proteins A and B. *Histopathology* 2000;36(1):8–16.

30. Fujita J, Ohtsuki Y, Bandoh S, et al. Expression of thyroid transcription factor-1 in 16 human lung cancer cell lines. *Lung Cancer* 2003;39(1):31–36.

31. Wu M, Wang B, Gil J, et al. p63 and TTF-1 immunostaining. A useful marker panel for distinguishing small cell carcinoma of lung from poorly differentiated squamous cell carcinoma of lung. *Am J Clin Pathol* 2003;119(5):696–702.

32. Ng WK, Chow JC, Ng PK. Thyroid transcription factor-1 is highly sensitive and specific in differentiating metastatic pulmonary from extrapulmonary adenocarcinoma in effusion fluid cytology specimens. *Cancer* 2002;96(1):43–48.

33. Chhieng DC, Cangiarella JF, Zakowski MF, et al. Use of thyroid transcription factor 1, PE-10, and cytokeratins 7 and 20

in discriminating between primary lung carcinomas and meta-static lesions in fine-needle aspiration biopsy specimens. *Cancer* 2001;93(5):330–336.

34. Reis-Filho JS, Carrilho C, Valenti C, et al. Is TTF1 a good immunohistochemical marker to distinguish primary from metastatic lung adenocarcinomas? *Pathol Res Pract* 2000; 196(12):835–840.

35. Rubin BP, Skarin AT, Pisick E, et al. Use of cytokeratins 7 and 20 in determining the origin of metastatic carcinoma of unknown primary, with special emphasis on lung cancer. *Eur J Cancer Prev* 2001;10(1):77–82.

36. Dennis JL, Vass JK, Wit EC, et al. Identification from public data of molecular markers of adenocarcinoma characteristic of the site of origin. *Cancer Res* 2002;62(21):5999–6005.

37. Milovic M, Popov I, Jelic S. Tumor markers in metastatic disease from cancer of unknown primary origin. *Med Sci Monit* 2002;8(2):MT25–MT30.

38. Bates SE. Clinical applications of serum tumor markers. *Ann Intern Med* 1991;115(8):623–638.

39. Abbruzzese JL, Raber MN, Frost P. The role of CA-125 in patients with unknown primary tumors. *Proc Am Soc Clin Oncol* 1991;10:(abst 39).

40. Mayordomo JI, Guerra JM, Guijarro C, et al. Neoplasms of unknown primary site: A clinicopathological study of autopsied patients. *Tumori* 1993;79(5):321–324.

41. Le Chevalier T, Cvitkovic E, Caille P, et al. Early metastatic cancer of unknown primary origin at presentation. A clinical study of 302 consecutive autopsied patients. *Arch Intern Med* 1988;148(9):2035–2039.

42. Culine S, Gazagne L, Ychou M, et al. [Carcinoma of unknown primary site. Apropos of 100 patients treated at the Montpellier regional center of cancer prevention]. *Rev Med Interne* 1998;19(10):713–719.

43. Stewart JF, Tattersall MH, Woods RL, et al. Unknown primary adenocarcinoma: Incidence of overinvestigation and natural history. *Br Med J* 1979;1(6177):1530–1533.

44. Schapira DV, Jaret AR. Cost of diagnosis and survival of patients with unknown primary cancer. *Proc Am Soc Clin Oncol* 1994;13:(abst 481).

45. Horning SJ, Carrier EK, Rouse RV, et al. Lymphomas presenting as histologically unclassified neoplasms: Characteristics and response to treatment. *J Clin Oncol* 1989;7(9):1281–1287.

46. McMillan JH, Levine E, Stephens RH. Computed tomography in the evaluation of metastatic adenocarcinoma from an unknown primary site. A retrospective study. *Radiology* 1982;143(1):143–146.

47. Karsell PR, Sheedy PF, O'Connell MJ. Computed tomography in search of cancer of unknown origin. *JAMA* 1982; 248(3):340–343.

48. Bedrosian I, Mick R, Orel SG, et al. Changes in the surgical management of patients with breast carcinoma based on preoperative magnetic resonance imaging. *Cancer* 2003;98(3): 468–473.

49. Podo F, Sardanelli F, Canese R, et al. The Italian multi-centre project on evaluation of MRI and other imaging modalities in early detection of breast cancer in subjects at high genetic risk. *J Exp Clin Cancer Res* 2002;21(3 suppl): 115–124.

50. Schelfout K, Kersschot E, Van Goethem M, et al. Breast MR imaging in a patient with unilateral axillary lymphadenop-

athy and unknown primary malignancy. *Eur Radiol* 2003; 13(9):2128–2132.

51. Henry-Tillman RS, Harms SE, Westbrook KC, et al. Role of breast magnetic resonance imaging in determining breast as a source of unknown metastatic lymphadenopathy. *Am J Surg* 1999;178(6):496–500.

52. Schorn C, Fischer U, Luftner-Nagel S, et al. MRI of the breast in patients with metastatic disease of unknown primary. *Eur Radiol* 1999;9(3):470–473.

53. Mantaka P, Baum RP, Hertel A, et al. PET with 2-[F-18]-fluoro-2-deoxy-D-glucose (FDG) in patients with cancer of unknown primary (CUP): Influence on patients' diagnostic and therapeutic management. *Cancer Biother Radiopharm* 2003; 18(1):47–58.

54. Lassen U, Daugaard G, Eigtved A, et al. 18F-FDG whole body positron emission tomography (PET) in patients with unknown primary tumours (UPT). *Eur J Cancer* 1999;35(7): 1076–1082.

55. Johansen J, Eigtved A, Buchwald C, et al. Implication of 18F-fluoro-2-deoxy-D-glucose positron emission tomography on management of carcinoma of unknown primary in the head and neck: A Danish cohort study. *Laryngoscope* 2002; 112(11):2009–2014.

56. Delgado-Bolton RC, Fernandez-Perez C, Gonzalez-Mate A, et al. Meta-analysis of the performance of 18F-FDG PET in primary tumor detection in unknown primary tumors. *J Nucl Med* 2003; 44(8):1301–1314.

57. Alberini JL, Belhocine T, Hustinx R, et al. Whole-body positron emission tomography using fluorodeoxyglucose in patients with metastases of unknown primary tumours (CUP syndrome). *Nucl Med Commun* 2003; 24(10):1081–1086.

58. Lenzi R, Kim EE, Raber MN, et al. Detection of primary breast cancer presenting as metastatic carcinoma of unknown primary origin by ^{111}In-pentetreotide scan. *Ann Oncol* 1998; 9(2):213–216.

59. Hainsworth JD, Greco FA. Poorly differentiated carcinoma and poorly differentiated adenocarcinoma of unknown primary tumor site. *Semin Oncol* 1993;20(3):279–286.

60. Soffietti R, Ruda R, Mutani R. Management of brain metastases. *J Neurol* 2002;249(10):1357–1369.

61. Ruda R, Borgognone M, Benech F, et al. Brain metastases from unknown primary tumour: A prospective study. *J Neurol* 2001;248(5):394–398.

62. Srodon M, Westra WH. Immunohistochemical staining for thyroid transcription factor-1: A helpful aid in discerning primary site of tumor origin in patients with brain metastases. *Hum Pathol* 2002;33(6):642–645.

63. Issing WJ, Taleban B, Tauber S. Diagnosis and management of carcinoma of unknown primary in the head and neck. *Eur Arch Otorhinolaryngol* 2003;260:436–443.

64. Randall DA, Johnstone PA, Foss RD, et al. Tonsillectomy in diagnosis of the unknown primary tumor of the head and neck. *Otolaryngol Head Neck Surg* 2000;122(1):52–55.

65. Kazak I, Haisch A, Jovanovic S. Bilateral synchronous tonsillar carcinoma in cervical cancer of unknown primary site (CUPS). *Eur Arch Otorhinolaryngol* 2003;260:436–443.

66. Yalin Y, Pingzhang T, Smith GI, et al. Management and outcome of cervical lymph node metastases of unknown primary sites: A retrospective study. *Br J Oral Maxillofac Surg* 2002; 40(6):484–487.

67. Iganej S, Kagan R, Anderson P, et al. Metastatic squamous cell carcinoma of the neck from an unknown primary: Management options and patterns of relapse. *Head Neck* 2002; 24(3):236–246.

68. Zuur CL, van Velthuysen ML, Schornagel JH, et al. Diagnosis and treatment of isolated neck metastases of adenocarcinomas. *Eur J Surg Oncol* 2002;28(2):147–152.

69. Garrow GC, Greco FA, Hainsworth JD. Poorly differentiated neuroendocrine carcinoma of unknown primary tumor site. *Semin Oncol* 1993;20(3):287–291.

70. Pignon JP, Bourhis J, Domenge C, et al. Chemotherapy added to locoregional treatment for head and neck squamous-cell carcinoma: Three meta-analyses of updated individual data. MACH-NC Collaborative Group. Meta-Analysis of Chemotherapy on Head and Neck Cancer. *Lancet* 2000; 355(9208):949–955.

71. Posner MR, Glisson B, Frenette G, et al. Multicenter phase I–II trial of docetaxel, cisplatin, and fluorouracil induction chemotherapy for patients with locally advanced squamous cell cancer of the head and neck. *J Clin Oncol* 2001;19(4): 1096–1104.

72. Olson JA, Jr., Morris EA, Van Zee KJ, et al. Magnetic resonance imaging facilitates breast conservation for occult breast cancer. *Ann Surg Oncol* 2000;7(6):411–415.

73. Ellerbroek N, Holmes F, Singletary E, et al. Treatment of patients with isolated axillary nodal metastases from an occult primary carcinoma consistent with breast origin. *Cancer* 1990;66(7):1461–1467.

74. Foroudi F, Tiver KW. Occult breast carcinoma presenting as axillary metastases. *Int J Radiat Oncol Biol Phys* 2000;47(1): 143–147.

75. Bugat R, Bataillard A, Lesimple T, et al. [Standards, Options and Recommendations for the management of patient with carcinoma of unknown primary site]. *Bull Cancer* 2002; 89(10):869–875.

76. Jackson B, Scott-Conner C, Moulder J. Axillary metastasis from occult breast carcinoma: Diagnosis and management. *Am Surg* 1995;61(5):431–434.

77. Ordonez NG. The immunohistochemical diagnosis of mesothelioma: A comparative study of epithelioid mesothelioma and lung adenocarcinoma. *Am J Surg Pathol* 2003;27(8): 1031–1051.

78. Gershenson DM, Silva EG. *Serous* ovarian tumors of low malignant potential with peritoneal implants. *Cancer* 1990; 65(3):578–585.

79. Strnad CM, Grosh WW, Baxter J, et al. Peritoneal carcinomatosis of unknown primary site in women. A distinctive subset of adenocarcinoma. *Ann Intern Med* 1989;111(3):213–217.

80. Briasoulis E, Kalofonos H, Bafaloukos D, et al. Carboplatin plus paclitaxel in unknown primary carcinoma: A phase II Hellenic Cooperative Oncology Group Study. *J Clin Oncol* 2000;18(17):3101–3107.

81. Porter AT, McEwan AJ, Powe JE, et al. Results of a randomized phase-III trial to evaluate the efficacy of strontium-89 adjuvant to local field external beam irradiation in the management of endocrine resistant metastatic prostate cancer. *Int J Radiat Oncol Biol Phys* 1993; 25(5):805–813.

82. Hogan BA, Thornton FJ, Brannigan M, et al. Hepatic metastases from an unknown primary neoplasm (UPN): Survival, prognostic indicators and value of extensive investigations. *Clin Radiol* 2002;57(12):1073–1077.

83. Ayoub JP, Hess KR, Abbruzzese MC, et al. Unknown primary tumors metastatic to liver. *J Clin Oncol* 1998;16(6): 2105–2112.

84. Greco FA, Johnson DH, Hainsworth JD. Etoposide/cisplatin-based chemotherapy for patients with metastatic poorly differentiated carcinoma of unknown primary site. *Semin Oncol* 1992;19(6 suppl 13):14–18.

85. Hainsworth JD, Johnson DH, Greco FA. Cisplatin-based combination chemotherapy in the treatment of poorly differentiated carcinoma and poorly differentiated adenocarcinoma of unknown primary site: Results of a 12-year experience. *J Clin Oncol* 1992;10(6):912–922.

86. Hainsworth JD, Erland JB, Kalman LA, et al. Carcinoma of unknown primary site: Treatment with 1-hour paclitaxel, carboplatin, and extended-schedule etoposide. *J Clin Oncol* 1997;15(6):2385–2393.

87. Greco FA, Vaughn WK, Hainsworth JD. Advanced poorly differentiated carcinoma of unknown primary site: Recognition of a treatable syndrome. *Ann Intern Med* 1986;104(4):547–553.

88. Richardson RL, Schoumacher RA, Fer MF, et al. The unrecognized extragonadal germ cell cancer syndrome. *Ann Intern Med* 1981;94(2):181–186.

89. Greco FA, Erland JB, Morrissey LH, et al. Carcinoma of unknown primary site: Phase II trials with docetaxel plus cisplatin or carboplatin. *Ann Oncol* 2000;11(2):211–215.

90. Culine S, Fabbro M, Ychou M, et al. Chemotherapy in carcinomas of unknown primary site: A high-dose intensity policy. *Ann Oncol* 1999;10(5):569–575.

91. Jeremic B, Zivic DJ, Matovic M, et al. Cisplatin and 5-fluorouracil as induction chemotherapy followed by radiation therapy in metastatic squamous cell carcinoma of an unknown primary tumor localized to the neck. A phase II study. *J Chemother* 1993;5(4):262–265.

92. Glisson BS, Murphy BA, Frenette G, et al. Phase II trial of docetaxel and cisplatin combination chemotherapy in patients with squamous cell carcinoma of the head and neck. *J Clin Oncol* 2002;20(6):1593–1599.

93. Hainsworth JD, Burris HA III, Calvert SW, et al. Gemcitabine in the second-line therapy of patients with carcinoma of unknown primary site: A phase II trial of the Minnie Pearl Cancer Research Network. *Cancer Invest* 2001;19(4):335–339.

94. Assersohn L, Norman AR, Cunningham D, et al. A randomised study of protracted venous infusion of 5-fluorouracil (5-FU) with or without bolus mitomycin C (MMC) in patients with carcinoma of unknown primary. *Eur J Cancer* 2003;39(8):1121–1128.

95. Culine S, Fabbro M, Ychou M, et al. Alternative bimonthly cycles of doxorubicin, cyclophosphamide, and etoposide, cisplatin with hematopoietic growth factor support in patients with carcinoma of unknown primary site. *Cancer* 2002; 94(3):840–846.

96. Macdonald AG, Nicolson MC, Samuel LM, et al. A phase II study of mitomycin C, cisplatin and continuous infusion 5-fluorourouracil (MCF) in the treatment of patients with carcinoma of unknown primary site. *Br J Cancer* 2002;86(8):1238–1242.

97. Greco FA, Burris HA III, Litchy S, et al. Gemcitabine, carboplatin, and paclitaxel for patients with carcinoma of unknown primary site: A Minnie Pearl Cancer Research Network study. *J Clin Oncol* 2002;20(6):1651–1656.

98. Saghatchian M, Fizazi K, Borel C, et al. Carcinoma of an unknown primary site: A chemotherapy strategy based on

histological differentiation—Results of a prospective study. *Ann Oncol* 2001;12(4):535–540.

99. Dowell JE, Garrett AM, Shyr Y, et al. A randomized phase II trial in patients with carcinoma of an unknown primary site. *Cancer* 2001;91(3):592–597.

100. Falkson CI, Cohen GL. Mitomycin C, epirubicin and cisplatin versus mitomycin C alone as therapy for carcinoma of unknown primary origin. *Oncology* 1998;55(2):116–121.

101. Warner E, Goel R, Chang J, et al. A multicentre phase II study of carboplatin and prolonged oral etoposide in the treatment of cancer of unknown primary site (CUPS). *Br J Cancer* 1998;77(12):2376–2380.

102. van der Gaast, Verweij J, Henzen-Logmans SC, et al. Carcinoma of unknown primary: Identification of a treatable subset? *Ann Oncol* 1990;1(2):119–122.

103. Eagan RT, Therneau TM, Rubin J, et al. Lack of value for cisplatin added to mitomycin-doxorubicin combination chemotherapy for carcinoma of unknown primary site. A randomized trial. *Am J Clin Oncol* 1987;10(1):82–85.

Supportive Care

INFECTION IN THE NEUTROPENIC PATIENT

Kenneth V. I. Rolston

Infection continues to be the most common complication associated with neutropenia (1). Bacterial infections predominate during the early phases of a neutropenic episode, whereas most fungal and some viral infections are more common in patients with persistent neutropenia (2). The spectrum of bacterial infection continues to change and is influenced by several factors, including the nature and intensity of chemotherapy, antimicrobial prophylaxis, and the use of catheters and other medical devices (3,4). Febrile neutropenic patients are a heterogeneous group. Risk prediction rules have been developed that can reliably identify a "low-risk" subset among febrile neutropenic patients (5,6). The administration of prompt broad-spectrum parenteral antibiotic therapy to a neutropenic patient who becomes febrile is the accepted standard of care (7). Oral and parenteral outpatient regimens have been successfully evaluated for the treatment of "low-risk" febrile neutropenic patients and represent new options in the management of such patients (8). Antimicrobial prophylaxis is useful for preventing infections in high-risk patients. Hematopoetic growth factors and granulocyte transfusions are useful in refractory infections. All these issues are discussed in this chapter, with an emphasis on strategies that have been developed at the University of Texas, M.D. Anderson Cancer Center (MDACC).

■ DEFINITIONS

Fever is defined as a single documented temperature ≥38.3°C (101°F). Some neutropenic patients may be unable to mount an adequate inflammatory response and may be afebrile or even hypothermic when infected. Neutropenia is defined as an absolute neutrophil count (ANC) of ≤ 500/mm^3, although the risk of infection begins to increase as the ANC falls below 1000/mm^3 (7,9).

■ SPECTRUM OF INFECTION

The epidemiology of bacterial infections in neutropenic cancer patients undergoes periodic changes, and it is important to conduct epidemiologic surveys in order to detect these changes in a timely manner (Fig. 36-1). Currently, in approximately 50% of febrile neutropenic patients no clinical site of infection (e.g., cellulitis, pneumonia) is identified, and all microbiological cultures are negative (Fig. 36-2). These are referred to as episodes of unexplained fever and probably represent low-grade or undetectable infection (2). The most common sites of infection include the respiratory tract, urinary tract, bloodstream, gastrointestinal tract, and skin/subcutaneous tissue infections (Fig. 36-3) (4).

Gram-positive organisms are the most frequent cause of bloodstream infections in neutropenic patients (3,10). Bloodstream infections however, account for only 20 to 35% of documented infections. Infections at most other sites are caused more often by gram-negative bacilli and are frequently polymicrobial (Fig. 36-4) (11). The most common fungal organisms causing infections in neutropenic patients are *Candida* and *Aspergillus* species, although the spectrum of opportunistic fungal pathogens keeps expanding (12). Certain subsets among neutropenic patients (hematopoetic stem cell transplant recipients and patients with hematologic

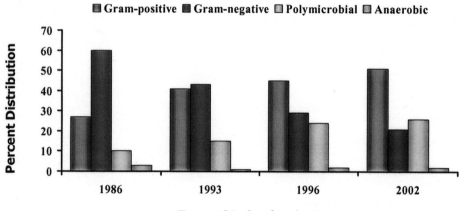

Type of Infection by Year

*Data are from the University of Texas M.D. Anderson Cancer Center Epidemiologic Surveys (1986–2002)

FIGURE 36-1 Changing epidemiology of bacterial infections in patients with cancer* (1986–2002).

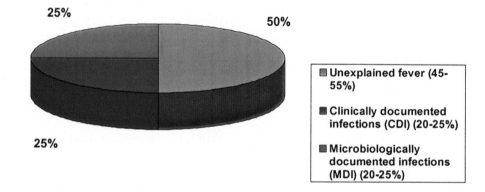

Data are from the University of Texas M.D. Anderson Cancer Center Epidemiologic Surveys in Febrile Neutropenic Patients (2002)

FIGURE 36-2 Nature of febrile episodes in neutropenic patients.

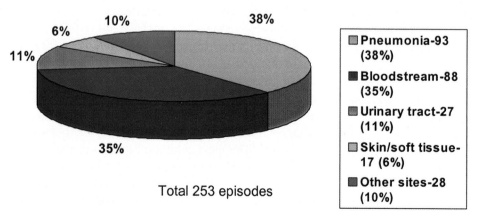

Total 253 episodes

Databases that focus only on bloodstream (EORTC, SCOPE) infections are incomplete and inaccurate

FIGURE 36-3 Breakdown of microbiologically documented infections in neutropenic patients.

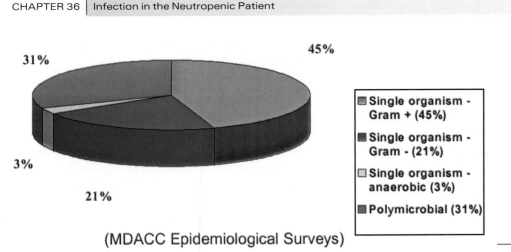

45%

31%

3%

21%

Single organism - Gram + (45%)

Single organism - Gram - (21%)

Single organism - anaerobic (3%)

Polymicrobial (31%)

(MDACC Epidemiological Surveys)

Databases that ignore polymicrobial infections are incomplete and inaccurate

FIGURE 36-4 Overall spectrum of bacterial infections in neutropenic cancer patients.

malignancies) are at increased risk of developing viral infections, predominantly those caused by the herpes groups of viruses [herpes simplex virus (HSV), varicella zoster virus (VZV), cytomegalovirus (CMV), Epstein-Barr virus (EBV), human herpesvirus 6 (HHV-6)] and the community respiratory viruses (RSV, influenza A and B, parainfluenza) (13). Table 36-1 lists the common pathogens causing infection in neutropenic patients.

vous system infection or septic arthritis. In institutions where resistant organisms such as methicillin-resistant *Staphylococcus aureus* (MRSA), vancomycin-resistant enterococci (VRE), or *Stenotrophomonas maltophilia* are common, surveillance cultures to detect colonization with these organisms for purposes of infection control, are indicated.

■ INITIAL EVALUATION

A detailed history and a careful and thorough physical examination are of paramount importance. Useful bits of historical information include the nature and intensity of antineoplastic therapy, travel history or environmental exposure, the use and nature of antimicrobial prophylaxis, history and nature of previous infection and/or surgical procedures, and drug allergies. A careful and systematic search for infected sites—including the oropharynx, upper and lower gastrointestinal tracts, skin (including scalp), perianal and genital regions, lungs, skin, nail beds, vascular access and biopsy sites—is mandatory. Blood cultures should be performed in all patients from a peripheral site and through each lumen of multilumen catheters to detect bacterial and fungal pathogens. Any drainage site should also be cultured and appropriate stains (Gram's, acid-fast, fungal, viral) should be performed. Stool cultures are recommended only for patients with diarrhea, and in these cases assays for *Clostridium difficile* toxin should also be performed. Urine cultures should be performed in symptomatic patients and those with urinary catheters in place. Testing of cerebrospinal fluid and joint fluid should be performed only in patients suspected to have central ner-

TABLE 36-1	ORGANISMS FREQUENTLY ISOLATED FROM NEUTROPENIC PATIENTS	
Gram-positive Bacteria	*Fungi*
Coagulase-negative staphylococci	*Candida* species
Staphylococcus aureus (including MRSA)	*Aspergillus* species
Enterococcus species (including VRE)	*Fusarium* species
Viridans streptococci	Zygomycetes
Corynebacterium species	*Trichosporon beigelii*
Bacillus species	
Micrococcus species	
Stomatococcus mucilaginosus	
Gram-negative Bacteria	*Viruses*
Escherichia coli	Herpes simplex virus I & II
Pseudomonas aeruginosa	Varicella zoster virus
Klebsiella species	Cytomegalovirus
Enterobacter species	Epstein-Barr virus
Citrobacter species	Human herpesvirus 6
Stenotrophomonas maltophilia	Respiratory syncytial virus
Acinetobacter species	Influenza A and B
Serratia species	Parainfluenza viruses
	Adenovirus

A baseline chest radiograph, although not considered mandatory, might provide useful information in some patients. Repeat studies should be obtained only if respiratory symptoms develop. Significant infiltrates may not develop in patients with pneumonia and severe neutropenia. All cutaneous lesions should be biopsied and sent for appropriate stains and cultures. All patients should have a complete blood count, liver and renal function tests, and a serum electrolyte panel at baseline with repeat studies every 3 to 4 days to screen for side effects (Table 36-2).

■ RISK ASSESSMENT

As our understanding of the clinical syndrome of febrile neutropenia has evolved, it has become quite evident that not all febrile neutropenic patients have the same risk for developing serious infection and/or complications during a particular neutropenic episode. It has only recently become possible to accurately predict different risk groups at the time of clinical presentation (8). The purpose of risk assessment is to stratify this heterogeneous population into meaningful subgroups based on clinical outcomes.

The initial observations made by Bodey and colleagues indicated that the risk and severity of infection were greatest in patients with severe neutropenia ($\leq 100/mm^3$) that lasted for 2 weeks or more (9). Several clinical trials conducted at MDACC also demonstrated significantly better response rates in patients with neutrophil recovery compared to those with persistent neutropenia (14). This was confirmed in a study from the National Cancer Institute (15). Patients with $\leq$ 7 days of neutropenia had a response rate to initial antibiotic therapy of 95%, with a 6.6 % rate of recurrent fever, compared to a response rate of only 32% and a 38% rate of recurrent fever in patients with $\geq$ 15 days of neutropenia. At greatest risk are patients with hematologic malignancies, particularly acute leukemia, and recipients of allogeneic hematopoietic stem cell transplants (HSCT), since the duration of severe neutropenia is likely to exceed 14 days in many of these patients. Various other factors—including damage to natural barriers (skin, mucosal surfaces), the presence of vascular access and other medical devices, and the general medical and nutritional status of the patient—have an impact on the risk and nature of infections in neutropenia patients.

Risk assessment can be performed using simple clinical criteria initially developed at MDACC and subsequently adopted by the National Cancer Institute (NCI) and the European Organization for the Research and Treatment of Cancer (EORTC) (16–18). These are outlined in Table 36-3 and include evidence of hemodynamic stability and lack of medical comorbidity. Two statistically derived risk prediction rules that can reliably identify low-risk patients have also been developed and validated (5,6,19). Details of these two prediction rules are outlined in Tables 36-4A and B. Most low-risk patients have solid tumors that are being treated in the outpatient setting with conventional chemotherapy. They generally have minimal comorbidity and have short-lived ($\leq$ 7 days) neutropenia. Regardless of which method is used for risk assessment, some patients will be misclassified, making close observation and monitoring of all neutropenic patients being treated for fever a necessity.

TABLE 36-2	INITIAL EVALUATION OF THE FEBRILE NEUTROPENIC PATIENT

Detailed history
Comprehensive physical examination (search for potential sites of infection (skin, nail, oropharynx, gastrointestinal and respiratory tracts, perianal and genital regions, vascular access and biopsy sites)
Blood cultures ×2 (for bacterial and fungal organisms), peripheral blood, and each catheter lumen
Drainage sites: stain and culture (bacteremia, AFB, fungi, viruses)
Chest radiograph: baseline and with symptoms
Urine cultures: symptoms or catheter in place
Cerebrospinal fluid, joint fluid: local infection suspected
Diarrheal stools: cultures, ova/parasites, *C. difficile* toxin assays
Cutaneous lesions: biopsy, stain, and culture
CBC, LFTs, RFTs, electrolyte panel: at baseline and every 3–4 days, as necessary
Surveillance cultures: for infection control purposes only (MRSA, VRE)

AFB = acid-fast bacilli; LFT = liver function test; MRSA = methicillin-resistant *Staphylococcus aureus*; RFT = renal function test; VRE = vancomycin-resistant enterococci.

■ EMPIRIC ANTIBIOTIC THERAPY

All febrile neutropenic patients need to be treated with empiric broad-spectrum antibiotic therapy based on local epidemiologic and susceptibility/resistance patterns (7). It has become customary to treat low-risk patients with oral or parenteral antibiotic regimens without admitting them to the hospital (8). Most oral regimens are quinolone based combinations, although newer broad-spectrum quinolones are being evaluated for monotherapy (16–18,20). Several parenteral regimens are also available for low-risk patients who might have some

TABLE 36-3	CLINICAL CRITERIA FOR RISK ASSESSMENT AND PARADIGM FOR RISK-BASED THERAPY FOR FEBRILE NEUTROPENIC PATIENTS	
Risk Group	*Clinical Criteria*	*Treatment Options*
Low-risk	Solid tumor (breast, sarcoma, etc.) on conventional chemotherapy; clinically/hemodynamically stable at onset of febrile episode; minimal medical co-morbidity; short lived neutropenia (≤ 7 days); favorable compliance profile	Outpatient therapy → parenteral, sequential (IV → PO), or oral
Moderate- risk	Solid tumor; high-dose chemotherapy ($\pm$) autologous PBSCT; clinically stable with minimal comorbidity; moderate duration of neutropenia (7–14 days); early response to initial antibiotic therapy	Hospital-based parenteral antibiotic therapy followed by early discharge on parenteral or oral antibiotics
High-risk	Hematologic malignancy, allogeneic SCT, substantial comorbidity, clinical and/or hemodynamic instability; prolonged neutropenia (> 14 days); slow response to initial therapy	Hospital-based parenteral antibiotics, close follow-up, appropriate modifications of initial regimen

mucositis or whose chemotherapy-induced emesis is not under full control. Commonly used outpatient regimens are listed in Tables 36-5A and B, which also outline the advantages and disadvantages of outpatient antibiotic therapy.

Patients who do not fall into the low-risk subset should receive parenteral, broad-spectrum antibiotics in the hospital so that they can be closely monitored for response, development of adverse events, or other complications. Two types of antibiotic regimens are used for empiric therapy in such patients: (1) combination regimens and (2) single-agent (monotherapy) regimens. Although a large number of prospective randomized trials have shown that monotherapy is as effective as combination therapy, some clinicians are still hesitant to prescribe monotherapy, particularly to high-risk patients with documented infections due to organisms such as *Pseudomonas aeruginosa*. This debate continues to rage and might never be settled by a definitive study, because it would take a single study of several thousand such high-risk patients to demonstrate a meaningful difference.

Since a large number of clinical trials of empiric therapy in febrile neutropenic patients have been considered at MDACC over the past three decades, we took a closer look at the outcomes of patients with bacteremic infection enrolled in these studies (14). In the 909 episodes studied, extensive tissue infection significantly

TABLE 36-4A	RISK-GROUPING IN FEBRILE NEUTROPENIC PATIENTS BASED ON THE TALCOTT SYSTEM	
Risk Group	*Characteristics*	*Percent Morbidity/ Mortality*
Group 1 (high-risk)	Hospitalized at onset of fever. Hematologic malignancy and/or BMT/HSCT	35/13
Group 2 (high-risk)	Outpatient at onset of fever: substantial concurrent comorbidity	40/12
Group 3 (moderate to high-risk)	Outpatient at onset of fever: no comorbidity but unresponsive/progressive tumors	25/18
Group 4 (low-risk)	Outpatient at onset of fever: Mainly solid tumor. Clinically/ hemodynamically stable. No comorbidity, responsive tumors.	3/0

BMT = bone marrow transplantation; HSCT = hematopoietic stem cell transplantation.
SOURCE: Data from Talcott et al. (5,19). With permission.

TABLE 36-4B	THE MASCC*[†] RISK-INDEX FOR IDENTIFICATION OF LOW-RISK FEBRILE NEUTROPENIC PATIENTS[†]	
Clinical Features		*Score*
Burden of illness*		
No symptoms		5
Mild symptoms		5
No hypotension		5
No chronic obstructive pulmonary disease		4
Solid tumor or no previous fungal infection		4
No dehydration		3
Moderate symptoms		3
Outpatient at fever onset		3
Age < 60 years		2

* Choose only one; maximum theoretical score is 26. A score ≥ 21 denotes low risk for severe complications or mortality.
[†] MASCC = Multinational Association of Supportive Care in Cancer.
SOURCE: MASCC Risk Index (6).

TABLE 36-5A	COMMONLY USED OUTPATIENT ANTIBIOTIC REGIMENS FOR LOW-RISK FEBRILE NEUTROPENIC PATIENTS

Parenteral regimens

   Aztreonam + clindamycin (or ampicillin/sulbactam)

   Ciprofloxacin + clindamycin (or ampicillin/sulbactam)

   Ceftazidime

   Cefepime

   Ceftriaxone (±) amikacin

Oral regimens

   Ciprofloxacin + amoxicillin/clavulanate

   Ciprofloxacin + clindamycin or a macrolide

   Gatifloxacin or moxifloxacin*

* Only pilot data for these agents as monotherapy are currently available (20).

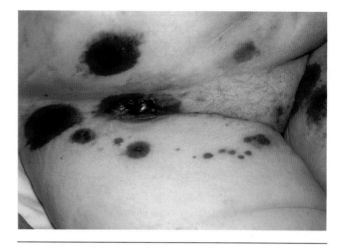

FIGURE 36-5 Typical cutaneous lesions (ecthyma gangrenosum) associated with *Pseudomonas aeruginosa* bacteremia.

compromised response to initial therapy (38 versus 74%), ultimate outcome of infection (73 versus 94%), median time to defervescence (5.3 versus 2.5 days), and survival. Other poor prognostic factors were shock and bacteremia caused by *Pseudomonas* or *Clostridium* spp. or a pathogen resistant to the initial antibiotic(s) (Fig. 36-5). Although the mortality rate was not significantly increased when patients with gram-negative bacteremia initially received monotherapy, this strategy increased the duration of therapy by 25 percent. It might be prudent to administer combination regimens initially to patients who have extensive tissue involvement or the other factors listed above and monotherapy to those who present with fever, hemodynamic stability, and no documented site of infection.

The various choices for combination therapy and monotherapy are listed in Table 36-6. Specific agents should be chosen based on local epidemiologic trends and susceptibility/resistance patterns. Periodic surveillance studies should be conducted in order to detect epi-

demiologic shifts and changes in susceptibility patterns (including the emergence of multidrug-resistant organisms) in a timely manner (21,22).

When opting for combination therapy, a decision regarding the initial administration of a glycopeptide (vancomycin) must be made. If a glycopeptide is not deemed necessary, combination therapy usually consists of an aminoglycoside (e.g., amikacin) with an extended spectrum cephalosporin (cefepime), and antipseudomonal penicillin (piperacillin ± tazobactam), or a carbapenem (imipenem, meropenem). The new carbapenem ertapenem should not be used for empiric

TABLE 36-5B	ADVANTAGES AND DISADVANTAGES OF OUTPATIENT ANTIBIOTIC THERAPY

Advantages

   Economic advantage (reduced costs)

   Enhanced quality of life (both for patient and caregivers)

   Reduced nosocomial infection rate

   More appropriate utilization of health care resources (material and personnel)

Disadvantages

   Potential for adverse events in an unmonitored setting

   Potential for poor compliance or noncompliance

   Need for adequate infrastructure to manage patients at home or in the clinic

   False sense of security

TABLE 36-6	OPTIONS FOR EMPIRIC ANTIBIOTIC THERAPY IN HIGH-RISK FEBRILE NEUTROPENIC PATIENTS*†

Combination regimens (without glycopeptide)

   Aminoglycoside + piperacillin/tazobactam

   Aminoglycoside + cefepime (ceftazidime?)

   Aminoglycoside + imipenem or meropenem

Combination regimens (with gylcopeptide)

   Vancomycin + piperacillin/tazobactam

   Vancomycin + cefepime (ceftazidime?)

   Vancomycin + imipenem or meropenem

   Vancomycin + aztreonam (±) aminoglycoside

   Vancomycin + ciprofloxacin (±) aminoglycoside

Single agents (monotherapy)

   Cefepime

   Imipenem

   Meropenem

   Piperacillin/tazobactam (?)

* Amikacin (used most often), tobramycin, or gentamicin,

† Choice of specific agent(s) depends on local susceptibility/resistance patterns.

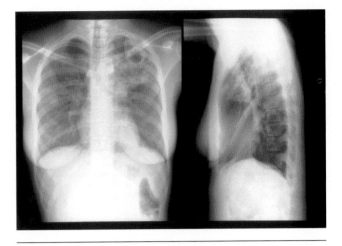

FIGURE 36-6 Cavitary pulmonary lesion located in the left upper lobe, caused by *Mycobacterium tuberculosis*.

monotherapy since its activity against *P. aeruginosa* and *Acinetobacter* spp. is suboptimal. When vancomycin is deemed necessary, any of the agents listed above can be combined with it (±) an aminoglycoside. Combinations which include a quinolone should only be considered in patients who have not received quinolone prophylaxis (Table 36-7).

Some antibiotic combinations are synergistic against both gram-positive and gram-negative pathogens and may be associated with better response rates. Combination therapy may also be associated with less emergence of resistant organisms, although data regarding this issue are conflicting. The major disadvantages are increased toxicity, drug-drug interactions, and cost.

Agents recommended for monotherapy include cefepime, imipenem, and meropenem. Recent studies have also indicated a potential role for piperacillin/tazobactam as monotherapy for febrile neutropenic patients. The quinolones are not currently recommended for use as single agents, although the potential of newer quinolones (gatifloxacin, moxifloxacin) for monotherapy in low-risk patients is being evaluated (20,23). Aminoglycosides should not be used as single agents in neutropenic patients under any circumstances (24).

■ SUBSEQUENT TREATMENT INCLUDING MODIFICATIONS AND DURATION OF THERAPY

Defervescence in febrile neutropenic patients does not happen overnight. It is customary to allow approximately 72 h to ascertain whether the initial regimen is effective or not. If fever persists unabated after 3 days, the patient should be reassessed. If initial cultures are negative and

there has been no clinical deterioration, the same regimen can be continued for an additional 3 to 4 days, since a substantial proportion of patients will defervescence by day 7. The initial regimen should be changed if there are signs of progressive infection or if microbiological cultures dictate the need for a change. The most frequent modifications include:

1. A specific gram-positive agent (vancomycin, linezolid, quinopristin-dalfopristin) for organisms such as MRSA, methicillin-resistant *Staphylococcus* epidermidis (MRSE), VRE, or other resistant gram-positive pathogens.
2. Additional gram-negative coverage (an agent belonging to a different class than the original regimens) particularly in some documented infections (*P. aeruginosa*, *Stenotrophomonas maltophilia*, *Acinetobacter* spp., *Enterobacter* spp., etc.).
3. Additional anaerobic coverage, particularly if an abdominal, pelvic, or perianal site of infection has been documented.
4. When fever persists beyond 5 to 7 days in the absence of a documented pathogen, empiric antifungal therapy should be initiated. Empiric antifungal therapy should be considered sooner in patients with hematologic malignancies, those with a focus of infection in the lungs or paranasal sinuses, and those with a previously documented fungal infection or fungal colonization at multiple sites.

The duration of therapy depends on several factors, including:

1. The nature of the febrile episode (i.e., unexplained fever versus documented infection)
2. The nature of the infection, if documented [bacteremia, urinary tract infection (UTI), pneumonia, perirectal infection, enterocolitis, etc.]
3. Recovery from neutropenia

In patients who did not have a documented infection, have been afebrile for approximately 48 h, and have an ANC that has risen above 500/mm^3, antibiotic therapy can safely be stopped by day 7. In patients who have defervescenced but are still neutropenic, opinion is divided regarding continuation or discontinuation of therapy. It has been our practice at MDACC to discontinue antibiotics in stable, afebrile, neutropenic patients, with the caveat that they be closely monitored while still neutropenic. In patients with documented infections, the duration of treatment will depend on the nature and site of infections (i.e., shorter for UTI, longer for bacteremia or pneumonia). Therapy may be safely discontinued in such patients when they have been afebrile for

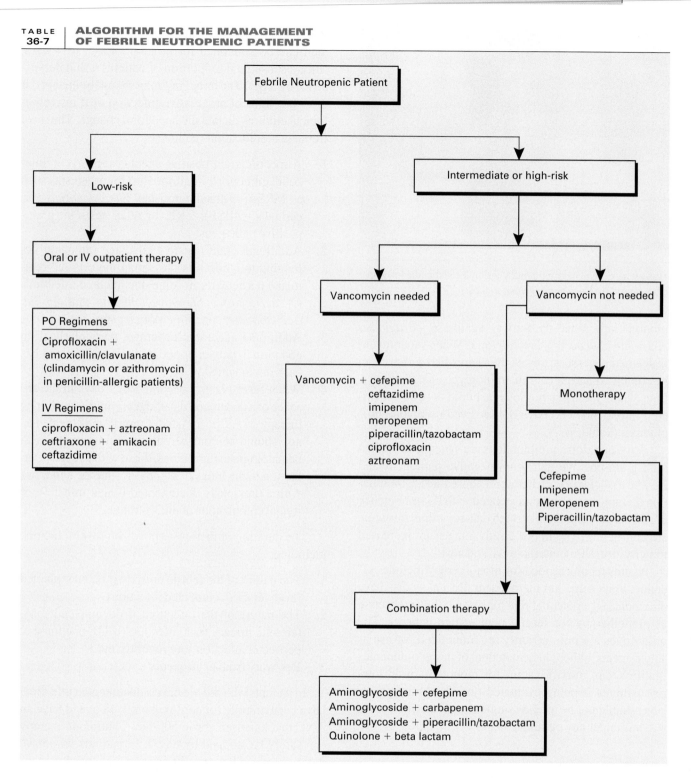

approximately 4 days and clinical, microbiological, and radiographic signs of infection have resolved. In the absence of a documented fungal infection, empiric antifungal therapy is also continued or discontinued using the criteria listed above, or for a total of 10 to 14 days. The management of specific fungal infections is discussed in Chap. 39.

In patients with persistent fever after recovery from neutropenia, a thorough investigation to look for a source, particularly a systemic fungal or mycobacterial infection, should be undertaken. This should include appropriate microbiological cultures, serologic studies, radiographic imaging, and invasive diagnostic procedures if indicated (Fig. 36-6).

■ OTHER CONSIDERATIONS

Empiric antiviral therapy is not recommended. A large number of antiviral agents are not available for the treatment of documented viral infections. The management of specific viral infections is discussed in Chap. 39. Granulocyte transfusions are not routinely recommended in patients with persistent fever and neutropenia. They have, however, been found to be useful in addition to appropriate therapy, in many patients with disseminated fungal infections (25). Interest in granulocyte transfusions has been rekindled after the availability of hematopoietic growth factors [(granulocyte colony-stimulating factor (G-CSF), granulocyte-macrophage colony-stimulating factor (GM-CSF)] to stimulate and facilitate the collection of large numbers of cells from normal donors (26,27).

Antibacterial prophylaxis remains controversial. Patients with short-lived neutropenia (<10 to 14 days) should not receive such prophylaxis. High-risk patients (severe neutropenia anticipated to last for >10 to 14 days) are generally given quinolone prophylaxis. This has been shown to result in fewer gram-negative infections, have a minimal impact on gram-positive infection, and have no impact on overall survival (28). The development of qionolone-resistant and/or multidrug-resistant organisms is the major drawback of this approach (29). Azole antifungal prophylaxis has had a significant impact on the frequency and severity of infections caused by *Candida* spp. (30). Prophylaxis against molds, primarily *Aspergillus* spp., has been much less successful, although the development of agents with better activity against many molds (voriconazole, posaconazole) is promising (31).

■ SUMMARY

The management of febrile neutropenic patients has evolved considerably over the past two decades. The spectrum of infection in such patients undergoes periodic changes that must be anticipated and monitored so that prophylactic/therapeutic strategies can be changed in a timely manner. The recognition of a low-risk subset has simplified management i.e., oral outpatient therapy of such patients. Conversely, the numbers of high-risk patients has actually increased as a result of widespread use of intensive chemotherapy and or peripheral blood stem cell transplantation, producing severe and prolonged myelosuppression. These patients still need prompt and sophisticated management in a hospital-based setting. Accurate and rapid diagnostic techniques must be developed, particularly for fungal infections. The prevention and treatment of many fungal and viral infections remains suboptimal. These issues will continue to challenge us for years to come.

References

1. Bodey GP. Infection in cancer patients: A continuing association. *Am J Med* 1986;81 (Suppl 1A):11–26.
2. Rolston KVI, Bodey GP. Infections in patients with cancer. In: Holland JF, Frei E (eds): *Cancer Medicine,* 6th ed. Montreal: BC Decker; 2003:2633–2658.
3. Wisplinghoff H, Seifert H, Wenzel RP, et al. Current trends in the epidemiology of nosocomial bloodstream infections in patients with hematological malignancies and solid neoplasms in hospitals in the United States. *Clin Infect Dis* 2003;36:1103–1110.
4. Yadegarynia D, Rolston KV, Tarrand J, et al. Current spectrum of bacterial infections in patient with hematological malignancies (HM) and solid tumors (st). 40th Annual Meeting of Infectious Diseases Society of America. Chicago, IL. Oct. 24–27, 2002 (abstr 139).
5. Talcott JA, Siegel RD, Finberg R, et al. Risk assessment in cancer patients with fever and neutropenia. A prospective, two-center validation of a prediction rule. *J Clin Oncol* 1992; 10:316–322.
6. Klastersky J, Paesmans M, Rubenstein E, et al. The MASCC Risk Index: A multinational scoring system to predict low-risk febrile neutropenic cancer patients. *J Clin Oncol* 2000;18: 3038–3051.
7. Hughes WT, Armstrong D, Bodey GP, et al. 2002 guidelines for the use of antimicrobial agents in neutropenic patients with cancer. *Clin Infect Dis* 2002;34:730–751.
8. Rolston K. New trends in patient management: Risk-based therapy for febrile patients with neutropenia. *Clin Infect Dis* 1999;29:515–521.
9. Bodey GP, Buckley M, Sathe YS, et al. Quantitative relationships between circulating leukocytes and infection in patients with acute leukemia. *Ann Intern Med* 1966;64:328–340.
10. Zinner SH. Changing epidemiology of infections in patients with neutropenia and cancer: Emphasis on gram-positive and resistant bacteria. *Clin Infect Dis* 1999;3:490–494.
11. Yadegarynia D, Tarrand J, Raad I, et al. Current spectrum of bacterial infections in cancer patients. *Clin Infect Dis* 2003;37: 1144–1145.
12. Anaissie EJ, Bodey GP, Rinaldi MG. Emerging fungal pathogens. *Eur J Clin Microbiol Infect Dis* 1989;8:323–330.
13. Whimbey E, Englund JA, Couch RB. Community respiratory virus infections in immunocompromised patients with cancer. *Am J Med* 1997;102:10–18.
14. Elting LS, Rubenstein EB, Rolston K, et al. Time to clinical response: An outcome of antibiotic therapy of febrile neutropenia with implications for quality and cost of care. *J Clin Oncol* 2000;18:3699–3706.
15. Rubin M, Hathorn JW, Pizzo PA. Controversies in the management of febrile neutropenic cancer patients. *Cancer Invest* 1988;6:167–184.

16. Rubenstein EB, Rolston K, Benjamin RS, et al. Outpatient treatment of febrile episodes in low risk neutropenic cancer patients. *Cancer* 1993;71:3640–3646.

17. Freifeld A, Marchigiani D, Walsh T, et al. A double-blind comparison of empirical oral and intravenous antibiotic therapy for low-risk febrile patients with neutropenia during cancer chemotherapy. *N Engl J Med* 1999;341:305–311.

18. Kern KV, Cometta A, De Bock R, et al. Oral versus intravenous empirical antimicrobial therapy for fever in patients with granulocytopenia who are receiving cancer chemotherapy. *N Engl J Med* 1999;341:312–318.

19. Talcott JA, Finbert R, Mayer RJ, et al. The medical course of cancer patients with fever and neutropenia. *Arch Intern Med* 1988;148:2501–2568.

20. Rolston KVI, Frisbee-Hume S, Manzullo E, et al. Once daily, oral, outpatient, quinolone monotherapy for low-risk, febrile neutropenic patients (FNP). 41st Annual Meeting of the Infectious Diseases Society of America. San Diego, CA, Oct. 9–12, 2003 (abstr 375).

21. Jacobson K, Rolston K, Elting L, et al. Susceptibility surveillance among gram-negative bacilli at a cancer center. *Chemotherapy* 1999;45:325–334.

22. Rolston KVI, Kontoyiannis DP, Raad II, et al. Susceptibility surveillance among gram-negative bacilli at a comprehensive cancer center. 103rd General Meeting American Society of Microbiology. Washington, DC, May 18–22, 2003 (abstr 2362).

23. Rolston KVI, Frisbee-Hume S, LeBlanc B, et al. In vitro antimicrobial activity of moxifloxacin compared to other quinolones against recent clinical bacterial isolates from hospitalization and community-based cancer patients. *Diagn Microbiol Infect Dis* 2003;47:441–449.

24. Bodey GP. Synergy: Should it determine antibiotic selection in neutropenic patients (editorial). *Arch Intern Med* 1985;145:1964–1966.

25. Dignani MC, Anaissie EJ, Hester JP, et al. Treatment of neutropenia-related fungal infections with granulocyte colony-stimulating factor-elicited white blood cell transfusions: A pilot study. *Leukemia* 1997;82:362–363.

26. Jendiroba DB, Lichtiger B, Anaissie E, et al. Evaluation and comparison of three mobilization methods for the collection of granulocytes. *Transfusion* 1998;38:722–728.

27. Hubel K, Dale DC, Engert A, et al. Current status of granulocyte (neutrophil) transfusion therapy for infectious diseases. *J Infect Dis* 2001;183:321–328.

28. Engels EA, Lau J, Barza M. Efficacy of quinolone prophylaxis in neutropenic cancer patients: A meta-analysis. *J Clin Oncol* 1998;16:1179–1187.

29. Rolston KVI. Commentary: Chemoprophylaxis and bacterial resistance in neutropenic patients. *Infect Dis Clin Pract* 1998;7:202–204.

30. Marr KA, Seidel K, Slavin MA, et al. Prolonged fluconazole prophylaxis is associated with persistent protection against candidiasis-related death in allogeneic marrow transplant recipients: Long-term follow-up of a randomized, placebo-controlled trial. *Blood* 2003;96:2055–2061.

31. Johnson LB, Kauffman CA. Voriconazole: A new triazole antifungal agent. *Clin Infect Dis* 2003;36:630–637.

CHAPTER
37

FUNGAL AND VIRAL INFECTIONS IN CANCER PATIENTS

Gerald P. Bodey
Roy F. Chemaly
Dimitrios P. Kontoyiannis

For many years, the major focus of attention was on the management of bacterial infections in cancer patients. It was recognized that some malignant diseases, such as chronic lymphocytic leukemia, were associated with viral infections, especially varicella zoster. Cytomegalovirus infection was reported sporadically, one of the largest early series being among children with acute leukemia (1). Likewise, small series of fungal infections were reported among patients with hematologic malignancies. One of the first large autopsy studies of fungal infections was a study in patients with acute leukemia demonstrating that most of these infections were caused by *Candida* spp. and *Aspergillus* spp. (2). Often they were not suspected and hence were never treated. In recent years, with more aggressive therapies, the widespread use of hematopoietic stem cell transplantation (HSCT), and the ability to control most bacterial infections, fungal and viral infections have emerged as a major cause of serious and fatal infections among cancer patients, especially patients with acute leukemia and HSCT recipients.

■ FUNGAL INFECTIONS

A multiplicity of factors affect susceptibility to fungal infections. The pathogenic fungi *Histoplasma capsulatam* and *Coccidioides immitis* are geographically restricted, but immunocompromised patients may experience reactivation of latent infections acquired at some earlier time. *Aspergillus* spp. and *Fusarium* spp. are ubiquitous in the environment. Although patients usually develop symptoms of infection due to these organisms while in the hospital, most infections are community-acquired except during periods of hospital construction or faulty air handling. Generally, patients are exposed to much lower concentrations of spores in the hospital than in the community. *Candida* spp., on the other hand, are often a component of the patient's endogenous microbial flora.

Most serious fungal infections occur in patients with prolonged and severe neutropenia. This is not surprising, since neutrophils are capable of ingesting and killing *Candida* spp. In animal studies, neutrophils were found to be the primary defense against the hyphae of *Aspergillus* sp. (3,4). The administration of high doses of adrenal corticosteroids, especially for protracted periods of time, predispose to aspergillosis and other mold infections. The macrophage ingests and kills *Aspergillus* spores and corticosteroids interfere with the fungicidal activity of macrophages (4).

Disruption of mucocutaneous barriers also predispose to fungal infections. Candidemias and, rarely, *Fusarium* fungemias are associated with intravascular catheters (5). Local *Aspergillus* and *Zygomycetes* infections have occurred at catheter insertion sites, often leading to disseminated infection (6). Disseminated fusariosis occasionally arises from paronychia due to skin trauma adjacent to sites of onychomycosis. Other sites of tissue damage may also facilitate fungal infections. Leukemic infiltrates and chemotherapy-induced ulcerations of the oropharynx and gastrointestinal tract may serve as the site of origin for disseminated candidiasis.

Cellular immunity, such as decreased numbers of CD4 T lymphocytes or cytokine production, play an important role in predisposing to some fungal infections such as oropharyngeal candidiasis. An increasing number of antitumor agents cause prolonged and severe CD4 lymphocytopenia. Impaired cellular immunity also predisposes to cryptococcosis and reactivation of histoplasmosis and coccidioidomycosis.

Broad-spectrum antibiotic therapy has been associated with fungal infections. This may be due to suppression of the normal flora, allowing for fungal overgrowth, as has been shown with *Candida* spp. in the oropharynx and gastrointestinal tract. Antibacterial and antifungal prophylaxis may be associated with fungal infection, the latter facilitating acquisition of fungi resistant to antifungal agents. For example, fluconazole prophylaxis has been associated with increased colonization and, in some studies, infection with *Candida krusei,* which is inherently resistant to fluconazole (7).

CANDIDIASIS

Candidiasis is the most common fungal infection in cancer patients, although its frequency has decreased substantially in recent years due to the widespread use of antifungal prophylaxis in highly susceptible populations. The ability of these organisms to adhere to mucosal surfaces is a critical factor in the initiation of infection. Chemoradiotherapy has been shown to reduce the inhibitory effect of saliva on *Candida* adhesion. Proteases and lipases are virulence factors for *Candida* spp. Other factors may include persorption (the ability to cross the intact epithelium), germ tube formation, and toxin production. These organisms can cause a wide variety of infections, ranging from mild but uncomfortable superficial infections to major organ invasion and widely disseminated infection.

Most candidal infections arise from the patient's endogenous microbial flora. Several studies have shown that most patients are colonized by a unique strain; it is uncommon for patients occupying the same hospital unit to be colonized by the same strain of *Candida* sp. Nevertheless, hospital epidemics have occurred due to contaminated equipment, solutions, and hospital personnel.

Most superficial infections are caused by *Candida albicans* and, until recent years, that was also true for most systemic infections. Although *C. albicans* still accounts for more than 50% of systemic infections, other species have emerged as relatively common pathogens. In a review of 36 studies reporting 1479 cancer patients, *C. albicans* accounted for only 54% (range 15 to 85%) of infections and *C. tropicalis* for 25% (range 0 to 83%) (8). In cancer patients when routine surveillance cultures have been collected at least once weekly, less than 10% of patients colonized by *C. albicans* have subsequently developed systemic infection, compared with 40 to 100% of patients colonized by *C. tropicalis* (9). *C. tropicalis* is more likely to cause the characteristic skin lesions associated with disseminated candidiasis and occasionally causes a syndrome of skin lesions and painful myositis.

C. glabrata has variable susceptibility to fluconazole; increased colonization and infection with *C. glabrata* has been associated with fluconazole prophylaxis. *C. parapsilosis* has been associated with parenteral alimentation and intravascular catheters. In a study of *C. parapsilosis* fungemia in cancer patients with intravascular catheters, only 10% responded to antifungal therapy without catheter removal (10). Fungemia persisted for more than a week in some patients despite appropriate therapy.

C. krusei is inherently resistant to fluconazole and has been isolated with increased frequency of colonization and infection in some institutions where fluconazole has been used prophylactically (7). *C. lusitaniae* is of concern because some strains may be inherently resistant to amphotericin B and others develop resistance during therapy associated with treatment failure. *C. dubliniensis*, which may be misidentified as *C. albicans*, can cause serious infections and may not be susceptible to fluconazole.

Superficial Candidiasis

Oral Infection

The most common superficial candidal infection occurring in cancer patients is acute pseudomembranous candidiasis of the oropharynx (thrush) (11). It occurs following mucosal damage by chemotherapy or radiotherapy. Lesions are creamy, whitish curd-like plaques or pseudomembranes on the buccal mucosa, palate, or tongue (Fig. 37-1). The exposed base is erythematous and painful; it may bleed. These lesions may be associ-

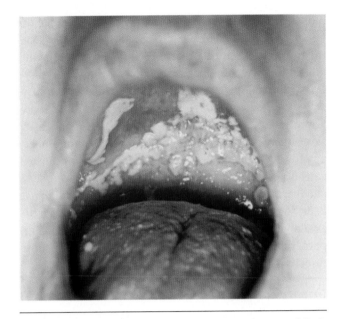

FIGURE 37-1 Typical appearance of oropharyngeal candidiasis on palatal and buccal mucosa.

ated with fissures in the angles of the mouth known as perleche. Rarely, patients may have nodular lesions on the tongue, which are a manifestation of disseminated infection. Some cancer patients with clinically significant thrush also have esophageal involvement that may cause only mild or moderate symptoms.

The diagnosis is confirmed by the demonstration of yeasts and pseudohyphae on a scraping of an infected area, along with a culture. Recovery of *Candida* sp. from a culture alone is insufficient evidence because these fungi are commonly found in the oropharynx, especially in patients receiving antibiotics. The most effective therapy has been fluconazole, which is well absorbed from the gastrointestinal tract, although some patients respond to topical agents (nystatin, clotrimazole).

Esophagitis

Cancer patients are also susceptible to esophageal candidiasis (11). Symptoms of esophageal candidiasis include dysphagia, retrosternal pain, and odynophagia. Serious complications of this infection can occur, including chronic esophageal strictures, bronchoesophageal fistulas, and mediastinitis. About 70% of patients with candidal esophagitis also have thrush; hence the diagnosis is usually easy to establish. A barium contrast roentgenogram may show peristaltic abnormalities, spasm, shaggy ulcerations, and a moth-eaten appearance of the mucosa. It is important to recognize that the symptoms and roentgenographic findings can be caused by other infectious agents, such as herpes simplex and cytomegalovirus. Esophagoscopy with brushings, biopsies, and cultures is the only way to confirm the diagnosis of candidal esophagitis. Since *Candida* spp. are the most common cause of infectious esophagitis and unless the patient has been receiving antifungal prophylaxis, it is usually appropriate to initiate therapy empirically with an antifungal agent and reserve esophagoscopy for those patients who fail to respond after several days of therapy. Fluconazole is the optimal therapy for most cases of esophageal candidiasis because it can be administered intravenously initially, if necessary, and then be replaced with oral therapy. Caspofungin has been shown to be as effective as fluconazole, but it is available only as an intravenous preparation (12). Amphotericin B preparations are rarely indicated for these infections.

Urinary Tract Infection

Cancer patients can develop primary infections of the urinary tract if they have urinary obstruction or urinary catheters in place (13). It is difficult to discriminate between colonization and infection in patients with urinary catheters. There is no concentration of organisms to indicate infection, and some patients may have a normal urinalysis. Candidal casts in the urine are diagnostic but are found infrequently. In addition to cystitis, in some patients (especially those with diabetes mellitus), the organism may migrate through the ureter to the renal pelvis and cause obstruction due to fungus ball formation or necrotizing papillitis. Candiduria in a febrile neutropenic patient may be a manifestation of disseminated infection. Fluconazole is the most appropriate agent for this infection.

▨ Disseminated Candidiasis

Disseminated candidiasis usually originates from lesions of the oropharynx or gastrointestinal tract or from intravenous catheters (9). Organs usually involved include the kidney, heart, muscle, gastrointestinal tract, lung, liver, and spleen.

Most patients with disseminated candidiasis have no unique signs or symptoms that would differentiate it from other infections. They are usually debilitated, have experienced a previous or concomitant bacterial infection, and have persistent or recurrent fever that may be associated with pulmonary infiltrates or deteriorating liver or renal function. Some patients present with the acute onset of fever and hypotension suggestive of endotoxin shock.

Eye lesions suggestive of this infection may develop, hence, a careful ophthamalogic examination should be performed when this infection is suspected (14). Typical lesions are single or multiple, whitish, fluffy exudates with indistinct margins, sometimes associated with hemorrhages and borders covered by a vitreous haze. Other types of lesions include Roth spots, uveitis, hypopion, iritis, and papillitis. Symptoms often are not present, but some patients complain of ocular pain, blurred vision, scotomas, or photophobia. These lesions are rarely found in neutropenic patients because they are unable to mount an adequate inflammatory reaction.

Characteristic skin lesions have been described in about 10% of patients (15). The lesions may be generalized or localized to the extremities and may be numerous or few. They are nontender, firm, raised nodules that are pink to red in color and do not blanch on pressure (Fig. 37-2). Some of these patients have an associated myositis (usually associated with *C. tropicalis* infection) manifest as diffuse severe muscle tenderness most pronounced in the legs. *Candida* spp. can be identified in the dermis and the organisms can be cultured from about half of the biopsies.

Diagnosis

The diagnosis of disseminated candidiasis may be difficult to establish because the organism may not be isolated from multiple blood culture specimens of as many as 40% of patients with widespread infection demonstrated at autopsy examination (16). The use of lysis centrifugation, the BacT-Alert system (which monitors CO_2 production), and the high-volume BACTEC system with infrared detection have improved the yield of positive blood cultures. A variety of methodologies have been developed to detect circulating candidal antigens or metabolites, including the polymerase chain reaction (PCR), but none has been entirely satisfactory. The

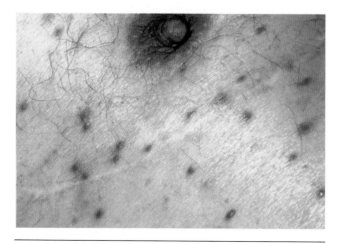

FIGURE 37-2 Widespread nodular skin lesions in a patient with disseminated candidiasis.

ability to culture *Candida* sp. from multiple other sites (sputum, urine, feces, etc.) does not establish the diagnosis of candidiasis. However, disseminated candidiasis is unlikely to be the cause of fever if the organism cannot be cultured from several body sites. Since the diagnosis may be difficult to establish, it is often appropriate to administer antifungal therapy empirically in neutropenic patients who fail to respond to broad-spectrum antibacterial agents, especially if they have not received antifungal prophylaxis.

Other Candidal Infections

Chronic Disseminated Candidiasis

A distinct syndrome known as chronic disseminated candidiasis has been described almost exclusively in patients with acute leukemia (17). Typically these patients develop fever unresponsive to broad-spectrum antibacterial antibiotics after prolonged periods of neutropenia. After the neutropenia resolves, the patients remain febrile with anorexia, progressive debilitation, and weight loss and may develop hepatosplenomegaly or pain in the right upper quadrant. The alkaline phosphatase is usually highly elevated, while other liver tests are only mildly elevated. Multiple small lesions can be detected in the liver and spleen by magnetic resonance imaging (MRI), computed tomography (CT), or ultrasound (Fig. 37-3). The disease can persist for several months despite therapy and may interfere with administration of cancer chemotherapy. The diagnosis can be confirmed by visualizing hyphae on liver biopsy, but the organism is cultured from only 50% of biopsy specimens. Occasional patients may develop hypersplenism. This form of candidiasis is rarely seen among leukemic patients at institutions where fluconazole prophylaxis is used routinely.

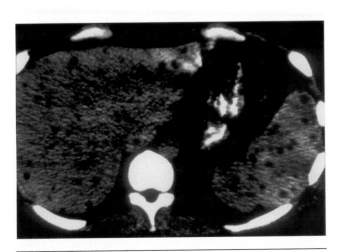

FIGURE 37-3 CT scan showing multiple lesions in liver and spleen of patient with chronic disseminated candidiasis.

Pneumonia

While the lung is usually involved in disseminated infection, primary candidal pneumonia occurs infrequently in cancer patients (18). It is possible that a patient may aspirate infected oral secretions and develop pneumonia. The isolation of *Candida* sp. in clinical specimens from a patient with a pulmonary infiltrate does not establish the diagnosis of candidal pneumonia. A recent autopsy study of cancer patients demonstrated that while many patients with pneumonia had *Candida* sp. cultured from sputum and bronchoalveolar lavage (BAL) specimens, the specificity and positive predictive values were low (19). Only histopathologic evidence is confirmatory, but it is often impossible to obtain from many of these patients. Empiric antifungal therapy may be indicated for susceptible patients with positive sputum cultures and progressive pulmonary infiltrates despite broad-spectrum antibacterial therapy.

Meningitis

Multiple small abscesses may be present in the brain in disseminated candidiasis and usually do not cause symptoms. Candidal meningitis occurs infrequently and is associated with disseminated infection in the majority of cases or with ventricular shunts. There are no specific clinical signs and symptoms to discriminate this infection from bacterial meningitis. Examination of cerebrospinal fluid (CSF) reveals decreased glucose and elevated protein concentrations as well as lymphocytosis. *Candida* spp. are rarely visualized by direct microscopic examination of CSF.

Therapy

Therapeutic agents available for treatment of candidiasis are listed in Tables 37-1 through 37-3. Mortality from candidemia and disseminated candidiasis has been especially high among cancer patients and HSCT recipients.

The mortality rates have been 70 to 77% among patients treated with amphotericin B deoxycholate (D-AMB) compared with 56 to 82% among patients who were not treated; very few neutropenic patients survive their infection unless their neutrophil counts recover (16). Although there are some laboratory and clinical data indicating that flucytosine and D-AMB interact synergistically and may be superior to D-AMB alone, especially against *C. tropicalis* infections, an adequate comparative trial has never been performed.

D-AMB has been compared with fluconazole in several prospective randomized trials, most of which have excluded neutropenic patients (20). All of these studies have shown these two drugs to be essentially

TABLE 37-1 | DOSAGE REGIMENS FOR SERIOUS FUNGAL INFECTIONS

Drug	Loading Dose	Daily Dose	Route
D-AMB	—	1–1.5 mg/kg	IV only
Lipid AMB	—	3–5 mg/kg	IV only
Fluconazole	800 mg	400–800 mg	IV, PO
Itraconazole IV	200 mg bid × 2 days	200 mg	IV
Itraconazole solution	200 mg bid × 2 days	200 mg	PO
Itraconazole capsules	200 mg tid × 3 days	200 mg bid	PO
Voriconazole IV	6 mg/kg q 12 h	4 mg/kg q 12 h	IV
Voriconazole tablets	—	200 mg q 12 h (>40 kg)	PO
		100 mg q 12 h (<40 kg)	
Caspofungin	70 mg	50 mg	IV

D-AMB = amphotericin B deoxycholate; IV = intravenous; PO = per os (oral).

equally efficacious, but fluconazole was substantially less toxic. In a single study that included patients with neutropenia at the onset their infection, the response rate was significantly higher with fluconazole, although the number of patients was not large (20). It is uncertain whether fluconazole is superior to D-AMB in patients with persistent neutropenia, but it is unlikely to be worse, since so few of these patients respond to D-AMB. Initiation of therapy with D-AMB plus fluconazole with subsequent discontinuation of D-AMB is more effective than fluconazole alone and is more appropriate in institutions where fluconazole is used extensively for prophylaxis (21). Also, it may be appropriate to use higher doses of fluconazole (800 mg/day), at least initially, in neutropenic patients.

Lipid formulations of AMB are less nephrotoxic, but there is no convincing evidence that they are more effective than D-AMB. Since most patients with candidiasis do not require prolonged therapy, the use of these more expensive preparations is usually not justified.

Caspofungin is a new agent with broad-spectrum activity against *Candida* spp. It has been compared to

TABLE 37-2 | MAJOR TOXICITIES OF ANTIFUNGAL AGENTS

Amphotericin B	Infusion-related (headache, chills, hypotension, etc); nephrotoxicity; hypo K, hypo/Mg; anemia
Fluconazole	Nausea, vomiting; headache; hepatotoxicity (rare); drug interactions
Itraconazole	Nausea, vomiting; headache; hepatotoxicity (rare); pulmonary edema; drug interactions
Voriconazole	Visual; rash; nausea, vomiting; headache; hepatotoxicity; drug interactions
Caspofungin	Fever; nausea; flushing; rash; some drug interactions; phlebitis

D-AMB for therapy of systemic candidal infections, 90% of which were candidemias (22). Caspofungin was at least as effective as D-AMB and considerably less toxic. In this study of invasive infections, very few patients were neutropenic.

The therapy of chronic disseminated candidiasis is often difficult and response to therapy has often been unsatisfactory (17). A small study showed that a lipid formulation of AMB was very effective. A larger experience indicated that fluconazole was effective even among patients who were failing to respond to D-AMB, and it should be considered the drug of choice for this form of candidiasis. Evidence of response may require several weeks of therapy, and duration of therapy should be determined by the rapidity of clinical improvement and lesions on roentgenographic examinations; in any event, it should last for 2 to 6 months. Patients can have residual lesions in the liver and spleen due to scarring.

A controversial issue is whether indwelling intravascular catheters should be removed routinely from patients with candidemia. These catheters are often vital to the management of seriously ill patients, and considerable expense is involved in removing and replacing catheters that have been surgically implanted. Nevertheless, some but not all studies have shown that catheter removal shortens the duration of candidemia and improves response rates to antifungal therapy (4,22). This is especially true if the infecting organism is *C. parapsilosis,* where fungemia can persist for more than a week despite appropriate therapy if the catheter is not removed (10). In vitro studies have shown that caspofungin and lipid formulations of AMB were more active against *Candida* spp. growing in the biofilms that characteristically form on catheters (23).

ASPERGILLOSIS

Invasive aspergillosis has emerged as an important infection, accounting for 20 to 40% of systemic fungal infections in patients with acute leukemia, 10 to 20% in HSCT recipients, and 5 to 15% of solid-organ transplant recipients (24,25). Most infections occur in patients with neutropenia or those who are receiving adrenal corticosteroids, which interfere with macrophage function (4). Several species are pathogenic, but *Aspergillus*

TABLE 37-3 | THERAPEUTIC OPTIONS FOR DISSEMINATED AND MAJOR ORGAN CANDIDIASIS

Regimen	Advantages	Disadvantages
Amphotericin B deoxycholate (D-AMB)	Broad-spectrum activity.	Acute chronic toxicities, minimally effective in patients with neutropenia and with chronic disseminated candidiasis, IV preparations only.
Lipid formulations of AMB	Broad-spectrum activity, reduced nephrotoxicity. Higher doses can be administered.	Only prospective randomized trial showed no advantage in efficacy over AMB deoxycholate despite higher doses. More expensive. IV preparations only.
Fluconazole	Oral and intravenous preparation. As effective as AMB in randomized trials of nonneutropenic. Minimal toxicity. More effective for chronic disseminated candidiasis. Little experience in neutropenic patients, but appears to be as effective as AMB.	Variable activity against *C. glabrata* and *C. dubliniensis,* inactive against *C. krusei.* Some drug-drug interactions.
Caspofungin	Broad-spectrum activity. Minimal toxicity. In randomized trials, as active as amphotericin B and fluconazole. Limited experience in neutropenic patients.	No oral preparation.
Flucytosine	Syngeristic with AMB and fluconazole. Combination of flucytosine and AMB may be superior to AMB alone for chronic disseminated candidiasis and *C. tropicalis* infection.	No IV preparation. Causes myelosuppression. Often need monitoring of serum concentrations. Emergence of resistance if used alone.

fumigatus causes most infections (24). Most infections are acquired by inhalation of spores, and epidemics have occurred in hospitals undergoing construction within them or at adjacent areas (3). *Aspergillus* spp. invade blood vessels, causing thrombosis and infarction, and can erode through facial planes, cartilage, and bone (26).

Pulmonary Infection

About 70% of infections involve the lung, and some patients may present with symptoms suggestive of pulmonary embolism, with sudden onset of pleuritic pain, fever, hemoptysis and a pleural friction rub. Other patients may present with fever unresponsive to antibacterial agents and may not have any abnormalities on chest roentgenography initially. A few patients develop acute fatal pulmonary hemorrhage.

The earliest abnormality on chest roentgenography is a single nodular lesion or multiple lesions (27). As the infection progresses, wedge-shaped infarcts, necrotizing bronchopneumonia, lobar consolidation, or diffuse infiltrates may be found. Patients with normal roentgenograms should have CT scans, which will usually reveal a nodular infiltrate surrounded by a halo of low attenuation (28) (Fig. 37-4). If the infection is controlled, the patient usually develops one or several cavitations, often containing fungus balls.

Sinusitis

About 15 to 20% of infections in neutropenic patients involve the sinuses. Signs and symptoms include fever, headache, retroorbital erythema and swelling, and rhinnorhea (26). Often a necrotic lesion can be found on the nose or palate (Fig. 37-5). A CT scan or MRI will show opacification of the sinuses and bony destruction. As

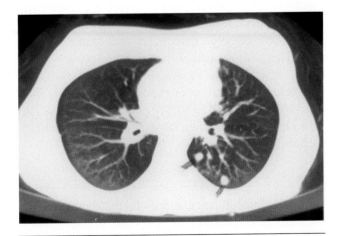

FIGURE 37-4 CT scan showing nodular lesions in lung of patient on high dose adrenal corticosteroid therapy who developed sudden onset of pleuritic chest pain and a pleural friction rub due to pulmonary aspergillosis. The chest roentgenogram was normal.

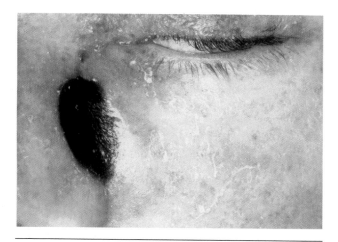

FIGURE 37-5   Black eschar on bridge of nose in a patient with aspergillus sinusitis.

the infection progresses, it causes proptosis, ophthalmoplegia, endophthalmitis, and cerebral infarction. Invasive oral infection involving the gingiva; spread of the infection to the facial muscle and bone has been described in leukemic patients (29).

Skin Infection

Primary invasive cutaneous infections have occurred, usually associated with venous access devices (6). Deposition of conidiae may occur during catheter insertion or from dressings impregnated with conidiae. The lesions begin as erythematous or violaceous plaques that progress to necrotic ulcers covered by black eschars.

Disseminated Infection

Hematogenous dissemination occurs in 30 to 40% of infections. The central nervous system is a common site of involvement, resulting in cerebral infarction, which then causes neurologic defects, seizures, stupor, or coma (30). The gastrointestinal tract is involved in 40% of cases, especially the esophagus and large bowel; this may lead to perforation or massive hemorrhage. Skin lesions are found in 5 to 10% of patients and evolve into well-circumscribed, often large ulcers covered by black eschars.

Diagnosis

One major impediment to successful management is the difficulty in establishing the diagnosis in patients with pulmonary or disseminated infection (31). For this reason most patients receive antifungal therapy for the presumed rather than proven diagnosis of aspergillosis. Tissue biopsies can be obtained from infected sinuses

or skin; these will reveal fungal hyphae, although the organism may not grow on culture media. Unfortunately the fungus is seldom isolated from blood cultures of patients with disseminated infection (32). *Aspergillus* spp. are seldom cultured from the sputum of patients with pulmonary infection, and bronchoscopy with BAL will often fail to establish the diagnosis. In a recent study, positive sputum cultures were obtained antemortem from only 30% of patients with histopathology-proven aspergillosis (33). Whenever *Aspergillus* spp. are cultured from respiratory secretions of susceptible patients, they are either already infected or likely soon to become infected.

A variety of noncultural methods have been attempted, but most are not entirely satisfactory. Serologic methods to detect circulating free antigens or immune complexes have been developed using enzyme linked immunosorbent assay (ELISA) and radioimmunoassay techniques (34). These procedures have focused on detecting galactomannan, carbohydrate antigens, and $1,3$-β-D-glucan (35,36). Attempts have been made to select those patients for therapy who are at high risk based on antigen detection and imaging techniques (37). It is anticipated that molecular approaches such as PCR (34) will become important diagnostic tools in the future.

Therapy

Table 37-4 lists the principles of management for aspergillosis. D-AMB was the only drug available for the treatment of aspergillosis until recently, and no prospective evaluations of this drug were attempted. A major obstacle was the difficulty in establishing the diagnosis; hence, most patients were treated empirically. Mortality rates were influenced by the fact that the diagnosis was most often determined at autopsy examination. Nevertheless, most infections occurred in neutropenic patients, and unless the neutropenia resolved,

TABLE 37-4	PRINCIPLES OF THERAPY OF ASPERGILLOSIS

Early, aggressive treatment with high doses of voriconazole or a lipid formulation of amphotericin B deoxycholate (D-AMB)

Rapid tapering of dose of adrenal corticosteroids if possible

Consideration for G-CSF-primed granulocyte transfusions in selected cases

Long-term antifungal therapy, which should be individualized based on response

Debridement of necrotic tissue of localized disease (onychomycosis, sinusitis, abscess)

the patient rarely responded to D-AMB. A more standardized approach to therapy has become possible with the recent introduction of uniform diagnostic criteria and categorization of infection into proven, probable, and possible asperigillosis (38).

The lipid formulations are an attractive alternative to AMB because of the reduced frequency of nephrotoxicity. Since many patients with aspergillosis require prolonged therapy, nephrotoxicity is a very frequent side effect with D-AMB, which requires dosage modifications. Many physicians believe that responses are more likely to occur with maximum tolerated doses and recommend initiating therapy with daily doses of D-AMB of 1.25 to 1.5 mg/kg, which inevitably leads to nephrotoxicity. The standard daily dose of lipid formulations is 5 mg/kg, although the most appropriate dose has not been determined. The lipid formulations of AMB have been shown in uncontrolled studies to have an efficacy rate of about 40 to 60% in patients with aspergillosis whose disease was refractory to D-AMB or who were intolerant to it (39). Although no comparative trials have been conducted, the lipid formulations appear to be equally efficacious, although their toxicities differ, as do their costs (39,40).

Itraconazole was the first azole introduced for the treatment of aspergillosis. All of the studies reported with this drug have been open trials. In a collated review of 269 cases reported in the literature, the complete and partial response rate was 63%, but it varied from 39 to 80% in the different series (41). Partial responses generally referred to patients whose infections were controlled but whose residual lesions persisted. The role of neutrophil recovery in the response of neutropenic patients is unclear in these presentations. Initially, only an oral capsule preparation was available, and it was not consistently well absorbed from the gastrointestinal tract. Recently an intravenous preparation and well-absorbed oral solution have become available. Unfortunately the oral solution is not well-tolerated by some patients. A small multicenter trial of the intravenous preparation demonstrated that adequate serum concentrations were achieved, the drug was well tolerated, and about half of the patients responded (42).

Voriconazole, another azole, has recently been introduced for the therapy of aspergillosis. It is available as both intravenous and oral preparations. In a large prospective randomized trial comparing voriconazole with D-AMB in patients with definite or probable aspergillosis, the response rates were 53 versus 32%, respectively, and survival at 12 weeks was 71 versus 58% (43). Patients who failed initial therapy received other medications. This happened more frequently among

the D-AMB population, primarily owing to the drug's toxicity.

Caspofungin is one of a new class of antifungal agents (echinocandins) that inhibit the synthesis of β-(1,3)-D-glucan, an essential component of the cell wall of many fungi. It is available only as an intravenous preparation. In a noncomparative trial of 90 patients with definite or probable aspergillosis who had failed other therapy, a complete or partial response occurred in 45% (44). Responses were observed in 50% of patients with pulmonary infection but in only 26% of those with neutropenia.

The lack of effective treatment of aspergillosis has made the concept of combination therapy theoretically appealing. To date, no clinical studies have convincingly determined whether antifungal combinations are more beneficial than therapy using AMB alone for aspergillosis (45). For instance, the sequence of administration of itraconazole in combination with AMB has produced a spectrum of responses ranging from synergy to antagonism. With the recent introduction of echinocandins, which have a different mechanism of action, it is important to determine whether new combinations (e.g., azoles plus echinocandins, AMB plus echinocandins, terbinafine plus azoles, AMB plus azoles and echinocandins), given either concomitantly or sequentially, would result in additive or synergistic effects (45). The sequence and timing of these combinations are important areas of future investigation (31).

The role of adjunctive surgery in the management of aspergillosis also has not been conclusively demonstrated. Pulmonary infarcts and tissue sequestration are common causes of antifungal therapy failure and fatal hemorrhage (46,47). Resection of infected pulmonary tissue is beneficial for some patients (48). After successful antifungal therapy, residual cavitary lesions, especially when they contain fungus balls, may cause late exsanguinating hemorrhage or reactivation of infection during subsequent myelosuppressive chemotherapy. Removal of these lesions, if surgically feasible, should be considered and may provide survival benefit (49). Surgical intervention may be lifesaving for acute pulmonary hemorrhage even when it occurs early in the disease process (46,48).

CRYPTOCOCCOSIS

Cryptococcus neoformans is found worldwide, especially in the excreta of pigeons (50). *C. neoformans* var. *gattii* is found in tropical and subtropical climates and is associated with eucalyptus trees. The infection is acquired by inhalation of organisms into the lungs. Patients at risk of developing this infection have impaired cellular immunity or are receiving adrenal corticosteroids; hence cancer patients at highest risk are those with chronic lymphocytic leukemia or lymphoma or are HSCT recipients.

Pneumonia

Although the lung is the primary site of infection, less than 40% of patients present due to symptoms of pneumonia (51). They may present with only minimal symptoms or with fever, chest pain, cough, or dyspnea. Sputum, the production of which is usually minimal, may be blood-stained. Chest roentgenographic abnormalities may include single or multiple nodules, lobar pneumonia, interstitial infiltrates, and occasionally pleural effusions. In the cancer patient, cryptococcal pneumonia can progress rapidly and cause death; hence an aggressive approach must be taken to make the diagnosis.

Sputum cultures may be negative in some patients. Also, C. neoformans can colonize the respiratory tract without causing infection. Nevertheless, isolation of this organism from respiratory specimens of a susceptible patient who has a pulmonary infiltrate on chest roentgenography should be considered sufficient indication for immediate therapy. The organism can be cultured from blood specimens of about 35% of patients with pneumonia.

Central Nervous System Infection

In most series, over 50% of infections in cancer patients involve the central nervous system (CNS), mainly as meningoencephalitis, but occasional patients have pure meningitis or a cryptococcoma (52). Meningoencephalitis is often an indolent process, but some patients may have an acute, rapidly progressive infection. The first symptoms are usually mild fever and headache. As the infection progresses, patients may develop nausea, vomiting, dizziness, somnolence, irritability, confusion, photophobia, or obtundation. Physical findings may include papilledema, cranial nerve palsies, motor or sensory defects, cerebellar abnormalities, hypereflexia, ankle clonus, and extensor plantar responses. Only about 15% have nuchal rigidity, which may be minimal. As many as 30% may develop blindness secondary to papilledema. Hydrocephalus can be a serious complication in some patients.

Examination of the CSF reveals an elevated opening pressure, decreased glucose and elevated protein concentration, and a mildly elevated white blood cell count, usually with lymphocyte predominance. Using the India ink preparation, cryptococci can be visualized in about

50% of infected patients. The cerebrospinal fluid may be normal in some patients with early disease. The latex agglutination test detects cryptococcal antigen in the CSF of 90% and in the blood of 70% of patients. Controls are used to detect nonspecific rheumatoid factor in serum. Cross-reactions can occur with *Trichosporon beigelii* and *Capnocytophaga canimorsus*.

Disseminated Infection

Disseminated infection may involve the bone, skin, liver, eye, and prostate. Painless skin lesions are found in about 10% of patients with disseminated infection and are most often located on the face, neck, and scalp (51). The lesions may be papules, ulcerations, plaques, draining sinuses, or acneiform lesions. Cellulitis with necrotizing vasculitis has cooccurred in transplant recipients. Occasional patients have developed primary skin infections due to local inoculation of organisms. Uncommon forms of cryptococcosis include panniculitis, epididymoorchitis, breast masses, otitis, sinusitis, ophthalmitis, myocarditis, endocarditis, peritonitis, and arthritis.

Therapy

D-AMB has been considered the mainstay of therapy for cryptococcosis, but the dosage has been variable (52). It may be more effective when combined with flucytosine, but the latter drug is available only as an oral preparation and has myelosuppressive toxicity (see Tables 37-1 and 37-2). The optimal regimen would appear to be D-AMB 0.7 to 1.0 mg/kg/day plus flucytosine 100 mg/kg/day for 2 weeks followed by fluconazole 400 mg for 8 weeks. Lipid formulations may be substituted for D-AMB to avoid nephrotoxicity, but there has been some concern about their equivalent efficacy, and nephrotoxicity is not generally a problem for such short courses of therapy. Because of its potential myelotoxicity, flucytosine can be omitted in severely neutropenic patients, or the duration of its use can be shortened. Experience with fluconazole alone is limited, but it appears to be an effective alternative in cancer patients (53). Many patients with pneumonia and other noncerebral infections can be treated with fluconazole 400 mg daily; however, patients with fulminant pneumonia should probably be treated with D-AMB, as in meningoencephalitis.

Neurologic complications and mortality from cryptococcal meningitis are strongly associated with a CSF pressure of >200 mmH$_2$O (54). This requires aggressive management, either with daily drainage by lumbar puncture or ventricular shunts. Such measures should be taken promptly, because neurologic damage may be irreversible and late onset of treatment may be ineffective in preventing a poor outcome. Initial drainage should be sufficient to reduce the CSF pressure by 50%, and thereafter sufficient fluid should be removed daily to maintain a normal CSF pressure.

FUSARIOSIS

Fusarium spp. are found in the air and soil throughout the world and are common plant pathogens. Several *Fusarium* spp. have been recognized as human pathogens, including *F. solani, F. moniliforme, F. oxysporum,* and *F. dimerum.* Some species produce mycotoxins and, when ingested, cause gastrointestinal disease (55,56). Continued ingestion of the toxin leads to aplastic anemia and death (alimentary toxic aleukia). Since *Fusarium* spores are recovered from environmental air samples and most systemic infections involve the lungs or sinuses, the predominant site of origin is the respiratory tract (57). Chronic superficial infection of the skin or nails may be the sources of some systemic infections (58). Most systemic infections occur in severely immunocompromised patients, such as HSCT recipients and patients with acute leukemia (59,60). The most important risk factors for infection are severe neutropenia and high-dose adrenal corticosteroid therapy.

The first sign of infection may be persistent fever that is unresponsive to antibacterial therapy, but signs of organ infection soon become apparent. Some infections originate in the sinuses, producing circumorbital erythema, retroorbital pain, or headache. The infection can progress to endophthalmitis. Like *Aspergillus* spp., *Fusarium* spp. have a propensity for invading blood vessels, causing thrombosis and infarction. Pulmonary infection may present with symptoms suggesting an acute pulmonary embolism.

About 75% of infections occurring in neutropenic patients disseminate, and the organism can be isolated from blood culture specimens in about 70% of these individuals (57). Organs involved in disseminated fusariosis include the lungs, liver, kidney, spleen, and brain. Multiple skin lesions are common in patients with disseminated fusariosis (61). A variety of other skin lesions may be found at the same time, including red or gray macules, papules (some with central necrosis or an eschar), or pustules (Fig. 37-6). Some patients develop significant myalgias or painful subcutaneous lesions. Occasional patients with less severely compromised host defenses may develop only localized infections of the skin, such as paronychia, erythematous nodules, hemorrhagic bullae, or tender, progressive necrotic lesions at a site of prior trauma.

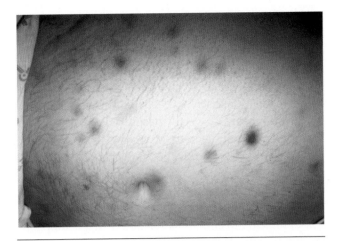

FIGURE 37-6 Skin lesions in a patient with disseminated fusariosis.

Therapy

The susceptibility of these fungi to antifungal agents in vitro has been variable; in one series, only 15% of isolates were susceptible to AMB (55,56). Some studies have shown that susceptibility to AMB depends on the species, whereas others have not shown this correlation. Some isolates are susceptible to new triazoles, such as voraconazole and posaconazole (62). At present, no antifungal agent is reliably effective, and most patients are treated with high doses ($\geq$5 mg/kg/day) of a lipid formulation of AMB. However, in neutropenic patients, recovery of neutrophil production is the most critical factor for a successful outcome (63).

TRICHOSPORONOSIS

Trichosporon asahi (beigelii) and *Blastochizomyces capitatus,* a related yeast, are widely distributed in air, soil, and decaying fruit. The majority of *Trichosporon* infections have been reported from the United States, whereas the majority of *Blastoschizomyces* infections have been reported from Europe (64,65). Infections occur predominantly in patients with acute leukemia and in HSCT recipients. These yeasts can cause endophthalmitis, meningitis, pneumonia, and osteomyelitis, but over 80% are disseminated (66,67). The organisms can be isolated from blood cultures of about 80% of patients with disseminated disease. The presenting symptoms of disseminated trichosporonosis depend on the predominant site of infection. Patients are usually acutely ill with fever and renal, cardiac, or pulmonary dysfunction. Renal involvement may be associated with azotemia, hematuria, proteinuria, and isolation of the organism from the urine. The lung is infected in up to 60% of patients with disseminated infection, and primary pneumonia may occur. These patients may have severe hypoxia but minimal abnormalities on chest roentgenography. The liver and spleen are frequently infected and a few patients have developed chronic infections similar to chronic disseminated candidiasis. About 30% of patients with disseminated infection develop skin lesions, which may begin as small maculopapular or nodular lesions that become necrotizing ulcerations.

Most *B. capitatus* infections are disseminated and occur in patients with acute leukemia. The liver is frequently infected, as is the CNS; the latter manifests as meningitis or brain abscess causing neurologic deficits. Disseminated infection is associated with maculopapular skin lesions in about 30% of cases.

A recent study indicated that 70% of *Trichosporon* infections were catheter-related fungemias without evidence of disseminated disease (68). Since fluconazole is active against *Trichosporon* spp., it is like that the widespread use of this drug for antifungal prophylaxis has prevented the development of disseminated infection.

Therapy

Fluconazole appears to be the most reliable therapeutic agent for trichosporonosis at present and to be more effective than AMB, based on both animal and human studies (69). There is limited clinical experience with voriconazole, but it may be the most effective agent currently available (70). Animal studies suggest that combination therapy with AMB plus an azole may represent optimal therapy for patients with disseminated infection (71). The mortality rate due to disseminated trichosporonosis has been reported to be as high as 80% in patients with disseminated infection who have persistent neutropenia despite antifungal therapy (65–68). Most patients with *B. capitatus* infections have been treated with D-AMB, so experience with azole therapy is limited (65).

ZYGOMYCOSIS

Zygomycosis is an infection caused by a variety of molds of the order Mucorales (72,73). Zygomycetes are widely distributed in the environment. Infection is usually acquired by inhalation of spores, but occasional cases are due to contamination of skin lesions or by ingestion of spores. Like *Aspergillus* spp., these fungi invade blood vessels, causing thrombosis and infarction. Macrophages and neutrophils are important host defenses against these infections. Patients susceptible to developing zygomycosis include those with acute leukemia, diabetic ketoacidosis, HSCT recipients, patients treated with adrenal corticosteroids, and those on he-

modialysis who are receiving deferoxamine. The presentations of zygomycosis are similar to those of aspergillosis, although infections caused by these fungi occur much less frequently. Types of infection are rhinocerebral, pulmonary, gastrointestinal, and cutaneous. Because of the similarities between aspergillosis and zygomycosis, they are not discussed in detail.

The mortality rate from these infections is high in patients with hematologic malignancies. The 3-month mortality was 71% in a study of cancer patients with definite or probable zygomycosis, and 75% of those who succumbed died within less than 4 weeks from the onset of their symptoms (74). The outcome of disseminated zygomycosis in patients with refractory neutropenia has been almost uniformly fatal despite aggressive antifungal therapy (75).

Therapy

For many years the only therapy available was D-AMB plus surgical excision (when possible). The ability to administer higher doses of the lipid formulations has made them the preferred treatment at present (76). Several new azoles, such as posaconazole, are undergoing investigation and may be more effective than existing therapies (77).

PATHOGENIC FUNGI

Acute infection caused by *Histoplasma capsulatum* or *Coccidioides immitis* usually presents as a severe pneumonia or disseminated infection in the severely immunocompromised cancer patient. Most of these infections occur in patients with hematologic malignancies, especially those with impaired cellular immunity. These patients are also susceptible to experiencing reactivation of latent infection acquired prior to the development of their malignancy.

Histoplasmosis

Most cases of histoplasmosis in patients with hematologic malignancies have been disseminated infections (78). Physical findings may include hepatosplenomegaly, mucocutaneous ulcerations (especially in the oral cavity), and signs of CNS involvement. The organism is visualized or cultured from infected tissues, respiratory secretions, and blood specimens. Therapeutic options include liposomal AMB (3 to 5 mg/kg/day) or intravenous itraconazole (200 mg twice daily for 2 days then 200 mg daily). Once the patient has improved substantially, oral itraconazole (200 mg daily) may be given. Therapy must be administered for 3 to 6 months.

Coccidiodomycosis

C. immitis may cause fulminant pneumonia in immuno-compromised hosts, with high fever, hypoxemia, and diffuse pulmonary infiltrates (78). Often these patients have disseminated infection that may involve the skin, bones, and meninges. Skin lesions may be papular, pustular, nodular, or ulcerative. While serologic tests are often positive, the fulminant nature of the infection usually requires a more aggressive diagnostic approach, with examination and culture of tissue specimens, sputum, or CSF. It is wisest to initiate therapy with D-AMB (0.7 to 1.0 mg/kg/day) plus fluconazole (400 to 800 mg/day) in most of these patients who have fulminant pneumonia, meningitis, or disseminated infection. Fluconazole (400 mg/day) or itraconazole (400 mg/day) should be continued for at least 1 year in most patients. Fluconazole (200–400 mg/day) should be continued for life in patients with chronic coccidial meningitis.

ADJUVANT THERAPY FOR FUNGAL INFECTIONS

White Blood Cell Transfusions

With the exception of superficial candidal infections, severely neutropenic patients seldom recover from fungal infections unless their neutropenia resolves. A variety of measures have been used to either provide neutrophils or expedite recovery. White blood cell (WBC) transfusions were introduced for neutropenic patients four decades ago (79). Although they have been shown to be effective in controlling experimental candidal infections in leukopenic dogs, their efficacy in patients has not been clearly demonstrated (80). A few clinical studies have suggested that they may be efficacious in fungal infections provided that adequate concentrations of neutrophils are transfused for an extended period, although the data are inconclusive (81). For many years, a major problem was the inability to collect sufficient numbers of neutrophils from normal donors. Recently, it has become possible to increase the collection of these cells by administering granulocyte colony-stimulating factor (G-CSF) to donors, which substantially increases the number of circulating neutrophils (82). This has been an effective adjuvant to antifungal therapy in some patients whose bone marrow recovers quickly; however, they are seldom effective in patients with prolonged neutropenia (primarily because there are insufficient donors available) or with advanced infection (83).

Cytokines

Colony-stimulating factors such as G-CSF (filgrastim) and granulocyte-macrophage colony-stimulating factor (GM-CSF) (sargramostim, molgramostim) reduce the severity and duration of neutropenia following intensive chemotherapy. GM-CSF is the most promising of these agents for use in fungal infections because it has effects on granulocyte production and function and macrophage function. There have been a few reports of the use of these agents as adjuncts to AMB therapy, but the data are insufficient to derive any conclusions (84). Proinflammatory cytokines have pleotrophic activating effects on effector immune cells, which may improve their function; these cytokines could therefore be useful adjunctive agents for the treatment of fungal infections (85). For example, gamma interferon enhances the ability of neutrophils and monocytes to cause hyphal damage to fungal pathogens (86). Further evaluations of cytokines are needed to define their role as adjunctive therapy.

■ VIRAL INFECTIONS

Some DNA viruses, such as herpes simplex, varicella, and cytomegalovirus, have been recognized for many years as causes of serious infections in patients with hematologic malignancies. The highly immunosuppressive regimens used for HSCT have created a population of recipients who are at risk for a variety of other serious viral infections, such as those due to adenoviruses, polyomavirus, and community respiratory viruses. Patients with other hematologic malignancies who receive intensive chemotherapeutic regimens are also at risk. Fortunately, rapid diagnostic techniques and effective therapies have become available that make it possible to manage some of these infections successfully.

HUMAN HERPESVIRUSES

Human herpesviruses are among the most common causes of viral infections in immunocompetent as well as in immunocompromised patients. Morbidity and mortality from these viruses are high among immunosuppressed patients. Herpesviruses are double-stranded DNA viruses. The herpesvirus group has eight members, six of which are important pathogens in immuno-suppressed patients (i.e., patients with hematologic malignancies and solid-organ or stem cell transplant recipients). This group of pathogens includes HSV 1 and 2, varicella zoster virus (VZV), cytomegalovirus (CMV), Epstein-Barr virus (EBV), and human herpesvirus 6 (HHV-6).

Herpesviruses establish a latent phase after primary infection. The reactivation of these DNA viruses can be triggered by several stimuli; this is perhaps best recognized in the recurrent blisters and ulcers associated with

HSV. The likelihood of reactivation of these viruses is increased during profound T-cell immunosuppression, as host defenses against these viruses are dependent on virus-specific helper and cytotoxic T lymphocytes. Over the past decade substantial improvements have been made in the techniques used to detect these infections, such as real-time PCR, as well as the development of effective antiviral agents and the use of different strategies for prophylaxis and treatment. Currently available drugs with activity against herpesviruses are acyclovir (with its prodrug valacyclovir), penciclovir (with the prodrug famciclovir), ganciclovir (GCV) (with its prodrug valganciclovir), cidofovir, and foscarnet. All these antiviral agents except foscarnet are nucleoside analogs that require phosphorylation by viral or cellular enzymes to become activated (Table 37-5).

HERPES SIMPLEX VIRUSES

Among the most common causes of mucocutaneous lesions in immunocompromised patients are HSV types 1 and 2 (87). Approximately 70 to 80% of seropositive patients undergoing induction chemotherapy for leukemia or conditioning for BMT will experience HSV reactivation, usually in early stages, when immunosuppression is most intense (88,89). HSV reactivation may cause severe disease during neutropenia. Oropharyngeal and esophageal disease is usually but not exclusively caused by HSV-1. The clinical manifestations of oropharyngeal HSV disease can range from gingivitis to stomatitis and cheilitis. HSV esophagitis may occur from local spread. Clinical presentation ranges from fever, malaise, myalgias, dysphagia, and bleeding to severe oral pain and odynophagia. Pneumonitis occurs rarely and requires a pulmonary biopsy for diagnosis. It

is acquired from aspiration of infected oropharyngeal secretions. HSV disease may progress and disseminate to the skin, gastrointestinal tract, liver (causing necrotizing hepatitis), and brain (causing meningoencephalitis). HSV-2 disease is more likely to cause genital and anal disease.

Diagnosis

The diagnosis of HSV infection can be made by isolating the virus in culture or by performing a biopsy showing the characteristic inclusions by immunohistochemistry. Direct detection methods of the virus in clinical specimens is generally not as sensitive as culture methods but offers the advantage of a rapid diagnosis. Direct or indirect immunofluorescence can be used to detect HSV-1, HSV-2, and VZV from specimens of cutaneous lesions.

Therapy

The available antiviral agents for the treatment of HSV disease include acyclovir, valacyclovir and famciclovir (see Table 37-5; Table 37-6). The bioavailability of oral valacyclovir and famciclovir is three to five times superior to that of oral acyclovir. All of these drugs are dependent on the virus-encoded thymidine kinase for their intracellular phosphorylation for activity.

Established HSV disease can be treated either orally or intravenously. The most commonly used drug is acyclovir. Immunosuppressed patients with disseminated or severe HSV disease should be treated with intravenous acyclovir (5 to 10 mg/kg every 8 h). Otherwise, an oral regimen can be used for milder HSV disease (famciclovir, 500 mg three times a day, or valacyclovir, 1 g three times a day).

TABLE 37-5	ANTIVIRAL COMPOUNDS		
Antiviral	*Dosage*	*Mechanism of Action*	*Active Against*
Acyclovir	5–10 mg/kg IV every 8 h	Inhibits DNA polymerase	HSV, VZV
Famciclovir	500 mg PO every 8 h	Inhibits DNA polymerase	HSV, VZV
Valacyclovir	0.5–1 g every 8–12 h	Inhibits DNA polymerase	HSV, VZV
Ganciclovir	5 mg/kg every 12 h	Inhibits DNA polymerase	CMV
Foscarnet	60 mg/kg IV every 8 h	Inhibits DNA polymerase	CMV, HSV, VZV
Cidofovir*	5 mg/kg IV once a week	Inhibits DNA polymerase	CMV, ADV, HSV, VZV
Ribavirin	PO or aerosolized	Inhibits viral replication	HCV, RSV
Oseltamivir	75 mg PO every 12 h	Neuraminidase inhibitor	Influenza A and B
Zanamivir	2 inhalations every 12 h	Neuraminidase inhibitor	Influenza A and B

* Licensed for CMV retinitis.
ADV = adenovirus; CMV = cytomegalovirus; HCV = hepatitis C virus; HSV = herpes simplex viruses; IV = intravenous; PO = oral; RSV = respiratory syncytial virus; VZV = varicella zoster virus.

TABLE 37-6	COMMON AND SERIOUS TOXICITIES OF ANTIVIRALS
Acyclovir	Transient renal insufficiency (IV), nausea, vomiting, agitation, confusion, TTP (rare)
Famciclovir	Headache, somnolence, nausea, diarrhea
Valacyclovir	Headache, nausea, vomiting, TTP (rare)
Ganciclovir	Anemia, neutropenia (more common), thrombocytopenia, fever, phlebitis, anorexia
Foscarnet	Nephrotoxicity (major toxicity), electrolyte disturbances (hypocalcemia, hypophosphatemia, hyperphosphatemia, hypomagnesemia, hypokalemia), diarrhea, nausea, vomiting
Cidofovir	Headache, rash, severe nephrotoxicity, metabolic acidosis, decreased intraocular pressure, neutropenia
Ribavirin	Fatigue, headache, nausea, rash, pruritus, conjunctivitis (inhalation, health-care workers administering ribavirin), hemolytic anemia (cardiac and pulmonary events have occurred), worsening respiratory status including death (inhalation)
Oseltamivir	Insomnia, vertigo, nausea, vomiting (most common), bronchitis
Zanamivir	Headache, nausea, diarrhea, cough, bronchospasm, decline in lung function (some fatal outcomes)

IV = intravenous; TTP = thrombotic thrombocytopenic purpura.

Prophylaxis

Antiviral prophylaxis should be strongly considered in HSV-seropositive patients at risk for reactivation as during intensive chemotherapy for acute leukemia and during early stages of HSCT (88,90). Finally, oral valacyclovir or famciclovir may be considered as alternative therapies for less serious manifestations of HSV disease.

VARICELLA ZOSTER VIRUS

VZV reactivation occurs primarily in elderly individuals, seropositive organ-transplant and HSCT recipients, patients with cancer, and those with AIDS. Disseminated VZV infection can be life-threatening in HSCT recipients and patients receiving intensive corticosteroid therapy.

VZV can be transmitted from person to person, and this can become problematic in a hospital or clinic setting. To prevent nosocomial transmission, immunocompromised patients with cutaneous lesions suspicious of VZV eruption and those with disseminated or dermatomal zoster should be placed under contact and respiratory isolation.

The clinical manifestations of VZV infection are primary varicella infection or chickenpox and herpes zoster. VZV infections are less common but usually more severe. The clinical presentation includes low-grade fever, malaise, and a vesicular rash that evolves to scabs. Constitutional symptoms usually develop after the onset of rash and include pruritus, anorexia, and listlessness. Primary VZV infection or chickenpox occurs mainly in children under 10 years of age. Children with acute leukemia who develop primary VZV infection are at particularly high risk for VZV pneumonia, which may occur in up to one-third of patients, with a mortality rate of about 10% (91).

Reactivation of latent VZV or herpes zoster is frequently observed among cancer patients, mainly patients with leukemia or lymphoma, as well as in HSCT recipients. Visceral herpes zoster may follow cutaneous dissemination in immunocompromised patients and can result in pneumonia, encephalitis, retinal necrosis, hepatitis, and small bowel disease. Cutaneous VZV eruption can be complicated by secondary bacterial infections, thrombocytopenia, and vasculitis (Fig. 37-7).

Diagnosis

The diagnosis of VZV reactivation in a single dermatomal distribution can usually be made on a clinical basis alone. On the other hand, immunocompromised patients usually develop multidermatomal or disseminated cutaneous disease, which can make the clinical diagnosis less certain on visual inspection alone. The diagnosis can be established within hours by the direct method of immunofluorescent staining on material collected from a skin lesion or from a skin biopsy. Viral

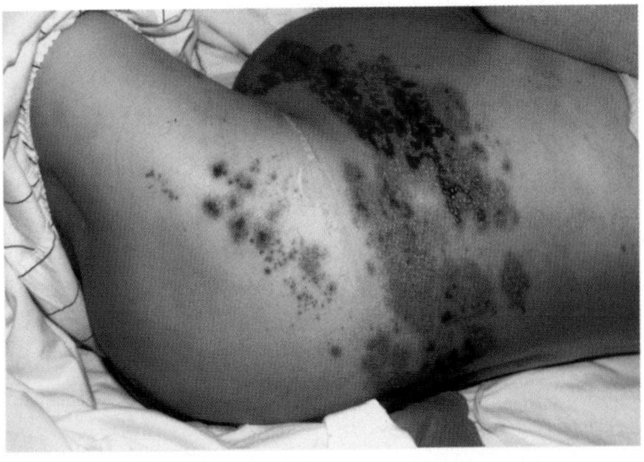

FIGURE 37-7 Hemorrhagic vesicular lesions of herpes zoster.

culture should also be performed. In some cases, a biopsy is required to establish the diagnosis, because other diseases can mimic VZV streptococcal impetigo and various noninfectious bullous diseases.

Therapy

The treatment of choice for chickenpox or VZV in immunocompromised patients is high-dose intravenous acyclovir (10 mg/kg every 8 h) (see Tables 37-5 and 37-6). Early initiation of acyclovir is paramount because it may reduce progression to end-organ disease and usually prevents death in patients with reactivated disease. Therapy can be changed to an oral agent once clinical improvement has occurred, such as resolution of fever or healing/crusting of lesions. The options for an oral regimen for treatment of localized herpes zoster among patients with mild immunosuppression include acyclovir, valacyclovir, and famciclovir (92).

Prevention of Infection

Immunosuppressed patients with negative VZV titers and no history of chickenpox should be offered varicella zoster immune globulin after being in close contact with individuals with either chickenpox or herpes zoster. Close contact includes prolonged face-to-face contact, a household or playmate contact, or exposure to a roommate in a shared hospital room. Varicella zoster immune globulin should be administered within 72 h of exposure to be most effective in preventing infection.

Active immunization with a live attenuated varicella vaccine using the live Oka strain (Merck) has been shown to be immunogenic, effective, and safe in children with leukemia (93,94). However, the American Academy of Pediatrics has warned about the use of the Oka vaccine in immunocompromised individuals except for children with acute lymphoblastic leukemia, to whom the vaccine may be administered (95). Immunocompromised persons should avoid contact with individuals who developed a rash after receiving varicella vaccine. No precaution is required if a rash has not developed.

CYTOMEGALOVIRUS

Cytomegalovirus (CMV) infection is commonly encountered in the recipients of solid-organ transplants and HSCT and may cause significant morbidity and mortality in these patients. Most of these cases represent reactivation of latent infection. Over the past decade, despite major advances in diagnosis, prophylaxis, and treatment of CMV, this viral infection remains a significant problem in immunocompromised patients. More-

over, CMV has an immunosuppressive effect that increases the risk for fungal and other opportunistic infections in immunocompromised patients. The development of preemptive therapy and prophylactic strategies decreased substantially the risk for development of CMV disease and especially pneumonia.

Primary CMV infection or its reactivation can range from asymptomatic viral shedding to a self-limited mononucleosis-like syndrome, to life-threatening end-organ disease. Signs and symptoms can range from fever, enlarged lymph nodes, splenomegaly, and lymphocytosis to hepatitis with increase liver enzymes, polyradiculopathy, and meningoencephalitis. CMV pneumonitis manifests as interstitial pulmonary disease resembling *Pneumocystis carinii* pneumonia; it may present with severe dyspnea (especially on exertion) and hypoxia and may progress to respiratory failure. Allogeneic HSCT recipients are at particular risk for CMV infection or disease. However, with the widespread use of prophylactic strategies and preemptive therapy against CMV, the number of seropositive patients developing CMV disease has decreased in frequency by half. In a seronegative recipient, CMV may be transmitted from the bone marrow allograft obtained from a seropositive donor or from infected blood products. Patients develop CMV disease mainly in the postengraftment period, between days 30 and 100 following transplantation. However, patients with graft-versus-host disease (GVHD) requiring intensive immunosuppressive therapy are at increased risk for CMV disease even after day 100 (96). The most common sites of CMV infection in the gastrointestinal tract are the esophagus and colon. CMV esophagitis is associated with pain and dysphagia. On upper gastrointestinal endoscopy, ulcerations can be seen in the esophagus and a biopsy must be obtained to rule out other infectious etiologies, such as HSV or candidal esophagitis. The hallmarks of CMV colitis are abdominal pain and diarrhea. A biopsy of the colon is necessary to diagnose this infection. CMV can also infect the liver, causing hepatitis with fever and elevations of liver enzymes.

Diagnosis

Several virologic and molecular detection methods are available for the diagnosis of CMV infection. Determination of antibodies against CMV is mainly used for screening for past infection or exposure. It is also used for donor selection, since CMV can be transmitted by blood, organ, and/or bone marrow donation. There are some limitations of serology in diagnosing primary CMV infection. Rheumatoid factor, antinuclear antibodies, and other cross-reactive factors can produce false-positive IgM antibody results. Moreover, persistence of IgM antibodies may occur in some patients with past CMV infection. Viral inclusions can be identified in biopsy samples of CMV-infected cells (liver, lungs) or, more efficiently, by immunohistochemistry (Fig. 37-8). In situ PCR or nucleic acid hybridization are also useful diagnostic tools.

The most commonly used assays for detection and quantitation of CMV load in blood include tests for antigenemia, DNA-emia, and mRNA-emia. The recent availability of molecular methods allows more rapid diagnosis and provides an important role in management of CMV infection.

Antigenemia assay by immunofluorescence consists of quantitation of leukocyte nuclei positive for CMV pp65 (lower matrix phosphoprotein) in a cytospin preparation of 2×10^5 peripheral blood leukocytes (97). This is a rapid assay and the result can be made available within a few hours. Although the correlation between high and low levels of antigen is not absolute in patients with CMV disease and asymptomatic infections, respectively, the test for antigenemia is known to be sensitive enough for monitoring infection and antiviral treatment in immunocompromised patients. On the other hand, this assay is semiquantitative and labor-intensive, and specimens must be processed within 6 h. Furthermore, the sensitivity of this assay is limited by the availability of sufficient numbers of WBCs.

Qualitative or quantitative PCR detects CMV DNA in clinical samples. One of the advantages of these PCR techniques is that they can detect a relatively stable double-stranded DNA present in the plasma or whole blood regardless of storage conditions or cell integrity. The drawback of the qualitative PCR assay is the lack of determination of viral load, which is useful for follow-up on therapy and for prognosis. Hence, the quantitative PCR assay is more useful clinically (98,99). Real-time quantitative PCR is a recently developed method. It holds promise for the rapid diagnosis of different pathogens. This technology, unlike traditional PCR, is completed in less than an hour. Many studies have demonstrated a good correlation between CMV DNA quantification in blood and pp65 antigenemia assay.

Newer methods have also been developed to detect RNA in blood, which may represent active CMV replication and disease. One promising technique, the nucleic acid sequence-based amplification (NASBA), has been studied for monitoring CMV infection in transplant recipients. Late pp67 CMV-specific mRNA can be detected by NASBA assay and should be indicative of replicating virus. Late CMV pp67 assay was found to be highly specific in a few studies (100,101). Its role in screening or diagnosing patients at risk for CMV infection is yet to be determined.

Therapy

Antiviral agents are used to treat or prevent CMV infection in immunocompromised patients (see Tables 37-5 and 37-6). In these patients, different strategies are currently employed to manage CMV infection and disease and also for prophylaxis, preemptive therapy, and treatment of an established disease. The nucleoside analog GCV and the pyrophosphate analog foscarnet have been used for the treatment or prophylaxis of CMV infection and disease in immunocompromised patients. The new nucleotide analog cidofovir has recently been approved for therapy of CMV retinitis in HIV patients. Its role in treatment or prophylaxis of CMV in immunocompromised patients is limited because of its major side effect, which is nephrotoxicity. GCV is a competitive inhibitor of viral DNA polymerase, and its antiviral activity requires monophosphorylation in the infected cell followed by diphosphorylation by cellular kinases. Intravenous GCV is considered the primary drug for the treatment of CMV infections (102). Its major side effect is myelosuppression; therefore periodic monitoring of blood counts is necessary during treatment. An oral formulation, valganciclovir, is a prodrug of GCV and is significantly better absorbed from the gastrointestinal tract than GCV in capsule form. Valganciclovir is useful for the treatment of CMV retinitis. Side effects are similar to those of intravenous GCV.

Foscarnet is a noncompetitive inhibitor of the pyrophosphate-binding site of CMV DNA polymerase, which

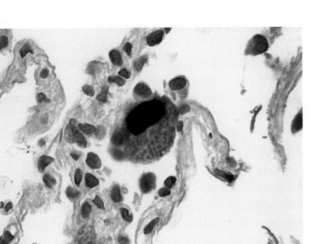

FIGURE 37-8 Typical cytomegalovirus inclusions in the lung parenchyma of a lymphoma patient with pneumonia.

does not require prior activation by a virally encoded enzyme. It is usually used as an alternative to GCV in patients whose infection is resistant to GCV or to avoid the side effects of GCV. Furthermore, foscarnet may have an advantage over GCV in patients with delayed engraftment or with GCV-associated neutropenia; it may also be used as a first-line antiviral in these instances. Its major side effects include nephrotoxicity, azotemia, and electrolyte abnormalities.

Cidofovir is a competitive inhibitor of the CMV DNA polymerase and can be used for the treatment of CMV retinitis. It has a long intracellular half-life, which makes once-weekly administration possible (103). High doses of probenecid and saline hydration are recommended with cidofovir to reduce the risk of nephrotoxicity. Cross-resistance with GCV is possible, since both antivirals share the same target; however, cidofovir remains effective against most foscarnet-resistant isolates of CMV studied in vitro.

HUMAN HERPESVIRUS 6

Human herpesvirus 6 is a beta herpesvirus with two variant groups (A and B). Primary infection with HHV-6 is very common in children. Exanthem subitum, the most common cause of fever and hospitalization of infants less than 1 year of age, is caused by HHV-6 subtype B. In addition to fever, children present with mild upper respiratory symptoms and a classic diffuse maculopapular exanthem. It is unclear whether HHV-6 subtype A causes any primary infection. In immunosuppressed individuals, typically AIDS patients and transplant recipients, HHV-6 may cause opportunistic viral infections. As this infection is very common early in life, positive titers are found in more than 95% of adults. In immunosuppressed individuals, especially HSCT recipients, this virus occasionally has caused interstitial pneumonia, encephalitis, hepatitis, and bone marrow suppression.

Therapy

Both ganciclovir and foscarnet should be effective therapy for HHV-6 infections, but this is based upon in vitro studies only, since clinical experience is minimal. Both ganciclovir and foscarnet have been reported to be effective against HHV-6 meningoencephalitis after HSCT in a small number of patients (104). Also, an epidemiologic study showed lower HHV-6 DNA levels in patients who received high-dose acyclovir, and these patients were less likely to experience delayed marrow engraftment (105).

EPSTEIN-BARR VIRUS

Epstein-Barr virus (EBV) infection is very common in the adult population. EBV is the cause of infectious mononucleosis and has also been linked to several geographically defined cancers. EBV-associated posttransplant lymphoproliferative disorder (PTLD) is an important cause of morbidity and mortality in HSCT and solid-organ transplant recipients. Although this EBV-related complication posttransplant is not common (< 1% after allogeneic HSCT), it can be fulminant and lethal. The disease is essentially the result of suppression of cytotoxic T-cell function. The first step in the management of PTLD is to reduce the dose of any immunosuppressive therapy if possible. Most of the antiherpesvirus drugs have antiviral effects in vitro against EBV. In HSCT recipients, no data are currently available concerning clinical efficacy of these antivirals against EBV. During the last few years, a new therapeutic approach using the anti-CD20 monoclonal antibody or rituximab has been tested for therapy of EBV-induced PTLD. It has been successful for the treatment or prevention of PTLD in solid-organ–transplant and HSCT-recipients as well as those with proven EBV lymphomas (106,107).

HEPATITIS VIRUSES

Hepatitis B

Hepatitis B (HBV) and C (HCV) infections are common in many countries. There is a global epidemic of HBV infections affecting more than 350 million people worldwide. Chronic HBV or HCV infections lead to progressive liver disease, cirrhosis, and hepatocellular cancer. The majority of HBV and HCV infections occur in individuals who use illegal drugs and/or engage in high-risk sexual behaviors. Hepatitis can be a serious problem in cancer patients for various reasons. Chemotherapy-induced immunosuppression may lead to reactivation and fulminant infection in patients with chronic HBV infection. Furthermore, the presence of hepatitis may require substantial delays in the administration of antineoplastic therapy.

Therapy

Although clinical experience is limited, lamivudine may potentially suppress HBV reactivation secondary to chemotherapy in patients with chronic HBV infection (positive HBV DNA and/or positive HBs Ag). It may also be beneficial for preventing reactivation in patients who have recovered from prior infection (positive hepatitis B core antibody with or without HBs Ab). Determining screening markers of chronic HBV infection or past exposure is important in immunosuppressed patients for determining the need for treatment of chronic infection or prophylaxis against acute reactivation (108, 109). Interferon alpha, lamivudine, and adefovir are antiviral agents with efficacy against HBV that can be used for prevention or treatment of HBV infection in seropositive patients undergoing chemotherapy for cancer or in HSCT recipients. Additional studies are needed to assess the usefulness of these agents to prevent HBV-associated complications in HSCT recipients. Preexposure vaccination of persons at risk using recombinant HBV vaccines offers protection against HBV infection. Postexposure prophylaxis includes the administration of HBV vaccine and HBV immunoglobulins.

Hepatitis C

Hepatitis C is the most common chronic blood-borne infection. In the United States, 4 million individuals (1.8% of the population) have been infected. It is the leading indication for liver transplantation, and about 8000 to 10,000 deaths occur per year. HCV transmission occurs primarily through exposure to infected blood. It can be acquired from intravenous drug abuse, blood transfusion before 1992, solid-organ transplantation from infected donors, unsafe medical practices, occupational exposure to infected blood, birth to an infected mother, sexual contact with an infected person, and possibly via intranasal cocaine use.

Several studies suggest an association between HCV infection and several B-cell lymphoproliferative disorders. Furthermore, epidemiologic studies from Italy, Japan, and California found a high prevalence of HCV among patients with non-Hodgkin's lymphoma (110, 111). Treatment of these lymphomas with chemotherapy can be complicated by viral reactivation and immune reconstitution hepatitis, which is more commonly encountered in cases of infection with HBV. In high-prevalence areas, screening for the virus should be performed when lymphoma is diagnosed. The combination of pegylated interferon alpha plus ribavirin produces sustained virologic responses in HCV infection in approximately 50% of genotype 1 infections and 80% of other genotypes. At present, no active or passive immunizations are available for HCV.

■ COMMUNITY RESPIRATORY VIRAL INFECTIONS

Infections caused by community respiratory viruses (CRV) were not considered to be a significant problem for cancer patients until the early 1990s. Since then it has been recognized that they represent a threat to patients undergoing chemotherapy for acute leukemia and to HSCT recipients, especially recipients of allogeneic transplants. Early surveys indicated that about 30% of respiratory illnesses occurring during the winter and spring among these patient populations were due to CRVs. Recent studies have reported CRVs as the cause of as few as 5% to as many as 48% of respiratory infections (112–114). Although many patients acquire only upper respiratory infections (URIs), some develop pneumonias, which may be fatal. Many of these pneumonias may be due to bacterial or fungal pathogens and not to the virus. For example, it has been recognized for many years that influenza can predispose to bacterial pneumonia. Epidemics of CRV have occurred on leukemia and transplant units, where the virus may be transmitted by patients, visitors, and hospital personnel. Clinics may serve as in important starting point for epidemics. Also, epidemics may occur among these susceptible patients in the absence of a recognized epidemic in the community. An additional problem is that these immunocompromised patients may have very prolonged viral shedding (in some cases >100 days) after resolution of symptoms (115).

The most commonly reported viruses causing infection are influenza A and B (predominantly influenza A), respiratory syncytial virus (RSV), and parainfluenza virus (almost entirely type 3). Rhinoviruses are the most common cause of community respiratory illnesses but are identified infrequently in most surveys of cancer patients, suggesting that they are underdiagnosed. It is uncertain whether these viruses can cause pneumonia. Influenza, RSV, and parainfluenza types 1 and 2 occur during the winter and spring, whereas parainfluenza 3 infection occurs throughout the year. Some patients may be infected by multiple viruses simultaneously or have multiple episodes of the same viral infection separated by only a few weeks. There is considerable variability in the relative frequency of the three major viruses in different geographical areas and in different years, most likely reflecting the relative prevalence of the infections within the community.

PREDISPOSING FACTORS

Several important predisposing factors for these infections have been identified in HSCT recipients and patients with hematologic malignancies. These include age >65 years, severe neutropenia, severe lymphopenia, allogeneic transplantation, transplant conditioning regimen, graft-versus-host disease (GVHD), and adrenal corticosteroid therapy. HSCT recipients are at greatest risk within the first 100 days posttransplant. Some of these predisposing factors are interrelated. For example, adrenal corticosteroids are used for therapy of GVHD.

The usual symptoms are the same as in normal hosts: cough, fever rhinorrhea, and sore throat. Some patients develop sinusitis or otitis media. Patients with pneumonia present with dyspnea and wheezing; they have rales on auscultation of the chest and hypoxemia. Chest roentogenography reveals diffuse interstial infiltrates with or without alveolar infiltrates.

PNEUMONIA

There is great variability in the frequency of pneumonia in different studies, ranging from 15 to over 70%, but most surveys have reported only small patient populations. In most series, pneumonia has occurred with equal frequency among the three predominant viruses, and it has occurred with approximately equal frequency among HSCT recipients and leukemic patients. Important predisposing factors for pneumonia include severe lymphopenia, adrenal corticosteroid therapy, allogeneic transplantation, and other concomitant infection (116, 117). Fatality rates from pneumonia vary widely in different reports, but most include only small numbers of cases. Fatality rates appear to be similar for the three viruses and are higher among leukemic patients than HSCT recipients. The same factors that predispose for pneumonia also predispose for death. Deaths have not been reported due only to URIs.

Diagnosis

The diagnosis of CRV infection is established from nasopharyngeal wash, sputum, or BAL specimens. Rapid antigen detection tests are available for influenza and RSV, whereas tissue cell cultures are used for detecting parainfluenza and rhinoviruses.

Therapy

Therapy for these infections has been limited (see Tables 37-5 and 37-6). At present, there is no demonstrably effective therapy for parainfluenza infection. Until recently, only amantidine and rimantidine were available for influenza, and they had activity only against influenza A. Experience with these agents was limited, but these drugs did not have a substantial effect on the mortality rate. Therapy was more effective if administered before the onset of symptoms of respiratory failure (116). Viral resistance to these agents developed in some patients during therapy. Recently oseltamivir has become available and has been found to have activity against both the A and B types of influenza. Among high-risk patients, administration of oseltamivir during the URI reduces the risk of progression to pneumonia, and our recent experience with HSCT recipients and leukemia patients is similar (118). There is insufficient evidence of its efficacy once pneumonia has occurred due to small numbers of cases reported.

Ribavirin is available for the therapy of RSV infection, but there is only limited experience in treating pneumonia in cancer patients (Fig. 37-9). Ribavirin is administered by aerosolization continuously for 18 h daily, requiring the patient to be confined in a tent. A few patients have been treated successfully with a higher dose administered over 2 h at 8-h intervals, but this cannot be recommended for routine practice at present. Most often ribavirin is combined with some type of immunoglobulin therapy. Initially, intravenous gamma globulin was used and then, more recently, preparations with high titers of RSV-neutralizing antibody. Palivizumab, a humanized monoclonal antibody directed against the F glycoprotein of RSV has become available. Most patients are being treated with combination therapy, but the limited numbers of patients reported make interpretation of results difficult. However, there is evidence that routine therapy of these immunocompromised patients with URIs significantly reduces the occurrence of pneumonia, which has been confirmed by recent extensive experience at our institution (119).

ADENOVIRUS

Adenoviruses are a common cause of self-limited respiratory and gastrointestinal infections in normal individuals. Transmission occurs by aerosolized droplets or the oral-fecal route. Adenovirus infections have been recognized in patients undergoing intensive chemotherapy for hematologic and occasionally other malignancies, but they are especially prevalent among HSCT recipients. The frequency of infection among HSCT recipients has varied from 3 to 21%, and it is more prevalent among children than adults (120,121). There is no seasonal variation, and the onset of infection from time of transplantation can be quite variable, although the median interval is about 50 days. The virus may persist for prolonged periods in normal individuals; hence, some infections in cancer patients represent reactivation.

Important risk factors have been identified for adenovirus infection, including childhood, allogeneic transplantation, GVHD, total-body irradiation (in children), T-cell depleting conditioning regimens, adrenal corticosteroid therapy, and lymphopenia (120,122). Use of antibody-positive donors may also be a predisposing factor for infection. About 50% of adenoviral infections occur in patients with other concomitant infections.

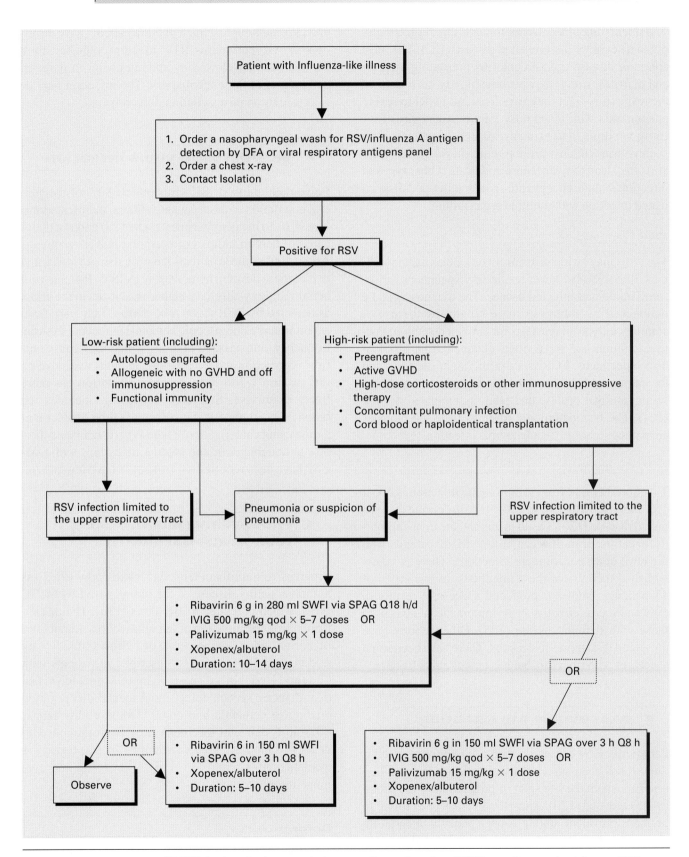

FIGURE 37-9 Management of RSV infection after hematopoietic stem cell transplantation. GVHD = graft-versus-host disease; RSV = respiratory syncytial virus.

Patients may have asymptomatic infection, single-organ disease, or disseminated disease (123). The most common disease is gastroenteritis presenting as fever and diarrhea, which may become bloody. Infections of the respiratory tract may vary from mild URI to severe pneumonitis with respiratory failure. Adenovirus may cause nephritis, and as many as 50% of patients with positive urine cultures develop hemorrhagic cystitis. Hepatitis may lead to liver failure and death. Other types of infection include encephalitis, pancreatitis, and disseminated infection with multiple organ failure.

Diagnosis

The virus may be identified from nasopharyngeal washings, throat swabs, lower respiratory specimens, urine, stool, blood and infected tissues. The diagnosis can be established by culture or more rapidly by the use of commercially available tests for antigen detection. Positive cultures are most often obtained from stool or urine specimens. PCR is a useful diagnostic tool, and the amount of DNA load detected can discriminate between nonfatal disease and fatal disseminated disease (124). The histopathologic findings in tissue biopsies are pathognomonic for adenovirus infection.

Outcome

The mortality rate from symptomatic infection is about 25%, but it is 60 to 75% in patients with definite disseminated disease (120). Death is mainly due to pneumonitis, hepatitis, or multiorgan failure. Many patients who die have other concomitant infections. There is no established therapy for these infections. In one series of 45 patients, cidofovir produced successful results in 69% and was as effective in asymptomatic patients as in those with definite disease (125). Other reports have presented less impressive results. There have been some successes with ribavirin, but it is not reliably effective.

■ PARVOVIRUS B19 INFECTION

Parvovirus B19 causes erythema infectiosum in children. It has been associated with aplastic crises in diseases in which the life span or production of red blood cells is reduced (126). Anti-B19 IgG has been found to be more prevalent among cancer patients undergoing chemotherapy than among the general population. In this study, 63% of the seropositive cancer patients had unexplained anemia (127). Prolonged erythroid aplasia in childhood acute lymphocytic leukemia was associated with detection B19 DNA in the bone marrow. Several chronic lymphocytic leukemia patients have developed severe parvovirus B19 infection, manifest by a flu-like illness followed by anemia owing to pure red cell aplasia in the bone marrow. The infection may be followed by an incapacitating polyarthritis.

■ BK (POLYOMA) VIRUS INFECTION

Polyoma hominis or BK virus infects 80% of the general population without causing clinical manifestations. It persists in the genitourinary tract (128) and is a major cause of hemorrhagic cystitis among HSCT recipients. About 50% of these patients have persistent viruria, and half of these develop hemorrhagic cystitis. Patients with hemorrhagic cystitis have higher viral loads in the urine, as detected by PCR (129). The disease may vary from asymptomatic microscopic hematuria to severe dysuria, frequency, and passage of clots, which may cause outflow obstruction and renal failure. Patients who develop this disease >100 days posttransplantation are more likely to survive. Symptomatic therapy includes red blood cell and platelet transfusions, saline bladder irrigations, and cauterization. There is no established therapy, although cidofir and bladder irrigations with GM-CSF have been reported to be of benefit in a few cases.

■ PROGRESSIVE MULTIFOCAL LEUKOENCEPHALOPATHY

Progressive multifocal leukoencephalopathy (PML) is a demyelinating disease of the brain caused by the JC virus, which is related to BK virus (130). The disease results from reactivation of latent infection. About 80% of normal adults demonstrate JC virus antibodies by middle age. PML was first described in patients with CLL and Hodgkin's disease. Symptoms include visual disturbances, speech defects, and mental deterioration leading to dementia and coma. The mortality rate is 80% at 1 year and the mean time from diagnosis to death is 4 months. No consistently effective therapy is available, but arabinosyl cytosine may bring improvement in some patients.

References

1. Bodey GP, Wertlake PT, Douglas G, et al. Cytomegalic inclusion disease in patients with acute leukemia. *Ann Intern Med* 1965;62:899–906.
2. Bodey GP. Fungal infections complicating acute leukemia. *J Chronic Dis* 1966;19:667–687.

3. Lehrer RI, Cline MJ. Leukocyte candidacidal activity and resistance to systemic candidiasis in patients with cancer. *Cancer* 1971;27:1211–1217.

4. Schaffner A, Douglas H, Braude A. Selective protection against *Conidia* by mononuclear and against *Mycelia* by polymorphonuclear phagocytes in resistance to *Aspergillus. J Clin Invest* 1982;69:617–619.

5. Raad II, Hanna H, Boktour M, et al. Management of central venous catheters in patients with candidemia. *Clin Infect Dis* 2004;38(8):1119–1127.

6. Allo MD, Miller J, Townsend T, et al. Primary cutaneous aspergillosis associated with Hickman intravenous catheters. *N Engl J Med* 1987;371:1105–1108.

7. Wingard JR, Merz WG, Rinaldi MG, et al. Increase in *Candida krusei* infection among patients with bone marrow transplantation and neutropenia treated prophylactically with fluconazole. *N Engl J Med* 1991;325:1274–1277.

8. Wingard JR. Importance of *Candida* species other than *C. albicans* as pathogens in oncology patients. *Clin Infect Dis* 1995;20:115–125.

9. Bodey GP. Hematogenous and major organ candidiasis. In: Bodey GP (ed): *Candidiasis: Pathogenesis, Diagnosis, and Treatment,* 2d ed. New York: Raven Press; 1993:279–329.

10. Girmenia C, Martino P, De Bernardis F, et al. Rising incidence of *Candida parapsilosis* fungemia in patients with hematologic malignancies: Clinical aspects predisposing factors, and differential pathogenicity of the causative strains. *Clin Infect Dis* 1996;23:506–514.

11. Roseff SA, Sugar AM. Oral and esophageal candidiasis. In: Bodey GP (ed): *Candidiasis: Pathogenesis, Diagnosis, and Treatment,* 2d ed. New York: Raven Press; 1993:185–203.

12. Villanueva A, Gotuzzo E, Arathoon EG, et al. A randomized double-blind study of caspofungin versus fluconazole for the treatment of esophageal candidiasis. *Am J Med* 2002;113:294–299.

13. Kauffman CA. Candiduria: Diagnostic and treatment conundrums. *Curr Treat Options Infect Dis* 2002;4:513–519.

14. Moyer DV, Edwards JE Jr. *Candida* endophthalmitis and central nervous system infection. In: Bodey GP (ed): *Candidiasis: Pathogenesis, Diagnosis, and Treatment,* 2d ed. New York: Raven Press; 1993:331–355.

15. Bodey GP, Luna M. Skin lesions associated with disseminated candidiasis. *JAMA* 1974;229:1466–1468.

16. Maksymiuk AW, Thongprasert S, Hopfer R, et al. Systemic candidiasis in cancer patients. *Am J Med* 1984;77:20–27.

17. Kontoyiannis DP, Luna MA, Samuels BI, et al. Hepatosplenic candidiasis: A manifestation of chronic disseminated candidiasis. *Infect Dis Clin North Am* 2000;14:721–739.

18. Haron E, Vartivarian S, Anaissie E, et al. Primary *Candida* pneumonia—Experience at a large cancer center and review of the literature. *Medicine* 1993;72:137–142.

19. Kontoyiannis DP, Reddy BT, Torres HA, et al. Pulmonary candidiasis in patients with cancer: An autopsy study. *Clin Infect Dis* 2002;34:400–403.

20. Bodey GP. Fungal infections in immunocompromised patients—Candidiasis (Part 1). *Infect Dis Rev* 1999;1:4–8.

21. Rex JH, Pappas PG, Karchmer AW, et al. A randomized and blinded multicenter trial of high-dose fluconazole plus placebo versus fluconazole plus amphotericin B as therapy for candidemia and its consequences in nonneutropenic patients. *Clin Infect Dis* 2003;36:1221–1228.

22. Mora-Duarte J, Betts R, Rotstein C, et al. Comparison of caspofungin and amphotericin B for invasive candidiasis. *N Engl J Med* 2002;347:2020–2029.

23. Kuhn DM, George J, Chandra PK, et al. Antifungal susceptibility of *Candida* biofilms: Unique efficacy of amphotericin B lipid formulations and echinocandins. *Antimicrob Agents Chemother* 2002;46:1773–1780.

24. Patterson TF, Kirkpatrick WR, White M, et al. Invasive aspergillosis: Disease spectrum, treatment practices, and outcomes. *Medicine* 2000;79:250–260.

25. Denning DW. Invasive aspergillosis. *Clin Infect Dis* 1998;26:781–803; quiz 804–805.

26. Bodey GP, Vartivarian S. Aspergillosis. *Eur J Clin Microbiol Infect Dis* 1989;8:413–437.

27. Libschitz HI, Pagoni J. Aspergillosis and mucormycosis: Two types of opportunistic fungal pneumonia. *Radiology* 1981;140:303–306.

28. Caillot D, Casasnovas O, Bernard A, et al. Improved management of invasive pulmonary aspergillosis in neutropenic patients using early thoracic computed tomographic scan and surgery. *J Clin Oncol* 1997;15:139–147.

29. Myoken Y, Sugata T, Kyo T-I, Fujihara M. Pathologic features of invasive oral aspergillosis in patients with hematologic malignancies. *J Oral Maxillofac Surg* 1996;54:263–270.

30. Pagano L, Ricci P, Montillo M, et al. Localization of aspergillosis to the central nervous system among patients with acute leukemia: Report of 14 cases. *Clin Infect Dis* 1996;23:628–630.

31. Kontoyiannis DP, Bodey GP. Aspergillosis in 2002: An update. *Eur J Clin Microbiol Infect Dis* 2002;21:161–172.

32. Kontoyiannis DP, Sumoza D, Tarrand J, et al. Significance of aspergillemia in patients with cancer. A 10 year study. *Clin Infect Dis* 2000;31:188–189.

33. Tarrand JT, Lichterfeld M, Warraich I, et al. Diagnosis of invasive septate mold infections: A correlation of microbiological culture and histologic or cytologic examination. *Am J Clin Pathol* 2003;119:854–858.

34. Erjavec Z, Verweij PE. Recent progress in the diagnosis of fungal infections in the immunocompromised host. *Drug Res Updates* 2002;5:3–10.

35. Bretagne S, Marmorat-Khuong A, Kuentz M, et al. Serum *Aspergillus galactomannan* antigen testing by sandwich ELISA: Practical use in neutropenic patients. *J Infect* 1997;35:7–15.

36. Miyazaki T, Kohno S, Mitsutake K, et al. (1–:3)-beta-D-glucan in culture fluid of fungi activates factor G, a limulus coagulation factor. *J Clin Lab Anal* 1995;9:334–339.

37. Maertens J, Verhaegen J, Lagrou K, et al. Screening for circulating galactomannan as a noninvasive diagnostic tool for invasive aspergillosis in prolonged neutropenic patients and stem cell transplantation recipients: A prospective validation. *Blood* 2001;97:1604–1610.

38. Ascioglu S, Rex JH, de Pauw B, et al. Defining opportunistic invasive fungal infections in immunocompromised patients with cancer and hematopoietic stem cell transplants: An international consensus. *Clin Infect Dis* 2002;34:7–14.

39. Arikan S, Rex JH. Lipid-based antifungal agents: Current status. *Curr Pharm Design* 2001;7:393–415.

40. Wingard JR. Lipid formulations of amphotericins: Are you a lumper or a splitter? *Clin Infect Dis* 2002;35:891–895.

41. Kreisel W. Therapy of invasive aspergillosis with itraconazole: Our own experience and review of the literature. *Mycoses* 1994;37(suppl 2):42–51.

42. Caillot D, Bassaris H, McGeer A, et al. Intravenous itraconazole followed by oral itraconazole in the treatment of invasive pulmonary aspergillosis in patients with hematologic malignancies, chronic granulomatous disease, or AIDS. *Clin Infect Dis* 2001;33:83–90.

43. Herbrecht R, Denning DW, Patterson TF, et al. Voriconazole versus amphotericin B for primary therapy of invasive aspergillosis. *N Engl J Med* 2002;347:408–415.

44. Keating G, Figgitt D. Caspofungin: A review of its use in oesophageal candidiasis, invasive candidiasis and invasive aspergillosis. *Drugs* 2003;63:2235–2263.

45. Lewis RE, Kontoyiannis DP. Combination chemotherapy for invasive fungal infections: What laboratory and clinical studies tell us so far. *Drug Resist Update* 2003;6:257–269.

46. Patterson PJ, Johnson EM, Ainscough S, et al. Treatment failure in invasive aspergillosis due to poor tissue penetration by antifungal agents. Abstract presented at the 41st Interscience Conference on Antimicrobial Agents and Chemotherapy, Toronto, Canada. 2000;133:1328 (abstr J 376).

47. Pagano L, Ricci P, Nosari A, et al. Fatal haemoptysis in pulmonary filamentous mycosis: An underevaluated cause of death in patients with acute leukaemia in haematological complete remission. A retrospective study and review of the literature. *Br J Haematol* 1995;89:500–505.

48. Salerno CT, Ouyang DW, Pederson TS, et al. Surgical therapy for pulmonary aspergillosis in immunocompromised patients. *Ann Thorac Surg* 1998;65:1415–1419.

49. Yeghen T, Kibbler CC, Prentice HG, et al. Management of invasive pulmonary aspergillosis in hematology patients: A review of 87 consecutive cases at a single institution. *Clin Infect Dis* 2000;31:859–868.

50. Powell KE, Dahl BA, Weeks, RJ, et al. Airborne *Cryptococcus neoformans*: Particles from pigeon excreta compatible with alveolar deposition. *J Infect Dis* 1972;125:412–415.

51. Pappas PG, Perfect JR, Cloud GA, et al. Cryptococcosis in human immunodeficiency virus–negative patients in the era of effective azole therapy. *Clin Infect Dis* 2001;33:690–699.

52. Gupta SK, Sarosi GA. Cryptococcal meningitis. *Curr Treat Options Infect Dis* 2002;4:503–511.

53. Kontoyiannis DP, Peitsch WK, Reddy BT, et al. Cryptococcosis in patients with cancer. *Clin Infect Dis* 2001;32:145–150.

54. Graybill JR, Sobel J, Saag M, et al. Diagnosis and management of increased intracranial pressure in patients with AIDS and cryptococcal meningitis. *Clin Infect Dis* 2000;30:47–54.

55. Nelson PE, Dignani MC, Anaissie EJ. Taxonomy, biology, and clinical aspects of *Fusarium* species. *Clin Microbiol Rev* 1994;7:479–504.

56. Torres H, Kontoyiannis DP. In: Dismukes W, Pappas P, Sobel J (eds): *Hyalohyphomycoses. Oxford Textbook of Clinical Mycology*. New York: Oxford University Press; 2003:252–270.

57. Boutati EI, Anaissie EJ. *Fusarium*, a significant emerging pathogen in patients with hematologic malignancy: Ten years' experience at a cancer center and implications for management. *Blood* 1997;90:999–1008.

58. Girmenia C, Arcese W, Micozzi A, et al. Onychomycosis as a possible origin of disseminated *Fusarium solani* infection in a patient with severe aplastic anemia. *Clin Infect Dis* 1992; 14:1167.

59. Girmenia C, Pagano L, Corvatta L, et al. The epidemiology of fusariosis in patients with haematological diseases. Gimema Infection Programme. *Br J Haematol* 2000;111:272–276.

60. Musa MO, Al Eisa A, Halim M, et al. The spectrum of *Fusarium* infection in immunocompromised patients with haematological malignancies and in non-immunocompromised patients: A single institution experience over 10 years. *Br J Haematol* 2000;108:544–548.

61. Bodey GP, Boktour M, Mays S, et al. Skin lesions associated with *Fusarium* infection. *J Am Acad Dermatol* 2002;47:659–666.

62. Consigny S, Dhedin N, Datry A, et al. Successsful voriconazole treatment of disseminated *Fusarium* infection in an immunocompromised patient. *Clin Infect Dis* 2003;37:311–313.

63. Kontoyiannis DP, Hanna H, Hachem R, et al. Risk factors of poor outcome of fusariosis in a tertiary care cancer center. *Leuk Lymph* 2004;45:141–143.

64. Walsh TJ, Newman KR, Moody M, et al. Trichosporonosis in patients with neoplastic disease. *Medicine* 1986;65:268–279.

65. Martino P, Venditti M, Micozzi A, et al. *Blastoschizomyces capitatus*: An emerging cause of invasive fungal disease in leukemia patients. *Rev Infect Dis* 1990;12:570–582.

66. Walsh TJ, Melcher GP, Rinaldi MG, et al. *Trichosporan beigelii*, an emerging pathogens resistant to amphoterioin B. *J Clin Microbiol* 1990;28:1616–1622.

67. Erer B, Galimberti M, Lucarelli G, et al. *Trichosporon beigelii*: A life-threatening pathogen in immunocompromised hosts. *Bone Marrow Transplant* 2000;25:745–749.

68. Chagua MR, Hachem R, Raad I, et al. Trichosporonosis in a tertiary care cancer center: Risk factors, spectrum and determinants of outcome. 40th Annual Meeting of the Infectious Diseases Society of America (IDSA), 2002. Abstract 100859.

69. Anaissie E, Gokaslan A, Hachem R, et al. Azole therapy for trichosporonosis: Clinical evaluation of eight patients, experimental therapy for murine infection, and review. *Clin Infect Dis* 1992;15:781–787.

70. Pournier S, Pavageau W, Feuillhade M, et al. Use of voriconazole to successfully treat disseminated *Trichosporon asahii* infection in a patient with acute myeloid leukaemia. *Eur J Clin Microbiol Infect Dis* 2002;21:892–896.

71. Anaissie EJ, Hachem R, Karyotakis NC, et al. Comparative efficacies of amphoteracin B, triazoles, and combination of both as experimental therapy for murine trichosporonosis. *Antimicrob Agents Chemother* 1994;38:2541–2544.

72. Ribes JA, Vanover-Sams CL, Baker DJ. Zygomycetes in human disease. *Clin Microbiol Rev* 2000;13:236–301.

73. Sugar AM. Agents of mucormycosis and related species. In: Mandel GL, Bennett JE, Dolin R (eds): *Principles and Practice of Infectious Diseases*, 5th ed. Vol. 2. Philadelphia: Churchill Livingstone; 2000:2685–2695.

74. Kontoyiannis DP, Wessel VC, Bodey GP, et al. Zygomycosis in the 1990s in a tertiary-care cancer center. *Clin Infect Dis* 2000;30:851–856.

75. Pagano L, Ricci P, Tonso A, et al. Mucormycosis in patients with haematological malignancies: A retrospective clinical

study of 37 cases. *Br J Haematol* 1997;99:331–336.

76. Walsh TJ, Hiemenz JW, Seibel N, et al. Amphotericin B lipid complex in patients with invasive fungal infections: Analysis of safety and efficacy in 556 cases. *Clin Infect Dis* 1998;26: 1383–1396.

77. Sun QN, Fothergill AW, McCarthy DI, et al. In vitro activities of posaconazole, itraconazole, voriconazole, amphotericin B, and fluconazole against 37 clinical isolates of zygomycetes. *Antimicrob Agents Chemother* 2002;46:1581–1582.

78. Kauffman CA. Endemic mycoses in patients with hematologic malignancies. *Semin Respir Infect* 2002;17:106–112.

79. Freireich EJ, Levin RH, Whang J, et al. The function and fate of transfused leukocytes from donors with chronic myelocytic leukemia in leukopenic recipients. *Ann NY Acad Sci* 1964;113:1081–1089.

80. Ruthe RC, Andersen BR, Cunningham BL, et al. Efficacy of granulocyte transfusions in the control of systemic candidiasis in the leukopenic host. *Blood* 1978;52:493–498.

81. Strauss RG. Clinical perspectives of granulocyte transfusions: Efficacy to date. *J Clin Aphersis* 1995;10:114–118.

82. Jendiroba DB, Lichtiger B, Anaissie E, et al. Evaluation and comparison of three mobilization methods for collection of granulocytes. *Transfusion* 1998;38:722–728.

83. Dignani MC, Anaissie EJ, Hester JP, et al. Treatment of neutropenia-related fungal infections with granulocyte colony-stimulating factor-elicited white blood cell transfusions: A pilot study. *Leukemia* 1997;11:1621–1630.

84. Bodey GP, Anaissie E, Gutterman J, Vadhan-Raj S. Role of granulocyte-macrophage colony-stimulating factor as adjuvant treatment in neutropenic patients with bacterial and fungal infection. *Eur J Clin Microbiol Infect Dis* 1994;13(Suppl 2): s18–s22.

85. Rodriguez-Adrian LJ, Grazziutti ML, Rex JH, et al. The potential role of cytokine therapy for fungal infections in patients with cancer: Is recovery from neutropenia all that is needed? *Clin Infect Dis* 1998;26:1270–1278.

86. Gaviria JM, van Burik JAH, Dale DC, et al. Comparison of interferon-γ, granulocyte colony-stimulating factor, and granulocyte-macrophage colony-stimulating factor for priming leukocyte-mediated hyphal damage of opportunistic fungal pathogens. *J Infect Dis* 1999;179:1038–1041.

87. Bustamante CI, Wade JC. Herpes simplex virus infection in the immunocompromised cancer patient. *J Clin Oncol* 1991; 9:1903–1915.

88. Saral R, Ambinder RF, Burns WH, et al. Acyclovir prophylaxis against herpes simplex virus infection in patients with leukemia. A randomized, double blind, placebo-controlled study. *Ann Intern Med* 1983;99:773.

89. Meyers JD, Flournoy N, Thomas ED. Infection with herpes simplex virus and cell-mediated immunity after marrow transplant. *J Infect Dis* 1980;142:338.

90. Wade JC, Newton B, Flournoy N, et al. Oral acyclovir for prevention of herpes simplex virus reactivation after marrow transplantation. *Ann Intern Med* 1984;100:823–828.

91. Feldman S, Lott L. Varicella in children with cancer: Impact of antiviral therapy and prophylaxis. *Pediatrics* 1987;80: 465–472.

92. Trying S, Barbarash RA, Nahlik JE, et al. Famciclovir for the treatment of acute herpes zoster: Effects on acute dis-

ease and postherpetic neuralgia. A randomized, double-blind placebo-controlled trial. Collaborative Famciclovir Herpes Zoster Study Group. *Ann Intern Med* 1995;123: 89–96.

93. Hardy I, Gershon AA, Steinberg SP, et al. The incidence of zoster after immunization with live attenuated varicella vaccine. A study in children with leukemia. Varicella Vaccine Collaborative Study Group. *N Engl J Med* 1991;325:1545–1550.

94. Gershon AA, Steinberg SP. Persistence of immunity to varicella in children with leukemia immunized with live attenuated varicella vaccine. *N Engl J Med* 1989;320: 892–897.

95. Peter G. *Red Book: Report of the Committee on Infectious Diseases.* Elk Grove Village, IL: American Academy of Pediatrics, 1997.

96. Miller W, Flynn P, McCullough J, et al. Cytomegalovirus infection after bone marrow transplantation: An association with acute graft-vs-host disease. *Blood* 1986;67(4):1162–1167.

97. van der Bij W, Schirm J, Torensma R, et al. Comparison between viremia and antigenemia for detection of cytomegalovirus in blood. *J Clin Microbiol* 1988;26:2531–2535.

98. Gerna G, Furione M, Baldanti F, et al. Quantitation of human cytomegalovirus DNA in bone marrow transplant recipients. *Br J Haematol* 1995;91:674–683.

99. Gerna G, Percivalle E, Baldanti F, et al. Diagnostic significance and clinical impact of quantitative assays for diagnosis of human cytomegalovirus infection/disease in immunocompromised patients. *New Microbiol* 1998;21:293–308.

100. Blok MJ, Goossens VJ, Vanherle SJV, et al. Diagnostic value of monitoring human cytomegalovirus late pp67 mRNA expression in renal-allograft recipients by nucleic acid sequence-based amplification. *J Clin Microbiol* 1998;36: 1341–1346.

101. Gerna G, Baldanti F, Middeldorp JM, et al. Clinical significance of expression of human cytomegalovirus pp67 late transcript in heart, lung and bone marrow transplant recipients as determined by nucleic acid sequence-based amplification. *J Clin Microbiol* 1999;37:902–911.

102. Crumpacker CS. Ganciclovir. *N Engl J Med* 1996;335:721–729.

103. Ho HT, Woods KL, Bronson JJ, et al. Intracellular metabolism of the antiherpes agent (S)-1-[3-hydroxy-2(phosphonylmethoxy) propyl] cytosine. *Mol Pharmacol* 1992;41:197–202.

104. Wang FZ, Dahl H, Linde A, et al. Lymphotropic herpesviruses in allogeneic bone marrow transplantation. *Blood* 1996;88:3615–3620.

105. Wang FZ, Linde A, Hagglund H, et al. Human herpesvirus 6 DNA in cerebrospinal fluid specimens from allogeneic bone marrow transplant patients: Does it have clinical significance? *Clin Infect Dis* 1999;28:562–568.

106. Milpied N, Vasseur B, Parquet N, et al. Humanized anti-CD20 monoclonal antibody (Rituximab) in post transplant B-lymphoproliferative disorder: A retrospective analysis on 32 patients. *Ann Oncol* 2000;11(suppl 1):113–116.

107. Esser JW, Niesters HG, van der Holt B, et al. Prevention of Epstein-Barr virus-lymphoproliferative disease by molecular monitoring and preemptive rituximab in high-risk patients after allogeneic stem cell transplantation. *Blood* 2002;99: 4364–4369.

108. Simpson ND, Simpson PW, Ahmed AM, et al. Prophylaxis against chemotherapy-induced reactivation of hepatitis B virus infection with lamivudine. *J Clin Gastroenterol* 2003; 37:68–71.

109. Picardi M, Selleri C, De Rosa G, et al. Lamivudine treatment for chronic replicative hepatitis B virus infection after allogeneic bone marrow transplantation. *Bone Marrow Transplant* 1998;21:1267–1269.

110. Zuckerman E, Zuckerman T, Levine AM, et al. Hepatitis C virus infection in patients with B-cell non-Hodgkin lymphoma. *Ann Intern Med* 1997;127(6):423–428.

111. Izumi T, Sasaki R, Tsunoda S, et al. B cell malignancy and hepatitis C virus infection. *Leukemia* 1997;11(suppl 3):516–518.

112. Whimbey E, Champlin RE, Couch RB, et al. Community respiratory virus infections among hospitalized adult bone marrow transplant recipients. *Clin Infect Dis* 1996;22:778–782.

113. Machado CM, Vilas Boas LS, Mendes AVA, et al. Low mortality rates related to respiratory virus infections after bone marrow transplantation. *Bone Marrow Transplant* 2003;31:695–700.

114. Martino R, Ramila E, Rabella N, et al. Respiratory virus infection in adults with hematologic malignancies: A prospective study. *Clin Infect Dis* 2003;36:1–8.

115. Couch RB, Englund JA, Whimbey E. Respiratory viral infections in immunocompetent and immunocompromised persons. *Am J Med* 1997;102:2–9.

116. LaRosa AM, Champlin RE, Mirza N, et al. Adenovirus infections in adult recipients of blood and marrow transplants. *Clin Infect Dis* 2001;32:871–876.

117. Ljungman P, Ward KN, Crooks BNA, et al. Respiratory virus infections after stem cell transplantation: A prospective study from the Infectious Diseases Working Party of the European Group for Blood and Marrow Transplantation. *Bone Marrow Transplant* 2001;28:479–484.

118. Kaiser L, Wat C, Mills T, et al. Impact of oseltamivir treatment on influenza-related lower respiratory tract complications and hospitalizations. *Arch Intern Med* 2003;163:1667–1672.

119. Small TN, Casson A, Malak SF, et al. Respiratory syncytial virus infection following hematopoietic stem cell transplantation. *Bone Marrow Transplant* 2002;29:321–327.

120. LaRosa AM, Champlin RE, Mirza N, et al. Adenovirus infections in adult recipients of blood and marrow transplants. *Clin Infect Dis* 2001;32:871–876.

121. Baldwin A, Kingman H, Darville M, et al. Outcome and clinical course of 100 patients with adenovirus infection following bone marrow transplantation. *Bone Marrow Transplant* 2000;26:1333–1338.

122. Chakrabarti S, Mautner V, Osman H, et al. Adenovirus infections following allogeneic stem cell transplantation: Incidence and outcome in relation to graft manipulation, immunosuppression, and immune recovery. *Blood* 2002;100: 1619–1627.

123. Kojaoghlanian T, Flomenberg P, Horwitz MS. The impact of adenovirus infection on the immunocompromised host. *Rev Med Virol* 2003;13:155–171.

124. Schilham MS, Claas EC, van Zaane W, et al. High levels of adenovirus DNA in serum correlate with fatal outcome of adenovirus infection in children after allogeneic stem cell transplantation. *Clin Infect Dis* 2002;35:526–532.

125. Ljungman P, Ribaud P, Eyrich M, et al. Cidofovir for adenovirus infections after allogeneic hematopoietic stem cell transplantation: A survey by the Infectious Diseases Working Party of the European Group for Blood and Marrow Transplantation. *Bone Marrow Transplant* 2003;31:481–486.

126. Chisaka H, Morita E, Yaegashi N, et al. ParvovirusB19 and the pathogenesis of anaemia. *Rev Med Virol* 2003;13: 347–359.

127. Kuo SH, Lin LI, Chang CJ, et al. Increased risk of parvovirus B19 infection in young adult cancer patients receiving multiple courses of chemotherapy. *J Clin Microbiol* 2002;40: 3909–3912.

128. Reploeg MD, Storch GA, Clifford DB. BK virus: A clinical review. *Clin Infect Dis* 2001;33:191–202.

ENDOCRINE MANIFESTATIONS OF NONENDOCRINE TUMORS

Mouhammed Amir Habra
Naifa L. Busaidy
Sai-Ching Jim Yeung
Rena Vassilopoulou-Sellin

In the past two decades, cancer research has rapidly advanced, spurred by the development of high-throughput technology and the maturation of genomic and proteomic research methods. These advances have resulted in treatments that have substantial effects on the outcomes of certain cancers. The continuous development of new antineoplastic agents adds increasing challenges to practicing physicians. Current cancer treatments include surgery, cytotoxic chemotherapy, hormonal therapy, bioimmunotherapy, and radiation therapy. Adverse effects of neoplastic agents on the endocrine system are caused by several different mechanisms and can range from a subtle laboratory abnormality to a fully developed clinical condition. Antineoplastic agents in general can be cytotoxic to endocrine cells and result in glandular dysfunction. Antineoplastic agents can also interfere with the synthesis or postsynthesis processing of hormones at different levels (i.e., transcription, translation, or posttranslation). An agent may inhibit or induce secretion of a hormone by interacting with receptors, perturbing intracellular second-messenger metabolism, or affecting hormone delivery by changing carrier protein levels in serum or competing for binding on the carrier protein. Finally, antineoplastic agents can interact with signal transduction pathways to inhibit or enhance hormonal action in the end organs.

In this chapter, we summarize the major and common endocrine complications of cancer therapy and discuss screening and surveillance of these complications in cancer survivors.

■ METABOLIC DISORDERS

GLUCOSE METABOLISM

Diabetes Mellitus

Serum glucose is under continuous complex regulation. Many processes can affect glucose levels, including gut absorption, cellular uptake, gluconeogenesis, and glycogenolysis. Multiple hormones—including insulin, glucagon, growth hormone (GH), cortisol, somatostatin, and incretins—also play important roles in overall glucose homeostasis.

Glucocorticoids are frequently used with many chemotherapy protocols and can have profound effects on glucose levels, even in patients without a history of diabetes. Corticosteroids can unmask preexisting diabetes mellitus or make diabetes more difficult to control. Patients can experience asymptomatic hyperglycemia or nonketotic hyperosmolar coma. Most patients taking glucocorticoids with elevated glucose will require insulin therapy to achieve blood glucose control, especially when given high-dose steroids. Long- and intermediate-acting insulin formulations are more effective at controlling glucose levels when they are combined with mealtime rapid- or short-acting insulins than are regimens that use short-acting insulin alone on the basis of sliding scales. A recent consensus conference on the inpatient management of diabetes recommended aban-

doning the practice of the sole use of sliding scales. The panel recommended more use of long- and intermediate-acting insulins.

L-asparaginase, streptozocin, and interferon-alpha (IFN-α) are other antineoplastic agents that have been associated with impaired glucose homeostasis or frank diabetes mellitus.

L-Asparaginase

An enzyme derived from *Escherichia coli* or *Erwinia* species, L-asparaginase inhibits protein synthesis by depleting L-asparagine. This drug is used mainly in the treatment of hematologic malignancies. Pegaspargase is formed by the linking of monomethoxypolyethylene glycol to *Escherichia coli* asparaginase in order to decrease immunogenicity. Pegylated *E. coli* asparaginase has been reported to have a similar risk of hyperglycemia compared with native asparaginase; in one study, the risk was about 5% in children with acute lymphoblastic leukemia treated with either agent (1). Hyperglycemia and glycosuria without ketonemia occurs in 1 to 14% of patients treated with L-asparaginase, an effect that is reversible on discontinuation of the drug (2–4). Insulin therapy is frequently required. One potential complication is hypoglycemia after cessation of L-asparaginase; thus, close monitoring of blood glucose is recommended. Diabetic ketoacidosis has been reported during L-asparaginase therapy (4,5). Long-term insulin therapy may not be needed in all cases of L-asparaginase–induced diabetes mellitus.

The exact mechanism of hyperglycemia is not known, although it has been postulated that inhibition of insulin, insulin receptor synthesis, or both may be the cause, leading to a combined insulin deficiency and resistance syndrome. Pancreatitis, which might occur with L-asparaginase therapy, is another possible mechanism for hyperglycemia through islet cell destruction.

Streptozocin

This is an *N*-nitrosourea derivative of glucosamide that is primarily used to treat malignant islet cell and other neuroendocrine tumors. Pancreatic beta cells exposed to streptozocin develop long-lasting impairment to the production and release of insulin, although other cell functions are better preserved. Streptozocin's effect on islet cells is species-specific and dose-related; rat islet cells appear to be more susceptible to the cytotoxic effects of streptozocin than do human islet cells. Most of streptozocin's effects are reversible upon discontinuation of the drug. Although the reported incidence of glucose intolerance varies from 6 to 60%, most cases are mild to moderate in severity (6–8).

Interferon Alpha

Use of recombinant IFN-α-2a and α-2b to treat malignancies has been associated with the development of hyperglycemia in patients without diabetes and deterioration of glycemic control in diabetics. Although the incidence of IFN-α–induced diabetes mellitus in patients with cancer is unclear, the incidence of diabetes mellitus is about 0.7% among patients who have received high-dose IFN-α for chronic active hepatitis C (9). Diabetic ketoacidosis has been reported in a variety of conditions treated with IFN-α-2 (10,11). The exact mechanism of IFN-α–induced diabetes is not well known. IFN-α acts as an immunomodulatory agent, inducing autoantibody production and the development of autoimmune disease in susceptible patients; but in a study of 58 patients who received IFN-α for the treatment of chronic, active hepatitis C, neither islet cell antibodies nor type I diabetes mellitus developed during therapy, though hemoglobin-A1c levels increased in two patients (12). IFNs may also directly inhibit preproinsulin synthesis in islet beta cells and thus contribute to insulin deficiency (13). Ironically some reports have postulated that IFN-α may preserve residual beta cell function in newly diagnosed type I diabetes (14). Insulin resistance is thought to contribute to diabetes mellitus in patients with hepatitis, and IFN-α therapy may improve insulin sensitivity.

Glucosuria

Some antineoplastic drugs (e.g., ifosfamide and mercaptopurine) cause a proximal tubular defect and lower the renal threshold for glucosuria without affecting glucose metabolism. To decrease the incidence of hemorrhagic cystitis, 2-mercaptoethane sulfonate sodium (MESNA) is often used with ifosfamide and has been reported to give a false-positive reaction for urinary ketones.

LIPID DISORDERS

Lipid disorders are seldom evaluated in the process of active anticancer therapy, as patients are often encouraged to maintain a positive metabolic balance via liberal oral intake. Investigation or treatment of mild lipid abnormalities is often overlooked because the focus is on maintaining a positive caloric balance during cancer treatment. Some lipid disorders may be short-lived and without clear clinical consequences, but some may be of clinical importance and need to be detected and treated. In general, triglyceride levels higher than 1000 mg/dL

increase the rate of complications, including pancreatitis and visual impairment, and must be treated urgently.

Hypertriglyceridemia

IFNs may induce hypertriglyceridemia by increasing hepatic and peripheral fatty acid production and suppressing hepatic triglyceride lipase. Elevation of serum triglyceride levels to more than 1000 mg/dL can occur. In one case, a controlled diet and gemfibrozil had therapeutic effects despite continued IFN-α therapy (15).

All-trans retinoic acid (tretinoin) and other retinoic acid derivatives have been used in the treatment of several malignancies, including, head and neck cancer and acute promyelocytic leukemia. They are well known to induce hypertriglyceridemia with elevated very low density lipoprotein (VLDL) (16–20) and hypercholesterolemia associated with increased low-density lipoproteins (LDL). Cerebrovascular accidents and pancreatitis have been described in association with retinoid-induced hypertriglyceridemia.

Bexarotene is a synthetic retinoid X receptor (RXR)–selective retinoid used in the treatment of cutaneous T-cell lymphoma. Hypertriglyceridemia is the most frequent drug-related adverse effect and occurred in 79% of patients (21,22). Hypertriglyceridemia is considered a dose-limiting toxicity, with three reported cases of pancreatitis during phase II/III trials. These three patients were taking 300 mg/m^2 or more of oral bexarotene per day and had triglyceride levels higher than 1300 mg/dL (22). Retinoid-induced hyperlipidemia has been successfully treated with fibrates or fish oil.

Hypercholesterolemia

Dose-related hypercholesterolemia has been described in patients with adrenocortical carcinoma treated with mitotane (23); inhibition of cholesterol oxidase is the likely mechanism. Patients with adrenocortical carcinoma usually have a poor prognosis, making mild to moderate elevation of cholesterol of less clinical importance, but in long-term (5- to 10-year) survivors, continued mitotane therapy can lead to early development of atherosclerotic disease. In long-term survivors, the benefits of treating mitotane-induced lipid abnormalities have not been established.

Hypercholesterolemia is the second most common side effect of bexarotene and has been reported in 48% of treated patients (22). The long-term significance of this drug-induced hypercholesterolemia is unclear; however, atorvastatin has been used successfully in treating patients at our institution.

Serum cholesterol and low-density lipoprotein cholesterol were increased in 41% of patients with germ cell tumors treated with cisplatin-containing chemotherapy regimens; the long-term significance of this is also not clear (24).

WATER AND ELECTROLYTE DISORDERS

Serum osmolality is tightly regulated, primarily by the interaction of the hypothalamic osmoreceptors that regulate secretion of antidiuretic hormone from cells in the paraventricular and supraoptic nuclei, the hypothalamic thirst center, and the kidneys. The disruption of any of the above-mentioned regulators may lead to a disturbance in free water clearance and subsequent abnormalities in serum sodium levels.

Syndrome of Inappropriate Antidiuretic Hormone Secretion (SIADH) and Hyponatremia

Hyponatremia is a relatively common electrolyte abnormality in patients with cancer. The syndrome of inappropriate antidiuretic hormone (SIADH) secretion is one of the most common underlying causes for hyponatremia in this patient population. This syndrome is characterized by hyponatremia, low serum osmolality, and an inappropriately high urine osmolality with elevated urine sodium in the absence of diuretics use, heart failure, cirrhosis, adrenal insufficiency, or hypothyroidism. In patients with cancer, SIADH may be caused by ectopic antidiuretic hormone (ADH) production by a variety of tumors. This is most commonly seen in patients with small cell lung cancer (SCLC). Other tumors are rarely described in association with SIADH; they include malignant thymoma, oral squamous cell carcinoma, prostate carcinoma, and pancreatic carcinoma. Chemotherapy-induced lysis of ADH-containing cancer cells may lead to more severe hyponatremia at the time of chemotherapy induction.

Other factors that may increase ADH secretion include nausea, pain, narcotics, nicotine, and antineoplastic agents such as high-dose intravenous cyclophosphamide, vincristine, vinblastine, and cisplatin.

SIADH is a diagnosis of exclusion after ruling out hypovolemia, adrenal insufficiency, hypothyroidism, renal insufficiency, congestive heart failure, cirrhosis, and, rarely, cerebral salt-wasting syndrome.

In cases of hyponatremia secondary to SIADH, urine osmolality is higher than plasma osmolality, and urine sodium is determined by sodium intake. Urine sodium is usually higher than 40 meq/L in patients with SIADH. Fluid restriction (usually 700 to 1200 mL of free water a day), increasing salt intake, and occasionally loop di-

uretics are usually attempted first in most cases of SIADH when the patient is asymptomatic or having mild symptoms. In the presence of severe symptoms (seizures or obtundation), hypertonic saline infusions might be needed, with close and frequent monitoring of sodium levels to avoid rapid correction and possible central pontine myelinolysis. Demeclocycline (600 to 1200 mg/day) can be used in the few cases in which hyponatremia does not respond to more conservative treatments. Vasopressin receptor (V2) antagonists are still being evaluated in clinical trials but carry the potential of being a more specific therapy for cases of SIADH.

Diabetes Insipidus and Hypernatremia

Central diabetes insipidus can happen after brain surgery and occasionally in cases of tumors invading the neurohypophysis or disrupting the pituitary stalk. These cases are often recognized by a clinical presentation of polyuria/polydipsia in patients who have undergone recent brain or pituitary surgery or who have known tumors near the sella or the hypothalamus. These cases are usually treated with 1-desamino-8-delta-arginine vasopressin (DDAVP) (subcutaneously, intranasally, or orally) to control the symptoms and correct the hypernatremia.

Nephrogenic diabetes insipidus (DI) can occur in patients with cancer, and multiple antineoplastic agents have been described in association with this syndrome. Ifosfamide is well known to induce renal tubular damage at the level of the proximal renal tubules and, to a lesser extent, the distal renal tubules, where it has been found to induce nephrogenic DI. Streptozocin has also been reported to cause nephrogenic DI.

Another common cause of hypernatremia in patients with cancer is the failure to deliver enough free water, especially when patients are on parenteral or tube feeding regimens or are too debilitated to obtain water for themselves.

■ DISORDERS OF BONE AND MINERAL METABOLISM

OSTEOPOROSIS

Normal bone remodeling requires a delicate balance between bone formation by osteoblasts and bone resorption by osteoclasts. Antineoplastic therapy may affect this balance by increasing the activity of osteoclasts (e.g., interleukin-2) and sometimes by having direct toxic effects on osteoblast function. Hormones and cytokines (i.e., ACTH, PTH, PTH-related peptide, and interleukin-1) can also affect the overall bone turnover rate. Malnutrition and poor calcium and vitamin D intake may be major factors affecting bone turnover in patients with cancer.

Antineolastic agents have been implicated in chemotherapy-associated osteoporosis. Prolonged therapy with oral methotrexate for acute lymphoblastic leukemia (ALL) has led to distal extremity pain, severe osteoporosis, and associated fractures, with significant improvement after cessation of methotrexate therapy (25).

Other agents reported to reduce bone density include cisplatin and carboplatin. In addition, many chemotherapy protocols include corticosteroids, which decrease bone density and increase the risk of fractures. Hypogonadism resulting from chemotherapy, hormonal therapy, or radiation therapy will also add to the reduced bone density in patients with cancer.

Patients who have undergone bone marrow transplantation have been reported to have low bone mass. The reduced bone density is likely to be secondary to the long-term side effects of bone marrow radiation, chemotherapy, corticosteroids, and hypogonadism.

Aromatase inhibitors, including anastrozole and letrozole, have been shown to decrease bone density and increase the rate of fractures in postmenopausal women. This is in sharp contrast to the positive effect on bone (both bone mineral density and fracture rates) seen with the alternative adjuvant hormonal treatment of breast cancer with tamoxifen, a selective estrogen receptor modulator (SERM) (Fig. 38-1).

In the Arimidex, Tamoxifen Alone or in Combination (ATAC) trial, 9366 postmenopausal women with invasive operable breast cancer who had completed primary therapy were randomly assigned to receive anastrozole, tamoxifen, or both. The anastrozole group had significantly more fractures of all kinds than did the tamoxifen-alone group (26). Patients treated with aromatase inhibitors should undergo bone mineral density prior to treatment with aromatase inhibitors and followed up annually thereafter. A bisphosphonate should be added to the treatment regimen if the patient's bone density is within the osteopenic or osteoporotic range before treatment or if a decline in bone mineral density is seen during follow-up.

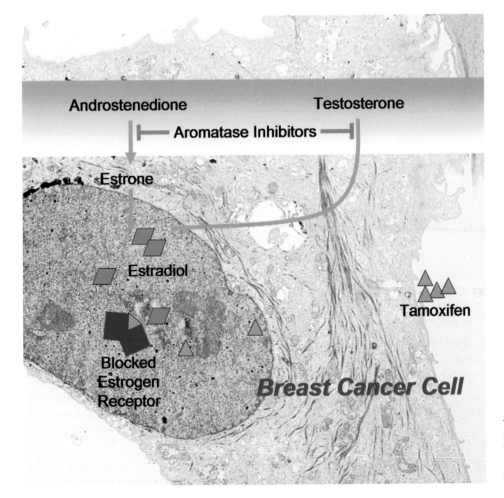

FIGURE 38-1 Mechanism of action of selective estrogen receptor modulators (SERMs) and aromatase inhibitors.

OSTEOMALACIA AND RICKETS

Osteomalacia results when normal mineralization of the organic bone matrix fails. In children, the abnormal mineralization and maturation of the growth plate at the epiphysis is called rickets. Nutritional deficiency (especially vitamin D) and renal wasting of phosphorus leading to hypocalcemia or hypophosphatemia are among the common causes of osteomalacia. Other contributing factors include drugs such as anticonvulsants or aluminum and systemic acidosis. Antineoplastic agents can also cause or worsen osteomalacia. Ifosfamide-induced tubular damage leads to renal phosphate wasting, hypophosphatemia, and rickets. Estramustine has also been used in prostrate cancer metastatic to bone and leads to hypocalcemia, hypophosphatemia, secondary hyperparathyroidism, and osteomalacia with normal vitamin D levels. Tumor-induced osteomalacia (TIO) is a rare form of hypophosphatemic rickets characterized by phosphaturia and hypophosphatemia. TIO has been reported mainly with benign tumors (especially hemangiopericytoma), but it has also been reported in a variety of malignant tumors (usually of mesenchymal origin). Fibroblast growth factor 23 (FGF23) is secreted from these tumors and causes hyperphosphaturia, with subsequent hypophosphatemia. Surgical removal of the tumor corrects the hyperphosphaturic abnormality and, subsequently, the hypophosphatemia and the bone mineralization defect. Radiolabeled octreotide has been reported to detect some of these tumors, and octreotide therapy has been used to treat these tumors with varying results (27,28).

HYPERCALCEMIA

Calcium homeostasis is normally maintained by the interplay of parathyroid hormone (PTH), calcitonin, phosphorus, and vitamin D metabolites on several target organs, including bones, parathyroid glands, intestines, and kidneys. In patients with cancer, multiple factors can affect this delicate balance, including nutritional status, medications, tumor secretion of cytokines, hormones, or other humoral factors.

Hypercalcemia occurs in 5 to 10% of all patients with advanced cancer, and severe hypercalcemia (calcium level >12 mg/dL) is seen in about 0.5% of all patients with cancer (29). Renal cell carcinoma, non–small cell lung carcinoma, breast carcinoma, leukemia, non-Hodgkin's lymphoma, and multiple myeloma are among the most common malignancies associated with hypercalcemia. Retinoic acid derivatives have been reported to induce hypercalcemia during the treatment of acute promyelocytic leukemia (30). Similarly, bexarotene has been reported to cause hypercalcemia in initial studies (31).

Hyperparathyroidism occurs 2.5 to 3 times more often in patients treated with low-dose (2 to 7.5 Gy) external radiation to the head and neck area than it does in the age-matched control population. Hyperparathyroidism after high-dose irradiation is uncommon. Radiation exposure from radioactive iodine treatment has also been reported in association with hyperparathyroidism.

HYPOCALCEMIA

Many factors can increase patients' risk of hypocalcemia. These include the patient's nutritional status, the antineoplastic agents used, and the type of surgical procedures performed (i.e., neck dissection). Cytotoxic chemotherapy can result in tumor lysis syndrome and its resultant hypocalcemia; this is more commonly seen in the treatment of hematologic malignancies. Hyperphosphatemia, hyperkalemia, hypocalcemia, and hyperuricemia can occur after induction chemotherapy; it is of vital importance to preempt this and prevent the complications of tumor lysis by hydration, alkaline diuresis, inhibition of uric acid synthesis, and administration of oral calcium or aluminum-based compounds to bind intestinal phosphate and enhance calcium absorption. Intravenous calcium administration can potentially cause calcium-phosphate precipitation in the presence of severe hyperphosphatemia and should be used with extreme caution. Dialysis may be needed in cases of symptomatic hypocalcemia and serum phosphorus levels higher than 10 mg/dL.

Cisplatin has been associated with hypocalcemia. One proposed mechanism of cisplatin's ability to induce hypocalcemia is through hypomagnesemia, resulting in a decreased PTH secretion. Other theories include the inhibition of 1,25-dihydroxy vitamin D formation by hypomagnesemia or cisplatin inhibition of mitochondrial function in the proximal renal tubules. Plicamycin (mithramycin) is an antitumor antibiotic that has a major effect on calcium metabolism. It inhibits bone resorption, resulting in lowered serum calcium concentrations within 24 to 48 h. The inhibitory effect of plicamycin on osteoclast function has made it useful in the treatment of Paget's disease of bone and osteoclast-mediated hypercalcemia associated with malignancy when other first-line agents have failed. Plicamycin carries a risk of hepatic and renal toxicity; therefore, it has limited usefulness in treating hypercalcemia of malignancy.

Other agents reported to induce hypocalcemia include dactinomycin, carboplatin, doxorubicin, and cytarabine. Hypocalcemia has been seen following bisphosphonate infusions (zolendronic acid and pamidronate) used to reduce skeletal complications in the treatment and prevention of advanced malignancies involving bone (32).

Serum calcium levels and 25-hydroxy vitamin D levels should be checked prior to and during therapy with bisphosphonates.

HYPOMAGNESEMIA

Hypomagnesemia is a well-known side effect in patients receiving platinum-based chemotherapy. Cisplatin has toxic effects on the kidney, causing morphologic changes and necrosis in the proximal tubule, a major site of magnesium reabsorption. Hypomagnesemia is a frequent complication of cisplatin chemotherapy, affecting up to 90% of patients; 10% of these patients have symptoms of muscle weakness, tremulousness, and dizziness. Vigorous hydration and the use of osmotic diuretics such as mannitol may prevent renal failure but have little effect on renal magnesium wasting, which can persist for long periods after cisplatin discontinuation.

Carboplatin is a second-generation platinum compound developed in an attempt to reduce the side effects of cisplatin. Hypomagnesemia following therapy with carboplatin is seen with increasing frequency and severity at higher doses of carboplatin and can be severe enough to cause clinical symptoms (33).

Oxaliplatin is a third-generation platinum derivative that has become an integral part of various chemotherapy protocols, particularly in advanced colorectal cancer. Oxaliplatin has dose-limiting cumulative sensory neurotoxicity similar to that of cisplatin (34). Renal toxicity was absent in phase I trials with doses up to $200 \, mg/m^2$ (35). It is felt to carry a much smaller risk, if any, for hypomagnesemia.

■ PITUITARY AND HYPOTHALAMIC DISORDERS

Hypothalamic-pituitary damage leading to single or multiple hormonal deficiencies can occur in patients treated with cranial or craniospinal irradiation or intracranial surgery (Fig. 38-2).

The hypothalamus appears to be more radiosensitive than the pituitary gland and may be damaged by lower radiation doses (<40 Gy), but higher radiation doses are likely to damage both hypothalamic and pituitary function. Deficiency of one or more pituitary hormones occurs following irradiation (about 40 Gy) of the

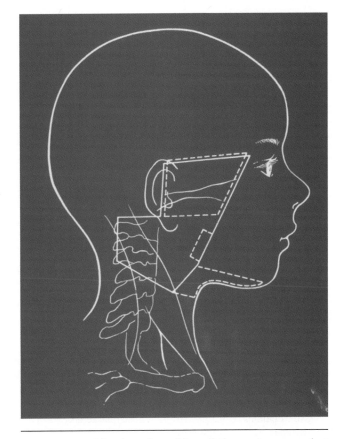

FIGURE 38-2 Mapping of possible radiation ports on a patient exposed during treatment for cancer of the head and neck region.

hypothalamic-pituitary areas in about 90% of patients 5 years after radiation treatment (Fig. 38-3).

GROWTH HORMONE DEFICIENCY

Growth hormone (GH) deficiency is frequently noted after cranial irradiation. In children, isolated GH deficiency can occur after lower radiation doses, but higher doses may produce panhypopituitarism. This side effect of radiation therapy appears to be dose-dependent. At lower doses (20 to 24 Gy), the only effect may be an altered pulsatile secretory pattern. At doses higher than 30 Gy, deficient GH secretion and growth retardation is observed in more than one-third of patients (36) (Fig. 38-4).

GH deficiency is also common in adults who have undergone cranial radiation therapy. In adults, GH deficiency is thought to cause decreased bone and muscle mass, fatigue, impaired sense of well-being, lowered exercise capacity, increased volume of adipose tissue, and altered myocardial function. In addition, patients with GH deficiency may have a higher occurrence of atherosclerotic plaques and an increased risk for cardiovascular diseases. GH replacement in these patients can

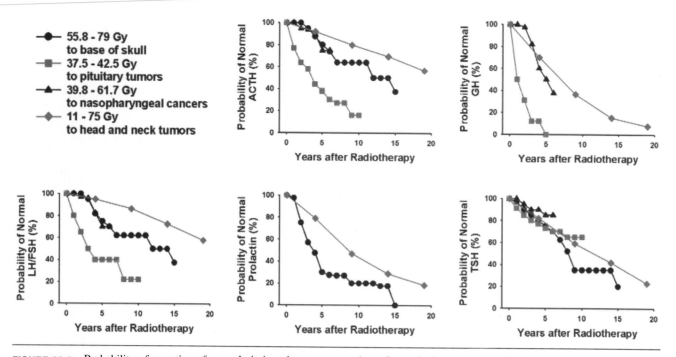

FIGURE 38-3 Probability of secretion of normal pituitary hormone over time after radiation exposure to the hypothalamic-pituitary areas. Data from four studies are replotted on this figure. The first set of values (*black circle*) is from Pai et al. (41), in which the patient received 55.8 to 79 Gy to the base of the skull. The second set of values (*red square*) is from Shalet et al. (36), in which patients with pituitary tumors were treated with 37.5 to 42.5 Gy. The third series (*blue triangle*), from Lam et al. (97), shows the effect of radiation treatment for nasopharyngeal carcinoma with 39.8 to 61.7 Gy. The final series (*green diamond*) shows data from Samaan et al. (42), in which 11 to 75 Gy was administered to treat head and neck tumors.

restore normal adipose tissue composition, bone metabolism, quality of life, sense of well-being, lipid profile, and cardiac function. Despite the apparent benefits, data about the effect of GH replacement in long-term cancer survivors are still lacking. GH replacement is contraindicated in any patient with an active malignant condition, but it can be initiated in an adult in whom malignant disease has been absent for at least 5 years.

Another treatment reported to result in GH deficiency includes long-term intrathecal opioids; patients receiving these have about a 15% risk of developing GH deficiency (37).

CENTRAL HYPOTHYROIDISM

Radiotherapy can cause immediate and long-term effects; central hypothyroidism may be a result of the possible effects of brain or head and neck irradiation on hypothalamic and pituitary regulation of thyroid-stimulating hormone (TSH) secretion. Some 15 to 20% of patients who had undergone cranial irradiation had diminished TSH secretion at 5 years after the treatment and approximately 35% after 10 years. The combined effect of irradiation on the thyroid gland and pituitary-hypothalamic area is so striking that we suggest routine

screening for this group of patients, with measurement of both serum-free thyroxine and TSH concentration at 2- to 4-year intervals.

Chemotherapy may exacerbate the deleterious effect of radiation. Children with brain tumors (not involving the hypothalamic-pituitary axis) who receive vincristine, carmustine or lomustine, procarbazine, and brain irradiation have a 35% incidence of hypothyroidism, compared with a 10% incidence for patients who undergo brain irradiation alone (38). Bexarotene was found to cause central hypothyroidism in 40% of patients with cutaneous T-cell lymphoma (22). Reversible retinoid X receptor–mediated suppression of TSH secretion is one explanation for this side effect (39). The fact that these patients often require twice the typical doses used to treat other causes of hypothyroidism suggests that bexarotene probably also increases thyroid hormone metabolic clearance (40).

HYPOGONADOTROPIC HYPOGONADISM

Brain surgery and irradiation of the skull carry the potential for hypothalamic-pituitary damage, including hypogonadotropic hypogonadism. Hyperprolactinemia is the most commonly reported hormonal abnormality

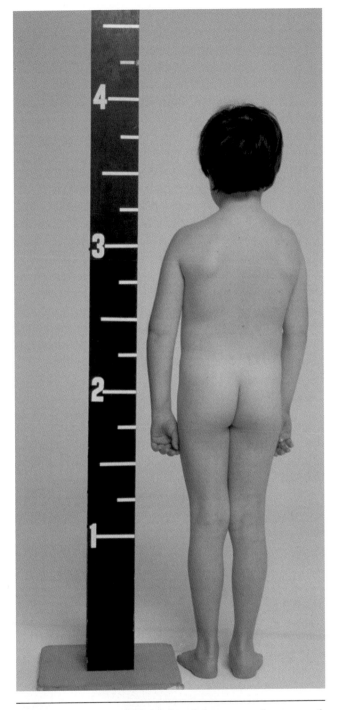

FIGURE 38-4 This patient developed short stature due to growth hormone deficiency from radiation treatment of a brain tumor.

in patients who have undergone head and neck irradiation, occurring in more than 66% of patients (41,42). Hyperprolactinemia inhibits gonadotropin secretion from the pituitary gland and decreases the responsiveness of the pituitary gland to gonadotropin-releasing hormone, causing secondary hypogonadism. Dopamine agonists can reverse this process, and it may be reasonable to proceed with a therapeutic trial if the other anterior pitu-

itary hormone axes are normal. Hypogonadism has been reported in 29% of patients following high-dose conformal fractionated proton-photon beam radiotherapy for tumors at the base of the skull (41). In children, inadequate sexual development, delayed puberty, and absent menarche are significant problems, whereas gonadotropin deficiency in adults may cause sex steroid hormone deficiency and infertility (Fig. 38-5). Sex steroid hormone deficiency lowers libido and may have deleterious effects on bone and lipid metabolism.

Early or even precocious puberty has also been reported in patients treated with combined chemotherapy and cranial irradiation for acute lymphoblastic leukemia (ALL) or cranial irradiation for brain tumors. This phenomenon is more common in girls. Coexisting GH deficiency is frequently noted. In a recent study of male cancer survivors (excluding those who had undergone treatment that may have otherwise affected gonadal function), chronic opioid therapy, given in morphine-equivalent daily doses of at least 200 mg daily, was associated with secondary hypogonadism (43).

■ THYROID DISORDERS

THYROID NEOPLASMS

Ionizing radiation is the only well-established etiology of thyroid cancer. Irradiation of the thyroid results in

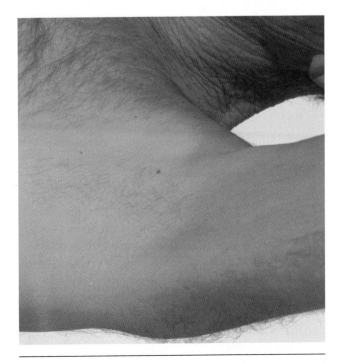

FIGURE 38-5 Loss of axillary hair in a patient who developed secondary hypogonadism after cranial irradiation.

DNA damage, with formation of chromosomal rearrangements involving the intracellular tyrosine kinase of *RET* fused with another gene product, typically *H4* or *ELE1*, creating *RET/PTC1* and *RET/PTC3* rearrangements respectively. There are different types of RET/PTC rearrangements, with *RET/PTC1* and *RET/PTC3* accounting for more than 90%. The prevalence of *RET/PTC* in papillary carcinomas shows significant geographic variation and is approximately 35% in North America. *RET/PTC* is more common in tumors in children and young adults and in papillary carcinomas associated with radiation exposure (44). A dose-response relationship between radiation exposure and relative risk of thyroid cancer is seen for radiation doses of ≤5 Gy (45). Female sex, age less than 15 years at radiation exposure, and 20 to 30 years post–radiation exposure are all associated with increased risk for thyroid cancer. Papillary thyroid carcinomas make up 90% of radiation-induced thyroid cancers; there is a higher incidence of local invasion, multicentric disease, and distant metastasis on presentation in radiation-induced thyroid cancer than there is in sporadic thyroid cancer (46). There is an increased prevalence of thyroid cancer among patients therapeutically irradiated in anatomic locations other than the head and neck because of unintended low-dose radiation exposure to the thyroid gland. Children tend to be more sensitive to these radiation doses (47). Thyroid carcinoma is most evident in long-term survivors of Hodgkin's disease and non-Hodgkin's lymphoma.

Chemotherapy is not a proven risk factor for thyroid carcinoma despite rare case reports to the contrary. The administration of iodine 131 (^{131}I) for diagnostic purposes does not seem to increase the risk of developing carcinoma of the thyroid.

HYPERTHYROIDISM

Radiation-induced hyperthyroidism has been described but is far less common than radiation-induced hypothyroidism.

Radiation-induced silent thyroiditis with transient thyrotoxicosis has been reported in patients treated with radiation therapy. Thyroiditis-induced thyrotoxicosis occurs within 2 years of radiation therapy in most cases; several months later, hypothyroidism occurs. There is an increased risk of Graves' disease following radiation therapy. Patients with lymphoma who have been treated with radiation therapy constitute the largest number of patients who have developed Graves' disease after radiation therapy; this raises the possibility of a relationship between the two clinical entities. Patients treated with radiation for nasopharyngeal, breast, and/or laryngeal carcinomas may also develop Graves' disease. Cytokines have also been reported to lead to Graves' disease. IFN-α is known to induce the production of autoantibodies and can lead to the occurrence of autoimmune thyroid disease, specifically autoimmune primary hypothyroidism, transient thyrotoxicosis, or, more rarely, Graves' disease. Women have a higher risk of developing autoimmune thyroid disease upon starting IFN-α treatment (48). It is important to distinguish the cases in which IFN-α induces transient thyrotoxicosis followed by hypothyroidism from the cases in which IFN-α induces Graves' disease (49). Thyroid scans showing increased homogeneous uptake in the presence of hyperthyroidism are highly suggestive of Graves' disease and warrant antithyroid medications (e.g., methimazole).

Interleukin-2 treatment alone causes transient hyperthyroidism followed by hypothyroidism in about 50% of patients (50). The mechanism of interleukin-2–induced autoimmune thyroid dysfunction is unclear, although interleukin-2–induced disruption of self-tolerance has been suggested as a mechanism.

HYPOTHYROIDISM

Head and neck irradiation is an important etiology of dysfunction of the thyroid gland. Radiation can induce primary hypothyroidism when given in doses higher than 25 Gy to the region near the thyroid gland (Fig. 38-6); secondary and tertiary hypothyroidism are seen with doses of 40 Gy or higher to the hypothalamic-pituitary area.

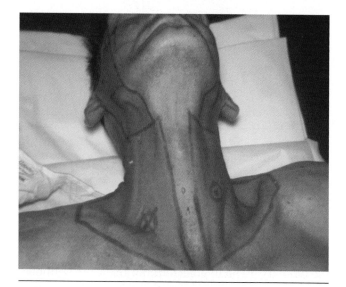

FIGURE 38-6 Mapping of radiation ports on a patient with squamous cell cancer of the head and neck. The patient developed primary hypothyroidism a few years after radiation therapy.

Most cases of primary hypothyroidism occur about 5 years after radiation therapy. The probability of hypothyroidism is dose-related and increases with longer duration of follow-up after radiation treatment. In a study of 1677 patients with Hodgkin's disease whose thyroid had been irradiated, the risk of thyroid disease was 52 and 67% after 20 and 26 years of follow-up, respectively. A total of 486 patients (29%) received thyroxine therapy because of elevated serum TSH concentrations and 27 (2%) had transient, untreated elevations of their serum (51).

A significant number of patients develop subclinical hypothyroidism (elevated TSH with normal thyroxine levels), not overt hypothyroidism, when less than 40 Gy of radiation are given (52). Multiple factors increase the risk for hypothyroidism, including high doses of radiation to the head and neck, combined radiation and surgical treatments, time interval since therapy, and failure to shield midline structures. Other risk factors include thyroid resection during a laryngectomy or disruption of the vascular supply of the thyroid gland during surgery.

The use of ^{131}I may result in thyroid dysfunction. ^{131}I-metaiodobenzylguanidine (MIBG) in the treatment of metastatic pheochromocytoma carries the possibility of inducing primary hypothyroidism and requires the routine use of potassium percholorate to block ^{131}I uptake by the thyroid.

IFN-α administration was reported to cause primary hypothyroidism in about 10% of treated patients and was not related to IFN dosage (53). The presence of pretreatment serum antithyroid antibodies in patients treated with IFN therapy increases the risk for the development of IFN-induced thyroid disease. During 6 years of observation after IFN therapy, the absence of thyroid autoantibodies at the end of IFN treatment was found to be a protective factor for the successive development of thyroiditis, whereas the positivity for thyroid antibodies at high titers at the end of IFN treatment was significantly related to chronic subclinical hypothyroidism. IFN-α–related thyroid autoimmunity is not a completely reversible phenomenon because some patients may develop chronic thyroiditis, especially in the presence of high autoantibody titers.

Interleukin-2 causes painless thyroiditis of acute onset, with initial hyperthyroxinemia followed by primary hypothyroidism. The hypothyroidism may last months but is occasionally permanent; 9% of these patients require replacement thyroid hormone therapy (54).

Patients treated with multiple drug regimens with antineoplastic agents (with or without radiation) also have a higher than normal incidence of primary hypothyroidism. Fifteen percent of patients who received a combination of cisplatin, bleomycin, dactinomycin, vinblastine, and etoposide developed elevated TSH levels with normal free T3 and free thyroxine (T4), compatible with subclinical primary hypothyroidism, in contrast to the control group (55).

ABNORMALITIES IN BINDING PROTEINS

Thyroid hormone is preferentially bound to thyroid hormone–binding globulin (TBG) (65 to 70%), transthyretin (15 to 20%), and albumin (10 to 15%) in serum. Multiple factors can affect the levels of these binding proteins and the subsequent levels of measured bound thyroid hormones. In patients with malignancies, changes in sex hormone levels, glucocorticoids, narcotics, nutritional status, and some antineoplastic agents are the major factors affecting the protein-binding properties. Overall, the level of total T3 and T4 may be affected, but in general the free (biologically active) hormone levels are normal. This effect on TBG synthesis or clearance is usually reversible. Estrogens are known to increase TBG and total thyroid hormone levels, but tamoxifen also causes elevated plasma concentrations of TBG in postmenopausal women with breast cancer after 6 months of therapy. Nonsteroidal aromatase inhibitors (anastrozole and letrozole) are known to lower estrogen levels, but the effect on TBG has still not been fully reported in the literature; when letrozole was given at 2.5 mg per day, however, there was a statistically significant decrease in total T4 but not total T3 levels (56).

Glucocorticoids are frequently used in combination with chemotherapy and are known to suppress TSH secretion and inhibit TBG synthesis. L-asparaginase has been shown to inhibit the synthesis of albumin and TBG, which, affects serum thyroid hormone levels (57,58). 5-Fluorouracil increases total T3 and T4 levels and maintains a normal free thyroxine index, suggesting that it an increases serum thyroid hormone–binding proteins, resulting in normal thyroid function (59).

Mitotane increases levels of hormone-binding globulins, but the increase in TBG is less remarkable than mitotane's effect on corticosteroid-binding globulin.

■ ADRENAL DISORDERS

PRIMARY ADRENAL INSUFFICIENCY

Mitotane is an insecticide derivative with selective toxicity for both normal and malignant adrenocortical cells. Adrenal insufficiency is commonly seen at the high doses used to treat adrenocortical carcinoma. It also causes a two- to threefold increase in serum levels of cortisol-binding globulin protein (60). Glucocorticoid replacement therapy is needed when mitotane is used; doses higher than usual are required because of the increased levels of binding globulin and enhanced metabolic clearance of dexamethasone by mitotane.

SECONDARY ADRENAL INSUFFICIENCY

Prolonged glucocorticoid treatment is the most common cause of adrenal dysfunction in patients with cancer. Secondary (central) adrenal insufficiency may develop after discontinuation of glucocorticoids and can persist for months. This can occur up to 2 years after discontinuation of therapy. Irradiation to the hypothalamic-pituitary region causes deficiency of ACTH, with resultant secondary adrenal insufficiency in 19 to 42% of these patients. The median time interval for the development of adrenal insufficiency after therapy is 5 years, but it can occur as early as 2 years after radiotherapy.

Prolonged therapy with busulfan was initially reported to cause a reversible clinical syndrome resembling central adrenal insufficiency, as evidenced by metyrapone testing (61). No recent reports have corroborated this. Long-term intrathecal opioid therapy for intractable nonmalignant pain (mean duration of treatment, 26.6 ± 16.3 months) resulted in central adrenal insufficiency in 15% of patients when they were tested with insulin-induced hypoglycemia (37).

Megestrol acetate is used to stimulate appetite in patients with cancer, but its prolonged use can lead to a Cushings-like syndrome, and sudden withdrawal of prolonged treatment may result in adrenal insufficiency. Megestrol shows glucocorticoid-like effects, with an acute depressing effect on the hypothalamic-pituitary-axis (HPA) and ACTH secretion, leading to central adrenal insufficiency as tested with the 1-μg ACTH stimulation test (62,63). Secondary adrenal insufficiency can be diagnosed by a variety of tests with varying sensitivity and specificity, but in our practices we tend to frequently use a combination of basal (8 a.m.) serum cortisol measurements and low-dose (1 μg) cosyntropin stimulation testing. Rarely, insulin-induced hypoglycemia is used to assess the overall cortisol and GH response to hypoglycemia in evaluating patients for panhypopituitarism.

■ GONADAL DISORDERS

Direct radiation exposure and cytotoxic chemotherapeutic agents are common causes of hypogonadism and infertility in cancer survivors. There are considerable differences between female and male gametogenesis, which results in a variety of effects of the cancer therapy on fertility and gonadal functions.

FEMALE GONADAL DISORDERS

Oogenesis occurs during embryonic life, and oocytes remain quiescent most of their lifespan; it is this property that makes them resistant to the adverse effects of cytotoxic chemotherapy. However, the combination of a limited number of oocytes and the inability to replace damaged ones results in a shortened reproductive period when oocytes have been damaged. The granulosa cells are also susceptible to these cytotoxic drugs, as shown by the results of ovarian biopsies performed after chemotherapy (Fig. 38-7). Infertility may occur as a result of either granulosa cell or oocyte impairment.

With advances in cancer treatment, an increasing number of women survive their malignancies to face reproductive disorders. It is of vital importance to discuss fertility issues before radiation or systemic chemotherapy, as these modalities carry significant risks for ovarian dysfunction and infertility. The effects of radiation treatment on the ovaries differ according to the patient's age, radiation dose, and field of treatment. With doses as low as 6 Gy, prepubertal girls can experience primary amenorrhea, and women above 40 years of age can develop ovarian failure and infertility (64,65). Permanent infertility in women below 40 years of age usually occurs after doses of 20 Gy or higher (64). Fractionated radiation seems to carry less risk for permanent sterility (66). When possible, fractionated radiation should be used; shielding of the gonads and restriction of the radiation fields reduce the risk of ovarian failure. Ovarian transposition (oophoropexy) to the paracolic gutters before pelvic irradiation has been suggested to preserve ovarian function in women below 40 years of age with cervical carcinomas less than 3 cm in diameter (67). It

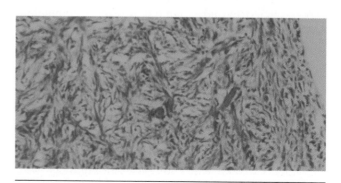

FIGURE 38-7 Hematoxylin and eosin staining of tissue from an ovarian biopsy showing atrophy of ovarian tissue after cytotoxic chemotherapy.

can also be used prior to pelvic irradiation in other diseases, including lymphoma. This procedure can be done by either laparotomy or laparoscopy with the intent of preventing radiation- but not chemotherapy-induced ovarian failure. Assisted fertilization is often needed after this procedure.

Oocyte cryopreservation has been proposed as a means of preserving fertility in women treated for cancer, but it has been less successful in humans than it has in animal models. Cryopreservation and transplantation of ovarian tissue has also been proposed for patients before cancer treatment.

The ethical issues behind these techniques are still being disputed, and there is still the concern of potential disease recurrence from residual disease in autografted ovarian tissue; obtaining unilaminar follicles from cryopreserved, thawed tissue and growing them in vitro has been proposed to reduce this risk of recurrence. The cytotoxic effects of chemotherapeutic agents are seen more in rapidly dividing cells than in cells at rest, which led to the hypothesis that gonadotropin-releasing hormone agonists would suppress the hypothalamic-pituitary-ovary axis and make the ovaries less susceptible to the cytotoxic effects of chemotherapy. In animal models, therapy with gonadotropin-releasing–hormone agonists lowered cyclophosphamide-induced but not radiation-induced ovarian toxicity. Some studies have reported encouraging results of the use of this approach in women with breast cancer, leukemia, and lymphoma (68,69).

In premenopausal women with breast cancer treated with regimens based on cyclophosphamide, methotrexate, and fluorouracil (CMF), the rate of chemotherapy-related amenorrhea is 68% (70). Alkylating agents are non-cell-cycle–specific drugs and are generally highly gonadotoxic.

Mechlorethamine is usually used in combination with vincristine, procarbazine, and prednisone (MOPP), a highly gonadotoxic combination; this makes the exact contribution of mechlorethamine to the gonadotoxicity of MOPP difficult to evaluate.

Chlorambucil appears to have a dose-dependent gonadotoxic effect, with infrequent ovarian failure at cumulative doses of 236 mg/m² (71,72). Melphalan, busulfan, and cyclophosphamide also carry a high risk of ovarian damage. The estimated odds ratio for ovarian failure with alkylating agents is 3.98 (73).

Procarbazine is also a non-cell-cycle–specific agent. Data regarding its gonadotoxic effects when used alone are unavailable; however, when used in combination regimens for Hodgkin's disease, gonadal toxicity was higher with procarbazine (74).

The nitrosoureas lomustine and carmustine, whether used alone or in combination with other agents, have been implicated in gonadal failure in prepubescent patients treated for brain tumors. These patients, however, also underwent craniospinal radiation and procarbazine, making the role of these agents in ovarian failure less clear (75,76).

The extent of cisplatin toxicity in women is less well defined, with an odds ratio of 1.77 (73). Temporary amenorrhea developed in 2 of 12 female patients in whom cisplatin (0.4 to 0.6 g/m²) was used in combination with bleomycin and vinblastine to treat ovarian germ cell tumors; the amenorrhea lasted from 12 to 15 months after the cessation of chemotherapy.

Transient and permanent ovarian failure had been reported with etoposide (VP-16) use (77,78).

Antimetabolites are cell-cycle–specific and may exert few toxic effects on the ovaries. As a single agent, doxorubicin has few if any adverse effects on ovarian function, although a synergistic effect of the combination of doxorubicin and cyclophosphamide is a concern.

Vinblastine has been known to cause reversible and dose-related amenorrhea when combined with alkylating agents (79).

MALE GONADAL DISORDERS

Spermatogenesis occurs in a continuous cycle of meiosis, mitosis, differentiation, and maturation. Germ cells and spermatogonia, in contrast to Leydig or Sertoli cells, are sensitive to cytotoxic agents. If sufficient germ cells remain after cytotoxic chemotherapy, resumption of spermatogenesis usually occurs; the longer the duration of azoospermia, the lower the likelihood of spermatogenesis recovery (80).

Radiation damage to the gonads is dose-dependent (81). Low-dose testicular irradiation leads to a transient suppression of sperm counts, with a recovery time proportional to the radiation dose (82). Permanent infertility was reported after fractionated radiation doses of more than 2 Gy, whereas clinically significant Leydig cell impairment occurs rarely with doses of less than 20 Gy (Fig. 38-8A and B) (83).

Therapy with alkylating agents such as cyclophosphamide and chlorambucil used as monotherapy may result in reversible but prolonged azoospermia. Chlorambucil also causes azoospermia at cumulative doses of 400 to 800 mg; recovery may take 3 to 4 years after a mean total dose of about 750 mg/m² (84).

Cyclophosphamide affects spermatogenesis more than Leydig cell function, causing reduced sperm count with normal testosterone levels.

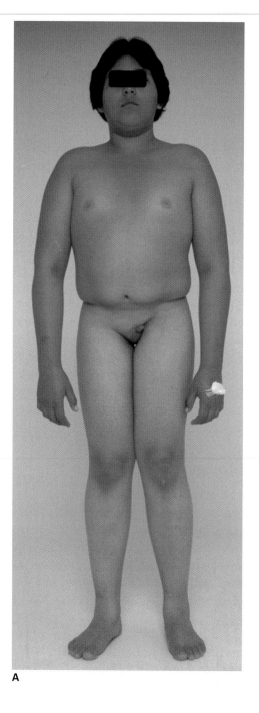

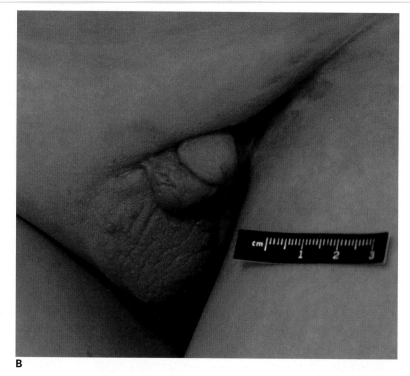

FIGURE 38-8 **A** and **B.** A young male patient after therapeutic irradiation to the left testicle for a testicular tumor. Note the loss of body hair, hypogonadal facial puffiness, decreased muscle mass, and increased body fat. The left testicle was small and firm. This patient was infertile.

A high rate of permanent testicular dysfunction has been reported with procarbazine use. Permanent sterility occurred in all 92 patients who received six or more cycles of cyclophosphamide, vincristine, procarbazine, and prednisone (85).

Dose-related impairment of spermatogenesis has been reported during testicular carcinoma treatment with cisplatin, etoposide, and bleomycin (PEB). Azoospermia was present in 19% of the patients who received a low-dose chemotherapeutic regimen (cisplatin 20 mg/m^2 × 5 every three weeks, etoposide 100 mg/m^2 × 5 every three weeks, and bleomycin 15 mg/m^2 every

week) compared with 47% of the high-dose–treated patients (cisplatin 40 mg/m^2 × 5 every 3 weeks, etoposide 200 mg/m^2 × 5 every three weeks, and bleomycin 15 mg/m^2 every week) (86). Only transient oligospermia was reported in 50% of patients treated with methotrexate plus leucovorin (87). The effect of doxorubicin as monotherapy on male gonadal function has not been well studied in humans, but in rats testicular toxicity can be detected at high doxorubicin doses (88). In patients with Hodgkin's disease treated with doxorubicin, bleomycin, vinblastine, and dacarbazine (ABVD), there was no evidence of long-term azoospermia (89). In patients with hairy cell leukemia, IFN seemed to have no significant effect on testicular function (90).

Multiple methods of preventing or reversing infertility in men treated for cancer have been suggested. In rats, fertility can be restored by suppressing testosterone with gonadotropin-releasing hormone (GnRH) agonists or antagonists, either before or after cytotoxic therapy. This approach does not protect the survival of the stem cells in the testes but enhances the ability of the testes to maintain the differentiation of the type A spermatogonia (91). It would be premature to apply this method to everyday clinical practice, as the limited data from human trials did not show this proposed benefit. Semen cryopreservation before starting gonadotoxic therapy followed by assisted fertilization is another strategy to preserve fertility in men with cancer.

In patients with Hodgkin's disease, different combination chemotherapies—including methotrexate, vincristine, prednisone, and procarbazine (MOPP); cyclophosphamide, vincristine, prednisone, and procarbazine (COPP); mechlorethamine, vinblastine, prednisolone, and procarbazine (MVPP); and a variety of combinations of chlorambucil, vinblastine, prednisolone plus procarbazine, doxorubicin, and vincristine plus etoposide (ChIVPP/EVA)—are known to cause substantial and considerable damage to gonadal function (92–94). Two different combinations—vincristine, epirubicin, etoposide, prednisolone (VEEP) and doxorubicin, bleomycin, vinblastine, and dacarbazine (ABVD)—are associated with much lower incidences of gonadal toxicity (95,96).

■ SURVEILLANCE FOR COMPLICATIONS IN CANCER SURVIVORS

Primary care physicians and oncologists should be aware of the major long-term consequences of cancer therapy for early detection and management. Long-term follow-up is, frequently, needed because many of these complications occur years after treatment and can have subtle clinical presentations.

For long-term cancer survivors who were treated with streptozocin, L-asparaginase, or partial pancreatectomy, screening for the delayed development of diabetes mellitus is recommended.

In children with a history of cranial irradiation or craniospinal irradiation, the growth rate should be assessed at 6-month intervals. A more detailed evaluation—including measurement levels of GH, insulin-like growth factor-1 (IGF-1), insulin-like growth factor binding protein 3, thyroid function tests, and bone-age assessments—should be performed where there is evidence of an abnormal growth pattern.

In adults who have undergone head and neck irradiation, clinical monitoring with measurement of serum IGF-1 (if the patient is a candidate for GH replacement) is appropriate, along with the measurement of serum testosterone levels and documentation of the menstrual history; this should be undertaken annually for 5 years and then at 5-year intervals for another 10 years.

If there is clinical suspicion of partial or complete pituitary failure in patients who have undergone total-body or head and neck irradiation, a thorough evaluation of pituitary-hypothalamic function—including assessment of GH levels, thyroid function, and the adrenal and gonadal axes—is appropriate. Dynamic testing may be performed to confirm hormone deficiencies prior to the initiation of replacement therapy. This detailed evaluation can be repeated in the future when there is a clinical presentation of radiation-related hormonal abnormality.

In children who have undergone either cranial or neck irradiation, T4 and TSH measurements should be performed annually for the first 5 years and every 2 years thereafter. Careful physical examination should be performed annually to detect thyroid nodules; if any are detected, a more detailed examination should be performed using ultrasound and, if necessary, fine-needle aspiration biopsy.

In survivors of childhood malignancies, bone mass may assessed in the early 30s, an age at which peak bone mass has been attained in most people. If bone mass is normal, no further evaluation is needed beyond the usual recommendations for prevention of osteoporosis.

It is also important to consider the possibility of bone loss in androgen- or estrogen-deficient adults. In those with low bone mass, an active program of calcium and vitamin D supplementation, exercise, and occasionally, medical therapy (bisphosphonates or recombinant parathyroid hormone) should be combined with assessment of bone mass every 12 to 18 months.

Patients who have been treated with chemotherapeutic agents that cause hypophosphatemia, hypomagnesemia, or hypocalcemia—such as ifosfamide, platinum compounds, fludarabine, or estramustine—are particularly at risk for osteomalacia and should undergo an evaluation of serum calcium, phosphorus, magnesium, alkaline phosphatase, and vitamin D metabolites levels.

Patients who have been treated with aromatase inhibitors should have their bone mineral density measured before and during treatment and should be given calcium and vitamin D. Patients can be given bisphosphonates if deemed necessary.

References

1. Avramis VI, Sencer S, Periclou AP, et al. A randomized comparison of native Escherichia coli asparaginase and polyethylene glycol conjugated asparaginase for treatment of children with newly diagnosed standard-risk acute lymphoblastic leukemia: A Children's Cancer Group study. *Blood* 2002;99(6): 1986–1994.

2. Whitecar JP Jr, Bodey GP, Harris JE, Freireich EJ. L-asparaginase. *N Engl J Med* 1970;282(13):732–734.

3. Whitecar JP Jr, Bodey GP, Hill CS Jr, Samaan NA. Effect of L-asparaginase on carbohydrate metabolism. *Metabolism* 1970;19(8):581–586.

4. Gillette PC, Hill LL, Starling KA, Fernbach DJ. Transient diabetes mellitus secondary to L-asparaginase therapy in acute leukemia. *J Pediatr* 1972;81(1):109–111.

5. Land VJ, Sutow WW, Fernbach DJ, et al. Toxicity of L-asparginase in children with advanced leukemia. *Cancer* 1972;30(2):339–347.

6. Sadoff L. Patterns of intravenous glucose tolerance and insulin response before and after treatment with streptozotocin (NSC-85998) in patients with cancer. *Cancer Chemother Rep* 1972; 56(1):61–69.

7. Schein PS, O'Connell MJ, Blom J, et al. Clinical antitumor activity and toxicity of streptozotocin (NSC-85998). *Cancer* 1974;34(4):993–1000.

8. Broder LE, Carter SK. Pancreatic islet cell carcinoma. II. Results of therapy with streptozotocin in 52 patients. *Ann Intern Med* 1973;79(1):108–118.

9. Okanoue T, Sakamoto S, Itoh Y, et al. Side effects of high-dose interferon therapy for chronic hepatitis C. *J Hepatol* 1996;25(3):283–291.

10. Guerci AP, Guerci B, Levy-Marchal C, et al. Onset of insulin-dependent diabetes mellitus after interferon-alfa therapy for hairy cell leukaemia. *Lancet* 1994;343(8906):1167–1168.

11. Murakami M, Iriuchijima T, Mori M. Diabetes mellitus and interferon-alpha therapy. *Ann Intern Med* 1995;123(4):318.

12. Imagawa A, Itoh N, Hanafusa T, et al. Autoimmune endocrine disease induced by recombinant interferon-alpha therapy for chronic active type C hepatitis. *J Clin Endocrinol Metab* 1995;80(3):922–926.

13. Rhodes CJ, Taylor KW. Effect of human lymphoblastoid interferon on insulin synthesis and secretion in isolated human pancreatic islets. *Diabetologia* 1984;27(6):601–603.

14. Brod SA, Atkinson M, Lavis VR, et al. Ingested IFN-alpha preserves residual beta cell function in type 1 diabetes. *J Interferon Cytokine Res* 2001;21(12):1021–1030.

15. Berruti A, Gorzegno G, Vitetta G, et al. Hypertriglyceridemia during long-term interferon-alpha therapy: Efficacy of diet and gemfibrosil treatment. A case report. *Tumori* 1992;78(5): 353–355.

16. Fujiwara H, Umeda Y, Yonekura S. Cerebellar infarction with hypertriglyceridemia during all-trans retinoic acid therapy for acute promyelocytic leukemia. *Leukemia* 1995;9(9): 1602–1603.

17. Vahlquist C. Effects of retinoids on lipoprotein metabolism. *Curr Probl Dermatol* 1991;20:73–78.

18. Kanamaru A, Takemoto Y, Tanimoto M, et al. All-trans retinoic acid for the treatment of newly diagnosed acute promyelocytic leukemia. Japan Adult Leukemia Study Group. *Blood* 1995;85(5):1202–1206.

19. Castaigne S, Chomienne C, Daniel MT, et al. All-trans retinoic acid as a differentiation therapy for acute promyelocytic leukemia. I. Clinical results. *Blood* 1990;76(9):1704–1709.

20. Marsden J. Hyperlipidaemia due to isotretinoin and etretinate: Possible mechanisms and consequences. *Br J Dermatol* 1986; 114(4):401–407.

21. Duvic M, Hymes K, Heald P, et al. Bexarotene is effective and safe for treatment of refractory advanced-stage cutaneous T-cell lymphoma: Multinational phase II–III trial results. *J Clin Oncol* 2001;19(9):2456–2471.

22. Duvic M, Martin AG, Kim Y, et al. Phase 2 and 3 clinical trial of oral bexarotene (Targretin capsules) for the treatment of refractory or persistent early-stage cutaneous T-cell lymphoma. *Arch Dermatol* 2001;137(5):581–593.

23. Vassilopoulou-Sellin R, Samaan NA. Mitotane administration: An unusual cause of hypercholesterolemia. *Horm Metab Res* 1991;23(12):619–620.

24. Raghavan D, Cox K, Childs A, et al. Hypercholesterolemia after chemotherapy for testis cancer. *J Clin Oncol* 1992;10(9): 1386–1389.

25. D'Angelo P, Conter V, Di Chiara G, et al. Severe osteoporosis and multiple vertebral collapses in a child during treatment for B-ALL. *Acta Haematol* 1993;89(1):38–42.

26. Baum M, Budzar AU, Cuzick J, et al. Anastrozole alone or in combination with tamoxifen versus tamoxifen alone for adjuvant treatment of postmenopausal women with early breast cancer: First results of the ATAC randomised trial. *Lancet* 2002;359(9324):2131–2139.

27. Seufert J, Ebert K, Muller J, et al. Octreotide therapy for tumor-induced osteomalacia. *N Engl J Med* 2001;345(26): 1883–1888.

28. Paglia F, Dionisi S, Minisola S. Octreotide for tumor-induced osteomalacia. *N Engl J Med* 2002;346(22):1748–1749; author reply 1748–1749.

29. Vassilopoulou-Sellin R, Newman BM, Taylor SH, Guinee VF. Incidence of hypercalcemia in patients with malignancy referred to a comprehensive cancer center. *Cancer* 1993;71(4): 1309–1312.

30. Sakamoto O, Yoshinari M, Rikiishi T, et al. Hypercalcemia due to all-trans retinoic acid therapy for acute promyelocytic leukemia: A case report of effective treatment with bisphosphonate. *Pediatr Int* 2001;43(6):688–690.

31. Miller VA, Benedetti FM, Rigas JR, et al. Initial clinical trial of a selective retinoid X receptor ligand, LGD1069. *J Clin Oncol* 1997;15(2):790–795.

32. Jones SG, Dolan G, Lengyel K, Myers B. Severe increase in creatinine with hypocalcaemia in thalidomide-treated myeloma patients receiving zoledronic acid infusions. *Br J Haematol* 2002;119(2):576–577.

33. English MW, Skinner R, Pearson AD, et al. Dose-related nephrotoxicity of carboplatin in children. *Br J Cancer* 1999; 81(2):336–341.

34. Grothey A. Oxaliplatin-safety profile: Neurotoxicity. *Semin Oncol* 2003;30(4 suppl 15):5–13.

35. Extra JM, Espie M, Calvo F, et al. Phase I study of oxaliplatin in patients with advanced cancer. *Cancer Chemother Pharmacol* 1990;25(4):299–303.

36. Shalet SM, Clayton PE, Price DA. Growth and pituitary function in children treated for brain tumours or acute lymphoblastic leukaemia. *Horm Res* 1988;30(2–3):53–61.

37. Abs R, Verhelst J, Maeyaert J, et al. Endocrine consequences of long-term intrathecal administration of opioids. *J Clin Endocrinol Metab* 2000;85(6):2215–2222.

38. Ogilvy-Stuart AL, Shalet SM, Gattamaneni HR. Thyroid function after treatment of brain tumors in children. *J Pediatr* 1991;119(5):733–737.

39. Sherman SI, Gopal J, Haugen BR, et al. Central hypothyroidism associated with retinoid X receptor–selective ligands. *N Engl J Med* 1999;340(14):1075–1079.

40. Sherman SI. Etiology, diagnosis, and treatment recommendations for central hypothyroidism associated with bexarotene therapy for cutaneous T-cell lymphoma. *Clin Lymph* 2003;3(4):249–252.

41. Pai HH, Thornton A, Katznelson L, et al. Hypothalamic/pituitary function following high-dose conformal radiotherapy to the base of skull: Demonstration of a dose-effect relationship using dose-volume histogram analysis. *Int J Radiat Oncol Biol Phys* 2001;49(4):1079–1092.

42. Samaan NA, Schultz PN, Yang KP, et al. Endocrine complications after radiotherapy for tumors of the head and neck. *J Lab Clin Med* 1987;109(3):364–372.

43. Rajagopal A, Vassilopoulou-Sellin R, Palmer JL, et al. Hypogonadism and sexual dysfunction in male cancer survivors receiving chronic opioid therapy. *J Pain Symptom Mgt* 2003;26(5):1055–1061.

44. Nikiforov YE. RET/PTC rearrangement in thyroid tumors. *Endocr Pathol* 2002;13(1):3–16.

45. Ron E, Lubin JH, Shore RE, et al. Thyroid cancer after exposure to external radiation: A pooled analysis of seven studies. *Radiat Res* 1995;141(3):259–277.

46. Samaan NA, Schultz PN, Ordonez NG, et al. A comparison of thyroid carcinoma in those who have and have not had head and neck irradiation in childhood. *J Clin Endocrinol Metab* 1987;64(2):219–223.

47. Tucker MA, Jones PH, Boice JD Jr, et al. Therapeutic radiation at a young age is linked to secondary thyroid cancer. The Late Effects Study Group. *Cancer Res* 1991;51(11):2885–2888.

48. Prummel MF, Laurberg P. Interferon-alpha and autoimmune thyroid disease. *Thyroid* 2003;13(6):547–551.

49. Wong V, Fu AX, George J, Cheung NW. Thyrotoxicosis induced by alpha-interferon therapy in chronic viral hepatitis. *Clin Endocrinol (Oxf)* 2002;56(6):793–798.

50. Vialettes B, Guillerand MA, Viens P, et al. Incidence rate and risk factors for thyroid dysfunction during recombinant interleukin-2 therapy in advanced malignancies. *Acta Endocrinol (Copenh)* 1993;129(1):31–38.

51. Hancock SL, Cox RS, McDougall IR. Thyroid diseases after treatment of Hodgkin's disease. *N Engl J Med* 1991;325(9):599–605.

52. Smith RE Jr, Adler AR, Clark P, et al. Thyroid function after mantle irradiation in Hodgkin's disease. *JAMA* 1981;245(1):46–49.

53. Dalgard O, Bjoro K, Hellum K, et al. Thyroid dysfunction during treatment of chronic hepatitis C with interferon alpha: No association with either interferon dosage or efficacy of therapy. *J Intern Med* 2002;251(5):400–406.

54. Krouse RS, Royal RE, Heywood G, et al. Thyroid dysfunction in 281 patients with metastatic melanoma or renal carcinoma treated with interleukin-2 alone. *J Immunother Emphasis Tumor Immunol* 1995;18(4):272–278.

55. Stuart NS, Woodroffe CM, Grundy R, Cullen MH. Long-term toxicity of chemotherapy for testicular cancer—The cost of cure. *Br J Cancer* 1990;61(3):479–484.

56. Bajetta E, Zilembo N, Dowsett M, et al. Double-blind, randomised, multicentre endocrine trial comparing two letrozole doses, in postmenopausal breast cancer patients. *Eur J Cancer* 1999;35(2):208–213.

57. Garnick MB, Larsen PR. Acute deficiency of thyroxine-binding globulin during L-asparaginase therapy. *N Engl J Med* 1979;301(5):252–253.

58. Heidemann PH, Stubbe P, Beck W. Transient secondary hypothyroidism and thyroxine binding globulin deficiency in leukemic children during polychemotherapy: An effect of L-asparaginase. *Eur J Pediatr* 1981;136(3):291–295.

59. Beex L, Ross A, Smals A, Kloppenborg P. 5-fluorouracil-induced increase of total serum thyroxine and triiodothyronine. *Cancer Treat Rep* 1977;61(7):1291–1295.

60. van Seters AP, Moolenaar AJ. Mitotane increases the blood levels of hormone-binding proteins. *Acta Endocrinol (Copenh)* 1991;124(5):526–533.

61. Vivacqua RJ, Haurani FI, Erslev AJ. "Selective" pituitary insufficiency secondary to busulfan. *Ann Intern Med* 1967;67(2):380–387.

62. Meacham LR, Mazewski C, Krawiecki N. Mechanism of transient adrenal insufficiency with megestrol acetate treatment of cachexia in children with cancer. *J Pediatr Hematol Oncol* 2003;25(5):414–417.

63. Raedler TJ, Jahn H, Goedeken B, et al. Acute effects of megestrol on the hypothalamic-pituitary-adrenal axis. *Cancer Chemother Pharmacol* 2003;52(6):482–486.

64. Lushbaugh CC, Casarett GW. The effects of gonadal irradiation in clinical radiation therapy: A review. *Cancer* 1976;37(2 suppl):1111–1125.

65. Howard GC. Fertility following cancer therapy. *Clin Oncol (R Coll Radiol)* 1991;3(5):283–287.

66. Thibaud E, Rodriguez-Macias K, Trivin C, et al. Ovarian function after bone marrow transplantation during childhood. *Bone Marrow Transplant* 1998;21(3):287–290.

67. Morice P, Juncker L, Rey A, et al. Ovarian transposition for patients with cervical carcinoma treated by radiosurgical combination. *Fertil Steril* 2000;74(4):743–748.

68. Recchia F, Sica G, De Filippis S, et al. Goserelin as ovarian protection in the adjuvant treatment of premenopausal breast cancer: A phase II pilot study. *Anticancer Drugs* 2002;13(4):417–424.

69. Blumenfeld Z. Ovarian rescue/protection from chemotherapeutic agents. *J Soc Gynecol Invest* 2001;8(1 suppl proc):S60–S64.

70. Bines J, Oleske DM, Cobleigh MA. Ovarian function in premenopausal women treated with adjuvant chemotherapy for breast cancer. *J Clin Oncol* 1996;14(5):1718–1729.

71. Freckman HA, Fry HL, Mendez FL, Maurer ER. Chlorambucil-prednisolone therapy for disseminated breast carcinoma. *JAMA* 1964;189:23–26.

72. Ezdinli EZ, Stutzman L. Chlorambucil therapy for lymphomas and chronic lymphocytic leukemia. *JAMA* 1965;191:444–450.

73. Meirow D, Nugent D. The effects of radiotherapy and chemotherapy on female reproduction. *Hum Reprod Update* 2001;7(6):535–543.

74. Bokemeyer C, Schmoll HJ, van Rhee J, et al. Long-term gonadal toxicity after therapy for Hodgkin's and non-Hodgkin's lymphoma. *Ann Hematol* 1994;68(3):105–110.

75. Ahmed SR, Shalet SM, Campbell RH, Deakin DP. Primary gonadal damage following treatment of brain tumors in childhood. *J Pediatr* 1983;103(4):562–565.

76. Clayton PE, Shalet SM, Price DA, Jones PH. Ovarian function following chemotherapy for childhood brain tumours. *Med Pediatr Oncol* 1989;17(2):92–96.

77. Choo YC, Chan SY, Wong LC, Ma HK. Ovarian dysfunction in patients with gestational trophoblastic neoplasia treated with short intensive courses of etoposide (VP-16-213). *Cancer* 1985;55(10):2348–2352.

78. Wong LC, Choo YC, Ma HK. Primary oral etoposide therapy in gestational trophoblastic disease. An update. *Cancer* 1986; 58(1):14–17.

79. Morgenfeld MC, Goldberg V, Parisier H, et al. Ovarian lesions due to cytostatic agents during the treatment of Hodgkin's disease. *Surg Gynecol Obstet* 1972;134(5):826–828.

80. Meistrich ML, Wilson G, Brown BW, et al. Impact of cyclophosphamide on long-term reduction in sperm count in men treated with combination chemotherapy for Ewing and soft tissue sarcomas. *Cancer* 1992;70(11):2703–2712.

81. Rowley MJ, Leach DR, Warner GA, Heller CG. Effect of graded doses of ionizing radiation on the human testis. *Radiat Res* 1974;59(3):665–678.

82. Clifton DK, Bremner WJ. The effect of testicular x-irradiation on spermatogenesis in man. A comparison with the mouse. *J Androl* 1983;4(6):387–392.

83. Howell SJ, Shalet SM. Effect of cancer therapy on pituitary-testicular axis. *Int J Androl* 2002;25(5):269–276.

84. Cheviakoff S, Calamera JC, Morgenfeld M, Mancini RE. Recovery of spermatogenesis in patients with lymphoma after treatment with chlorambucil. *J Reprod Fertil* 1973;33(1):155–157.

85. Charak BS, Gupta R, Mandrekar P, et al. Testicular dysfunction after cyclophosphamide-vincristine-procarbazine-prednisolone chemotherapy for advanced Hodgkin's disease. A long-term follow-up study. *Cancer* 1990;65(9):1903–1906.

86. Petersen PM, Hansen SW, Giwercman A, et al. Dose-dependent impairment of testicular function in patients treated with cisplatin-based chemotherapy for germ cell cancer. *Ann Oncol* 1994;5(4):355–358.

87. Shamberger RC, Rosenberg SA, Seipp CA, Sherins RJ. Effects of high-dose methotrexate and vincristine on ovarian and testicular functions in patients undergoing postoperative adjuvant treatment of osteosarcoma. *Cancer Treat Rep* 1981;65(9–10):739–746.

88. Adachi T, Nishimura T, Imahie H, Yamamura T. Collaborative work to evaluate toxicity on male reproductive organs by repeated dose studies in rats 9). Testicular toxicity in male rats given Adriamycin for two or four weeks. *J Toxicol Sci* 2000; 25(spec no):95–101.

89. Bonadonna G, Santoro A, Viviani S, et al. Gonadal damage in Hodgkin's disease from cancer chemotherapeutic regimens. *Arch Toxicol Suppl* 1984;7:140–145.

90. Schilsky RL, Davidson HS, Magid D, et al. Gonadal and sexual function in male patients with hairy cell leukemia: Lack of adverse effects of recombinant alpha 2-interferon treatment. *Cancer Treat Rep* 1987;71(2):179–181.

91. Meistrich ML, Shetty G. Suppression of testosterone stimulates recovery of spermatogenesis after cancer treatment. *Int J Androl* 2003;26(3):141–146.

92. Whitehead E, Shalet SM, Blackledge G, et al. The effects of Hodgkin's disease and combination chemotherapy on gonadal function in the adult male. *Cancer* 1982;49(3):418–422.

93. Clark ST, Radford JA, Crowther D, et al. Gonadal function following chemotherapy for Hodgkin's disease: A comparative study of MVPP and a seven-drug hybrid regimen. *J Clin Oncol* 1995;13(1):134–139.

94. Shafford EA, Kingston JE, Malpas JS, et al. Testicular function following the treatment of Hodgkin's disease in childhood. *Br J Cancer* 1993;68(6):1199–1204.

95. Hill M, Milan S, Cunningham D, et al. Evaluation of the efficacy of the VEEP regimen in adult Hodgkin's disease with assessment of gonadal and cardiac toxicity. *J Clin Oncol* 1995; 13(2):387–395.

96. Viviani S, Santoro A, Ragni G, et al. Gonadal toxicity after combination chemotherapy for Hodgkin's disease. Comparative results of MOPP vs ABVD. *Eur J Cancer Clin Oncol* 1985;21(5):601–605.

97. Lam KS, Tse VK, Wang C, et al. Effects of cranial irradiation on hypothalamic-pituitary function—A 5-year longitudinal study in patients with nasopharyngeal carcinoma. *Q J Med* 1991;78(286):165–176.

CHAPTER
39

ONCOLOGIC EMERGENCIES

Stephanie B. Mundy
Ellen Manzullo

Oncologic emergencies can result from either the cancer or its treatment. Whereas the patient without cancer commonly presents in an emergency setting with one chief complaint, cancer patients are often immunocompromised, have metabolic and hematologic defects, and can have more than one source for their complaints. In addition, certain emergencies occur predominantly in cancer patients. It is important for practitioners who treat patients with cancer to be aware of the various oncologic emergencies that might arise so that they can be recognized and treated promptly. This chapter discusses many of these emergencies, including their signs and symptoms, causes, and management.

■ NEUROLOGIC EMERGENCIES

SPINAL CORD COMPRESSION

Spinal cord compression is a serious complication of cancer progression, affecting 5 to 10% of cancer patients (1–4). It is not immediately life-threatening unless it involves vertebra C3 or above but can otherwise lead to significant morbidity (2). The spinal cord is compressed at the thoracic vertebrae in 70% of patients, cervical vertebrae in 10% of patients, and lumbar vertebrae in 20% of patients (5). In 10 to 38% of cases, spinal cord compression occurs at multiple levels (6). Such compression is predominantly due to metastatic tumors, with lung, breast, and prostate cancer comprising 50% of these (7). Other tumors that commonly metastasize to the spine are multiple myeloma, renal cell carcinoma, melanoma, lymphoma, sarcoma, and gastrointestinal cancers (3,7). The mechanisms by which tumors can appear in the spine are hematogenous spread of tumor cells to the vertebral bodies, metastasis of primary lesions to the posterior spinal elements, and direct extension of paraspinal tumors (4). Spinal cord compression is caused by epidural metastases in 75% and bony collapse in 25% of cases (8).

The most common presentation of spinal cord compression is back pain, occurring in 90 to 96% of patients (2,6,7). Compression at the level of the lumbar and cervical vertebrae can cause unilateral radicular pain. Tumor involvement at the level of the thoracic vertebrae can cause bilateral pain (3). In particular, pain from compression at the level of the thoracic vertebrae usually produces a band-like sensation around the patient's chest or abdomen, whereas pain from the cervical and lumbar levels usually radiates down the respective dermatomes (6). Patients typically report that their pain is worse when they are recumbent and better when they are standing. Some patients present with ataxia, which is due to compression of the spinocerebellar tracts. Ataxia can be confused with cerebellar metastasis, overmedication with analgesics, or other disorders. Metastasis to the spinal cord can precede spinal cord compression by weeks or months. The patient may also note sensory symptoms, including numbness or tingling in the toes, which can progress proximally. Preexisting peripheral neuropathy must be differentiated from spinal cord compression due to tumor, and the patient should be asked if he or she has experienced any new numbness

or tingling. Motor symptoms are the second most common complaint after pain; difficulty walking, buckling under of the legs, and a feeling of heaviness in the legs are all frequent symptoms. In this case, compression of the spinal cord must be distinguished from dehydration, anemia, and orthostatic hypotension. The last symptoms to appear are autonomic symptoms, such as an inability to urinate, urinary retention, and constipation. Autonomic symptoms are late findings in spinal cord compression and must be distinguished from the effects of chemotherapy, pain medicines, and antihistamines (7). It is important to remember that the patient may present with intractable pain only, so a high level of suspicion for spinal cord compression is important in treating cancer patients.

The physical examination usually reveals tenderness to percussion over the affected level of the spine, but the spine might not be tender if there is no bone involvement (9). Other possible findings are urinary retention, decreased rectal sphincter tone, and muscle weakness. The patient might have pain at a referred site; for instance, patients with L1 compression might have pain in the sacroiliac area. Sensory effects are more difficult to diagnose than motor effects and can either precede or accompany motor effects. The patient might have decreased sensation in the lower extremities, which may ascend to the level of spinal cord involvement with dorsal column deficits, including loss of light touch sensation, proprioception, and position sense. When the cauda equina is compressed, the sensory changes are dermatomal, with loss of sensation in the perineal area, the posterior thigh, or lateral leg (6). The patient might also exhibit decreased deep tendon reflexes.

The diagnosis of spinal cord compression can be made from careful history taking, physical examination, and diagnostic imaging. The differential diagnosis of spinal cord compression includes osteoarthritis, degenerative disk disease, spinal abscess, bleeding, hemangioma, chordoma, meningioma, and neurofibroma. A standard x-ray is generally ordered first to analyze the area of the spine within which compression is suspected. However, simple roentgenography yields false-negative results in 10 to 17% of cases, in part because approximately 30 to 50% of the bone must be destroyed before bony lesions can be seen on x-ray films (4). If plain films or bone scans reveal abnormalities at the level from which the patient's symptoms seem to emanate, there is a 60% chance that the patient will have underlying epidural disease; the chance is even greater if these findings are coupled with vertebral collapse (1). Magnetic resonance imaging (MRI) is the imaging technique of choice today for suspected spinal cord compression (Fig. 39-1).

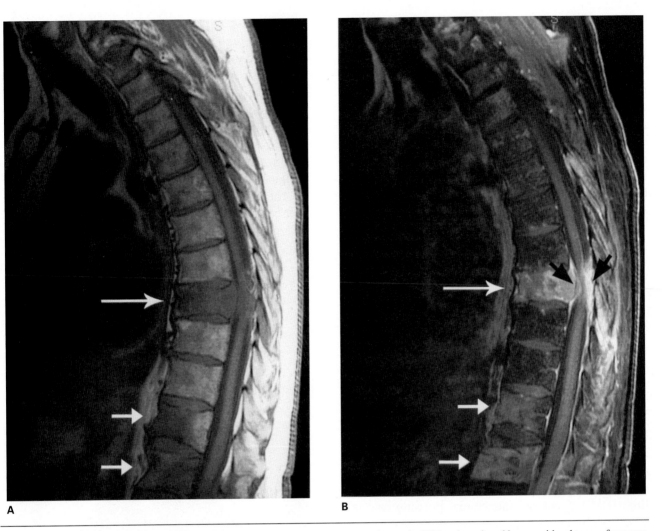

FIGURE 39-1   **A.** Pre-contrast T1-weighted MR image of thoracic cord compression at the T8 level produced by an epidural tumor from vertebral body metastasis (*large arrow*). Smaller arrows point to other sites of bony metastasis. The patient is a 67-year-old man with melanoma and back pain. **B.** Post-contrast T1-weighted MR image of the same patient. The epidural tumor is visualized better with contrast (*black arrows*). (*Images courtesy of Dr. Ashok Kumar, M.D. Anderson Cancer Center.*)

Previously, myelography was the "gold standard" in diagnosing spinal cord compression, but this technique is invasive, requires the use of intravenous dye, is time-consuming, and can be painful for the patient. Patients who are not able to undergo MRI can undergo computed tomography (CT) of the spine, although, like myelography, this technique is more time-consuming and tedious than MRI, requiring multiple images. Nevertheless, these options are available for use on patients who cannot tolerate MRI because of the presence of cerebral aneurysm clips, cardiac pacemakers, magnetic implants, or severe claustrophobia. For patients with suspected spinal cord compression, physicians should consider imaging the entire spine, as spinal cord compression is commonly multifocal. Findings for the whole spine can help the physician optimize the type and extent of therapy needed. For any patient with rapidly progres-sive neurologic symptoms, diagnostic imaging should be performed on an emergency basis.

Treatment of spinal cord compression includes the use of dexamethasone, initially 10 to 100 mg intravenously and then 4 to 24 mg every 4 h, with the dosages dependent on the degree of compression and the speed of neurologic deterioration (1–3,5,7,9). It is important to taper such high doses of steroids rapidly to prevent complications of steroid use. Surgery is indicated for patients who have already undergone maximal radiotherapy to the affected area of the spine, for progressive symptoms during radiotherapy, spine instability, an unknown diagnosis, or for bony compression of the spinal cord, as in the case of vertebral collapse (2,6). Currently, anterior decompression with spinal stabilization is the surgery of choice, allowing removal of the affected vertebral body and stabilization above and below the vertebrae by metal hardware. If surgery is not indicated, radiation therapy can be used; the most common dosage is 3000 cGy delivered in 10 fractions (6). The incidence of myelopathy, which can occur as a complication of radiation therapy, increases with increasing total dosage of therapy and can appear from months to several years after such therapy is given (1). Chemotherapy is occasionally used for chemosensitive tumors, such as those of Hodgkin's disease, neuroblastoma, non-Hodgkin's lymphoma, germ cell tumors, and breast cancer. Hormonal therapy can benefit some patients with hormone-responsive tumors, such as prostate and breast cancers (4).

One of the most important prognostic factors at diagnosis is the patient's neurologic function. Of patients who are ambulatory at the time of presentation, approximately three-fourths will be able to regain their strength with treatment. By contrast, only a small percentage of patients who are paralyzed at the time of presentation are likely to walk again (1). This difference illustrates why it is imperative to diagnose spinal cord compression at an early stage.

INCREASED INTRACRANIAL PRESSURE

Increased intracranial pressure in cancer patients is commonly due to hemorrhage (from thrombocytopenia or tumor bleeding), brain metastasis with cerebral edema, mass effect, or obstruction of the flow of cerebrospinal fluid (CSF). Increased intracranial pressure can also be caused by tumor treatments, such as radiation therapy and surgery. The normal CSF pressure is less than 10 mmHg. As intracranial pressure increases, herniation syndromes may develop, including uncal, central, and tonsillar herniation. Uncal herniation is caused by unilateral supratentorial lesions that push brain tissue through the tentorial notch. Signs and symptoms include ipsilateral pupil dilation, decreased consciousness, and hemiparesis, first contralateral and then ipsilateral to the mass. Central herniation involves bilateral supratentorial lesions that displace tissue symmetrically and bilaterally. Signs and symptoms of central herniation include decreased consciousness leading to coma and Cheyne-Stokes respiration, followed by central hyperventilation, midposition unreactive pupils, and posturing. Tonsillar herniation involves increased pressure in the posterior fossa, which forces the cerebellar tonsil through the foramen magnum, thereby compressing the medulla. Signs and symptoms of tonsillar herniation include decreased consciousness and respiratory abnormalities leading to apnea. Headache is the most frequent symptom reported in increased intracranial pressure. Headache is a common symptom in any patient popula-

tion, but in cancer patients the clinician must always maintain a high index of suspicion for increased intracranial pressure. Headaches due to increased intracranial pressure are typically present on waking in the morning, recur throughout the day, are increased with Valsalva maneuver; they can be associated with nausea and vomiting, altered mental status, vision changes, seizures, or focal neurologic deficits. On physical examination, the patient might have papilledema, focal neurologic deficits, or a decreased level of consciousness.

The diagnosis of increased intracranial pressure can be ascertained from CT scans of the brain. Noncontrast CT imaging of the brain is superior to MRI in detecting acute hemorrhage (Fig. 39-2).

CT scans with contrast will usually reveal cerebral metastasis and occasionally leptomeningeal disease. Contrast-enhanced MRI is more sensitive than CT in revealing cerebral neoplasms and metastases as small as 3 mm (Fig. 39-3), leptomeningeal disease (Fig. 39-4), and early strokes (Fig. 39-5). Lumbar puncture should

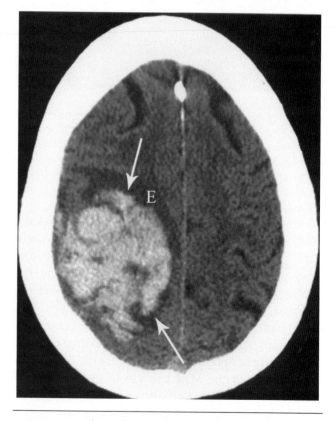

FIGURE 39-2 Acute intracranial hemorrhage within the right frontoparietal lobe (*arrows*) with edema (E) in a 79-year-old woman with ovarian cancer. The hemorrhage was revealed by noncontrast CT imaging. This modality is superior to MRI in detecting acute hemorrhage. (*Image courtesy of Dr. Ashok Kumar, M.D. Anderson Cancer Center.*)

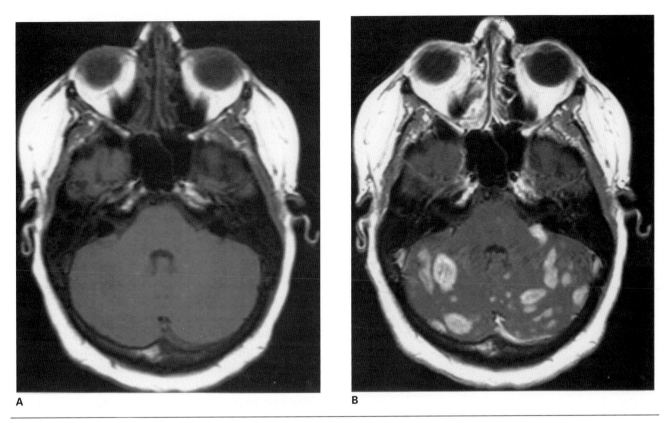

FIGURE 39-3 **A.** Pre-contrast T1 weighted MR images in a 40 year-old woman with breast cancer and multiple cerebellar metastases. **B.** Post-contrast images of the same patient reveal dramatic enhancement of the cerebellar metastases.

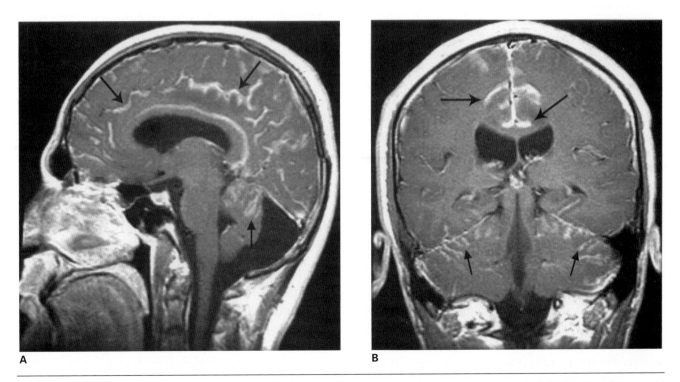

FIGURE 39-4 **A.** Sagittal postcontrast T1-weighted MRI showing subarachnoid spread of melanoma metastasis to the brain in a 29-year-old man. Abnormal enhancement of the cortical sulci (*large arrows*) and cerebellar sulci (*small arrows*) is noted. **B.** Coronal postcontrast T1-weighted MRI in the same patient. (*Images courtesy of Dr. Ashok Kumar, M.D. Anderson Cancer Center.*)

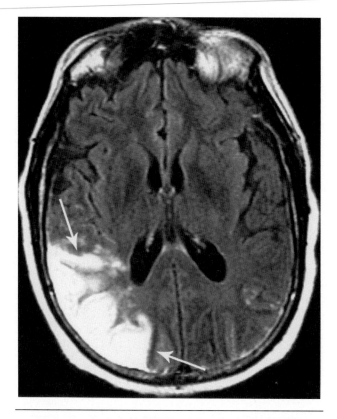

FIGURE 39-5 Acute infarction involving the territory of the right middle cerebral artery in a 58-year-old patient with renal cell carcinoma. MRI [fluid-attenuated inversion recovery (FLAIR) image] demonstrates abnormal thickening, with a T2–weighted increase in signal intensity (*arrows*) involving the right temporooccipital lobe cortex and subcortical white matter. MRI is more sensitive than CT in detecting early stroke. (*Image courtesy of Dr. Ashok Kumar, M.D. Anderson Cancer Center.*)

not be used to diagnose increased intracranial pressure, as this can lead to brain herniation.

The differential diagnosis of increased intracranial pressure includes bleeding, tumor edema, hydrocephalus, postradiation effects, postradiosurgery effects, brachytherapy-induced changes, benign tumor effects, subdural hematomas, meningitis, encephalitis, and abscess formation.

Brain metastases may develop in 10 to 40% of cancer patients (3,10). Previously, half the identified brain metastases were felt to be solitary lesions, but with increased use of MRI, which is more sensitive in detecting brain metastasis, two-thirds to three-quarters of brain metastases are recognized as multiple (3). Lung cancer is the neoplasm that most frequently metastasizes to the brain, followed by breast cancer and melanoma. Other cancers that commonly metastasize to the brain are colorectal, kidney, prostate, testicular, and ovarian cancers and sarcomas, although any systemic cancer can metastasize to the brain (11). Melanomas have the highest

propensity to metastasize to the brain, with up to 40% of cases behaving in this manner at some point (3). Cancers that commonly present as single metastatic lesions in the brain are kidney, colon, breast, thyroid, and adenocarcinoma of the lung, whereas melanoma and small cell cancer of the lung commonly present as multiple metastases (12). Tumors most commonly metastasize to the gray-white junction where the vessels are small and narrow and tumor emboli can be trapped. Eighty percent of tumors metastasize to the cerebral hemispheres, 15% to the cerebellum, and 5% to the brainstem (3). Pelvic tumors have an increased propensity to metastasize to the posterior fossa, possibly by means of venous drainage of these tumors through Batson's plexus (11). Metastatic brain tumors usually do not involve the corpus callosum, although malignant gliomas can (13). The tumors that are most often hemorrhagic include melanoma, renal cell carcinoma, and choriocarcinoma (12).

The treatment for increased intracranial pressure depends on the underlying etiology. Infectious sources, such as meningitis, should be treated with antibiotics, and brain abscesses should be drained. Hydrocephalus should be treated with surgical shunting or ventriculostomy, and subdural hematomas should be either drained or, if small, monitored under the guidance of a neurosurgeon. Edema associated with brain tumors is initially treated with oral dexamethasone at a dosage of 16 mg/day or 4 mg every 6 h (13,14). For patients with impending herniation, very large doses of intravenous dexamethasone can be used, initially 40 to 100 mg intravenously and subsequently 40 to 100 mg/day (6). Dexamethasone is the steroid of choice because of its lack of mineralocorticoid effect and therefore minimal effects on blood pressure, protein binding, and potential for infection. Steroid myopathy is a possible complication of corticosteroid use, which increases in incidence in chronically ill patients with low albumin levels and is due to higher than normal levels of unbound steroids. Dexamethasone is believed to decrease endothelial permeability and possibly have a stabilizing effect on the tumor, thereby decreasing edema (4,10). Steroids should not be used to treat asymptomatic brain lesions (15).

For life-threatening edema, mannitol can be used to decrease intracranial pressure in patients with an intact blood-brain barrier. Mannitol is a hyperosmotic agent that can draw fluid out of the brain and into the vessels; its effect can be augmented by the use of diuretics. The recommended dose of mannitol is a 20 to 25% solution at 0.5 to 2.0 g/kg administered intravenously over 10 to 30 min. Mannitol has a rapid onset of action and lasts for hours, but it can lead to hyperosmolarity and an inadvertent increase in intracranial pressure (6,9). Hyperventilation can be used to decrease intracranial pressure, but it must be kept within the modest range of a P_{CO_2} of 25 to 30 mmHg so as to prevent acidosis. The onset of action is immediate and its effect will last for several minutes (6).

Radiation therapy can be used to treat brain metastasis. The dosage for whole-brain radiation therapy (WBRT) typically ranges between 20 Gy over 1 week to 50 Gy over 4 weeks. WBRT can increase survival in patients by 3 to 6 months relative to no treatment (14). Asymptomatic brain lesions can also be treated except for metastases from renal cell cancer, which are often erratic and not treated until they become symptomatic (10). Increased intracranial pressure should be treated before WBRT is instituted, as radiotherapy can further increase pressure. Common side effects of WBRT are nausea and vomiting, alopecia, headache, hearing loss, loss of taste, and fever. Possible delayed complications of WBRT are progressive leukoencephalopathy with dementia, ataxia, apraxia, and incontinence syndrome, which can mimic normal-pressure hydrocephalus. This dreaded side effect can occur as much as 1 year after therapy, and elderly patients are more susceptible (12,13).

Surgery can be used to treat accessible brain metastases. A stereotactic biopsy can be performed for the patient with multiple brain metastases, which are then generally treated with radiation (16). Surgery is generally not indicated for patients with widespread systemic disease, poor functional status, or tumors in critical or hard-to-access locations (14,16). The experience at the University of Texas M.D. Anderson Cancer Center (MDACC) has been that for select patients with good functional status, even when multiple brain metastases are present, survival time is longer for those patients who have all tumors removed than for those who do not. Consequently, it is common for the neurosurgeons at our institution to remove up to four metastatic lesions at a time (15). Patchell and colleagues found that patients with single brain metastases who underwent WBRT after surgery had longer survival than those who had surgery alone (17).

For patients with brain lesions that are not amenable to surgery, stereotactic radiosurgery can be used in single doses as high as 1400 cGy. This approach is typically used for brain tumors less than 4 cm in diameter and has the benefit of being noninvasive and relatively fast-acting (3,4,13). Brachytherapy can be used on larger tumors, but this approach requires that radioactive seeds be invasively implanted in the designated area and left for 5 or 6 days, delivering approximately 6000 cGy to the area. One common side effect of brachytherapy is radiation necrosis, which develops in up to 50% of patients 6 months after treatment. This adverse effect can mimic tumor recurrence, is not distinguishable from tumor on MRI, and often requires biopsy to determine the etiology. Positron emission tomography (PET) scanning can be helpful, typically revealing decreased uptake in radiation necrosis and increased uptake in recurrent tumor. Radiation necrosis is not often found after stereotactic radiosurgery, perhaps because of the relatively small size of the irradiated area (13). No treatment exists for radiation necrosis, although the symptoms may respond to corticosteroids.

Chemotherapy can be used in some patients with brain metastasis. Dexamethasone, which is thought to aid in reestablishing the blood-brain barrier, should not be used if possible, so that the selected chemotherapeutic agent(s) can reach the tumor cells. Cancers for which chemotherapy has been used include choriocarcinoma, small cell cancer of the lung, and breast cancer (9,13,14,18).

LEPTOMENINGEAL DISEASE

Leptomeningeal disease (LMD) can involve invasion of the brain, the spinal parenchyma, the nerve roots, and blood vessels of the nervous system. The cancers that most commonly result in LMD are breast and lung cancer, melanoma, non-Hodgkin's lymphoma, and leukemia. Patients present with a variety of symptoms depending on the location of the leptomeninges affected, but they can include headache, altered mental status, cranial nerve palsies (in about 50% of patients), incontinence, back pain, sensory changes, seizures, isolated neurologic findings, and even a stroke-like presentation (1,4,19). Leptomeningeal metastases occur in 0.8 to 8% of all cases of cancer (4). The mechanism of LMD spread can be hematogenous, as in leukemias, by direct extension or bone marrow metastasis.

The diagnosis of LMD can be difficult to make. CT scans will occasionally be suggestive of LMD. MRI scanning has better sensitivity than CT for detecting LMD, including leptomeningeal enhancement, hydrocephalus, and cortical nodules. However, MRI results are not diagnostic (1). Inflammation of the meninges can also be found in cases of meningitis, trauma, infection, and hematoma formation (20). Lumbar puncture and evaluation of the CSF is the gold standard for diagnosing LMD, although multiple lumbar taps may be required to make the diagnosis, as only 50% of patients will have positive cytologic evidence of LMD on the first CSF evaluation (4,20). CSF findings consistent with LMD include a high opening pressure, low glucose and high protein levels, and a mononuclear pleocytosis (4). Among patients with normal values for CSF protein, glucose, opening pressure, and cytology negative for LMD, less than 5% will have LMD (20).

The treatment of LMD can include chemotherapy through an implanted subcutaneous reservoir and ventricular catheter (SRVC) or through lumbar puncture instillation. Lumbar tap administration does not require placement of a catheter, but 10 to 15% of the subarachnoid space might be missed using this technique. Chemotherapeutic agents frequently used are methotrexate and thiotepa. Cytarabine can also be used in patients with leukemias and lymphomas, but it is generally not effective against solid tumors. Radiation therapy is commonly used for localized LMD or in areas of nerve root involvement where intrathecal chemotherapy is not likely to reach adequate concentrations. Fixed neurologic deficits caused by LMD are not likely to improve

with therapy, but encephalopathy may (20). The prognosis of patients with LMD is very poor, with a median survival of 3 to 6 months and only a 15 to 25% chance of surviving more than 1 year (4).

SEIZURES

Seizures are the presenting symptom in 15 to 20% of patients with brain metastases (19). In cancer patients presenting with seizures, metabolic, infectious, and coagulopathic causes should also be considered. The initial laboratory work should include analysis of glucose level, electrolytes, blood urea nitrogen (BUN), creatinine, liver enzymes, calcium, urine analysis, prothrombin time (PT), activated partial thromboplastin time (PTT) and toxicology screening if indicated (Fig. 39-6) (21).

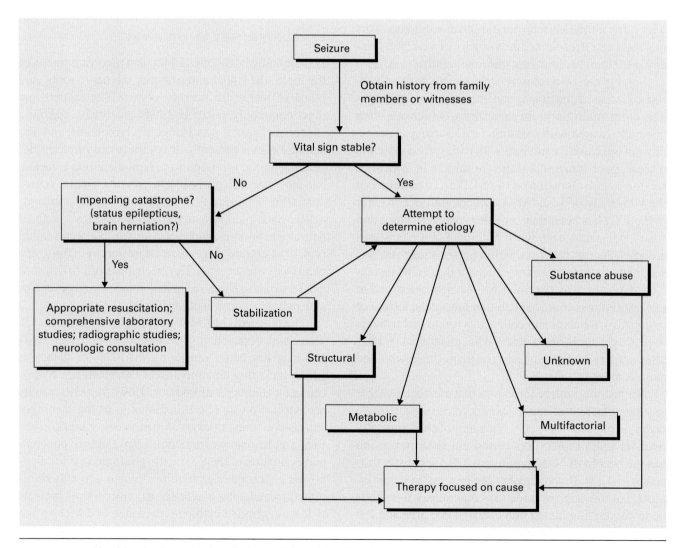

FIGURE 39-6 Algorithm for the evaluation of seizure. (*Adapted from Escalante CP, Hwang JP, Grover TS, et al. Major presenting symptoms. In: Yeung SJ, Escalante CP, eds.* Oncologic Emergencies. *Hamilton, Ontario, Canada: BC Decker; 2002, with permission.*)

Patients can have seizures during withdrawal from high-dose, short-acting benzodiazepines (such as alprazolam), alcohol withdrawal, antibiotics (such as the carbapenems), pain medicines (such as meperidine), and many other medicines. The patient's family can be helpful in sorting out the etiology of seizures by providing information about the patient's medications, social history, and preceding symptoms, such as fever or headache. CT without and with contrast is also helpful and can identify increased intracranial pressure, bleeding, or brain metastasis. Electroencephalography (EEG) is also helpful in the evaluation of seizures and can determine whether an epileptic focus is present. Lumbar tap can be helpful if the seizures are believed to be secondary to infection or LMD, but this procedure should not be performed in patients with suspected increased intracranial pressure because of the risk of cerebral herniation.

Status epilepticus occurs when a patient has prolonged seizures lasting more than 30 min or recurrent seizures without full recovery of consciousness between seizures (22). Initial care for patients with status epilepticus includes placing the patient in a safe environment, administering 100% oxygen by nonrebreather mask, monitoring with a continuous-pulse oximeter providing suction, and administering intravenous fluids (normal saline). Priority should be placed on protecting the airway and extinguishing the seizure, which can be treated initially with intravenous benzodiazepines (such as diazepam, 0.2 mg/kg at 5 mg/min, up to 10 mg, or lorazepam, 0.1 mg/kg at 2 mg/min, up to 4 mg). For persistent seizures, fosphenytoin or phenytoin can be administered intravenously. Fosphenytoin can be given more rapidly and causes less hypotension than phenytoin, but continuous cardiac and blood pressure monitoring should be instituted during intravenous administration of 15 to 20 mg phenytoin equivalents (PE) per kilogram. Patients with persistent seizures might require intubation and sedation with phenobarbital (20 mg/kg intravenously at 100 mg/min) or other agents, such as pentobarbital or a midazolam drip. At this point, the patient will require careful monitoring and intensive care unit (ICU) care.

It is the general consensus of the American Academy of Neurology that routine use of prophylactic antiepileptic drugs (AEDs) for patients with brain metastases who have not experienced a seizure is not indicated (16). In certain instances prophylactic AEDs should be considered, including cases of metastatic melanoma with more than one brain metastasis, brain metastases involving the motor cortex, and cases involving both brain metastases and LMD. These three conditions have a high propensity for seizure development (4,10,19,23). Prophylactic AEDs might also be considered for patients in whom the brain metastases and edema are so large that a seizure would increase intracranial pressure, predisposing the patient to cerebral herniation (13).

Once seizures have been controlled, the patient should be placed on an AED. Several drugs can be used, among them phenytoin, carbamazepine, clonazepam, gabapentin, lamotrigine, phenobarbital, primidone, topiramate, and valproate. For many of the newer AEDs, the appropriate serum levels are not monitored. For those medicines in which effective and safe levels have been defined, such as phenytoin, carbamazepine, phenobarbital, and valproate, the levels should be monitored carefully to limit toxic effects and maintain an effective preventive drug concentration.

ALTERED MENTAL STATUS

Altered mental status is a common neurologic complaint in cancer patients, with metabolic encephalopathy being the most common cause (1,12). Altered mental status can range from a slight decrease in normal intellectual functioning to coma. A cancer patient's mental status may change in response to several factors, such as infections, metabolic derangements, bleeding, medications, hypoxemia, cancer therapies, paraneoplastic neurologic syndromes, and intracranial events, such as brain metastases. Organ failure whether hepatic, renal, adrenal, thyroid, or pulmonary, can also produce fluctuations in mental status. The most common metabolic deficiencies causing such alterations are hyponatremia, hypercalcemia, hypoglycemia, and vitamin B_1 deficiency (1). The causes of altered mental status are numerous; an extensive history and physical examination can help to identify the underlying cause and determine appropriate therapy (Fig. 39-7) (21). The differential diagnosis and diagnostic evaluation are beyond the scope of this chapter, but a few entities are unique to cancer patients.

For instance, cancer therapy is a common cause of altered mental status. Many neurologic manifestations, such as dementia, cognitive decline, and encephalopathy, can result from chemotherapy. Table 39-1 highlights some of the common neurologic complications of chemotherapy (1,4,15,24).

Radiation therapy can also cause complications, among them leukoencephalopathy, radiation necrosis, and decreased memory and mental functioning. (The preceding section on increased intracranial pressure provides a fuller discussion of the cognitive side effects

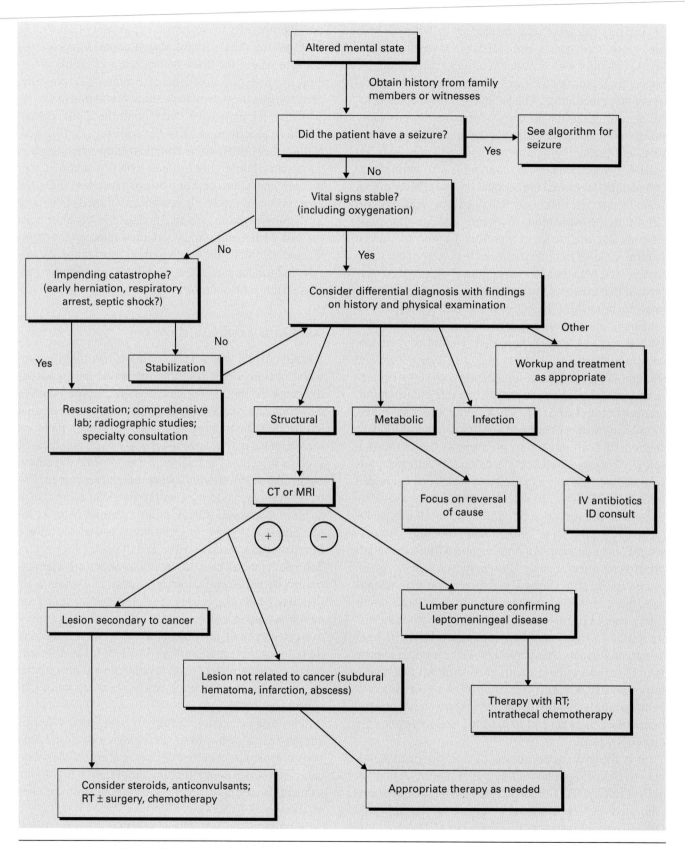

FIGURE 39-7 Algorithm for the evaluation and treatment of altered mental status. CT = computed tomography; ID = infectious disease; IV = intravenous; MRI = magnetic resonance imaging; RT= radiation therapy. (*Adapted from Escalante CP, Hwang JP, Grover TS, et al. Major presenting symptoms. In: Yeung SJ, Escalante CP, eds.* Oncologic Emergencies. *Hamilton, Ontario, Canada: BC Decker; 2002, with permission.*)

TABLE 39-1 | NEUROLOGIC COMPLICATIONS OF CHEMOTHERAPY

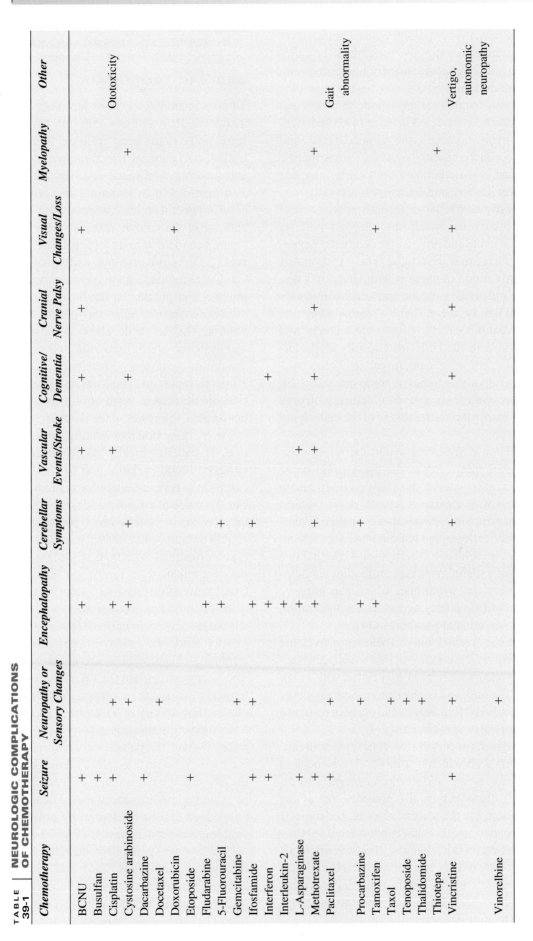

Chemotherapy	Seizure	Neuropathy or Sensory Changes	Encephalopathy	Cerebellar Symptoms	Vascular Events/Stroke	Cognitive/ Dementia	Cranial Nerve Palsy	Visual Changes/Loss	Myelopathy	Other
BCNU	+		+		+	+	+	+		
Busulfan	+									
Cisplatin	+	+	+		+					Ototoxicity
Cystosine arabinoside		+	+	+		+			+	
Dacarbazine	+									
Docetaxel		+								
Doxorubicin	+							+		
Etoposide										
Fludarabine			+							
5-Fluorouracil			+	+						
Gemcitabine		+								
Ifosfamide	+	+	+	+						
Interferon	+		+							
Interleukin-2			+			+				
L-Asparaginase	+		+		+					
Methotrexate	+	+	+	+	+	+	+		+	
Paclitaxel	+									Gait abnormality
Procarbazine		+	+	+						
Tamoxifen			+					+		
Taxol		+								
Tenoposide		+								
Thalidomide		+								
Thiotepa									+	
Vincristine	+	+		+		+	+	+		Vertigo, autonomic neuropathy
Vinorelbine		+								

of radiation therapy.) Other possible causes of cognitive decline are narcotics (commonly prescribed for pain), infections (pneumonia, sepsis, urinary tract infection), and cerebral infarction.

Paraneoplastic syndromes are unique to cancer patients and should be considered in cases of altered mental status. In many instances, the paraneoplastic syndrome will precede the cancer diagnosis. Paraneoplastic syndromes must be differentiated from cancer, the side effects of cancer therapy, and disease progression.

Paraneoplastic cerebellar degeneration is the most common paraneoplastic syndrome; affected patients present with subacute and progressive cerebellar degeneration with ataxia and dysarthria. This syndrome is most commonly found in patients with Hodgkin's disease, ovarian and breast cancers, and small cell cancer of the lung. It can be diagnosed by lumbar puncture, which can reveal pleocytosis, high protein levels, and oligoclonal bands in the CSF. MRI results might initially be normal, but later scans reveal cerebellar atrophy. Anti-Yo antibody is found in some patients' CSF and blood. This syndrome can be debilitating, with only some patients responding to treatment of the underlying tumor (4).

Lambert-Eaton myasthenic syndrome is an autoimmune disorder that involves the presynaptic nerve terminals and is associated with small cell lung cancer. Patients present with weakness, cranial nerve palsies, and autonomic symptoms. Physical examination reveals decreased tendon reflexes and muscle weakness, which, however, improves with use. Neurophysiologic findings and detection of anticholinesterase antibodies are helpful in diagnosing this syndrome, which can improve with treatment of the underlying cancer, administration of corticosteroids, and plasmapheresis (4).

Paraneoplastic opsoclonus-myoclonus syndrome presents as involuntary, erratic eye movements and saccades. This syndrome has been associated with small cell cancer of the lung and breast cancer. Some patients have anti-Ri antibody. Remissions can occur in response to cancer treatment or spontaneously (4).

Dermatomyositis occurs in 10% of patients with cancer. The cancers with which it is most often associated are lung, ovarian, breast, and stomach cancers. The diagnosis of this disorder typically precedes that of the underlying cancer, but the search for a cancer diagnosis in patients with dermatomyositis is not often revealing. Diagnosis is based on skin changes, elevation of creatinine phosphokinase (CPK), electromyelographic (EMG) changes, and muscle biopsy results revealing myositis. Dermatomyositis responds to treatment of the underlying tumor and to immunosuppressive drugs.

■ CARDIAC EMERGENCIES

CARDIAC TAMPONADE

Tumors involving the heart are much more frequently metastatic than primary. The tumors that most often metastasize to the heart are lung, breast, and gastrointestinal tract cancers, leukemia, lymphoma, melanoma, and sarcoma. Metastatic involvement of the heart has also been noted in leukemia and lymphoma patients (7). Certain therapies can also affect the myocardium and cause pericardial disease, especially cyclophosphamide and ifosfamide at high doses, all-*trans* retinoic acid (ATRA), doxorubicin, and radiation therapy (25). Cardiac tamponade occurs when pericardial fluid accumulates and presses on the heart, increasing diastolic pressure in the ventricles and thereby decreasing stroke volume. The patient develops decreased cardiac output and systemic arterial pressure and can present with a shock-like syndrome. Most patients with pericardial effusions report no symptoms, but patients with cardiac tamponade present with shortness of breath, cough, hoarseness, epigastric pain, or chest pain that is made worse by lying down or leaning forward. On examination, the patient typically has distended neck veins, low systemic blood pressure and low pulse pressure, and can have a pericardial rub or decreased heart sounds. The presence of pulsus paradoxus, which is an inspiratory decline in systolic blood pressure of >10 mmHg, should be ruled out. Pulsus paradoxus can also occur in chronic obstructive pulmonary disease (COPD), pulmonary embolism, right ventricular infarction, and shock. Chest x-ray often reveals a "water bottle" configuration if the effusion has accumulated slowly, but the cardiac silhouette can appear normal if the effusion accumulates rapidly. Prior chest x-ray images can be useful in determining changes in the size of the cardiac silhouette. The electrocardiogram (ECG) might reveal electrical alternans (a variation of voltage in individual QRS complexes), low-voltage or ST-segment and T-wave changes. Transthoracic echocardiography is the best test to determine whether tamponade exists. If cardiac tamponade is present, echocardiography can help determine whether the effusion is localized or loculated, and it can also aid in planning pericardiocentesis. On echocardiograms, tamponade can be evidenced by collapse of the right ventricle and atria in diastole (Fig. 39-8).

Treatment of tamponade includes the administration of oxygen, intravenous fluids, and vasopressors if necessary. Pericardiocentesis can be performed under ultrasound guidance and is relatively safe. Data collected from 1127 consecutive cases at the Mayo Clinic between

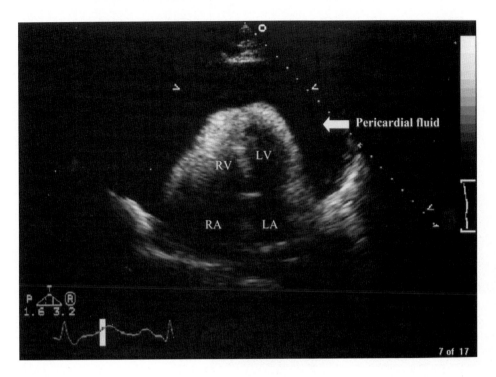

FIGURE 39-8 Two-dimensional echocardiogram in the apical four-chamber view demonstrating a large pericardial effusion. The right ventricle is not well visualized because of acoustic shadowing, which commonly occurs with large effusions. (*Image courtesy of Dr. Joseph Swafford, M.D. Anderson Cancer Center.*)

1979 and 2000 revealed a success rate of 97% and a complication rate of 4.7% in patients with significant pericardial effusions (26). At MDACC, a drainage catheter is commonly placed in patients with tamponade, with drainage performed daily. When the total volume of fluid drained is less than 50 mL/day, the catheter can be removed (27). A pericardial window can also be created to prevent reaccumulation of fluid. Radiation therapy and chemotherapy can also be used to prevent reaccumulation of fluid, as can sclerosis of the pericardial sac.

SUPERIOR VENA CAVA SYNDROME

Superior vena cava (SVC) syndrome is characterized by low blood flow from the SVC to the right atrium. Malignancy is by far the most common cause of SVC syndrome, although nonmalignant causes, such as indwelling central venous catheters, aneurysms, and goiters, can also cause this (2). Lung cancer is the most common malignant neoplasm causing SVC syndrome, but lymphoma, breast and gastrointestinal cancers, sarcomas, melanomas, prostate cancer, and any mediastinal tumor can also cause this disorder (28). Among mechanisms that can lead to this syndrome are extrinsic compression by tumor, intrinsic compression by tumor or clot, or fibrosis. Patients may present with headache; dizziness; confusion; swelling of the upper extremities, face, and neck; shortness of breath; and dysphagia. Physical examination often reveals engorgement of veins and collaterals in the upper extremities due to elevated pressure in the venous system.

Diagnosis of SVC syndrome requires imaging. Routine chest x-rays will often reveal mediastinal widening, a right-side chest mass, or a mediastinal mass. CT scanning of the chest using intravenous contrast is an excellent means of delineating the cause of the obstruction and any associated finding (Fig. 39-9). MRI, Doppler ultrasound, and radionuclide venography can be used to exclude the presence of a clot.

The treatment of SVC syndrome depends on the nature of the obstruction. Patients might respond to elevation of the head, corticosteroids if the intracranial pressure is increased, and occasionally diuretics. If thrombosis is present, local lytic therapy or anticoagulation can be used. It is important to obtain a tissue specimen of the tumor if its type is not known, so that it can be treated adequately. For patients with tumors that are chemosensitive, such as small cell lung cancer, chemotherapy can be instituted. Patients with non–small cell lung cancer will often respond to radiation therapy. Intravascular stenting with metallic stents can be used, as can angioplasty. Stent placement has been associated with a faster resolution of symptoms relative to radiation therapy (28,29) (Fig. 39-10).

MYOCARDIAL ISCHEMIA

Patients with cancer can present to the emergency center with myocardial ischemia. A full discussion of ischemic

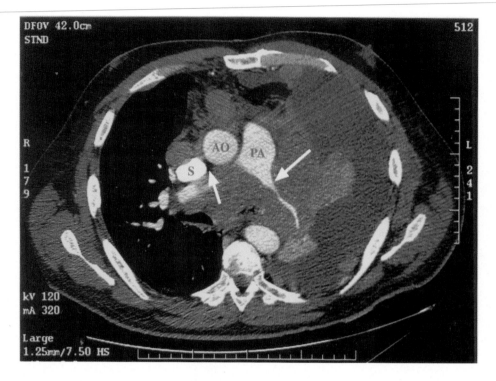

FIGURE 39-9 CT scan revealing superior vena cava (SVC) syndrome from extrinsic compression of the SVC in a patient with non–small cell lung cancer. Large arrow indicates compression of the left pulmonary artery; small arrow indicates obliteration of the right pulmonary artery. T = tumor; AO = aorta; S = superior vena cava; PA = main pulmonary artery. (*Image courtesy of Dr. Joel Dunnington, M.D. Anderson Cancer Center.*)

heart disease is beyond the scope of this chapter, but there are special considerations in cancer patients that should be mentioned.

Many cancer patients have thrombocytopenia due to chemotherapy, radiation therapy, or bone marrow infiltration with tumor. Despite platelet counts in the single or double digits, these patients can still present with acute cardiac syndrome. Although the practitioner might feel uncomfortable giving aspirin to these patients, cardiologists at MDACC have found that patients with platelet counts less than $50,000/\mu L$ who have cardiac ischemia and are treated with aspirin have a better 24-h survival rate than those patients who are not given aspirin (27).

Certain chemotherapeutic agents can predispose patients to myocardial ischemia, including 5-fluorouracil (5-FU), interferons, and presumably capecitabine, which is a metabolite of 5-FU. Radiation therapy can also be a predisposing factor (25). It is important to consider myocardial ischemia in patients who have undergone any of these therapies, especially those who otherwise have no risk factors for ischemic heart disease.

The cardiac markers troponin, CPK, and CPK-MB are useful in diagnosing myocardial infarction. Cardiac troponins are more sensitive and specific markers for ischemic heart disease than CPK-MB, which can be influenced by skeletal muscle injury; however, cardiac troponin levels can also be raised by chronic renal insufficiency (CRI), cardiomyopathy with severe congestive heart failure, myocarditis, and massive pulmonary embolism. In one small study evaluating 24 patients with submassive pulmonary embolism, troponin levels were higher than normal in five patients (30). In this study, those patients who presented with chest pain and for whom a ventilation/perfusion scan revealed a high probability of submassive pulmonary embolism were analyzed. High troponin was defined as a level $>0.4 \mu g/L$, and myocardial infarction was evidenced by a level $>2.3 \mu g/L$. It was found that 4 of the 5 patients with submassive pulmonary embolism had slightly elevated troponin levels and the fifth had a troponin level of 11.1 $\mu g/L$. The study was limited in that it did not investigate the possibility of underlying ischemia in patients with documented pulmonary embolism. Such patients commonly present with chest pain, and pulmonary embolism and ischemic heart disease are both in the differential diagnosis of myocardial infarction. In patients with small increases of troponin, pulmonary embolism (even submassive) can be the cause, rather than ischemic heart disease; this possibility should be considered in patients presenting with chest pain (30).

■ HEMATOLOGIC EMERGENCIES

HYPERVISCOSITY SYNDROME

Hyperviscosity syndrome is due to abnormally high concentrations of paraproteins in the serum, which increase viscosity and cause red blood cell (RBC) sludging and

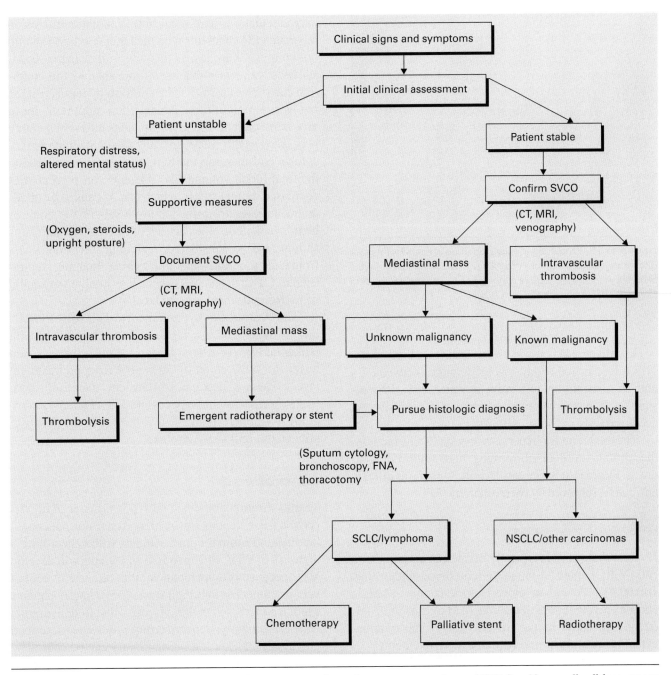

FIGURE 39-10   Algorithms for the diagnosis and management of superior vena cava syndrome. NSCLC = Non–small cell lung cancer; SCLC = small cell lung cancer; SVCO = superior vena cava obstruction. (*Adapted from Gao S, Shannon VR. Vascular emergencies. In: Yeung SJ, Escalante CP, eds.* Oncologic Emergencies. *Hamilton, Ontario, Canada: BC Decker; 2002, with permission.*)

low oxygen delivery to the tissues. This disorder occurs in 15% of patients with Waldenstrom's macroglobulinemia, which is characterized by the presence of high molecular-weight (IgM) macromolecules and thus predisposes patients to this syndrome. Aggregation of IgG macromolecules and polymerization of IgA macromolecules, as well as purely light-chain myeloma are also capable of causing this syndrome (31). Other conditions that can cause hyperviscosity syndrome are polycythemia vera, dysproteinemias, and occasionally leukemias.

Hyperviscosity syndrome can present with either bleeding due to abnormal platelet functioning or thrombosis due to hyperviscosity. Visual complaints, headache, dizziness, alterations in mental status, and mucosal bleeding are all symptoms of hyperviscosity syndrome. Patients can also develop retinal hemorrhages, congestive heart failure due to increased plasma volume, peripheral neuropathy, weakness, and fatigue (31). Funduscopic examination can reveal venous dilitation, retinal vein occlusion, or papilledema (Fig. 39-11).

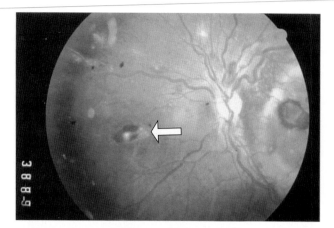

FIGURE 39-11 Funduscopic examination revealing a Roth's spot (the white-centered retinal hemorrhage). The Roth's spot is the hallmark of leukemic retinopathy. (*Image courtesy of Dr. Bita Esmaeli, M.D. Anderson Cancer Center.*)

The diagnosis is made on the basis of a high serum viscosity. Normal serum viscosity ranges between 1.4 and 1.8 Ostwald units (relative to water, at 1). Patients start to develop symptoms when serum viscosity exceeds 4.0 Ostwald units (31–33).

The treatment for hyperviscosity syndrome includes the administration of intravenous fluids followed by diuresis. Plasma exchange can decrease symptoms quickly and can be followed by chemotherapy (31).

HYPERLEUKOCYTOSIS

Hyperleukocytosis is typically defined as a white blood cell (WBC) count in the peripheral blood higher than 100,000/L. Acute myelogenous leukemia (AML), chronic myelogenous leukemia (CML), and less frequently (because of the smaller size of the lymphocytes) acute and chronic lymphocytic leukemia (CLL) are associated with hyperleukocytosis. The WBC count in acute lymphocytic leukemia (ALL) typically must be greater than 400,000/μL before hyperleukocytosis will develop (6). The highest rate of mortality is in patients with AML who have high blast counts.

Symptoms of hyperleukocytosis are headache, dizziness, vertigo, shortness of breath, altered mental status, and hemoptysis. WBCs are poorly deformable and can become lodged in the microvasculature of the kidneys, lungs, brain, and other organs. The pulmonary and neurologic systems are most critically affected in hyperleukocytosis syndrome. In the lungs, WBCs can get caught in the pulmonary circulation, causing adult respiratory distress syndrome (ARDS), or can mimic pulmonary embolism because of WBC stasis in the pulmo-

nary vasculature, thereby causing a ventilation/perfusion mismatch (34). Patients with the latter condition should not be given diuretics, as this will further increase stasis. Most patients with leukemia are anemic; this condition can offset the WBC elevation, so hyperviscosity is not as common in these patients. It is important not to give these patients blood transfusions unless absolutely necessary, as this treatment can exacerbate hyperleukocytosis and increase the RBC mass without changing the total blood volume (24). Patients can present with decreased mental status, which can be caused by endothelial leakage from the small vessels of the brain or hemorrhage, but other causes of altered mental status should also be considered, including infection, LMD from leukemia, and metabolic sources. Imaging studies, such as CT scan and MRI, as well as lumbar tap should be performed when indicated (6,10).

The treatment of hyperleukocytosis involves lowering the WBC count, which can be accomplished with leukapheresis or chemotherapy. Leukapheresis can lower the WBC count by 30 to 60% from pretreatment levels. These effects can be transient; therefore repeat leukapheresis might be necessary (33). Patients undergoing leukapheresis should also be monitored closely to prevent tumor lysis syndrome.

THROMBOSIS

Venous thromboembolism (VTE) is influenced by Virchow's triad: venous stasis, higher-than-normal coagulability, and intimal injury. Patients with cancer have a high risk of VTE, and up to 15% of patients will develop VTE because of hypercoagulability, the use of central venous catheters, and high stasis (35). Cancer patients can have increased serum viscosity due to dehydration or, less frequently, hyperviscosity syndrome (described previously). Stasis and intimal injury can be caused by numerous events—for example, tumor encroachment on blood vessels or indirect effects of cancer, such as spinal cord compression, brain metastasis, dehydration, or impaired ambulation. Some chemotherapeutic cancer agents can also induce VTE, among them tamoxifen, cisplatin, cyclophosphamide, methotrexate, and 5-FU (35).

Symptoms of pulmonary embolism (PE) include chest pain, shortness of breath, palpitations, fever up to 102°F, and syncope in the case of massive PE. ECG findings can include T-wave inversion in the precordial leads, sinus tachycardia, right bundle branch block, or rightward movement of the QRS axis. Chest roentgenograms can be normal or might reveal a pleural effusion or elevation of the diaphragm on the involved side. Physical examination can reveal tachypnea, tachycardia, and leg edema or erythema in the case of associated deep vein thrombosis.

Diagnosis of PE can be made by ventilation/perfusion scanning, spiral CT angiography, pulmonary angiography, or MRI (Fig. 39-12).

Ventilation perfusion scans are noninvasive and the results are useful in patients with a high probability of PE, which can be treated as VTE; normal results on ventilation/perfusion scans can rule out PE. Clinical suspicion based on the patient's risk factors and results of other tests can guide the clinician regarding the patient's pretest probability of PE. Patients with indeterminate result from ventilation/perfusion scans who are strongly suspected of having a PE can undergo further testing, such as spiral CT angiography, pulmonary angiography, or MRI. Spiral CT scanning and MRI can detect segmental PE but not necessarily subsegmental PE. Both of these tests are useful in that they give further information about the condition of the lung, such as whether pneumonia is present, tumor size, and impingement on the bronchial airways; this additional information is helpful in determining the cause of the patient's symptoms. Pulmonary angiography remains the gold standard in detecting PE, although it requires more dye than other contrast methods and a greater risk of renal complications. The alveolar-arterial gradient (A-a gradient) from an arterial blood gas (ABG) can serve to corroborate the diagnosis of PE, but a normal A-a gradient does not rule out a PE. The upper limit of normal of

an A-a gradient is equal to patient age/4 + 4, but this value can also increase when the patient is supine. In the PIOPED study, ABGs were normal in 14% of patients with preexisting cardiopulmonary disease and in 38% of patients with no underlying cardiopulmonary disease despite the presence of pulmonary emboli (28,36) (Fig. 39-13).

The diagnosis of peripheral VTE can be made by Doppler ultrasound, impedance plethsmography (IPG), venography, nuclear venogram, or magnetic resonance (MR) venography (Fig. 39-14) (28).

The D-dimer test can also be used in the evaluation of VTE; normal results are associated with a significantly lower likelihood of VTE than high values. A normal D-dimer level does not rule out VTE, however (35). Because D-dimer is commonly high in patients with cancer, an elevated D-dimer is not useful in diagnosing VTE.

First-line treatment for VTE consists of either unfractionated heparin (UFH) or low-molecular-weight heparin (LMWH). LMWH has the advantage that factor Xa levels usually do not have to be monitored because protein binding is low. LMWH also has a longer half-life than UFH and thus can be given less frequently (once or twice per day). The LMWHs enoxaparin, tinzaparin, and dalteparin are all different and cannot be used interchangeably. Monitoring may be required for patients with obesity and renal insufficiency, because LMWH is cleared by the kidneys. When monitoring is necessary, the Xa level should be measured 4 h after the

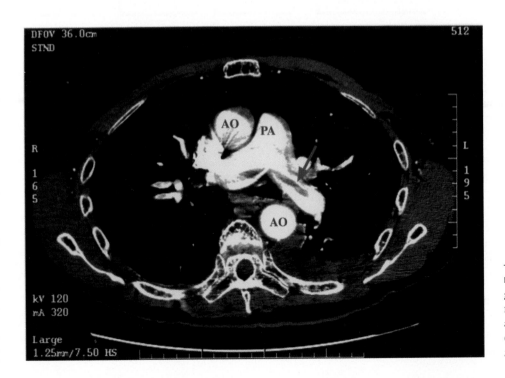

FIGURE 39-12 Spiral CT angiogram in a patient with a saddle pulmonary embolism (*arrow*). AO = aorta; PA = main pulmonary artery. (*Image courtesy of Dr. Joel Dunnington, M.D. Anderson Cancer Center.*)

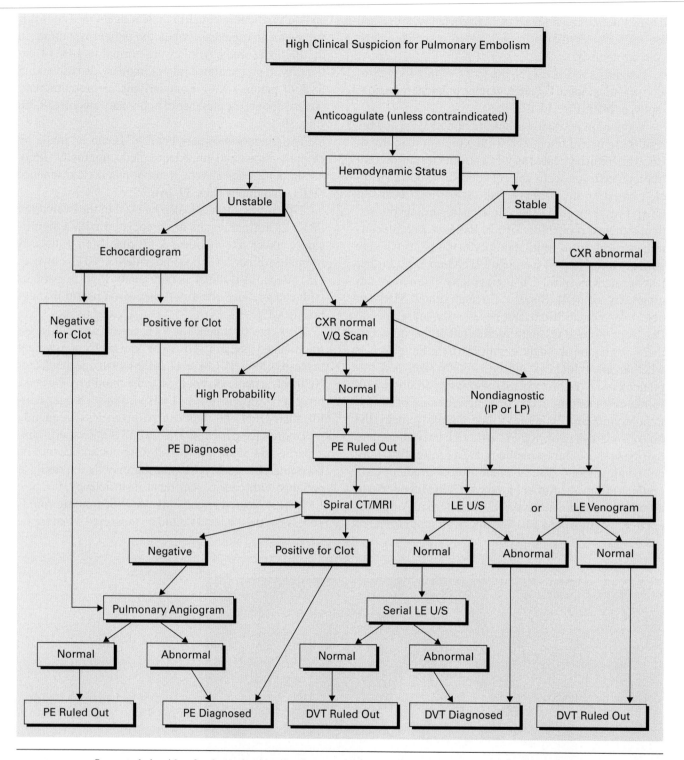

FIGURE 39-13 Suggested algorithm for the evaluation of pulmonary embolism. IP = intermediate probability; LP = low probability; LE US = lower extremity ultrasound; LE venogram = lower extremity venogram; V/Q scan = ventilation perfusion scan; PE = pulmonary embolism; DVT = Deep venous thrombosis. (*Adapted from Shannon VR, Ng A. Noninfectious pulmonary emergencies. In: Yeung SJ, Escalante CP, eds.* Oncologic Emergencies. *Hamilton, Ontario, Canada: BC Decker; 2002, with permission.*)

injection, with a target level ranging from 0.6 to 1.0 IU/mL for twice-daily dosing. For daily dosing, the Xa level should range between 1.9 and 2.0 IU/mL (37). For patients who will be transitioned to warfarin treat-

ment, there should be an overlap of at least 5 days with LMWH.

Levine and colleagues recently presented the results of a study involving VTE in cancer patients at the 44th

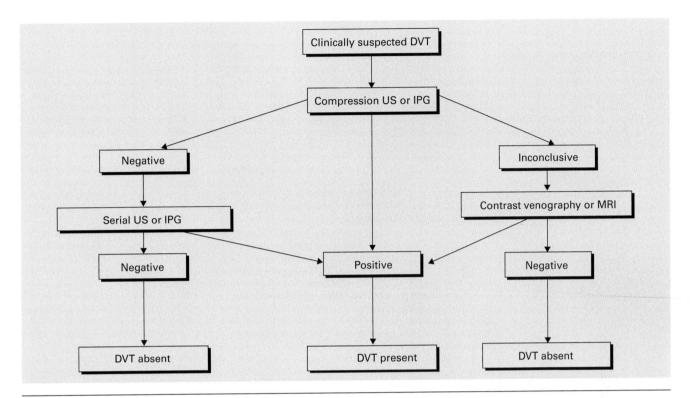

FIGURE 39-14   Diagnostic approach to patients with suspected acute deep venous thrombosis. DVT = deep venous thrombosis; IPG = impedance plethysmography; MRI = magnetic resonance imaging; US = ultrasonography. (*Adapted from Gao S, Shannon VR. Vascular emergencies. In: Yeung SJ, Escalante CP, eds. Oncologic Emergencies. Hamilton, Ontario, Canada: BC Decker; 2002, with permission.*)

American Society of Hematology Meeting. In their study, 672 cancer patients with VTE were randomized to dalteparin with oral anticoagulation versus dalteparin alone. The oral anticoagulation (OA) group were given warfarin and dalteparin 200 IU/kg subcutaneously every day for 5 to 7 days until the international normalized ratio (INR) reached 2 to 3. At that point, dalteparin was discontinued and the warfarin continued for 6 months. In the OA group, the goal INR was 2.5. The dalteparin group was given dalteparin 200 IU/kg subcutaneously every day for 1 month and then 150 IU/kg subcutaneously every day for the remaining 5 months. The patients in the dalteparin group had a lower rate of recurrent VTE at 6 months (8.8%) than the OA group (17.4%). There were no significant differences in major or minor bleeding between the two groups. The study investigators concluded that the occurrence of recurrent VTE can be decreased by the use of dalteparin rather than warfarin (38).

Although VTE can often be treated on an outpatient basis, patients not eligible for outpatient treatment are those with active bleeding, major comorbid illnesses, a history of heparin-induced thrombocytopenia, hypertensive emergencies, major surgery or trauma within the previous 2 weeks, recent gastrointestinal bleeding, stroke or transient ischemic attack, severe renal dysfunction, or a platelet count below 100,000/μL (39). Figure 39-15 shows the dosing schedule.

Most patients are treated for at least 3 to 6 months. Patients from whom the central venous catheter has been removed can undergo repeat testing using such techniques as Doppler ultrasound or nuclear venous flow study to determine whether the clot has resolved, so that cessation of anticoagulation therapy may be considered. For patients with small clots at the distal tip, manifested by the inability of the central line to work, tissue plasminogen activator (t-PA) can be given carefully provided that there are no contraindications.

Inferior vena cava (IVC) filters can be used for patients who cannot tolerate anticoagulation therapy. IVC filters do not decrease peripheral edema from deep venous thrombosis (DVT) and, in fact, can serve as a nidus for further clot formation. IVC filters can prevent life-threatening pulmonary emboli. Patients with massive pulmonary emboli may require thrombolysis or embolectomy. See Fig. 39-16 for a synopsis of the relative and absolute contraindications for thrombolytic therapy (40) and Fig. 39-17 for thrombolytic doses.

Patients with cancer and VTE should be treated indefinitely if the cancer remains active or for at least 3 to

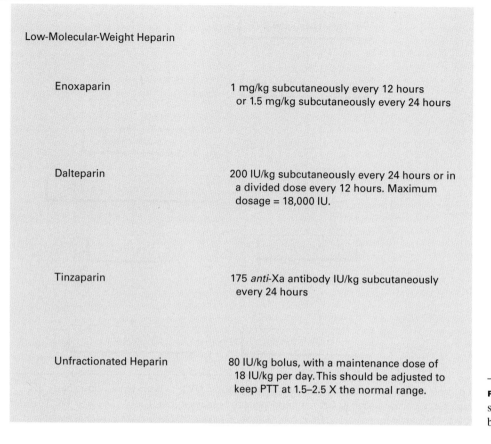

Low-Molecular-Weight Heparin

Enoxaparin   1 mg/kg subcutaneously every 12 hours
                           or 1.5 mg/kg subcutaneously every 24 hours

Dalteparin   200 IU/kg subcutaneously every 24 hours or in
                           a divided dose every 12 hours. Maximum
                           dosage = 18,000 IU.

Tinzaparin   175 *anti*-Xa antibody IU/kg subcutaneously
                           every 24 hours

Unfractionated Heparin   80 IU/kg bolus, with a maintenance dose of
                           18 IU/kg per day. This should be adjusted to
                           keep PTT at 1.5–2.5 X the normal range.

FIGURE 39-15 Heparin dosage schedule for venous thromboembolism.

6 months after resolution of the VTE if the cancer is no longer active (41,42). For patients who are treated with warfarin but who experience warfarin failure as evidenced by the recurrence or progression of clot formation, the INR range can be increased from 2 to 3, to 3 to 3.5, the patient can be switched to twice-daily UFH, or the patient can be switched to LMWH (42). Thrombectomy should be used only for patients with massive PE who are hemodynamically unstable and who either have contraindications for thrombolytic therapy or have previously failed thrombolytic therapy (35).

BLEEDING

Bleeding in cancer patients is most commonly due to thrombocytopenia induced by chemotherapy, marrow infiltration, disseminated intravascular coagulopathy (DIC), extensive radiation therapy, splenic sequestration, peripheral destruction, or infection. Thrombocytopenia usually manifest as mucocutaneous bleeding, such as gum oozing, epistaxis, and gynecologic or gastrointestinal bleeding (35). At MDACC, all patients generally receive platelet transfusions if their platelet count falls to 10,000/μL or below. If the patient has active bleeding

and the platelet count is between 20,000 and 50,000/μL, a platelet transfusion will also be given. A patient will also receive a platelet transfusion if an invasive procedure is planned and his or her platelet count is below 50,000/μL. The American Society of Clinical Oncology (ASCO) recommends prophylactic platelet transfusions for patients being treated for leukemia and those receiving bone marrow transplants if their platelet counts are below 10,000/μL. Transfusion thresholds may be higher for patients with fever, hyperleukocytosis, a rapid fall in platelet count, coagulation abnormalities, or active bleeding. ASCO recommends that patients with chronic stable thrombocytopenia who are not undergoing active treatment, such as those with aplastic anemia and patients with myelodysplastic syndrome (MDS), be monitored and given platelets only for active bleeding, even if their platelet count is below 10,000/μL. For patients with solid tumors, prophylactic platelet transfusions should be given if the platelet counts are below 10,000/μL unless the tumor is necrotic or is located in the bladder and undergoing treatment; in those cases the threshold for transfusion should be 20,000/μL. According to ASCO's guidelines, platelet counts of 50,000/μL should be sufficient for invasive procedures, such as surgery.

Absolute Contraindications to Thrombolysis

Major intracranial surgery or trauma within prior 2 months

Cerebrovascular hemorrhage within prior 3–6 months

Active intracranial neoplasm

Major internal hemorrhage within prior 6 months

Severe bleeding diastheses, including those associated with severe liver or renal disease

Relative Contraindications to Thrombolysis

Prolonged cardiopulmonary resuscitation

Pregnancy or postpartum period within prior 10 days

Nonhemorrhagic stroke within prior 2 months

Major trauma or surgery (excluding that of the central nervous system) within prior 10 days

Thrombocytopenia (platelet count <100,000/mm^3)

Hemorrhagic retinopathy

Allergies to thrombolytic agents

Minor surgery to noncompressible vessels within prior 10 days

Tissue biopsy within prior 10 days

Peptic ulceration within prior 3 months

Infective endocarditis/pericarditis

Uncontrolled hypertension (systolic BP ≥200 or diastolic BP ≥110 mmHg)

Aortic aneurysm

FIGURE 39-16 Absolute and relative contraindications to thrombolysis. (*Adapted from Shannon VR, Ng A. Noninfectious pulmonary emergencies. In: Yeung SJ, Escalante CP, eds.* Oncologic Emergencies. *Hamilton, Ontario, Canada: BC Decker; 2002, with permission.*)

For lumbar puncture, the platelet count should be above 20,000/μL. Patients with AML commonly receive multiple transfusions and can develop alloimmunization against human leukocyte antigens (HLA). Approximately 25 to 35% of patients with AML will become alloimmunized and refractory to nonhistocompatible platelet transfusions, predominantly through their exposure to leukocytes. Random-donor platelets are derived from pooled platelet concentrates from whole-blood donations, whereas single-donor platelets are obtained from one donor by platelet pheresis. The likelihood of alloimmunization can be decreased by using single-donor platelets, leukocyte-depleted platelets, leukocyte filters, and UV-irradiated platelets. ASCO recommends that patients who are platelet-refractory not receive platelet transfusions unless they are hemorrhaging or HLA-compatible platelets are available (43).

DIC can cause bleeding and thrombosis. DIC should be suspected in a patient who has an unexplained elevation in PT, PTT, or thrombocytopenia with associated bleeding or thrombosis. Although bleeding is most often noted in patients with DIC, it is the thrombosis of small (and occasionally large) blood vessels that leads to the most serious complications (44). Collaborative laboratory findings are high D-dimer and fibrin split product (FSP) levels, low levels of fibrinogen and thrombin-antithrombin III (TAT), or the presence of schistocytes (44,45). It is important to remember that DIC is a clinical diagnosis based on the entire clinical scenario, and results for these laboratory tests might not

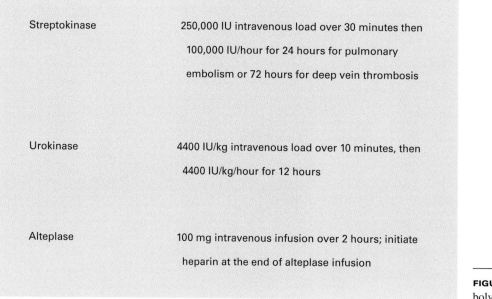

Streptokinase	250,000 IU intravenous load over 30 minutes then 100,000 IU/hour for 24 hours for pulmonary embolism or 72 hours for deep vein thrombosis
Urokinase	4400 IU/kg intravenous load over 10 minutes, then 4400 IU/kg/hour for 12 hours
Alteplase	100 mg intravenous infusion over 2 hours; initiate heparin at the end of alteplase infusion

FIGURE 39-17 Dosages of thrombolytics.

be abnormal. Patients can also have mildly abnormal test results in cases of subclinical DIC, and these patients should be monitored closely for conversion to overt DIC.

Tumors can cause DIC, especially adenocarcinomas of the breast, prostate, stomach, lung, and colon. In this instance, the disorder is believed to be stimulated by mucin produced from these cancers. Leukemia, especially acute promyelocytic leukemia (APL), is associated with DIC in up to 85% of patients because of a tissue factor in APL that has procoagulant activity. Other tumors associated with DIC are melanoma, lymphoma, and ovarian and pancreatic cancers. Other causes of DIC are sepsis, acidosis, extensive burns, the use of Denver catheters or Laveen shunts in patients with malignant ascites, hemolytic blood transfusion reactions, polycythemia rubra vera, and amniotic fluid embolism (35,44).

Patients who have both DIC and bleeding can present with oozing from multiple sites, such as arterial or venous punctures or the mucous membranes, with gastrointestinal hemorrhage, or with epistaxis. Thrombotic complications can be visible on the skin in the form of hemorrhagic bullae, acral cyanosis, or even gangrene (44). Microvascular thrombosis most commonly affects the lungs, brain, and kidneys. The patient may develop shortness of breath, pleuritic chest pain, and ARDS. The kidneys can become clogged with microemboli, in which case patients often present with oliguria, anuria, hematuria, or proteinuria. The small vessels of the brain also can receive microemboli, causing strokes, seizures, altered mental status, or coma. As the patient deterio-

rates, hypotension, acidosis, and hypoxia can develop (44,45).

The treatment of DIC should focus on reversing the underlying cause or trigger, such as treating an underlying infection. Acidosis, high catecholamine release, vasoconstriction, and corticosteroid use can exacerbate thrombosis associated with DIC (44). Additional therapeutic measures for thrombosis can include heparin administration at 15 U/kg/h by continuous infusion. When the patient is bleeding, blood components (including platelets) can be transfused to correct coagulation abnormalities. Platelet transfusions are indicated to maintain platelet counts of at least 50,000/µL. Cryoprecipitate should only be used for severe hypofibrinogenemia <50 mg/dL, or <100 mg/dL if patient is actively bleeding (45). Cryoprecipitate can be given at 0.2 bags per kilogram of body weight, and the fibrinogen level should be tested 20 to 60 min after the infusion and every 6 h thereafter until the bleeding has stopped. Fresh frozen plasma (FFP) can be transfused at 10 to 15 mg/kg to correct abnormalities in PT. Other products that might be needed are prothrombin complex, antithrombin concentrates, or washed RBCs. For patients with persistent bleeding, fibrinolytic inhibitors, such as epsilon-aminocaproic acid (EACA), can be given. EACA should always be given with heparin to prevent thrombosis; because EACA can cause hypotension, ventricular arrythmias, and hypokalemia, it should be used with caution. Tranexamic acid is a newer fibinolytic inhibitor that has fewer side effects and has been used successfully in DIC associated with APL (45).

■ GENITOURINARY EMERGENCIES

HEMORRHAGIC CYSTITIS

Hemorrhagic cystitis is inflammation or bleeding of the bladder; it can be due to radiation therapy, viral infection, or chemotherapy. Radiation-induced bladder bleeding can present as early as 3 months or as late as 5 years after the termination of radiation therapy (46). Chemotherapeutic agents associated with hemorrhagic cystitis are cyclophosphamide and ifosfamide (because of the liver metabolites secreted during use of these compounds, namely acrolein and chloroacetaldehyde). The mechanism by which cyclophosphamide and ifosfamide metabolites are toxic to the urinary bladder is not known, but they have been implicated as the cause of hematuria in some patients (46,47). Mesna is a thiol compound that binds acrolein, chloroacetaldehyde, and other metabolites of cyclophosphamide and ifosfamide; when it is administered before the patient receives the chemotherapeutic agents, the incidence of bladder toxicity can be decreased (46,47). Forced diuresis and adequate hydration complement mesna administration (46,47).

In addition to radiation therapy and chemotherapy-inducing hemorrhagic cystitis, the BK virus (a polyomavirus) can become activated in immunocompromised patients undergoing bone marrow transplantation and cause hematuria (47).

Treatment of hemorrhagic cystitis involves gentle bladder irrigation to remove any clots and decompress the bladder. Any coagulopathy, such as thrombocytopenia, should be corrected, as should manifestations of DIC, such as low fibrinogen levels or an elevated PT or PTT. For patients with persistent bleeding, prostaglandins E2 or F2, 1% alum, or formalin can be instilled. Formalin instillation is painful and requires general or spinal anesthesia. To correct continued bleeding, some patients require surgery, hypogastric artery embolization, or open surgical intervention (46).

URINARY TRACT OBSTRUCTION

Obstructive uropathy can be secondary to outflow obstruction or impingement on the ureters or kidneys; it can also be due to tumor invasion, radiotherapy-induced changes, or indirect effects of the tumor, such as ascites, lymphadenopathy, or fibrosis. A patient who is unable to urinate should have a small Foley catheter, such as a 14F placed. In patients with benign prostatic hypertrophy (BPH), a coudé catheter can often be inserted more easily (46,47). The catheter should not be forced, and if the bladder cannot be accessed, a suprapubic catheter can be used. A lack of residual urine in the absence of severe dehydration usually indicates either obstruction at a more proximal level in the urinary system or acute anuric renal failure. Patients who have residual urine may be unable to urinate because of a mechanical cause, such as BPH, urethral stricture, tumor impingement, or stone obstruction. Other possible causes of acute urinary retention are infection, spinal cord compression, viral radiculomyelitis, postsurgical effects interrupting bladder innervation, or medicines such as pain medications and antihistamines (47). In each case, the underlying disorder should be treated. Patients with BPH can undergo a trial of alpha blockers, such as terazosin, prazosin, oxazosin, or finasteride, a type II 5-alpha-reductase inhibitor. Transurethral resection of the prostate (TURP) can be considered for patients who do not respond to medical treatments.

Laboratory values are also useful in differentiating prerenal, postrenal and renal failure. Patients with prerenal failure typically have a high ratio of blood urea nitrogen (BUN) to creatinine of more than 20:1, although upper tract gastrointestinal bleeding, corticosteroid use, and high protein intake can also increase the BUN-to-creatinine ratio. Acute urinary obstruction can present as flank pain, whereas chronic obstruction is often painless, with patients presenting with anuria or decreased urine output. The tumors most likely to cause ureteral obstruction are cervical, prostate, bladder, ovarian, breast, and gastrointestinal cancers as well as lymphoma (47). Patients with infected urine and obstruction may also present with symptoms of urosepsis, including fever, confusion, and a high WBC count.

CT scanning of the abdomen is good for evaluating the cause of ureteral obstruction in that it can elucidate the nature of the obstruction. Other tests that can be used are MRI, renal ultrasound, intravenous urography, retrograde pyelography, and radionuclide renography (46,47). Helical CT scanning of the abdomen has the added benefit of avoiding the use of intravenous contrast (46). Urinary obstruction can be managed with ureteral stents or percutaneous nephrostomy tubes with or without internal stents; the stents or tubes are typically placed under guidance by interventional radiology. Many patients with stents develop infection, which often requires hospitalization, intravenous antibiotics, and stent replacement. Other possible complications are stent clogging and stent migration. The "double J" stent, which is now most frequently used, is anchored in the bladder and the renal pelvis, so that stent migration is less common than it once was. Open surgical procedures are much less frequently performed now than in the past and are generally reserved for patients in whom endourologic procedures have failed (47).

■ RESPIRATORY EMERGENCIES

AIRWAY OBSTRUCTION

Airway obstruction can be caused by intraluminal tumor growth or compression of the airway by an extraluminal tumor. Rigid or flexible bronchoscopy can be used to both diagnose and treat airway obstruction. Patients with severe respiratory distress and airway obstruction should undergo endotracheal intubation distal to the obstruction before the obstruction is treated. Once the airway has been stabilized, the obstruction can be treated. The methods that can be used to provide expedient relief of airway obstruction include laser treatment, argon plasma coagulation (APC), electrocautery, endobronchial balloon dilation, and stent placement. APC can be achieved through flexible or rigid bronchoscopy, at a relatively low cost and degrades the obstructive tissue by increasing its temperature. Electrocautery is also relatively inexpensive and can provide immediate relief of the obstruction, but side effects can include fire, hemorrhage, and electrical shock. Rigid bronchoscopy can be used to treat extraluminal tumors

by metal or silicone stent placement; this technique is most useful for tracheal or main bronchial disease. Metal stents can promote the growth of granulomatous tissue, whereas silicone stents are more likely to develop mucous plugging and to migrate. Laser therapy can also be used for endobronchial lesions, with the possible side effects of hemorrhage, pneumothorax, and pneumomediastinum. Laser therapy is more expensive than the other techniques and requires a skilled technician. Other methods that can be used for airway obstruction are cryotherapy, brachytherapy, and photodynamic therapy, although in many cases these do not provide rapid relief (29) (Table 39-2).

HEMOPTYSIS

Massive hemoptysis is defined as bleeding into the airway at a rate of 100–600 mL/day, although any amount of blood that compromises the airway can be considered massive. Some 7 to 10% of patients with lung cancer will develop massive hemoptysis, which carries a poorer prognosis than massive hemoptysis associated with other cancers (29). In addition to structural abnormalities in the lungs, bleeding can be due to chemotherapy or other medications, sepsis, fungal infections, and thrombocytopenia. Death from this type of hemorrhage usually results from asphyxiation rather than anemia or blood loss.

TABLE 39-2 | BRONCHOSCOPIC METHODS OF TREATING DYSPNEA FROM TUMOR OBSTRUCTION

Tumor Type	Tumor Location (I) Intraluminal (E) Extraluminal	Rate of Relief of Dyspnea Symptoms (I) Immediate (D) Delayed	Complications/ Disadvantages	Advantages/Uses
Argon plasma coagulation	I	I		Low cost Ease of use Rapid coagulation
Brachytherapy	I	D	Fistula Hemoptysis	Best used in small epithelial tumors
Cryotherapy	I	D		Less expensive
Electrocautery	I	I	Fire Hemorrhage Shock	Less expensive
Laser	I	I	Bleeding Pneumothorax Pneumomediastinum	Special training; expensive equipment
Photodynamic therapy	I	I	Phototoxicity Hemoptysis Bronchial obstruction due to debris	
Stent placement	I/E	I	Migration of stent	Used in tracheal or main bronchial disease

The most important aspect of managing massive hemoptysis is protecting the airway. If the right lung is affected, the left lung can be selectively intubated through bronchoscopy. Use of a rigid bronchoscope allows removal of the tumor or clots, whereas flexible bronchoscopy allows access to the more distal airways. If the left lung is affected, the right lung should not be selectively intubated because inadvertent collapse of the right upper lobe can ensue. A single-lumen endotracheal tube is easier to place than a double-lumen tube and allows a larger area for evacuation of blood and clots. The patient should lie on the side of the bleeding lung to promote aeration of the unaffected lung. Any coagulopathy should be corrected, and cough suppressed with codeine or other agents. If a tumor is causing the bleeding and it can be localized, the patient can undergo bronchial artery embolization or tumor resection. If the tumor is unresectable external beam radiation therapy (EBRT) can be used. If only the location of the bleeding can be determined, a solution of 1:10,000 epinephrine can be injected. Other means of halting bleeding are laser treatment, electrocautery, APC, photocoagulation, balloon tamponade, or iced-saline lavage (40).

TOXIC LUNG INJURY

ARDS is a serious condition that can be a complication of infection or chemotherapy. ATRA is a chemotherapy used in APL, and it has been found to cause ARDS in 26% of patients starting 2 to 47 days after treatment. Cytarabine (Ara-C) can cause diffuse lung injury, capillary leakage, and pulmonary edema, usually after 6 days of therapy. These effects can be treated with diuresis and corticosteroids. Bleomycin can cause pulmonary fibrosis and increased sensitivity to intraoperative oxygen administration. Other chemotherapeutic agents that can cause pulmonary edema are mitomycin C, gemcitabine, cyclosporine, interferon, tumor necrosis factor, interleukin-2, and granulocyte–macrophage colony-stimulating factor (GM-CSF) (25).

Interstitial lung disease can be caused by bleomycin, carmustine, lomustine, busulfan, cyclophosphamide, methotrexate, doxorubicin, and actinomycin D. Bleomycin toxicity is usually dose-related and most often occurs when the cumulative dose is greater than 450 U. It can be treated with corticosteroids. Busulfan's toxic effects can occur after 3 weeks of therapy, but they sometimes emerge as late as 3 years after treatment. Busulfan toxicity is associated with a high mortality rate, but corticosteroids can be used with some response. Cyclophosphamide complications present differently depending on whether they are early or late. The early-

onset effect is pneumonitis, which can be treated with corticosteroids. The late-onset symptoms include a progressive fibrosis that is not responsive to steroids. Methotrexate can also produce pulmonary fibrosis, which can appear from several days to years after treatment. Doxorubicin and actinomycin D can present with pulmonary fibrosis characterized by a "recall" effect after radiation therapy, even in areas of the lung not exposed to radiation (25). Radiation can cause pneumonitis or fibrosis, the occurrence of which is most closely related to the rate of delivery of radiation. Pneumonitis is an acute-phase reaction that occurs 2 to 6 months after irradiation and may respond to corticosteroids. The late-phase response to radiation toxicity, fibrosis of the lungs, does not respond to corticosteroids.

Pulmonary venoocclusive disease can be caused by bleomycin, mitomycin C, or carmustine. Patients present with shortness of breath, pulmonary hypertension, pleural effusions, or respiratory failure. Patients with this disorder have a poor prognosis.

■ CHEMOTHERAPY-INDUCED EXTRAVASATIONS

Extravasation injuries due to chemotherapy can produce a variety of symptoms ranging from skin irritation to skin ulceration, tissue necrosis, nerve damage, and (rarely) loss of limbs. Vesicant chemotherapy agents, including the alkylating agents (mechlorethamine, cisplatin, mitomycin C), DNA intercalating agents (doxorubicin, daunorubicin), and plant alkaloids (vinblastine, vincristine, vinorelbine), can cause the most severe reactions. Irritant chemotherapy extravasations are generally not severe, causing only pain, erythema, and inflammation at the extravasated site (48).

The goal is to prevent chemotherapy extravasations. The patient should be told to inform the staff of any discomfort, swelling, or erythema over the infusion site. Nursing staff should evaluate the intravenous infusion site carefully by administering intravenous fluids before chemotherapy agents are infused. and they should monitor the patient frequently for any evidence of extravasation. Intravenous lines should be placed carefully; areas that have a poor blood supply or overlie a joint should be avoided. If an extravasation does occur, the infusion should be stopped immediately with the catheter left in place, and the staff should attempt to withdraw any remaining chemotherapy agents. Cold compresses should then be placed on the involved site except when the agents are plant alkaloids, in which case warm compresses should be applied (49–51).

Topical dimethylsulfoxide (DMSO) in a 50% solution can relieve extravasations when applied at a volume of 1.5 mL to the site every 6 h for 7 to 14 days. DMSO is commonly used to treat extravasations caused by mitomycin C and the anthracyclines (49–53).

For extravasations caused by plant alkaloids (vinblastine, vincristine, vinorelbine) and epidophyllotoxins (etoposide, teniposide), a solution of 150 U of hyaluronidase in 1 to 3 mL of saline can be injected into the needle and subcutaneously around the extravasated site (50,51,53).

A 0.17-mol/L solution of sodium thiosulfate can be injected into mechlorethamine-induced extravasation sites (2). Sodium thiosulfate is thought to work by creating an alkaline-rich site to which the vesicant binds instead of the skin. The by-product is then excreted in the urine (51). There is some evidence that sodium thiosulfate can also be used for extravasations caused by carmustine, cisplatin, carboplatin, cyclophosphamide, dacarbazine, and oxaliplatin (49,52,53). Table 39-3 lists selected chemotherapeutic agents and their antidotes (48–53).

If local measures fail to contain symptoms in all patients with anthracycline-induced extravasations, a plastic surgeon should be consulted. Surgery can consist of debridement, excision of dead tissues, and, in severe cases, skin graft placement. In patients with doxorubicin-induced extravasation, the drug remains in the tissue for a long period, perhaps being released by dying or dead cells and spreading over time (50).

Patients who have had previous extravasation reactions can also experience a "recall reaction" when the same chemotherapy is received later, causing ulcerations or burns to reappear at the previously affected area (49).

■ METABOLIC EMERGENCIES

SYNDROME OF INAPPROPRIATE ANTIDIURETIC HORMONE SECRETION

Hyponatremia is the most common electrolyte abnormality, present in approximately 2% of hospitalized patients. The syndrome of inappropriate antidiuretic

TABLE 39-3 CHEMOTHERAPEUTIC EXTRAVASATIONS AND THEIR ANTIDOTES

Chemotherapy Agent	Irritant/Vesicant	Sodium Thiosulfate	DMSO	Hyaluronidase	Cool	Warm
Carboplatin	I	+			+	
Carmustine	I/V	+			+	Dry warm
Cisplatin	I/V	+			+	
Cyclophosphamide	I	+			+	
Dacarbazine	I/V	+				
Dactinomycin	I/V				+	
Daunorubicin	I/V		+		+	
Docetaxel	I				+	Warm soaks
Doxorubicin	I/V		+		+	
Epirubicin	I/V		+		+	
Etoposide	I/V			+		+
Idarubicin	I/V		+		+	
Ifosfamide	I				+	
Mechlorethamine	I/V	+				
Mitomycin C	V		+		+	
Oxaliplatin	I/V	+				
Paclitaxel	I/V			+		
Plicamycin	I/V					
Streptozocin	I/V					
Teniposide	I/V			+		+
Topotecan					+	
Vinblastine	I/V			+		+
Vincristine	I/V			+		+
Vindesine	I/V			+		+
Vinorelbine	I/V			+		+

DMSO = dimethylsulfoxide.

hormone secretion (SIADH) is a paraneoplastic syndrome in which antidiuretic hormone (ADH) is secreted inappropriately from the posterior pituitary gland, despite lower serum osmolality. Typically ADH is secreted in response to hypernatremia, hypotension, or hypoxemia to increase the permeability of the collecting ducts so that water can be reabsorbed and the blood pressure and sodium level restored to normal values. In patients with cancer, a protein similar to ADH, atrial natriuretic factor (ANF), is secreted by the cardiac atria, which increases the renal excretion of sodium. The pituitary gland does not respond to feedback from ANF. Thus SIADH can be characterized by inappropriate ADH secretion despite normal blood volume, with hyponatremia, serum osmolality less than 260 mOsm/L, inappropriate sodium secretion in the urine of greater than 20 meq/L, and high urine osmolality (54).

SIADH can be caused by various cancers, including small cell lung cancer, pancreatic cancer, and primary brain cancers. Other causes of SIADH are pulmonary infections, postoperative effects, central nervous system disorders (meningitis, stroke, hemorrhage), and chemotherapeutic agents (vincristine, cisplatin and cyclophosphamide) (5).

Symptoms of SIADH depend upon the sodium level and the rate at which the sodium level declines. The patient can present with confusion, seizures, headache, or weight gain without edema. In evaluating hyponatremia, the patient's volume status should be addressed, and the plasma osmolality, urine osmolality, and urine sodium and chloride levels should be determined. Hyponatremia should be distinguished from pseudohyponatremia, in which plasma osmolality is normal (hyperlipidemia, hyperproteinemia) or even high (hypertriglyceridemia, hyperglycemia, and mannitol use).

Most patients with hyponatremia have low serum osmolality, which can be grouped by type: primary sodium loss, primary sodium gain, and primary water gain. Patients with sodium gain present with volume overload, which occurs in congestive heart failure, liver disease, and nephrotic syndrome. Patients with primary sodium loss present with dehydration; sodium deficits can be due to gastrointestinal loss (nausea, vomiting, diarrhea, bowel obstruction), renal loss (thiazide diuretics), and skin loss (severe burns). Patients with SIADH can also have primary water gain, although other sources of primary water gain (primary polydipsia, decreased solute intake, beer potomania, chronic renal insufficiency, adrenal or thyroid deficiency, or increased ADH secretion in response to pain, nausea, vomiting, or drugs) should be distinguished. Some patients appear to have SIADH based on laboratory test results but actually

have a reset osmostat. This adjustment can occur in patients with quadriplegia, tuberculosis, psychosis, chronic illness, volume contraction, encephalitis, malnutrition, or malignancy and in elderly or pregnant patients. Other rare causes of euvolemic hyponatremia are an incomplete pituitary stalk and increased sensitivity to ADH secretion. SIADH is diagnosed by low plasma osmolality, urine osmolality greater than 100 mOsm/kg, and urine sodium level greater than 20 mmol/L. Patients with SIADH typically have low uric acid levels (54).

Treatment of SIADH involves restricting water to 500 to 1000 mL/day from all sources and treating the underlying disorder. If this combination is not effective, demeclocycline (600 to 1200 mg/day) can be used in divided doses two to four times per day (54). Patients whose symptoms include coma or seizure can be treated by slow infusion of 3% normal saline; care must be taken not to increase serum sodium by more than 0.5 to 1 meq/h. Too-rapid correction of serum sodium level can lead to central pontine myelinolysis (Fig. 39-18) (55).

TUMOR LYSIS SYNDROME

Tumor lysis syndrome (TLS) is a result of excessive tumor breakdown, causing hypocalcemia, hyperphosphatemia, hyperkalemia, elevated uric acid, and occasionally acute renal failure. Risk factors for TLS include high tumor burden, chronic renal insufficiency, and certain tumor types (Burkitt's lymphoma, lymphoblastic lymphoma, diffuse large cell lymphoma, undifferentiated lymphoma, and leukemia) (2,5). TLS usually presents during chemotherapy, but it can also occur after radiation therapy, corticosteroid treatment for sensitive tumors, or administration of hormonal agents (55).

Patients with TLS can present with nausea and vomiting, diarrhea, constipation, low urine output, weight gain, acute renal failure, weakness, cramps, seizures, tetany, or arrhythmias.

Prophylaxis is very important in preventing TLS and consists of intravenous hydration, oral allopurinol (100 to 600 mg day), and occasionally alkalinization of the urine with sodium bicarbonate to maintain a urine pH greater than 7.5. Alkalinizing the urine decreases uric acid crystallization in the kidneys. Because allopurinol use is now common before chemotherapy, hyperphosphatemia, rather than hyperuricemia, is now the predominant cause of acute renal failure in TLS (55). To prevent TLS, patients with leukemia and high WBC counts should be treated with leukapheresis or hydroxyurea before chemotherapeutic agents are administered (5). Some patients with refractory electrolyte

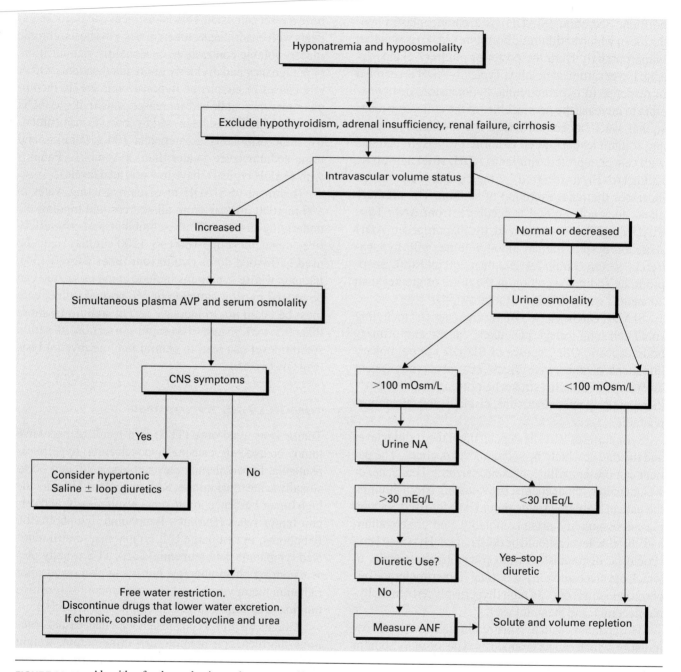

FIGURE 39-18   Algorithm for the evaluation and treatment of hyponatremia. ANF = atrial natriuretic peptide; AVP = arginine vasopressin; CNS = central nervous system. (*Adapted from Yeung SJ, Diaz GL, Gagel RF. Metabolic and endocrine emergencies. In: Yeung SJ, Escalante CP eds.* Oncologic Emergencies. *Hamilton, Ontario, Canada: BC Decker; 2002, with permission.*)

abnormalities might require dialysis if conservative measures fail (2).

HYPERCALCEMIA

Hypercalcemia is present in 10 to 20% of patients with advanced cancer (2). The most common cancers include squamous cell cancer of the lung, breast cancer, multiple myeloma, and lymphoma (2). The two major

mechanisms of hypercalcemia include the secretion of a parathyroid-related peptide (PTHrP) and abnormal 1,25-vitamin D production (which occurs in Hodgkin's disease and non-Hodgkin's lymphoma).

Symptoms of hypercalcemia are altered mental status, polyuria, polydipsia, nausea, vomiting, anorexia, constipation, and seizures (2,7). Measured serum calcium levels should be adjusted according to the albumin level for accurate estimation. A low albumin level should be subtracted from 4, and the difference should be multiplied by 0.8. This product should be added to the serum calcium level to arrive at the estimated calcium. Alternatively, ionized calcium can be measured, which assesses the active calcium in the serum and is more accurate.

The choice of treatment for hypercalcemia depends on the patient's calcium level and symptoms. Calcium is a potent diuretic, and patients with mild hypercalcemia can be treated by intravenous fluids. Patients with a calcium level greater than 14 mg/dL should be treated with additional measures. Patients who have symptoms of hypercalcemia and a calcium level between 12 and 14 mg/dL should also receive additional treatment to lower the calcium level (7).

Bisphosphonates are the drugs of choice in treating hypercalcemia. Pamidronate can be given intravenously over 2 to 24 hours. A 60-mg dose corrects hypercalcemia 60% of the time, and a 90-mg dose does so 100% of the time (2). Bisphosphonates do not work immediately but have an onset of action after 12 to 48 h (2). Zoledronic acid, a relatively new agent, can be infused more rapidly than pamidronate; the recommended dose is 4 mg intravenously over 15 min. Bisphosphonates are useful not only in reducing serum calcium levels but can also help to decrease bone pain and treat skeletal complications in cancer patients with bone metastases (56).

Calcitonin can also be used to treat hypercalcemia; it has an onset of action of 2 to 4 h, but its effects are transient because tachyphylaxis develops after 3 days. Patients may develop nausea, abdominal cramps, or hypersensitivity reactions to calcitonin (2,7).

Corticosteroids can be helpful in some patients with hypercalcemia—for instance, those with lymphoma and myeloma. Dialysis is reserved for patients who are unable to tolerate hydration. Furosemide can be used, but only after the patient has been hydrated adequately. Gallium nitrate and plicamycin are rarely used because of the high risk of toxic effects.

■ GASTROINTESTINAL EMERGENCIES

GASTROINTESTINAL BLEEDING

Patients with cancer can present with gastrointestinal (GI) bleeding due to direct tumor invasion, effects of chemotherapy agents or corticosteroids, thrombocytopenia, coagulopathy, side effects of radiation therapy, or Mallory Weiss tears from intractable nausea and vomiting. Other possible causes of GI bleeding are gastritis, peptic ulcer disease, duodenal ulcers, arteriove-

nous malformations, and diverticulosis. Patients who have undergone bone marrow transplantation can present with GI bleeding as a manifestation of graft-versus-host disease, which typically presents as ulcerations in the small intestine. For patients bleeding from the upper GI tract, a nasogastric tube should be inserted and the tract lavaged with normal saline until the bleeding clears. If the bleeding does not clear, the patient should undergo upper GI endoscopy. Gastroenterologists at MDACC report that upper GI tract endoscopy is not often helpful for patients who have primary tumors in the GI tract. Patients with small tumors rarely have significant bleeding, and patients with large tumors tend to ooze and bleed. However, relief of bleeding by endoscopic measures is usually temporary, and these tumors tend to bleed repeatedly (57). Endoscopic interventions can include electrocoagulation, epinephrine injections, and argon plasma laser treatment. For patients with persistent bleeding, arteriography and embolization is occasionally successful. If all other interventions have failed, surgery can be considered. Patients with bleeding should have any coagulopathy corrected, including deficits in the platelet count, which should be greater than 60,000/μL and preferably greater than 100,000/μL (57). Somatostatin or vasopressin can be used to control bleeding of esophageal varicies. The patient should receive either an H2 blocker or a proton pump inhibitor intravenously. Nausea should be controlled using intravenous antiemetics, and the patient should receive nothing by mouth. The patient should also receive normal saline if his or her blood pressure is low.

TYPHLITIS

Typhlitis is a syndrome of bowel inflammation, edema, and wall thickening involving the proximal large bowel in patients with neutropenic fever. It commonly affects the cecum but can also affect the ascending colon and occasionally the transverse colon. Typhlitis can occur in conjunction with any cancer but is most common in patients with leukemia (25). The organisms most often isolated in cases of typhlitis are *Clostridium* and gram-negative bacilli (58).

Patients with typhlitis present with fever, pain in the right lower quadrant of the abdomen, and sometimes diarrhea, which may be bloody. The patient with typhlitis is neutropenic, and plain abdominal x-ray films are often inconclusive. The diagnosis of typhlitis is made based on clinical suspicion and CT or MRI findings that reveal bowel inflammation, edema, wall thickening, and possibly air formation or, in severe cases, free air (Fig. 39-19).

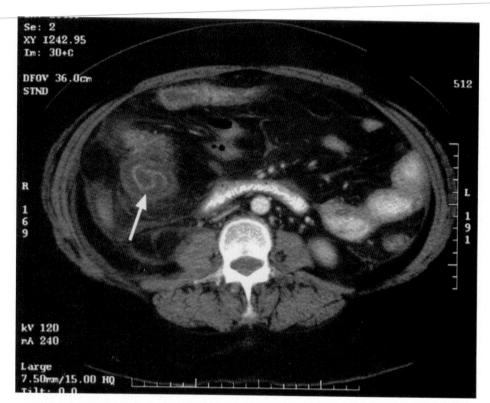

Se: 2
XY I242.95
Im: 30+C

DFOV 36.0cm
STND

512

R

1
6
9

L

1
9
1

kV 120
mA 240

Large
7.50mm/15.00 HQ
Tilt: 0.0

FIGURE 39-19. Inflammation of the cecum and ascending colon in a 45-year-old patient with typhlitis. The arrow points to inflammation and edema of the cecum. (*Image courtesy of Dr. Stephanie Mundy, M.D. Anderson Cancer Center.*)

Typhlitis is managed by bowel rest and intravenous administration of broad-spectrum antibiotics, including anaerobic coverage. Patients rarely require surgery unless they develop intractable bleeding or bowel perforation or do not respond to conservative measures.

References

1. Cascino TL. Neurologic complications of systemic cancer. *Med Clin North Am* 1993;77(1):265–278.
2. Krimsky WS, Behrens RJ, Kerkvliet GJ. Oncologic emergencies for the internist. *Cleve Clin J Med* 2002;69(3):209–210, 213–214, 216–217.
3. Rude M. Selected neurologic complications in the patient with cancer. Brain metastases and spinal cord compression. *Crit Care Nurs Clin North Am* 2000;12(3):269–279.
4. Schiff D, Batchelor T, Wen PY. Neurologic emergencies in cancer patients. *Neurol Clin* 1998;6(2):449–483.
5. Tan SJ. Recognition and treatment of oncologic emergencies. *J Infus Nurs* 2002;25(3):182–188.
6. Quinn JA, DeAngelis LM. Neurologic emergencies in the cancer patient. *Semin Oncol* 2000;27(3):311–321.
7. Neilan BA. Oncologic emergencies. Treating acute problems resulting from cancer and chemotherapy. *Postgrad Med* 1994;95(1):125–128, 131–132.
8. Saarto T, Janes R, Tenhunen M, et al. Palliative radiotherapy in the treatment of skeletal metastases. *Eur J Pain* 2002;6(5):323–330.
9. Cher LM. Cancer and the nervous system. *Med J Aust* 2001;175(5):277–282.
10. Vecht CJ. Clinical management of brain metastasis. *J Neurol* 1998;245(3):127–131.
11. Soffietti R, Ruda R, Mutani R. Management of brain metastases. *J Neurol* 2002;249(10):1357–1369.
12. O'Neill BP, Buckner JC, Coffey RJ, et al. Brain metastatic lesions. *Mayo Clin Proc* 1994;69(11):1062–1068.
13. DeAngelis LM. Management of brain metastases. *Cancer Invest* 1994;12(2):156–165.
14. Arnold SM, Patchell RA. Diagnosis and management of brain metastases. *Hematol Oncol Clin North Am* 2001;15(6):1085–1107 vii.
15. Sawaya R. Considerations in the diagnosis and management of brain metastases. *Oncology* (Huntingt) 2001;15(9):1144–1154, 1157–1158; discussion 1158, 1163–1165.
16. Wen PY, Loeffler JS. Brain metastases. *Curr Treat Options Oncol* 2000;1(5):447–458.
17. Patchell RA, Tibbs PA, Regine WF, et al. Postoperative radiotherapy in the treatment of single metastases to the brain: A randomized trial. *JAMA* 1998;280(17):1485–1489.
18. Ewend MG, Carey LA, Morris DE, et al. Brain metastases. Central nervous system malignancies. *Curr Treat Options Oncol* 2001;2(6):537–547.
19. Davey P. Brain metastases: Treatment options to improve outcomes. *CNS Drugs* 2002;16(5):325–338.
20. Grossman SA, Krabak MJ. Leptomeningeal carcinomatosis. *Cancer Treat Rev* 1999;25(2):103–119.
21. Escalante CP, Hwang JP, Grover TS, et al. Major presenting symptoms. In: Yeung SJ, Escalante CP, eds. *Oncologic Emergencies.* Hamilton, Ontario, Canada: BC Decker, 2002:48–50
22. Treatment of convulsive status epilepticus. Recommendations of the Epilepsy Foundation of America's Working Group on Status Epilepticus. *JAMA* 1993;270(7):854–859.

23. Posner JB. Management of brain metastases. *Rev Neurol (Paris)* 1992;148(6–7):477–487.

24. Demopoulos A, DeAngelis LM. Neurologic complications of leukemia. *Curr Opin Neurol* 2002;15(6):691–699.

25. Shanholtz C. Acute life-threatening toxicity of cancer treatment. *Crit Care Clin* 2001;17(3):483–502.

26. Tsang TS, Enriquez-Sarano M, Freeman WK, et al. Consecutive 1127 therapeutic echocardiographically guided pericardiocenteses: Clinical profile practice patterns and outcomes spanning 21 years. *Mayo Clin Proc* 2002;77(5):429–436.

27. Ewer MS, Duran JB, Swofford J, et al. Emergency cardiac problems. In: Yeung SJ, Escalante CP, eds. *Oncologic Emergencies.* Hamilton, Ontario, Canada: BC Decker, 2002:304–314.

28. Gao S, Shannon VR. Vascular emergencies. In: Yeung SJ, Escalante CP, eds. *Oncologic Emergencies.* Hamilton, Ontario, Canada: BC Decker, 2002:315–336.

29. Kvale PA, Simoff M, Prakash UB. Lung cancer. Palliative care. *Chest* 2003;23(1 suppl):284S–311S.

30. Douketis JD, Crowther MA, Stanton EB, et al. Elevated cardiac troponin levels in patients with submassive pulmonary embolism. *Arch Intern Med* 2002;162(1):79–81.

31. Blumenthal DT, Glenn MJ. Neurologic manifestations of hematologic disorders. *Neurol Clin* 2002;20(1):265–281 viii.

32. Drew MJ. Plasmapheresis in the dysproteinemias. *Ther Apher* 2002;6(1):45–52.

33. Weiser MA, O'Brien S, Narvios AB. Hematologic emergencies. In: Yeung SJ, Escalante CP, eds. *Oncologic Emergencies.* Hamilton, Ontario, Canada: BC Decker, 2002:337–354.

34. Kaminsky DA, Hurwitz CG, Olmstead JI. Pulmonary leukostasis mimicking pulmonary embolism. *Leuk Res* 2000;24(2):175–178.

35. DeSancho MT, Rand JH. Bleeding and thrombotic complications in critically ill patients with cancer. *Crit Care Clin* 2001;17(3):599–622.

36. Tissue plasminogen activator for the treatment of acute pulmonary embolism. A collaborative study by the PIOPED Investigators. *Chest* 1990;97(3):528–533.

37. Nazario R, Delorenzo LJ, Maguire AG. Treatment of venous thromboembolism. *Cardiol Rev* 2002;10(4):249–259.

38. Levine MN. Can we optimize treatment of thrombosis? *Cancer Treat Rev* 2003;29 Suppl 2:19–22.

39. Spyropoulos A. Venous thromboembolism. Outpatient-based treatment protocols using LMWH. *J Respir Dis* 2001;22 (suppl 12):23–28.

40. Shannon VR, Ng A. Noninfectious pulmonary emergencies. In: Yeung SJ, Escalante CP, eds. *Oncologic Emergencies.* Hamilton, Ontario, Canada: BC Decker, 2002.

41. Levine M. Managing thromboembolic disease in cancer patient: Efficacy and safety of antithrombotic treatment options in patients with cancer. *Cancer Treat Rev* 2002;28:145–149.

42. Lee AY. Treatment of venous thromboembolism in cancer patients. *Thromb Res* 2001;102(6):V195–V208.

43. Schiffer CA, Anderson KC, Bennett CL, et al. Platelet transfusion for patients with cancer: Clinical practice guidelines of the American Society of Clinical Oncology. *J Clin Oncol* 2001;19(5):1519–1538.

44. Bick RL. Disseminated intravascular coagulation: A review of etiology, pathophysiology, diagnosis, and management: Guidelines for care. *Clin Appl Thromb Hemost* 2002;8(1):1–31.

45. Maxson JH. Management of disseminated intravascular coagulation. *Crit Care Nurs Clin North Am* 2000;12(3):341–352.

46. Johnson EK, Klotz AD, Vaze AA, et al. Nephrology and urologic emergencies. In: Yeung SJ, Escalante CP, eds. *Oncologic Emergencies.* Hamilton, Ontario, Canada: BC Decker, 2002.

47. Russo P. Urologic emergencies in the cancer patient. *Semin Oncol* 2000;27(3):284–298.

48. Alley E, Green R, Schuchter L. Cutaneous toxicities of cancer therapy. *Curr Opin Oncol* 2002;14(2):212–216.

49. Bertilli G. Prevention and management of extravasation of cytotoxic drugs. *Drug Safety* 1995;12(4):245–255.

50. Dorr RT. Antidotes to vesicant chemotherapy extravasations. *Blood Rev* 1990;4(1):41–60.

51. Kassner E. Evaluation and treatment of chemotherapy extravasation injuries. *J Pediatr Oncol Nurs* 2000;17(3):135–148.

52. Fenchel K, Karthaus M. Cytotoxic drug extravasation. *Antibiot Chemother* 2000;50:144–148.

53. Susser WS, Whitaker-Worth DL, Grant-Kels JM. Mucocutaneous reactions to chemotherapy. *J Am Acad Dermatol* 1999;40(3):367–398; quiz 399–400.

54. Milionis HJ, Liamis GL, Elisaf MS. The hyponatremic patient: A systematic approach to laboratory diagnosis. *CMAJ* 2002;166(8):1056–1062.

55. Yeung SJ, Diaz GL, Gagel RF. Metabolic and endocrine emergencies. In: Yeung SJ, Escalante CP, eds. *Oncologic Emergencies.* Hamilton, Ontario, Canada: BC Decker, 2002.

56. Janjan N. Bone metastases: Approaches to management. *Semin Oncol* 2001;28(4 suppl 11):28–34.

57. Gagneja HK, Sinicrope FA. Gastrointestinal emergencies. In: Yeung SJ, Escalante CP, eds. *Oncologic Emergencies.* Hamilton, Ontario, Canada: BC Decker, 2002.

58. Casariego I, Vincente A, Greene J. Neutropenic enterocolitis in leukemia. *Infect Medicine* 2002;19(A):410.

Palliative Care and Symptom Management

PRINCIPLES OF PALLIATIVE CARE

Michael J. Fisch
Kay Swint

■ CASE VIGNETTE: STRIVING TO LIVE BETTER DESPITE SERIOUS ILLNESS

Randy, 49 years old, was until recently a strapping, 6-ft 1-in. 230-lb man able to handle his physically demanding job as an oilfield supervisor. When he began having shoulder pain, he was not especially worried, but he consulted a doctor anyway. He and his family were stunned to learn the actual cause of the pain: lung cancer that had metastasized to bone—a condition with a poor prognosis.

Randy began palliative radiation treatment in his home community, but the pain was so severe and the side effects of the pain medication so debilitating that his quality of life plummeted. Within a few months, he was too weak and fatigued to leave the house, and he had such severe nausea that he lost 40 lb. His physical condition forced him to miss his son's high school graduation ceremony.

That was when Randy and his wife, Alicia, were referred to the University of Texas M. D. Anderson Cancer Center (MDACC), where he hoped to participate in a clinical trial. Unfortunately, when he was first evaluated at MDACC, his thoracic oncologist could not enter him into a trial because he was too sick to meet the criteria for inclusion. Fortunately, though, she did not have to say, "There's nothing more we can do for you."

Randy was then referred to the palliative care outpatient center, where he was thoroughly assessed and treated for his complex symptoms, which included pain, nausea, fatigue, and depression. The palliative care physician and nursing staff helped him manage his medication schedule and helped him and his wife with making decisions, including advance directives. Within a few visits over a 10-day period, Randy's symptoms diminished dramatically and he was able to resume some pleasurable activities, such as going out to a restaurant with his three children or taking a stroll around the mall with his wife. "They gave me back my life," Randy said.

Palliative care cannot directly change the odds of survival for someone like Randy, but it can and does change patients' quality of life during the time they have left—time that is more precious than it ever was before. And better control of symptoms improves the chances that this kind of patient can receive the best available standard treatment and the opportunity to enroll in a clinical trial.

Ultimately, Randy was well enough to take part in a study of a new antiangiogenic agent. The novel treatment at the very least helped give some meaning to Randy's experience with cancer because he knew that it would help researchers understand the effects of the new treatment. In a sense, it was as if good symptom control and palliative care had provided him and his treating oncologist with elbow room to explore a broader set of choices. Unfortunately, Randy did not respond to the novel therapy. Shortly after his cancer progressed, he returned home with good symptom control as a starting point for hospice enrollment and care toward the end of his life.

■ MEETING A CRITICAL NEED: THE "SPONGE" MODEL

At MDACC, the mission is to eliminate cancer in Texas, the nation, and the world. The staff at our institution feel a pressing need and duty to develop newer, more advanced treatments that will save more lives. Many people have been cured of cancer here; many others have had long-term remissions. But the hard reality is that many patients do die of cancer. About 7500 patients at MDACC die each year—roughly half the number of new patients we see in a given year and a figure consistent with national statistics.

Oncologists here are members of multidisciplinary teams organized by disease site and configured toward crafting curative treatment strategies. Although they recognize the value of diminishing suffering and caring for the whole person, achieving that goal consistently while balancing the demands of their specialties can be challenging. Patients and their families, on the other hand, often have increasingly complex physical and psychological needs over time as a cure begins to look less realistic. Understandably, they want to remain connected with the institution they have come to trust. One oncologist summarized the role of palliative care as follows:

Years ago, my father-in-law had colon cancer. When all curative treatment was exhausted, his oncologist told him to go somewhere else for his care, literally telling him that he didn't have time for him. That was so traumatic for him and his family that 15 years after his death, during the Christmas holidays, his widow is still traumatized when she recalls that experience. I don't ever want to be the doctor that people remember that way ... but the oncologists here cannot continue to care for all of these patients and their complex needs after we are no longer realistically able to find a cure. Palliative care has made it possible for us to feel good about how we handle these needs.

As this physician suggests, palliative care can help oncologists stay in stride as their efforts are configured in a very specific way toward the care of patients who are most likely to benefit from the comprehensive approach of a multidisciplinary treatment team organized by disease type. These patients might be considered "high multiplier" patients, in the sense that they are more likely to use laboratory and radiology services, enroll in clinical trials, and receive complex treatments. These multidisciplinary teams are not perfectly designed to provide complex care to patients with very advanced disease and poor performance status.

Currently, roughly 55,000 patients each year receive care at MDACC, and nearly 60% of new patients die within 2 years of registration (1). Overall, 1300 patients receive palliative care (900 in the inpatient setting and 700 in the palliative care outpatient clinic and 300 in both settings). Over the past 2 years, 277 physicians out of 650 active staff (43%) have referred patients for palliative care. The patients who receive palliative care are often, but not always, "low multiplier" patients. The palliative care team is able to respond to the unmet needs of these patients, serving as a "sponge" that absorbs from the primary team some of the excess burden of caring for these patients without forcing those providers to abandon their patients or their role in disease management. The overall effect of this sponge model, ideally, is better patient outcomes, including patient and family satisfaction and gratitude expressed for the primary teams. There is also less burnout on the part of oncologists and better overall system efficiency. The effect of the sponge model on the overall operation of a comprehensive cancer center is shown in Fig. 40-1.

■ PALLIATIVE CARE DEFINITIONS AND FUNCTIONAL MODELS

Palliative care is often misunderstood as an approach to be taken when there are no other options left. In reality, the World Health Organization's definition of palliative care, which follows, is much broader: "Palliative care is an approach that improves the quality of life of patients and their families facing problems associated with life-threatening illness, through the prevention and relief of suffering by means of early identification and impeccable assessment and treatment of pain and other problems, physical, psychosocial, and spiritual (2)." Thus, palliative care is both comprehensive and interdisciplinary in its scope and it is also applicable early in a serious illness such as cancer. Figure 40-2 shows models that summarize how palliative care is integrated with disease management (curative care).

The early models involved a vertical separation of curative and palliative care. In more recent models, however, palliative care is incorporated more linearly over

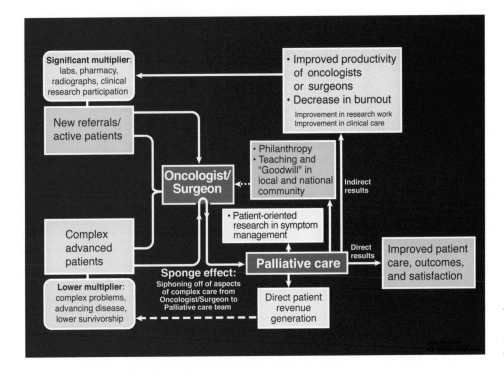

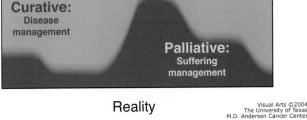
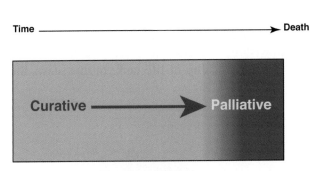
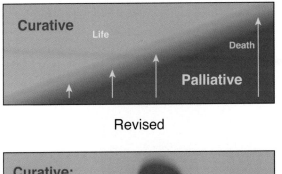
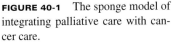

FIGURE 40-2 Models of palliative care and curative care in the trajectory of illness. [*From Fisch (4). With permission.*]

time, but this is oversimplified and unrealistic. The reality is that there are limitless possible ways to integrate optimal disease management and palliative care. The most appropriate plan for any given patient depends on many factors, including the trajectory of the patient's illness, the way the patient expresses his or her subjective experience of the symptoms, the patient's access to personal and professional care, and personal preferences.

The early integration of disease treatment and palliative care in patients with cancer has been described by Meyers and Linder (3) as "simultaneous care." Many of our patients who receive palliative care are still actively receiving curative treatment. A much larger percentage, however, are receiving simultaneous care that involves the integration of local or systemic anticancer therapies being delivered with palliative intent. These patients and their primary oncologists are supported by the palliative care team in the inpatient or outpatient setting. This team provides expert symptom assessment and management, assistance with medical decision making, and assessments to determine needs for interdisciplinary care (such as the involvement of physical or occupational therapy, speech therapy, and the chaplaincy). Perhaps most important, we give patients time to tell their story and help us understand how to work with them and their primary team to identify and attain their quality-of-life goals.

One model often used to explain to patients and families the approach of the palliative care team is the "quality-of-life tank model," as shown in Fig. 40-3 (4).

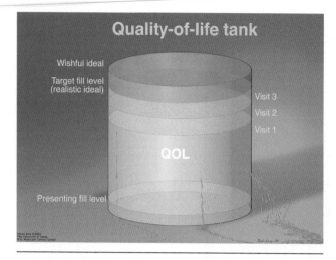

FIGURE 40-3   Model of the quality-of-life tank. [*From Fisch (4). With permission.*]

A typical discussion of this model with a patient might sound as follows:

Imagine your quality of life as if it could be contained in a tank. I have a vision for you of what would be the realistic ideal in terms of the level of fill for your quality-of-life tank. Of course, I recognize that there is a level of fill even higher than the "realistic ideal." It is what I call the "wishful ideal." This is to acknowledge that the presence of this cancer is unspeakable and unwelcome.... I wish it were different for you. Nevertheless, I'm focused on the fact that your quality-of-life tank has leaked down much too far. My goal is to identify the leaks and find a way to stop the leaks such that your quality-of-life tank fills back up to where it should be. I'm very optimistic about how well you should feel and live, even given the circumstances regarding your cancer.

Of course, using this metaphor is effective only for patients who are able to focus, concentrate, and use abstract reasoning. However, physicians in various specialties frequently use analogies to help make complex clinical concepts more understandable to lay people (5). This quality-of-life tank model can be explained in words alone or along with a visual image of the tank and its leaks. Particularly useful in this discussion is the notion of the wishful ideal. It allows the patient room to talk about how unfair and dreadful their situation is. The model has a place for those feelings. The use of "wish" expressions can be very helpful in scenarios such as breaking bad news, responding to hopes and fears, deal-

ing with feelings of loss and grief, dealing with unrealistic demands for aggressive treatment, or even responding to disappointments or errors regarding medical treatment (6). This "wishful" space toward the top of the tank gives providers a place to put their empathy and use words that help build empathy, such as, "Let me see if I have this right" or "It sounds like it is very difficult for you to have to take so many pills" (7). The wishful ideal can also be conceptualized as an ideal that may be achievable but is not guaranteed. It can be a space where the patient and provider confront the tyranny of uncertainty. In turn, counseling can be directed toward hoping for the best (the wishful ideal) and preparing for the worst, while at the same time identifying the important short-term goal of living as well as possible (8).

To best understand an individual's sense of quality of life and what is missing, one must have as complete an understanding of the person as possible. More than 20 years ago, Cassell (9) described suffering as that which threatens the integrity of the person. Figure 40-4 summarizes the many things that make a person what he or she is.

These are also the broad dimensions of understanding that palliative care providers can use to identify both the wishful ideals and the leaks in an individual's highly personal quality-of-life tank. In this sense, the

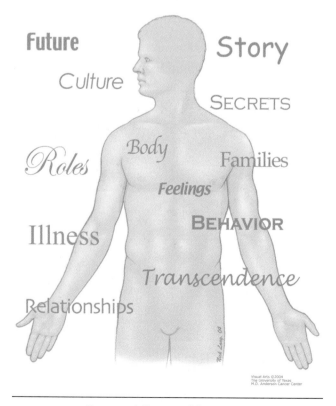

FIGURE 40-4   Conceptual diagram of the person.

quality-of-life tank model is enhanced by skillful techniques of communicating with patients, such as the use of the patient-centered interview and open-ended questions, such as "tell me about yourself" (10).

Finally, the quality-of-life tank model can be a rich metaphor for incorporating aspects of dignity-preserving care. Chochinov (11) described living in the moment, maintaining normalcy, and finding spiritual comfort as examples of dignity-preserving practices. Following is an example of a way to communicate this message:

> *Despite the fact that your cancer has spread to your bones and is causing considerable pain, you continue to hold up very well. You are as dignified as ever! How do you find the strength to endure these things? [The patient might mention faith or family support.] It is as if you had an extra reservoir, perhaps a spiritual well-being reservoir, that helps fill your tank despite the various leaks. I admire that a lot. You are very fortunate. Nevertheless, I try not to let that distract me from doing my part to find and fix the leaks. That way, you get the very best quality of life, and you can fully benefit from all of your blessings that buoy you each day.*

Figure 40-5 shows an adapted quality-of-life tank model that incorporates a spiritual well-being reservoir, which might be evident for certain patients. By showing these patients how to fit their spirituality into the model in an integrative fashion, it allows them to accept the full package of palliative care (including the palliative use of local or systemic anticancer therapies) and preserve their dignity.

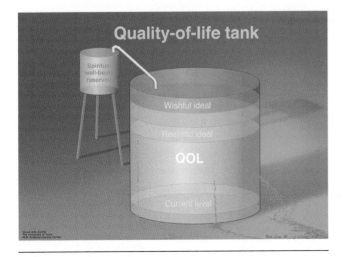

FIGURE 40-5 The quality-of-life tank with spiritual well-being reservoir.

■ AUTHENTIC, BENEVOLENT, AND ACCESSIBLE CARE

Often, the first point of contact for a patient with our palliative care team is during a time of acute distress, such as when an MDACC physician has just delivered bad news. To meet their needs, we focus on "just in time" care, often seeing patients on the same day as the referral. Our mobile team (a palliative care physician and sometimes a fellow and/or advanced practice nurse) goes where it is called, either to the referring physician's outpatient clinic or to the bedside of an inpatient.

After a consultation is completed and the patient's needs are identified, the referring team has multiple options. The palliative care team can work in a consulting role, it may incorporate palliative care as an ongoing part of the treatment team, or—in the event of more advanced or end-of-life needs—it may request that the palliative care team become the primary care team. In this last scenario, the patient is not abandoned by the primary team; rather, it is as if the palliative care is dialed to the foreground and the primary team is still present but more in the background. In essence, palliative care for patients with cancer at MDACC is often rooted in being flexible enough to deal with whatever unmet needs confront our patients, with providers dialed to the foreground or background, depending on what is most fitting at each point in time. Whereas many subspecialty referrals are very specific in terms of the nature of the request (e.g., "Please evaluate this patient for the cause of tachypalpitations and presyncope"), palliative care referrals are often appropriately vague. The nature of the problem may be unclear. At times, the palliative care team is able to discern a virtual "symptom masquerade," whereby, for example, a patient with nociceptive pain and inadequate pain treatment describes the problem exclusively in terms of fatigue or some other symptom because of unmet needs. By recognizing this masquerade, the palliative care team may be able to fix the patient's quality-of-life problems by initiating the proper treatment for pain, with the expectation that the unbearable fatigue will thus be relieved. In other cases, what is described as unrelieved pain may turn out to be somatization. The key to successful palliative care is proper assessment followed by careful and timely reassessment in the context of an excellent rapport with the patient and family along with fidelity to the continuity of care. Major themes in the delivery of our services are authenticity, benevolence, and accessibility. *Authenticity* refers to that which conforms to fact and is genuine and trustworthy. In this case, authenticity is based on our experience, training, and expertise in the field of palliative medicine, which is now a distinct specialty in the United States (12,13). *Benevolence* is demonstrated by putting patient and family needs at the forefront, and *accessibility* refers to our acknowledgment that timing is paramount in palliative care—the window of opportunity to make a difference in the lives of a patient and family can be very narrow, and appropriate care must be delivered on a just-in-time basis.

■ OUTPATIENT CENTER

About one-third of our patients are first seen in the Palliative Care and Rehabilitation Medicine outpatient center, which is staffed by a medical director and three registered nurses and supported by four department physicians. Like that of the mobile consultation team, their commitment is to prompt response, with the staff striving to provide same-day appointments whenever possible.

Although outpatients average 2.5 visits to our center, it is not unusual for us to follow patients for months to years. The key to success in outpatient palliative care is ensuring continuity of care and concentrating on responding to patient and family needs wherever they happen to be and whenever the need arises. The existence of a palliative care outpatient clinic also allows ill patients to be assessed without putting an undue burden on the emergency center and in a setting that preserves dignity. More important, the outpatient part of the comprehensive palliative care program allows the early integration of palliative care with the usual oncologic approaches to cancer treatment (3).

The palliative care product line in the outpatient setting is extremely diverse, and there are innumerable examples of excellent referrals. It is easier to describe the patient who does not need a referral: the patient whose symptoms and medical problems are readily manageable, whose suffering is minimal, and whose care lacks enormous complexity. However, many patients are lacking in one of these areas. Most such patients can still receive good care, but the care takes extraordinary energy and resources from multiple providers. Such patients not only take time and create inefficiency for the primary team but also use time and resources in unpredictable amounts at unpredictable times. For such complex patients, the palliative care team not only provides another level of expertise and multidisciplinary care but also has the sponge effect described earlier. Common scenarios that have provided the basis for palliative care referrals are listed in Table 40-1.

TABLE 40-1 | COMMON REASONS FOR REFERRAL TO PALLIATIVE CARE

Cognitive impairment leading to misleading results on symptom assessment

Patient overwhelmed with unexpected bad news about cancer ("hit by a truck," as they say)

Opioid toxicity or phobia, creating poor pain control

Patient too debilitated for systemic chemotherapy, but could benefit from treatment if rehabilitation is achieved

Patient needs immediate anticancer therapy and concomitant intensive symptom management

Complex pain syndrome (neuropathic plus somatovisceral) due to uncontrolled pelvic involvement of tumor

Patient (or family) with magical thinking or extreme denial about health status

Severe chronic dyspnea-triggering anxiety crises and difficult disposition

Patient wants hospice with a link to M. D. Anderson

Somatization: Patient with chronic, stable, and unchangeable levels of extreme symptom expression

Aberrant drug-taking behaviors or known addiction

Patient cannot get hospice care because of special needs or preferences but needs end-of-life care

Primary team wants patient to leave hospital, but patient will not or cannot go

Need to distinguish terminal delirium from potentially reversible delirium (dying from "not quite dying yet")

Indolent, advanced cancer or prolonged survivorship but debilitating psychological distress

Difficult symptoms compounded by overwhelming family conflict

Difficult symptom control compounded by severe communication barriers (physical or cultural)

One symptom masquerading as another (nausea due to anxiety, fatigue due to pain or depression, pain due to delirium, anxiety due to dyspnea, etc.)

Serious medical or psychiatric comorbidities and advanced cancer symptoms in need of careful coordination of care

Particularly high expectations for care or VIP status and some bothersome symptoms

Difficult or surprising acute or chronic complications of cancer treatment

Chronic nonmalignant pain causing distress and confusion in the context of advanced cancer

Acute, reversible medical problems that must be distinguished from chronic cancer problems

Patient's preference (or the preference of the referring doctor) for early integration of palliative care with cancer care

Cancer pain not responding to first-line opioids—hence need opioid dose titration, administration of coanalgesics, and management of expected opioid side effects

Patient who is actively dying and needs suffering management, family counseling, and "peeling back" of care not specifically contributing to comfort at the end of life

The most painstaking aspect of initiating secondary palliative care in the outpatient center at a cancer center is establishing a trusting relationship between the treating cancer experts and the palliative care team. The ideal palliative care outpatient physician strives to help the patient feel better and maximize overall quality of life while at the same time enhancing the reputation and effectiveness of the primary team of providers. If the patient feels better but the reputation or the effectiveness of the primary oncologist is diminished, then in some respects palliative care has failed. The essence of successful secondary palliative care in a cancer center is finding a win-win situation for the patient and the treating team of cancer experts. To accomplish this, the palliative care physicians need to establish credibility by demonstrating sufficient internal medicine expertise to manage a wide array of clinical problems and sufficient knowledge in oncology to recognize and manage common oncologic problems and to understand the natural history and treatment paradigms for various malignancies.

In addition, the palliative care physicians must have great flexibility in their expectations. That is, the palliative care team must recognize that elegant and artful oncology care takes many forms, and the specific approach being recommended by the primary oncologist has to be understood and supported. The palliative care physician can also expect to be asked by some patients and/or family members to explain some of the nuances of cancer management choices. This can happen for several reasons. First, some patients do not feel comfortable asking their oncologist to carefully explain treatment choices. Often, this is because they have great trust in the oncologist and do not want to appear as if they are questioning the plan of care. Sometimes, superb oncologists are able to craft highly effective management plans, but they have some difficulty explaining the basis of the plan in layman's terms, or they may not have sufficient time to go into as much detail as patients would like.

One example of a subtle aspect of the reasoning behind oncology care that is commonly misunderstood by patients with a refractory solid tumor is that the oncologist is planning to deliver therapeutic maneuvers in sequence and does not expect to achieve cure with the first chosen regimen. Indeed, systemic anticancer therapy is most often prescribed in an effort to improve quality of life over time. In essence, the treatment goal is to maximize the area under the curve if quality of life were plotted over time. One oncologist summarized it in an e-mail to a palliative care physician as follows: "Oral etoposide will be a consideration at some time along the way. There is no real priority in this patient at this stage; rather, it is likely that the patient will exhaust all options in sequence as long as he is prepared to continue and I am prepared to offer something."

In the palliative care clinic, we generally have more time to explain this type of approach to patients. One way to explain this treatment approach is by using the analogy of a hitchhiker making his way from Houston to Los Angeles. First, we acknowledge that the trip is most unwelcome; given the choice, nobody would hitchhike. But if one were to face this type of trip, one would not expect to be picked up by one driver who would take them the entire distance. Rather, the traveler would expect to take a series of rides, making every effort to choose safe and smooth rides and hoping that each ride goes a long distance in the right direction. When a ride runs out, or if it takes the traveler in the wrong direction, then the hitchhiker jumps off and waits for the next driver who is going in the right direction. In this analogy, the oncologist is someone with special expertise in guiding the patient through the series of therapeutic maneuvers (rides). Each treatment has a certain probability of producing a response (the chance that it takes the traveler in the correct direction), and each response has a certain duration (the length of the ride). If one considers stable disease as one of the acceptable responses in a given situation, then the notion that a treatment pause is one type of "ride" that could be appropriate becomes understandable. Like any other chosen ride, a "pause maneuver" would need to be monitored carefully and, when appropriate, abandoned in favor of a different approach. The hitchhiker model is illustrated in Fig. 40-6.

Overall, the outpatient palliative care center provides a safe setting where patients can have their treatment plans explained further. Of course, it is also a safe place to discuss other difficult issues, such as pain, fatigue, nausea, anxiety, depression, loss of appetite, dyspnea, sexual dysfunction, spiritual distress, or whatever else is affecting function or quality of life. In this setting, the care is both comprehensive and interdisciplinary. With regard to the latter, various disciplines (physical therapy, occupational therapy, nutrition care, wound/ostomy care, chaplaincy, social work, speech therapy, clinical psychology, etc.) are incorporated into the individual care plans as needed in a sequence deemed most helpful by the palliative care physician.

■ INPATIENT UNIT (TERTIARY LEVEL PALLIATIVE CARE)

Sally, a 27-year-old woman with acute lymphoblastic leukemia, had intensive chemotherapy followed by al-

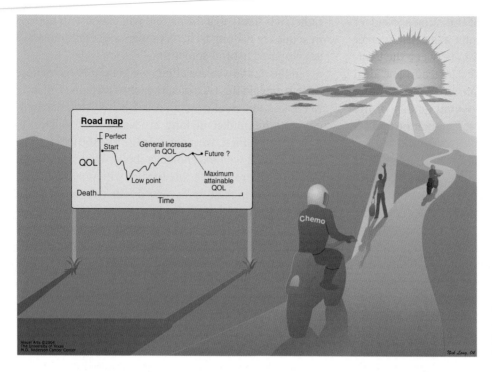

Road map

Perfect
Start
General increase
in QOL
Future ?
QOL
Low point
Maximum
attainable
QOL
Death
Time

Visual Arts ©2004
The University of Texas
M.D. Anderson Cancer Center

Nick Long, 04

FIGURE 40-6 The hitchhiker metaphor in describing care for a refractory solid tumor.

logeneic bone marrow transplantation. About 6 months after the transplantation, progressive paraparesis developed as a result of treatment-related cervical myelopathy. One year later, she was referred to the palliative care outpatient clinic for the management of painful decubitus ulcers and depression. Within 2 months, she experienced progression of chronic graft-versus-host disease, requiring hospitalization. On day 22 of this hospital admission, she was transferred from the bone marrow transplant service to the palliative care inpatient unit for the management of progressive nausea, vomiting, and jaundice. The patient received aggressive symptom management, and she and her family received supportive counseling with the help of nurses, the unit social worker, and a psychiatry nurse liaison in addition to the palliative care physicians. Before the hospitalization, Sally had lived with her elementary school–aged daughter and her common-law husband. During her illness, she elected to be married in a ceremony in the inpatient unit before her discharge home. She chose to receive intravenous medications for graft-versus-host disease as directed by the bone marrow transplant team in addition to the comprehensive management of her symptoms. Within 12 days of returning home, she developed acute renal failure and delirium and was readmitted to the palliative care inpatient unit, where she received care directed toward her comfort and dignity at the end of life. She died 7 days after this second admission, with her family at her bedside.

A fully designated symptom control and palliative care inpatient unit is available at MDACC for the care of patients with advanced cancer and complex, intractable symptoms. This unit opened in May 2003 and has 12 beds with a 96% occupancy rate and often an additional 1 to 3 patients awaiting transfer to the unit from another floor. Typical patients, such as Sally, have an overwhelming symptom burden, medically complex conditions, and possibly other needs that can be met only in a tertiary palliative care environment. Sally was an appropriate candidate for home hospice care at the conclusion of her first hospital admission, but she did not choose to receive hospice care. A particular advantage of the tertiary palliative care unit is that it offers a scope of interdisciplinary care and other options that are not typically offered by hospices (such as blood transfusions, palliative radiotherapy, and immunosuppressive therapies directed by other specialists). In many cases, the palliative care unit is an optimal transition to hospice care. Other times, patients' conditions are stabilized before they are discharged to home.

Roughly one-quarter of teaching hospitals have established palliative care programs (12), and the number with tertiary palliative care units is growing (13). One of the most successful palliative care programs in the United States opened a dedicated inpatient unit about 11 years after the program was founded (14), but newer programs are moving toward inpatient units much earlier in their history. One program has been able to demonstrate a reduction in the in-hospital end-of-life care costs associated with a tertiary palliative care unit (15), but more data are needed to fully understand the net benefits of these units in terms of both health outcomes and the use of resources. One source of trepidation related to the opening of the tertiary palliative care unit at our cancer center was that it would increase the number of inpatient deaths as a proportion of all hospital discharges. This has not been the case, however, as this proportion of deaths has remained at 3% to 4%. Roughly 20% of all inpatient deaths occur in the palliative care inpatient unit, and about 25% of the patients admitted to the palliative care inpatient unit die during the admission.

The median age of patients admitted to our inpatient unit is 57 years, and the most common cancer diagnoses are thoracic/head and neck (40%), gastrointestinal (19%), hematologic (11%), and genitourinary or gynecologic (10%) malignancies (16). The most common symptoms prompting referral are pain (50%), dyspnea (18%), and delirium (14%).

A recent process improvement on our inpatient unit changed the way we conduct rounds. In recognition of the fact that the nursing staff has the most extensive and timely information from the patient and family—but has heavy constraints on its time because of direct patient care duties—our interdisciplinary team conferences are now scheduled around the availability of the nursing team. The cases of patients assigned to a specific nurse are reviewed at one time, allowing all of the nurses to rotate through and participate fully in the discussions about their patients. This has allowed us to make significant improvements in care planning and provides daily opportunities for education and consultation.

THE INTERDISCIPLINARY TEAM

A hallmark of our program is a diverse team that is well prepared to consider the total person and family. Our physicians include three oncologists, one family practitioner, two internists, and an anesthesiologist. All our physicians are board-certified in palliative medicine. We also have three medical fellows who are board-certified internists. Our advanced-practice nurses include two nurses with acute medical certifications and one with psychiatric nursing certification. The inpatient nurse manager is certified in palliative care and brings years of hospice experience to our team. In addition, we have a social worker, chaplain, case manager, and pharmacist who participate in the program daily; other team members include a nutritionist, physical therapist, and

occupational therapist. The team reflects the principle that palliative care is comprehensive and interdisciplinary, with care directed toward both patients and their families.

An important decision has been staffing the program with nurses who have a special interest in palliative care. Initially, inpatient nurses were assigned to palliative care, incorporating these duties into their broader oncology practice. However, in reviewing nursing satisfaction through surveys and frank discussions, we determined that the typical oncology nurse felt particularly stressed by having to shift rapidly between palliative and curative goals—and many were not comfortable with or prepared to deal intensely with end-of-life issues. The survey data provided important support for the decision to designate a separate inpatient unit and staff for palliative care. Now, all the nurses in our program have chosen palliative care and have completed a special orientation; we also maintain a 1:3 nurse-to-patient ratio for this high-need patient group. We are now administering a survey to confirm whether this has improved nurse satisfaction, but spontaneous feedback and empiric observation support the philosophy that palliative nursing is a specialty that should be chosen, not assigned.

SUPPORTING FAMILIES AND CAREGIVERS

Caregivers and other family members are an important focus of care. In the outpatient unit, a member of the nursing staff routinely spends 20 minutes at each outpatient visit assessing the needs of the patient and caregiver. Caregivers are regularly offered an opportunity to discuss concerns privately with the nurse, who may then make referrals to social services, schedule a family meeting, or request support from appropriate members of the team.

A 1 hour family meeting is scheduled for all inpatients, typically about 3 days after admission. This meeting is coordinated by our social worker and attended by the physician and other members of the team. Although considerable communication occurs during a social work assessment before the meeting, the team uses this structured meeting to ensure that the family is encouraged to fully express their concerns, identify their preferences, and ask questions of any team member. The initial discharge plan is reviewed and modified. The case manager assumes leadership after this meeting to work with the entire team to attain a successful discharge. This is a very hands-on process, as she spends most of her time on the unit and meets daily with the team and often with the family.

■ ADDRESSING GRIEF, SPIRITUALITY, AND BEREAVEMENT

A psychosocial team composed of a social worker, chaplain, and nurse therapist is particularly important for palliative care patients and their families. Confronting a life-threatening illness can involve grief, depression, and questions about spirituality. The social worker does comprehensive grief assessments with patients and their families to identify areas of need. She also determines when someone needs more intensive support. Depending on the unique situation, she may be the primary support person, or she may involve the chaplain or the nurse therapist. The center's nondenominational chaplain works with patients of all faiths and cultures to support and guide their own spiritual and emotional journeys, helping them review their lives and find meaning and closure. Prayer, ritual, music, journal writing, and meditation are some of the tools offered to patients. The nurse therapist works most closely with children and adults with complicated grief.

When a patient dies on our unit, cards are sent to the family to support and honor their experience. The family receive a packet of information about the grieving process to help them understand the emotions they are going through and direct them to appropriate support groups and other bereavement services in their community. The special needs of grieving children are considered, and a recommended reading list is provided for children and adults. Our patients come from all parts of the world; therefore, when return visits are not feasible, we equip the family with information, resources, and contact information for support groups when they return home. Support groups for families in our area also meet at MDACC.

Because palliative care can be stressful for direct care staff, we offer support through a clinical supervision program. Individually and in groups, staff members can discuss therapeutic relationships with patients, families, and one another. This program is led by a highly experienced psychiatric advanced practice nurse assigned full time to the palliative program, the inpatient nurse manager who is certified in palliative nursing, and a licensed counselor who is assigned to the Division of Nursing. Every nurse in the clinic participates at least monthly in the clinical supervision program. All palliative care volunteers and other direct care staff are encouraged to access these services on an as-needed basis.

■ MEASURING SUCCESS

A key measure of the success of our palliative care program is the patient satisfaction reports obtained quarterly by the Department of Quality Improvement through telephone surveys conducted by Press Ganey Associates, Inc. We have taken specific steps to improve and achieve high ratings and have found that they correlate with process improvements to ensure just-in-time scheduling rather than scheduling around a fixed weekly clinic for each faculty member, more consistent follow-up with "no-show" patients to determine how we can accommodate each individual, the professional development and specialization of our nursing staff, and growth in the comprehensiveness of our service.

An indirect but nevertheless meaningful measure of effectiveness is the growth in the number of referrals. In the fiscal year from September 2001 to August 2002 (FY02), we treated 703 inpatients and 656 outpatients. The number of unique patients—eliminating overlap between outpatient and inpatient numbers—was 1113. After completing data analysis of the first 9 months of FY03, we are projected to treat 938 inpatients, 761 outpatients, and a total of 1397 unique patients, representing a 26% growth in patient referrals in 1 year. In addition, we have grown dramatically in the diversity of referring physicians, with referrals received from all eligible clinical departments in the institution.

Benchmarked data from other palliative care services are difficult to interpret because of the differences in the populations and missions of the programs. However, our most recent discharge data (now reflecting our experience in the first 6 months of operation of our dedicated inpatient unit) shows that 30% of our inpatients were discharged at the time of death; 38% were discharged to a hospice; 24% were discharged to home with outpatient care; 5% were discharged to subacute care, nursing homes, or other hospitals; and 2% were discharged to other arrangements. We had a mean length of stay of 10 days, with a median stay of 9 days. The average daily charges for a palliative care stay, including technical and professional services, were 63% of the average for the institution.

Measures of symptom improvement in a study of 184 discharged palliative care inpatients found that 67% achieved improvement in their target symptoms during hospitalization. This was a retrospective study, examining data routinely collected by the staff on a variety of symptom assessment scales (16). This symptom improvement rate might seem low, given the expertise and resources applied to the patients, but it reflects the referral bias that exists. That is, palliative care inpatients have very challenging and complex conditions; often multiple maneuvers have failed to control their symptoms by the time they are admitted. It is also important to recognize that outcome assessment extends beyond symptom measures; there are several different concepts and domains around which success can be measured. Such domains were summarized by Patrick and colleagues (17); an adapted summary is outlined in Table 40-2.

■ CHALLENGES WE HAVE MET

In instituting our program, we overcame a number of hurdles, including these:

Misconceptions about the needs and preferences of our patient population.

Assumptions that hospices had broader capabilities and fewer limitations than actually exist, thus minimizing the need for hospital-based palliative care programs.

The slow process of determining the best way to serve the needs of referring clinicians.

A nursing staffing model that fostered "scattered beds" versus specialty medical units.

There are many challenges as we work to continually improve our program. We have seen substantial changes in the mindsets and clinical practices of the clinicians who consult with us, but there is much more to be done. Our goal is to reach a much greater percentage of MDACC patients and families and their providers who would benefit from palliative care services. The pace of growth is a major challenge as the palliative care team struggles to find balance in their personal lives and works to respond to the rapidly growing demand. In addition, we are working to form more strategic relationships with the institution's other leaders in end-of-life care, particularly social work and case management, capitalizing on all our strengths and roles to improve decision making, discharge planning, and followup.

■ ADVICE WE CAN OFFER

Our program is individualized for a comprehensive cancer center, and our advice would be most applicable in that setting. It is as follows:

An individualized assessment of the needs of your particular center is the most essential step.

Although utilization statistics and financial analyses are necessary to concretely illustrate the need for a palliative care program, interviews with key physicians, representatives of social work, case management, and

TABLE 40-2 | CONCEPTS AND DOMAINS TO ASSESS PALLIATIVE CARE

Quality of life
Physical
  Self-care
  Activities of daily living
  Walking
  Mobility
  Eating
  Sleeping
  Thinking, remembering, speaking
Psychosocial
  Interaction with family
  Giving and receiving help
  Contributing to the community
  Recreation
  Sexual life
  Income
  Respect
  Variety in life
Symptom-related
  Pain
  Fatigue
  Nausea
  Dyspnea
  Anxiety
  Depression
  Anorexia
  Sleep disturbance

Quality of death and dying
  Symptoms and personal care
  Preparation for the end of life
  Moment of death
  Family
  Treatment preferences
  Spiritual well-being (meaning and purpose)

Quality of end-of-life care
  Continuous healing relationships through death and after death
  Focus on the dying patient's needs and preferences
  Providing the patient with locus of control and loved ones with involvement
  Shared knowledge about prognosis and all important aspects of care
  Shared decision making based on evidence
  Transparency in care and decision processes
  Anticipation of individual needs both inside and outside of the care settings
  Cooperation and communication among providers
  Coordination among caregivers, patients, and families

SOURCE: Adapted from Patrick et al. (17). With permission.

the chaplaincy will clarify how they currently manage palliative care and what their needs and goals are. Similarly, structured focus groups with patients and families will also help pinpoint areas of need.

From interviews and focus groups, you can identify potential program champions and goals.

We recommend beginning with a consulting service, structured as a mobile team, that travels to outpatient or inpatient settings.

For an inpatient program, recruit team members who have chosen palliative care rather than having been assigned to it.

Ensure that there is a strong medical competency in your palliative care team with the ability to serve as the primary treatment team for patients with acute medical needs.

Insurers tend to equate palliative care with hospice and try to negotiate a "step-down" or hospice rate. Be prepared to clearly identify your unit as acute care and to demonstrate the differences. The clinical team will need strong discharge planning support to transition patients to hospice, nursing home, or subacute care as appropriate.

The program's justification must include a major focus on several key factors, including providing a full spectrum of care for patients and families, reducing burnout of clinical team members with a curative focus, improving patient and community goodwill, and increasing the productivity of the institution as it more effectively and efficiently deploys its resources.

■ ACKNOWLEDGMENT

Graphic illustrations were done by Nick Lang.

References

1. Bruera E, Russell N, Sweeney C, et al. Place of death and its predictors for local patients registered at a comprehensive cancer center. *J Clin Oncol* 2002;20:2127–2133.

2. Sepulveda C, Marlin A, Yoshida T, et al. Palliative care: The World Health Organization's global perspective. *J Pain Symptom Manage* 2002;24:91–96.

3. Meyers FJ, Linder J. Simultaneous care: Disease treatment and palliative care throughout illness. *J Clin Oncol* 2003;21: 1412–1415.

4. Fisch MJ. Principles of palliative chemotherapy. In: Fisch MJ, Bruera E (eds): *Handbook of Advanced Cancer Care*. Cambridge, UK: Cambridge University Press; 2003:12–22.

5. Arroliga AC, Newman S, Longworth DL, et al. Metaphorical medicine: using metaphors to enhance communication with patients who have pulmonary disease. *Ann Intern Med* 2002;137:376–379.

6. Quill TE, Arnold RM, Platt F. "I wish things were different": expressing wishes in response to loss, futility, and unrealistic hopes. *Ann Intern Med* 2001;135:551–555.

7. Coulehan JL, Platt FW, Egener B, et al. "Let me see if I have this right...": words that help build empathy. *Ann Intern Med* 2001;135:221–227.

8. Back AL, Arnold RM, Quill TE. Hope for the best, and prepare for the worst. *Ann Intern Med* 2003;138:439–443.

9. Cassell EJ. The nature of suffering and the goals of medicine. *N Engl J Med* 1982;306:639–645.

10. Platt FW, Gaspar DL, Coulehan JL, et al. "Tell me about yourself": The patient-centered interview. *Ann Intern Med* 2001; 134:1079–1085.

11. Chochinov HM. Dignity-conserving care—a new model for palliative care: helping the patient feel valued. *JAMA* 2002; 287:2253–2260.

12. von Gunten CF. Secondary and tertiary palliative care in US hospitals. *JAMA* 2002;287:875–881.

13. von Gunten CF, Muir JC. Palliative medicine: an emerging field of specialization. *Cancer Invest* 2000;18:761–767.

14. Walsh D. The Harry R. Horvitz Center for Palliative Medicine (1987–1999): development of a novel comprehensive integrated program. *Am J Hosp Palliat Care* 2001;4:239–250.

15. Smith TJ, Coyne P, Cassell B, et al. A high volume specialist palliative care unit and team may reduce in-hospital end-of-life care costs. *J Palliat Med* 2003;6:699–705.

16. Elsayem A, Swint K, Fisch MJ, et al. Palliative care inpatient service in a comprehensive cancer center: clinical and financial outcomes, *J Clin Oncol* 2004;22:2008–2014.

17. Patrick DL, Curtis JR, Engelberg RA, et al. Measuring and improving the quality of dying and death. *Ann Intern Med* 2003; 139:410–415.

CHAPTER
41

PAIN MANAGEMENT AND SYMPTOM CONTROL

Suresh K. Reddy
Ahmed Elsayem
Rudranath Talukdar

Patients with cancer develop a number of devastating physical and psychosocial symptoms that may arise during different phases and stages of cancer (1). These patients need optimal control of symptoms in order to continue receiving anticancer treatment as well as to improve their quality of life in advanced stages. They need access to multidisciplinary palliative care services in order to achieve optimal symptom control. Symptoms in patients with advanced incapacitating illness include fatigue, pain, anorexia, nausea, dyspnea, constipation, anxiety, depression, and cachexia (Table 41-1).

■ PAIN

Pain is one of the most common symptoms experienced by cancer patients. It was the most common symptom (82%) among patients referred to a palliative care ser-

vice (2). Pain may be the only symptom before the diagnosis of cancer and may indicate the recurrence and spread of cancer. It can occur both during active treatment as well as in the advanced and terminal stages of cancer. Generally as many as 30 to 50% of patients in active anticancer therapy and as many as 60 to 90% of those with advanced disease have pain (3–7).

Most pain in cancer is caused by direct involvement of tumor with body structures, most notably neural structures. Pain associated with direct tumor involvement occurs in 65 to 85% of patients with advanced cancer (7). Cancer therapy accounts for pain in approximately 15 to 25% of patients receiving chemotherapy, surgery, or radiation therapy, and 3 to 10% of cancer patients have pain syndromes of the sort commonly observed in the general noncancer population—for example, low back pain secondary to degenerative disk disease.

TABLE 41-1	SYMPTOMS IN ADVANCED CANCER
Pain (80–85%)	
Fatigue (90%)	
Weight loss (80%)	
Lack of appetite (80%)	
Nausea, vomiting (80–90%)	
Anxiety (25%)	
Shortness of breath (50%)	
Confusion/agitation (80%)	

SOURCE: Elsayem et al. (131). With permission.

PATHOPHYSIOLOGY

The pathophysiologic classification of pain forms the basis for therapeutic choices. Pain states may be broadly divided into those associated with ongoing tissue damage (nociceptive) and those resulting from nervous system dysfunction (neuropathic), due either to tissue damage or in the absence of damage in some situations. Nociceptive pain can be of the somatic or visceral type. It results from the activation of nociceptors in cutaneous and deep tissues and is described as well localized aching, throbbing, and gnawing. Visceral pain is caused by activation of nociceptors resulting from distention, stretching, and inflammation of visceral organs. It is described as poorly localized, deep aching, cramping, and as a sensation of pressure. Sometimes it is referred pain; e.g., pancreatic cancer pain in the abdomen with referral to back.

Breakthrough pain is a common entity in cancer patients and is defined as "transitory exacerbation of pain that occurs on a background of otherwise stable persistent pain"; it is caused by activity or end-of-dose failure or can occur spontaneously. It tends to be moderate to severe and, according to one study, it is less than 3 min in duration in 43% of such cases (8). It tends to be of relatively short duration with frequency of one to four episodes per day. Breakthrough pain tends to be an adverse prognosticator for the successful treatment of pain, as per Bruera et al. (9).

ASSESSMENT

It is crucial to assess and monitor the intensity of pain. This can be measured by simply using visual analog scales, verbal scales, numerical scales, or more complex pain questionnaires (10). The most popular tool used generally is a scale of 0 to 10, where 0 is the best pain and 10 is the worst pain. Most instruments and techniques are very reliable for the assessment of the intensity of pain. The assessment can be made more effective by graphic ongoing display of pain and other symptoms in the patient's chart, along with other vital signs monitoring. This forms a basis for outcomes as well as helping to administer appropriate care (Fig. 41-1). Pain assessment should always be done in the context of other symptoms in cancer.

In 1984, the World Health Organization (WHO) proposed a simple analgesic ladder for the pharmacologic management of cancer pain (11). Experience with the application of this ladder in several countries worldwide has shown that the simple principles of escalating from nonopioid to strong opioid analgesics is safe and effective (Fig. 41-2). In addition to the WHO guidelines, a number of other guidelines have been published (12).

PRINCIPLES OF MANAGEMENT

Assess pain syndromes and other symptoms accurately.
Respect and accept the complaint of pain as real.
Treat pain appropriately.
Treat underlying disorder(s).
Address psychosocial issues.
Utilize a multidisciplinary approach.

■ PHARMACOTHERAPY

PRINCIPLES OF PHARMACOTHERAPY

Match drug to pain syndrome.
Have low threshold to prescribe opioids.
Sustained-release formulations for constant pain and short-acting ones for breakthrough pain are commonly used.
Add adjunct medications where appropriate.
The oral route should be the route of choice.
Use the intravenous route for acute titration.
Treat side effects before switching opioids.
Sequential opioid trials should be done, including methadone.
Familiarize yourself with equianalgesic dosing.
Familiarize yourself with the pharmacokinetics of opioids.
Differentiate between tolerance, physical dependence, and addiction.
Be aware of renal failure and analgesic drugs.

Pharmacotherapy is the most simple and very effective way to control cancer pain. The class of medications used includes opioids as well as nonopioids and adjuvant medications.

Referral Date:		Referring Physician:															
Date:																	
Pain	(0–10)*																
Fatigue	(0–10)*																
Nausea	(0–10)*																
Depression	(0–10)*																
Anxiety	(0–10)*																
Drowsiness	(0–10)*																
Shortness of Breath	(0–10)*																
Appetite	(0–10)*																
Sleep	(0–10)*																
Feeling of Well-Being	(0–10)*																
Mini Mental State Score (0–30)																	
Assessment from: Pt/SO/HCP (If SO or HCP – use red ink)																	
Total Opioid MEDD:_____mg/day																	
Staff Initials (Signature & Title Below)																	

*0 = No Symptom/Best   10 = Worst Imaginable

FIGURE 41-1 Edmonton symptom assessment scale (ESAS). [*From El-sayem et al. (131). With permission.*]

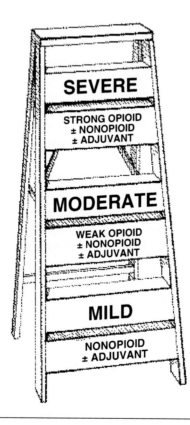

FIGURE 41-2 World Health Organization (WHO) three-step ladder oral analgesic program for managing cancer pain.

OPIOIDS

Opioid medications form the basis for the management of cancer pain regardless of its pathophysiology. Opioids are the drugs of choice for somatic pain, but there is good evidence that they are effective in neuropathic pain also, contrary to earlier belief (13,14).

Opioids are pharmacodynamically classified into pure agonists, mixed agonist-antagonists, and antagonists. As a rule in our practice, only pure agonists are used. Partial agonists and agonist-antagonists are not used because they exhibit a "ceiling effect" and have an unfavorable side-effect profile. Table 41-2 lists the most commonly used opioids in cancer pain with their equianalgesic dose ratios.

LOW-POTENCY OPIOID AGONISTS

This list includes codeine, propoxyphene, hydrocodone, and dihydrocodeine, with a potency about one-quarter to one-tenth that of morphine sulfate. Indications for drugs from this group include mild to moderate pain not responsive to nonopioids. A good example is mild bone pain and an early visceral pain. They are also occasionally used for in-between breakthrough pain for patients with constant pain on sustained-release opioids. Drugs

TABLE 41-2	OPIOID ANALGESICS	

Drug	*Usual Starting Dosages*
Full opioid agonists	
Morphine*	15–30 mg PO q 3–4 h
	30–60 mg PO q 8–12 h
Hydromorphone (Dilaudid)	2–4 mg PO q 4–6 h
Levorphanol (Levo-Dromoran)	2–4 mg PO q 4–6 h
Fentanyl (Duragesic)	25–50 mcg/h TD every 3 days
Codeine	15–30 mg PO q 3–4 h
Oxycodone (Percodan and others)	5–10 mg PO q 3–4 h
Meperedine (Demerol hydrochloride)	75–100 mg IM q 3–4 h
Methadone Hydrochloride (Dolophine)[†]	5–10 mg PO q 3–4 h
Propoxyphene (Darvon and others)	100 mg PO q 4–6 h
Partial agonists and mixed agonists/antagonists[‡]	
Nalbuphine (Nubain)	10 mg IV q 3–4 h
Butorphanol (Stadol)	0.5–2 mg IV q 3–4 h
	1–2 mg SL three times a day
Dezoncine (Dalgan)	10 mg IV q 3–4 h
Pentazocine (Talwin)	50 mg PO q 4–6 h

Equianalgesic Dosing[#]	*From Parenteral Opioid to Parental Opioid*	*From Same Parenteral Opioid to Oral Opioid*	*From Oral Opioid to Oral Morphine*	*From Oral Morphine to Oral Opioid*
Opioid				
Morphine	1	2.5	1	1
Hydromorphone	5	2	5	0.2
Meperidine	0.13	4	0.1	10
Levorphanol	5	2	5	0.2
Codeine	NA	NA	0.15	7
Oxycodone	NA	NA	1.5	0.7
Hydrocodone	NA	NA	0.15	7

* Morphine can be given as an immediate-release or sustained-release preparation. It is recommended that a relatively rapid onset, short-acting opioid preparation (such as immediate-release morphine) be given to patients who take sustained-release morphine to provide rescue medication for breakthrough pain.

† Methadone is 10–15 times more potent than morphine. Expertise is needed to use it.

‡ This class of drugs is *not* recommended for the management of chronic cancer pain because they will reverse analgesia when coadministered with full opioid agonists and precipitate withdrawal in physically dependent individuals.

(1) Take the total amount of opioid that effectively controls pain in 24 h. (2) Multiply by conversion factor in table; give 30% less of the new opioid to avoid partial cross tolerance. (3) Divide by the number of doses per day.

NA = not applicable.

SOURCE: Modified from Elsayem et al. (131). With permission.

in this group are formulated with acetaminophen; hence the dose escalation of these drugs is limited by the maximum allowable dose of acetaminophen. However, formulations without acetaminophen can be prepared by some pharmacies.

HIGH-POTENCY OPIOID AGONISTS

These classes of drugs are used for all pain types. Available in short- and long-acting formulations, *morphine* is the standard drug most widely used and is the prototype drug of its class. It is a μ agonist, working in the spinal cord and brain receptors. It is converted to morphine-3-glucoronide and morphine-6-glucoronide (M3G and M6G, respectively) by glucuronyl transferase in the liver. These compounds may contribute to the opioid side effects, mostly excitatory side-effects by M3G (15). Caution should be exercised in patients with renal impairment, as these compounds are excreted by the kidney. They are available for oral, rectal, intramuscular, intravenous, and sublingual use as well as in intrathecal preparations. Other strong opioid-class drugs include oxycodone, hydromorphone, meperidine, fentanyl, and methadone.

OXYCODONE

Once classified as a low-potency opioid when its dosage was limited by its combination with acetaminophen or aspirin, oxycodone is now gaining widespread popularity as an alternative to morphine in the treatment of cancer pain. According to recent studies, oxycodone is 1½ times more potent than morphine. It is available only in the oral form in the United States and has a higher bioavailability than morphine. It is available in the sustained-release as well as the short-acting form.

HYDROMORPHONE

Commercially known as Dilaudid (Knoll AG, Listeral, Switzerland), hydromorphone is a useful short-acting opioid that is six to seven times as potent as morphine. It is available for administration via all routes including the neuroaxial route. Hydromorphone is commonly used as a "rescue" agent in patients on longer-acting opioid preparations, as the sustained-release form is not yet commercially available in the United States. Hydromorphone is used as an alternative to morphine when dose-limiting side effects necessitate opioid rotation to a more potent opioid.

MEPERIDINE

Meperidine (Demerol) is a commonly used opioid analgesic throughout the world, but it is not used as often as morphine. In the oral form, its potency is one-tenth that of morphine, which makes it less efficacious in most patients. The increase in dosing to get to morphine's equianalgesic level on a chronic basis is associated with the risk of accumulation of the metabolite normeperidine, produced by the liver. Both compounds cause central nervous system (CNS) excitability and may result in frank convulsions, especially in renally impaired and elderly patients (16). Hence the use of meperidine has been rapidly declining in the cancer patient population. It continues to enjoy a good reputation in surgery circles as the drug of choice for postoperative pain.

FENTANYL

Fentanyl is a semisynthetic opioid available in parenteral as well as transdermal form. Its rapid onset and relatively short duration of action make it a good choice for control of acute pain. A sustained-release, transdermal form has been developed and used successfully for stable pain. Each patch is changed every 72 h and hence was found to be convenient in patients whose pain is stable. Recently an oral transmucosal fentanyl (OTFC) has been approved for use in breakthrough pain (17,18).

METHADONE

Methadone is a synthetic opioid that has recently re-emerged and is being used beneficially to treat cancer pain. Recent updates (19) and research on the equianalgesic dosing (20,21) coupled with its lower cost, absence of active opioid metabolites, excellent bioavailability, and possible N-methyl-D-aspartate antagonist action (22) have enabled many to use methadone safely and effectively to treat cancer pain. The potency of methadone seems to be 10 to 15 times that of morphine. Hence caution should be exercised when switching from an opioid to methadone. Methadone is characterized by a long plasma half-life and low cost, making it suitable for most pain syndromes. Close monitoring at the time of commencement is warranted secondary to the cumulative side effects of methadone. The half-life seems to be 15 to 190 h. Drug interactions with methadone involve the same pathway of the cytochrome P-450 system common to antifungals, antiretroviral agents, and selective serotonin reuptake inhibitors (SSRIs) (23).

Opioid medications exhibit a wide interindividual variation, possibly because of differences in intrinsic activity and action at different receptors of different subtypes (24,25). Hence opioid rotation is a worthwhile exercise when dose-limiting side effects are encountered. Some groups treat side effects of opioids before embarking on opioid rotation. But the generally accepted method is to treat side effects before opioid switching. There is no general consensus as to the number of opioid rotations, but in the authors' experience at least two to three opioid rotations, which should include methadone at some stage, need to be attempted.

ADJUVANT MEDICATIONS

These groups of drugs are used mostly in conjunction with opioid medications in cancer pain. The categories include nonsteroidal anti-inflamatory drugs (NSAIDs), tricyclic antidepressants (TCAs), antiepileptic drugs (AEDs), and a miscellaneous group (Table 41-3).

NONSTEROIDAL ANTI-INFLAMMATORY DRUGS

NSAIDs are essentially limited to the inhibitors of the enzyme cyclooxygenase (COX), thus inhibiting the synthesis of prostaglandin, the pain and inflammation mediator. This group is now subdivided into nonspecific COX

TABLE
41-3

TABLE 41-3	ADJUVANT ANALGESICS

Tricyclic antidepressants
   Amitriptyline
   Nortriptyline
   Doxepin
   Doxepram
Antiepileptic drugs
   Gabapentin
   Topiramate
   Levetiracetam
   Tiagabine
   Oxcarbazepine
   Lamotrigine
   Felbamate
Local anesthetics
   Lidocaine
N-methyl-D-aspartate (NMDA) receptor antagonists
   Ketamine
   Methadone
   Dextromethorphan
Topical analgesics
   Capsaicin
   Lidocaine patches

Miscellaneous drugs (psychotropic drugs, benzodiazepines, bisphosphonates, steroids, radiopharmaceuticals).

inhibitors and selective COX-2 inhibitors. The nonselective inhibitors, which are also referred to as NSAIDs, are medications such as ibuprofen and naproxen. However these drugs continue to cause concern with regard to the integrity of gastric mucosa and alteration in renal function. COX-2 inhibitors block COX-2 enzyme with little effect on COX-1, thereby offering an advantageous effect on the integrity of gastric mucosa and platelet aggregation (26). After initial approval by the US Food and Drug Administration (FDA), rofecoxib (Vioxx), a leading COX-2 inhibitor, has been withdrawn from the market secondary to increasing incidents of heart attacks and strokes (27).

TRICYCLIC ANTIDEPRESSANTS

TCAs are the main group of antidepressants currently being used to treat neuropathic pain syndromes. They probably act by inhibiting reuptake of serotonin and norepinephrine at the nerve endings in the spinal cord as well as in the brain. Recently it has been widely accepted that their action is independent of their mood-altering effects and that they exert either an inherent influence over the nervous system or modulate the opioid pathways (28,29).

TCAs are not universally tolerated, especially at the initiation of therapy, and they often have to be discontinued or decreased due to dose-limiting side effects, most commonly the anticholinergic and sedative effects. Amitriptyline and nortriptyline (which have lower cardiovascular side-effect profiles) are felt to be the most efficacious agents and thus are more often used.

ANTICONVULSANTS

Anticonvulsants are traditionally used in the treatment of diabetic neuropathy, postherpetic neuralgia, trigeminal neuralgia, and similar syndromes with good results (29). These conditions can definitely coexist in cancer patients; however, AEDs are useful in treating brachial and lumbosacral plexopathies (Table 41-4).

Medications such as phenytoin, valproate, carbamazepine, and clonazepam have been used. Owing to concerns over safety and side effects, their use has been strictly limited. Gabapentin has become the "gold standard" and prototypical drug in this category to treat neuropathic pain (30,31). With its wide therapeutic window and a level of efficacy comparable to that of other anticonvulsants, gabapentin is preferred by many clinicians, especially as it does not require the monitoring of blood levels or other clinical tests. Sedation is a noted side effect, which can be reduced by starting therapy at 100 mg tid and adding 100 mg to each dose every second or third day until the desired effect is achieved. If necessary, dose escalation up to 3600 mg/day is recommended.

Recently newer AEDs are gaining in popularity (see Table 41-4).

MISCELLANEOUS

In refractory pain situations, drugs from other classes have been tried; some have been tried with a good response and others with only a minimal response. They include: psychotropic drugs (32,33), benzodiazepines (34), bisphosphonates (35–37), steroids (in spinal cord compression) (38), lidocaine, intravenous and patch (39–41), ketamine (42,43), capsaicin (44), and radiopharmaceuticals (strontium 89, samarium) (45,46).

■ STEPS TO TREAT CANCER PAIN

The successful formula to treat cancer pain involves some simple rules. Pain management is governed by factors such as pain syndrome (somatic versus neuropathic), pain severity, previous opioid use, dosing and side effects, the presence of other symptoms such as delirium, anxiety, depression, and preexisting conditions.

TABLE 41-4	ANTIEPILEPTIC DRUGS		
Drug	*Action*	*Uses*	*Dose*
Carbamazepine	Anticonvulsant decreases abnormal CNS neuronal activity	Useful for neuropathic pain; hematologic monitoring suggested	Start with 100 mg daily, increase by 100 mg q4d to 500–800 mg/day
Phenytoin	Anticonvulsant decreases abnormal CNS activity	Useful for neuropathic pain; hematologic monitoring suggested	Start with 100 mg/day, increase by 25–50 mg q4d to 250–300 mg/day
Gabapentin	Anticonvulsant decreases abnormal CNS neuronal activity	Useful for neuropathic pain; better toxicity profile	300–3200 mg
Lamotrigine	Treatment of trigeminal analgesia, migraine headaches, diabetic neuropathy	Inhibitor of voltage gated Na^+ channels, suppresses glutamate release and inhibits serotonin reuptake	25–50 mg/day, increased by 50 mg/week until max 900 mg bid or tid
Topiramate	Treatment of cluster headaches, diabetic neuropathy	Increases CNS GABA levels, blocks AMPA kainite excitatory receptors	200–400 mg/day with bid dosing Start at 25 mg bid increasing 50 mg every week
Oxcarbezapine	Treatment of trigeminal neuralgia, neuropathic pain states	Blockade of voltage gated Na^+ channels	300–600 mg/day, up to a max 1200–2400 mg/day
Zonisamide	Trials ongoing	Na^+ channel blockade T-type Ca^{2+} channel blockade	
Tiagabine	Neuropathic pain therapeutic effects	GABA reuptake inhibitor	Dosage

SOURCE: Modified from Elsayem et al. (131). With permission.

PAIN SYNDROME

Pain syndromes in cancer can be somatic, neuropathic, or mixed. Based on the predominance of one versus the other, medications are chosen accordingly. If the pain is predominantly somatic but mild, an NSAID with a mild opioid is initiated. The medication can be advanced to a strong opioid based on the pain's severity. A short-acting opioid may be tried first to test its tolerability; the medication may then be advanced to a sustained-release form once the pain stabilizes. If the pain is predominantly neuropathic, either a TCA or an AED is started, possibly with a mild opioid. Again, titration to a strong opioid is undertaken based on the severity of the pain. But most often cancer pain is of a mixed type, in which case a balanced analgesic approach which involves drugs with different mechanism of action are chosen.

PAIN SEVERITY

Pain severity will serve as a guide in the decision-making process with regard to choosing a low-potency opioid versus a high-potency drug such as morphine. Most low-potency opioids are less suitable for high-grade pain due to dose limitations and the presence of the ceiling effect

or a plateau effect seen with increasing doses. Most cancer pain situations need high-potency opioids. If the patient had an optimal trial with oral opioids, including rotation to a different opioid, or has experienced dose-limiting side effects, an alternative route (e.g., intravenous or neuroaxial) may be tried. Pain severity reported on a verbal numerical scale should be interpreted in the context of associated psychosocial symptoms.

OPIOID HISTORY AND SIDE EFFECTS

Patient-to-patient variability in the response to a specific opioid has been widely appreciated and documented (24). Some patients may respond surprisingly well to one opioid after failing or not tolerating others, possibly due to how a given drug acts on different opioid receptors and also owing to genetic factors. This phenomenon will obviously influence drug selection within the same class (24,25).

PREVIOUS OPIOID DOSING AND PHARMACOKINETICS

This reflects the degree of tolerance to opioids, as "opioid naive" patients will obviously require lower doses, at least initially. Furthermore, opioid-tolerant patients may require stronger opioids from the beginning and also higher than conventional doses.

PRESENCE OF OTHER SYMPTOMS

Sometimes symptoms of delirium, anxiety, and depression may be interpreted as physical pain, and opioid dosages are escalated with worsening of delirium. Hence assessment of these symptoms is mandatory to avoid overdosing of opioids.

■ SIDE EFFECTS OF OPIOIDS

Diminution or elimination of side effects is an important part of effective opioid therapy. With few exceptions, dose readjustment whenever possible should be the first measure in managing adverse reactions. Some of the common opioid side effects are as follows:

Sedation
Nausea and vomiting
Constipation
Cognitive impairment
Urinary retention
Myoclonus
Respiratory depression
Pruritus

■ NONPHARMACOLOGIC TREATMENT

Many nonpharmacologic approaches are available for the treatment of cancer pain and are widely employed. These include nerve blocks, neurosurgical procedures, physical modalities to control pain, behavioral therapy, and others.

NERVE BLOCKS

A small percentage of patients who fail to respond to oral therapy may be helped with appropriate nerve blocks (Table 41-5).

It is not known which patients might benefit from interventions done earlier in the course of the disease (47,48). Somatic nerve blocks are effective for nociceptive somatic pain in the territory of a root, plexus or peripheral nerve. Blocks can be short-lasting when a local anesthetic is employed. These temporary blocks have a limited role in cancer pain management but may act as precursors to permanent neurolysis. Examples include root block, brachial plexus block, and psoas compartment block.

TABLE 41-5	USEFUL ANESTHETIC PROCEDURES
Celiac plexus/splanchnic block for abdominal visceral pain, e.g., pancreatic cancer pain
Subarachnoid neurolytic block for extremity and thoracic wall pain in terminally ill patients
Epidural/intrathecal opioids ± local anesthetic, e.g., for neuropathic or plexopathy pain
Cordotomy for intractable lower extremity pain
Vertebroplasty (injection of cement into a vertebral body) for metastatic spinal pain involving one or two vertebrae

SOURCE: Modified from Elsayem et al. (131). With permission.

Neurolytic blocks generally have a favorable risk-benefit ratio in patients with advanced cancer whose life expectancy is limited. Sympathetic blocks such as celiac plexus block have been demonstrated to be effective for pancreatic cancer pain and other abdominal visceral pain syndromes (49). Contrary to a previous study demonstrating improved survival (50), Wong et al. showed that although pain is better relieved with a celiac plexus block, there was no significant difference in survival or quality of life (51). Occasionally a subarachnoid neurolytic block (52), and a neurolytic intercostal block may be employed. The risks of neurologic deficits that may result from these blocks must be weighed against the possible benefits. A recent study by Smith et al. (53), randomizing intrathecal and comprehensive medical management, favored intrathecal opioid therapy and found improved survival in the intrathecal group; however, a number of concerns, particularly about the comprehensive medical management group, were raised (54,55). Perhaps more studies with more carefully selected cohorts are needed to confirm the findings.

Surgical ablation (56) may be accomplished by rhizotomy (section of a nerve root) or dorsal root entry zone lesions. Spinal anterolateral tractotomy or cordotomy, midline myelotomy, and cingulotomy should be reserved for carefully selected cases. Percutaneous cordotomy employed for intractable pain of the lower extremity has been shown to be useful in selected patients (57). Recently a procedure called vertebroplasty, which involves injecting cement into metastatic compression fractures, has been employed successfully and it is gaining wide popularity (58,59). Radiofrequency lesioning of bone metastasis has recently been shown to be another way of treating bone pain (60).

Other principles of symptom management are routinely employed. These include counseling, psychotherapy, relaxation techniques, massage therapy, music therapy, addressing psychosocial and spiritual needs, and bereavement counseling for family members.

■ FATIGUE

Fatigue is one of the most common symptoms in cancer patients (61), experienced by 70 to 100 % of those receiving cancer treatment (62). The term *fatigue* refers to a subjective sense of decreased vitality in physical and/or mental functioning; it usually occurs in the setting of medical disease. The physical dimension is usually described as a perception of muscle weakness or a tendency to tire rapidly. Physical activity is difficult to sustain and in some cases dyspnea accompanies minimal exertion. Rest or sleep does not return perceived strength or stamina to normal. The mental component is described as lack of interest or motivation in objects or activities. Other symptoms include difficulty in concentrating or maintaining attention. Mood may be flat or depressed. Lethargy or tendency to somnolence may be noted, but there is no need for excessive sleep. Rest or sleep may improve symptoms but does not eliminate them. Fatigue is experienced both during treatment as well as during terminal stages. For patients with advanced cancer, however, fatigue may be a severe symptom that either decreases their capacity for physical and mental work or renders them completely unable to function normally. Fatigue gets worse as the disease progresses toward the end stage. The presence of fatigue may also magnify other symptoms affecting the patient. The causes of fatigue are multifactorial and interrelated. These include problems related to the cancer itself, side effects or toxicities of treatment, underlying systemic pathophysiologic disorders, and other causes (Fig. 41-3).

ASSESSMENT

The severity of fatigue can be measured on a scale of 0 to 10 (where 0 equals no fatigue and 10 equals the worst fatigue imaginable), as in the Edmonton Symptom Assessment System (ESAS) or by other numerical or verbal rating scales (see Fig. 41-1). Like other symptoms in cancer, the assessment of fatigue should focus on the multidimensional aspect. The impact of fatigue on activities, function, and quality of life should be assessed. Laboratory investigations and imaging studies should be based on indications derived from the patient's history and physical examination.

MANAGEMENT

As with other problematic symptoms in advanced cancer patients, management of fatigue should address possible underlying etiologies as well as the patient's expression of symptoms (63,64).

Underlying problems such as pain, depression, anxiety, stress, and sleep disturbances must be treated. Dehydration should be corrected and an attempt made to treat cachexia in appropriate cases. Medication regimes can be simplified; infections treated; well as anemia relieved by transfusions where appropriate or by administering epoetin alfa 10,000 U subcutaneously three times weekly or as indicated (65). Low-dose steroids may alleviate some of the symptoms of fatigue in patients with advanced cancer (66,67). Psychostimulants, such as methylphenidate 5 to 10 mg in the morning and at noon, may be useful if the patient is experiencing concomitant problems such as depression, hypoactive delirium, or drowsiness due to opioids (68–70). Some antidepressants, such as the SSRIs, may improve energy levels in some fatigued patients, though their benefit is unproven. Recently there is increasing evidence that cancer patients with hypogonadism who are on chronic opioid

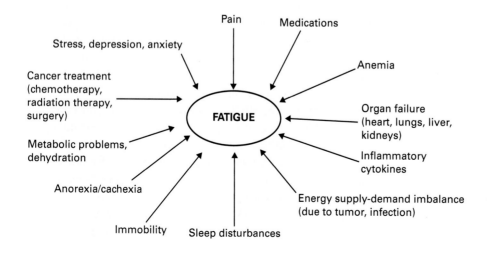

FIGURE 41-3   Multifactorial etiologies of fatigue. [*From Elsayem et al.* (131). *With permission.*]

therapy may suffer from fatigue (71). Replacement therapy with testosterone may improve fatigue in these patients but needs further study. Bruera et al. showed that patient-controlled methylphenidate administration rapidly improved fatigue and other symptoms (72).

■ DYSPNEA

Dyspnea is defined as the "uncomfortable awareness of breathing" (73). It is described in terms of air hunger, suffocation, choking, or heavy breathing. It is a subjective sensation, associated with and affected by factors such as the location and progression of the tumor, psychosocial phenomena (74), and pre-existing chronic lung pathology such as chronic obstructive pulmonary disease (COPD), asthma, and congestive heart failure. The frequency and severity of dyspnea depends on the stage of the disease; it increases in frequency when death is imminent.

Dyspnea as an isolated symptom or in association with other parameters is an adverse prognostic indicator of survival (75, 76). Dyspnea is a multidimensional symptom influenced by factors such as anxiety, tumor location, fatigue, and others. It can be caused by a number of clinical conditions, but the causes fall into two main categories: (1) dyspnea with abnormal mechanics of ventilation, e.g., cachexia, asthenia, myasthenic syndrome, Eaton-Lambert syndrome, and so on, and (2) dyspnea with normal mechanics of ventilation. This category may be subdivided into respiratory and nonrespiratory causes of dyspnea (Table 41-6).

ASSESSMENT

Dyspnea is a complex symptom caused by various factors, some not well understood. But a thorough history, with physical examination and appropriate laboratory and imaging studies should be undertaken to assess it. Some of the factors that contribute to dyspnea include anxiety, phobia, pain, and fatigue.

TREATMENT

The aim of the dyspnea treatment is a subjective improvement in the patient's perception. Treatment involves treating the cause and the symptoms as well as managing psychosocial issues contributing to dyspnea.

TABLE 41-6 | CAUSES OF DYSPNEA IN CANCER PATIENTS*

Dyspnea with Abnormal Mechanisms of Ventilation	Dyspnea with Normal Mechanisms of Ventilation
☐ Asthenia	Direct effect of the tumor
☐ Cachexia	☐ Primary or metastatic tumor
☐ Myasthenia gravis	☐ Pleural effusion/pericardial infusion
☐ Eaton-Lambert syndrome	☐ Superior vena cava syndrome
☐ Rib fracture	☐ Carcinomatous lymphangitis
☐ Chest wall deformity	☐ Atelectasis
☐ Neuromuscular disease (motor neuron disease)	☐ Phrenic nerve palsy
	☐ Tracheal obstruction
	☐ Tracheal-esophageal fistula
	☐ Carcinomatous infiltration of the chest wall (carcinoma en cuirasse)
	Effect of therapy
	☐ Postactinic fibrosis
	☐ Postpneumectomy
	☐ Mitomycin-vinca alkaloid (acute dyspnea syndrome)
	☐ Bleomycin-induced fibrosis
	☐ Doxorubicin- and cyclophosphamide–induced cardiomyopathy
	Not directly related to the tumor or therapy
	☐ Anemia
	☐ Ascites
	☐ Metabolic acidosis
	☐ Fever
	☐ Chronic obstructive pulmonary disease
	☐ Asthma
	☐ Pulmonary embolism
	☐ Pneumonia
	☐ Pneumothorax
	☐ Heart failure
	☐ Obesity
	☐ Thyrotoxicosis
	☐ Psychosocial distress (i.e., anxiety, somatization)
	☐ Unknown

* The physician is to check off all the causes of dyspnea in a given patient.
SOURCE: Modified from Elsayem et al. (131). With permission.

Treatment of the Cause

Treatment of the underlying cause is attempted as an initial step: thoracentesis for pleural effusion, blood transfusion for anemia, corticosteroids for carcinomatosis lymphangitis, anticoagulants for pulmonary embolism, and antibiotics for pneumonia where appropriate.

Symptomatic Treatment

Oxygen Therapy

Long-term oxygen therapy has been shown to have beneficial effects on the outcome of patients with COPD (77,78). Crossover trials with cancer patients suffering from dyspnea suggest beneficial effects of oxygen (79,80). Oxygen may be given by nasal cannula and should be humidified whenever feasible. Oxygen treatment toward the end of life may lead to anxiety among family members, who sometimes interpret this as a way of prolonging life and suffering. Counseling of family members with regard to this issue is of paramount importance.

Drug Therapy

A number of pharmacologic agents have been tried effectively to relieve the perception of dyspnea in terminally ill cancer patients. The major drugs are opioids, corticosteroids, and benzodiazepines. Many studies have found that opioids of different types, doses, and routes of administration are capable of relieving dyspnea (81, 82). Nebulized opioids have also been shown to be effective in some studies (83–87). There are some conflicting studies about the use of nebulized opioids to treat dyspnea (88). Opioids may act by reducing the subjective sensation of dyspnea without reducing respiratory rate or oxygen saturation. They may also cause venodilation of pulmonary vessels, thereby reducing preload to the heart and improving breathing. Corticosteroids are useful only if dyspnea is caused by carcinomatosis lymphangitis or in superior vena cava syndrome. They may also play a role if associated COPD or asthma coexists (89). Benzodiazepines have a limited role in dyspnea except when anxiety and apprehension are underlying causes. Consequently benzodiazepines are commonly used medications for terminal dyspnea in hospice settings. Bronchodilators play a role if dyspnea is caused by bronchospasm. Both nebulized and oral agents are used. In a study by Congleton and Muers, bronchodilators provided significant relief of dyspnea in patients with lung carcinoma and airflow obstruction (90). Sometimes phenothiazines, such as chlorpromazine may help in drying secretions and help in reducing anxiety (91).

General Supportive Measures

A number of measures can be implemented for the support of both the patient and the family. Relaxation techniques or guided imagery provide relief in patients with anticipatory or anxiety-driven dyspnea. Assist devices can be used to minimize muscle effort. Maneuvers such as postural drainage and incentive spirometry can help in special situations.

■ DELIRIUM

Delirium is defined as a transient organic brain syndrome characterized by the acute onset of disordered attention (arousal) and cognition, accompanied by disturbances of psychomotor behavior and perception (92). Delirium is common with progressive disease and is common in patients with pancreatic cancer who are near death. It may signal a new and serious medical complication, markedly impair the function and comfort of the patient, and increase the family's distress (93). The prevalence of delirium in hospitalized medical and surgical patients is approximately 10%, and the prevalence in hospitalized cancer patients ranges from 8 to 40% (94–96). Causes of delirium are listed in Fig. 41-4.

CLINICAL FEATURES

The symptoms and signs of delirium fluctuate; therefore careful attention should be paid to the mental status examination. The diagnosis is established by a new onset of cognitive dysfunction accompanied by a disturbance of arousal or clouding of consciousness. Three clinical variants have been described based on the type of arousal disturbance: Hypoalert-hypoactive, hyperalert-hyperactive, and mixed type (97,98). The presenting features include memory impairment or confusion, dysphoria, hypomania, illusions, hallucinations, and altered arousal state. The criteria for delirium presented in the fourth edition of the *Diagnostic and Statistical Manual of Mental Disorders* (DSM-IV) (99) have been considered the gold standard for its diagnosis. These include impairment in responsiveness and alertness as manifest by fluctuating inability to maintain or shift attention to external stimuli; cognitive dysfunction of recent onset; development of the disturbance over a short period of time; and evidence from history, physical examination, or laboratory findings that are etiologically related to the disturbance.

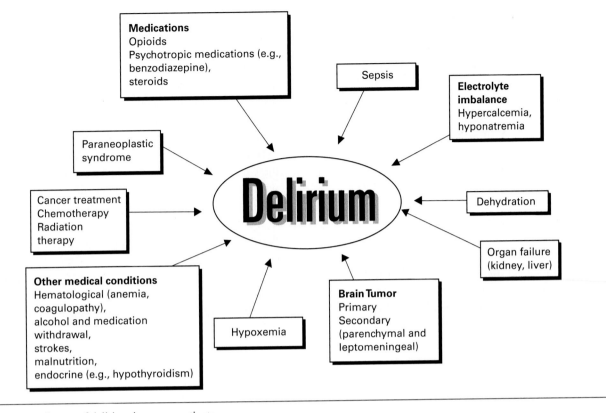

FIGURE 41-4 Causes of delirium in cancer patients.

ASSESSMENT

Delirium is a frequently missed diagnosis and is more often misdiagnosed as insomnia, anxiety, or depression because the presenting symptoms may mimic any of these conditions. Understanding the patient's baseline and listening to the observations of family members and nurses will help pick up the diagnosis of delirium before the condition is florid and out of control. The cause of the delirium should be investigated, if possible, since the treatment will depend on correction of the cause. The history is of utmost importance, especially when this condition has an acute onset. Medications—particularly opioids, benzodiazepines, some antiemetics and corticosteroids—are frequent causes of delirium. Physical examination may reveal signs of dehydration or increased intracranial pressure. Laboratory examinations may show hypercalcemia, hyponatremia, and renal or hepatic failure.

TREATMENT

If the diagnosis of delirium is suspected, the clinician should act immediately to establish the diagnosis and remove inciting medication if this is the likely cause. Safety is of paramount importance, especially in the ag-

itated (hyperactive) type, since patients may endanger themselves by removing intravenous lines, fall, or walk out. Educating family members and nurses is important. The appropriate management includes identifying and treating the underlying causes. Other reversible causes should be identified and corrected. If opioids are the cause, dosage reduction or rotation to a different opioid should be attempted. Treating infection, hydrating a dehydrated patient, or correcting hypercalcemia may be all that is needed in the way of treatment. Symptomatic treatment to control agitation is achieved by the use of neuroleptics. Haloperidol remains the drug of choice for the treatment of delirium. It is a dopamine blocker with useful sedative effects and a low incidence of cardiovascular and anticholinergic side effects. Mostly haloperidol in the dosage of 1 to 3 mg/day is effective in treating agitation, paranoia, and fear. A higher dose may be needed in special circumstances. Sometimes acute dystonias and extrapyramidal side effects are seen with haloperidol, in which case benztropine can be administered. Methotrimeprazine is sometimes used effectively to control agitation. It has also been shown to be an analgesic. Newer antipsychotics such as olanzapine (100) are as effective and may be more sedating in the control of agitated patients, but unfortunately they are more expensive. Sometimes a combination of haloperidol and a benzodiazepine is useful. In a study by Brietbart (101), lorazepam alone was ineffective in the treatment of delirium and, in fact, contributed to the worsening of delirium and increased cognitive impairment. In severe cases, consultation with a palliative care physician is important; if, in terminal cases, the condition proves to be refractory to antipsychotic medication, sedation should be considered. Figure 41-5 indicates treatment algorithm for delirium.

■ DEPRESSION

Depression is a common and devastating problem for patients with cancer and other terminal diseases. Major depression can affect from 25 to 35% of cancer patients (102). This prevalence touches 77% in those with advanced disease (103). Pancreatic cancer is more likely to be associated with depression, in which case it will be associated with an even greater loss of appetite, weight loss, low energy, and so on. Thus it can be critically important to diagnose and treat depression early, thereby ameliorating some of the physiologic changes that are inevitable with advanced cancer. The cause of depression in pancreatic cancer is unclear. It may be caused by an indirect effect of cancer on the serotoninergic function of brain, or it may result from a psychological reaction to the cancer itself (104). Pain has a close correspondence with psychiatric illness. It is very likely that patients reporting pain will also have a psychiatric diagnosis (105).

As per the DSM-IV (106), the cardinal features of depression include loss of interest or pleasure; impaired decision-making ability; changes in appetite, sleep, and psychomotor activity; decreased energy, as well as feelings of guilt and/or worthlessness. Mild episodes of depression may be masked by increased effort on the patient's part.

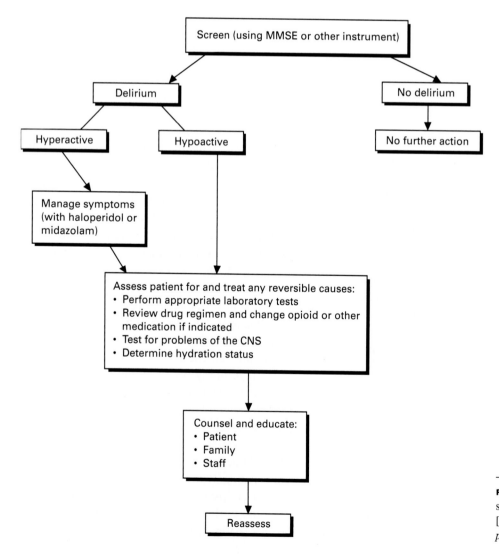

FIGURE 41-5 Algorithm for the assessment and treatment of delirium. [*From Elsayem et al. (131). With permission.*]

ASSESSMENT

Diagnosis is confounded by the presence of normal sadness and grief and also by delirium. Anhedonia can be mistaken for the fatigue that occurs in cancer patients. Assessing depression quickly and accurately is important. There are no clear-cut guidelines on assessing depression in terminal cancer patients. A recent report by Fisch et al. (107) suggested the usefulness of a brief two-question assessment of depression in advanced cancer patients, with the primary objective being to measure the quality of life after intervention with fluoxetine and the secondary objective being to assess the reduction in depression. Other validated measures of assessing depression in the primary care setting include the WHO-5 well-being index (108), the PHQ-9 screening test (109), Hamilton Rating Scale for Depression (HAM-D) (110), and the Montgomery Asberg Depression Rating Scale (111) (MADRS). The patient should be evaluated for depressive episodes and substance abuse, family history of depression and suicide, concurrent life stressors, losses secondary to cancer, and availability of social support.

Delirium, particularly in the early stages, is often misidentified as depression and treated as such, with poor effects (112). The key is to diagnose the clinical problem accurately. In doubtful situations, a consultation with a palliative care physician or psychiatrist should be obtained.

TREATMENT

A combination or a balanced approach of supportive psychotherapy and pharmacotherapy is key to the optimal treatment of depression. Individual or group counseling has been shown to be useful. Other methods include relaxation techniques, guided imagery (113), and music therapy (114). Counseling of both patients and their families is crucial to the successful treatment of depression. This helps to reduce anxiety, allows patients to express their fears and disappointments in a "safe" way, and enhances well-being.

PHARMACOTHERAPY

The mainstay of the treatment of depression is pharmacotherapy.

The agents commonly employed include the newer SSRIs (115), TCAs (116), and psychostimulants (117). The SSRIs fluoxitene hydrochloride, sertraline hydrochloride, paroxetine hydrochloride, citalopram, and recently escitalopram have gained popularity due to their improved side-effects profiles compared with the TCAs.

For mild depression, SSRIs are very useful. However, they take weeks to become effective. Some, such as escitalopram, have a lower side-effects profile and work a little faster than the first-generation SSRIs, such as fluoxetine. The side effects are generally mild, but others are problematic, such as reduced appetite, nausea, and anxiety. These effects tend to be of limited duration and have not prevented their application in cancer patients. Other problems arise from their mechanism of action; these include diarrhea, fatigue, and sexual dysfunction (115). If a switch from an SSRI to another medication, especially a monoamine oxidase inhibitor (MAOI), is considered, the washout period of various SSRIs will have to be taken into account. It may be therefore useful to have a patient take SSRIs such as sertraline or escitalopram, which have a shorter washout period than older drugs such as fluoxetine. Our experience has shown methylphenidate to be particularly useful, especially in patients with a limited life expectancy where a few weeks could be too much to ask. Methylphenidate also helps to reduce the symptoms of fatigue, a common problem in cancer patients; this makes it a particularly useful medication (72).

TCAs have been widely used and work faster than SSRIs; however, they have more side effects, some of which (like their anticholinergic effects) can be a major problem for older cancer patients. They do offer additional benefits for patients suffering from neuropathic pain. For that reason, these medications should be started at a low dose and slowly escalated as tolerated. Desipramine and nortriptyline are generally better tolerated than amitriptyline and imipramine in the older population.

In a recent study, mirtazapine was found to be effective in ameliorating symptoms of depression in cancer patients (118). Some additional benefits of mirtazapine may accrue from its beneficial effects on chemotherapy-induced nausea/vomiting (CINV) and insomnia (Table 41-7) (119).

■ CONSTIPATION

Constipation is the infrequent and difficult passage of hard stool. It is a very common cause of morbidity in the palliative care setting and is thought to affect the overwhelming majority (>95%) of patients consuming opioids for cancer-related pain syndromes (120,121). Constipation can be a difficult condition to assess and treat because of the wide variety of presenting symptoms. Patients may report a feeling of incomplete evacuation, bloating, decreased appetite, or generalized abdominal

TABLE 41-7	COMMON ANTIDEPRESSANT DOSAGES

The following are common initial doses:

Nortriptyline 25 mg/day (at bedtime)

Amitriptyline 25 mg/day (at bedtime)

Fluoxetine 10–20 mg/day

Paroxetine 10 mg/day

Sertraline 20 mg/day

Citalopram 20 mg/day

Venlafaxine 37.5 mg/day

Mirtazapine 15 mg/day (at bedtime)

Methylphenidate 5–10 mg in the morning and 5 mg at noon

SOURCE: Modified from Elsayem et al. (131). With permission.

discomfort or pain. Due to the wide variability in normal bowel movement patterns in individual patients, the diagnosis of constipation can be made only in comparison with an individual's normal pattern (122).

CAUSES

The most common causes of constipation include opioid medication and progressive disease. Other causes include anorexia/cachexia, bowel obstruction, immobility, hypercalcemia, and dehydration. In the palliative care setting, careful attention must be given to the multifactorial nature of constipation. The common causes of constipation are outlined in Table 41-8.

COMPLICATIONS

Although constipation is often overlooked in the setting of other comorbid conditions, it is not necessarily a benign condition; some of the complications of unrelieved constipation can indeed be life-threatening (123). Severe constipation can lead to bowel obstruction, with attendant issues of severe morbidity. In patients who are neutropenic, severe constipation can lead to bacterial transfer across the colon, with bacteremia and sepsis.

DIAGNOSIS

The diagnosis of constipation begins with a careful history of the patient's recent bowel movements. Specific topics to be queried include the date of the last bowel movement, the characteristics of the stool (hard versus soft, loose versus formed, "ribbon-like" versus "pellet-like"), the degree of straining and pain involved, and whether or not the movement felt complete. Related questions include whether or not there was blood in the stool (possibly identifying tumor mass or a hemorrhoid)

TABLE 41-8	CAUSES OF CONSTIPATION IN PATIENTS WITH ADVANCED CANCER

Structural abnormalities

  Obstruction

  Pelvic tumor mass

  Radiation fibrosis

  Painful anorectal conditions

    Anal fissure, hemorrhoids, perianal abscess

Drugs

  Opioids

  Agents with anticholinergic actions

    Anticholinergics

    Antispasmodics

    Antidepressants

    Antipsychotics (e.g., phenothiazines, haloperidol)

    Antacids (aluminum-containing)

    Antiemetics (e.g., ondansetron)

  Diuretics

  Anticonvulsants

  Iron

  Antihypertensive agents

  Anticancer drugs (e.g., vinca alkaloids)

Metabolic disturbances

  Dehydration (vomiting, fever, polyuria, poor fluid intake, diuretic use)

  Hypercalcemia

  Hypokalemia

  Uremia

  Diabetes

  Hypothyroidism

Neurologic disorders

  Cerebral tumors

  Spinal cord compression

  Sacral nerve infiltration

  Autonomic failure

SOURCE: Modified from Elsayem et al. (131). With permission.

or an urge to defecate at all (suggesting colonic inertia) (120,122).

After the history, a careful physical examination should include the abdominal examination (distention, firmness, tenderness, the presence or absence of bowel sounds) and a rectal examination. The rectal examination should assess the presence of hard stool in the vault and may reveal the presence of masses, hemorrhoids, fissures, or fistulas. Caution should be exercised in performing a rectal examination on anyone with neutropenia or thrombocytopenia.

In addition to the history and physical examination, a simple "constipation score" (124) may also be obtained. A flat abdominal radiograph of the abdomen is obtained whereby the colon is divided into four quadrants (ascending, transverse, descending, and sigmoid) by drawing a large "X" with the umbilicus in the middle. Each quadrant is assigned a score from 0 to 3 based on the degree of stool in the lumen. A score of zero indicates no stool, a score of 1 indicates less than 50% occupancy, a score of 2 indicates greater than 50% occupancy, and a score of 3 indicates complete occupancy of the lumen with stool. Scores may range from 0 to 12 and score of 7 (or greater) indicates severe constipation (Fig. 41-6).

PREVENTION AND TREATMENT

Prevention of constipation includes patient education on the various reasons for constipation, encouragement of adequate fluid intake, and the prescription of stool softeners and laxatives. In addition, a high degree of vigilance should be maintained regarding the patient's other medications that may cause constipation.

Initial treatment of constipation includes starting the patient on a stool-softening agent (e.g., docusate 100 to 240 mg by mouth twice daily) with a laxative agent (e.g., senna 1 to 2 tablets twice daily). Refractory constipation may be managed with lactulose 30 mL by mouth every 6 h until a large bowel movement occurs. Intractable cases may require a bisacodyl suppository, milk-and-molasses enema, or Fleet enema. Proximal impaction may require magnesium citrate. In rare cases where hard stools are present in the vault, manual dis-

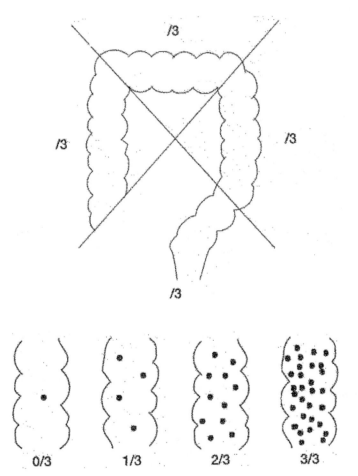

On a flat abdominal x-ray, draw 2 diagonal lines intersecting at the umbilicus as shown here. This transects the abdomen into 4 quadrants corresponding to the ascending, transverse, descending, and rectosigmoid colons. Then, assess the amount of stool in each of the 4 quadrants using the following scoring system: 0 = no stool; 1 = stool occupying <50% of the lumen of colon; 2 = stool occupying >50% of the lumen; 3 = stool completely occupying the lumen. The total score will therefore range from 0 to 12. A score of 7 indicates severe constipation and requires immediate intervention.

FIGURE 41-6 How to calculate a "constipation score" using a flat abdominal x-ray.

impaction may be necessary. In refractory cases, the opioid antagonist naloxone, given orally, may produce laxation (125–127). Mild opioid withdrawal may be seen with naloxone. Recently methylnaltrexone, given parenterally, has been showing promising effects in the treatment of opioid-induced constipation (128,129).

■ CHRONIC NAUSEA

Nausea and vomiting are highly unpleasant symptoms that affect between 40 and 70% of patients in the palliative care setting (130–132). In the cancer setting, nausea is prevalent in patients under the age of 65, females, and patients with breast, stomach, or gynecologic cancers. The etiology of chronic nausea is often multifactorial and could be due to the underlying disease, its treatment, or as a side effect of medications that treat cancer-related pain (e.g., opioids). The underlying cause of nausea should be ascertained if possible, and the selection of the antiemetic agent should be tailored to maximize therapeutic value (130). Figure 41-7 lists the common causes of nausea in the cancer setting.

Medication side effects and chronic constipation are the most common causes. As shown in the figure below, the experience of nausea and vomiting is generated as a result of the complex interrelationship between the chemoreceptor trigger zone (CTZ) and the vomiting center (VC). The CTZ can be affected directly by drugs, toxins, or metabolites or may receive afferent impulses from chemoreceptors and mechanoreceptors originating in the gastrointestinal tract, chest, or pelvis, which will subsequently influence the vomiting center. The VC also receives direct input from the cerebral cortex (Fig. 41-9).

ASSESSMENT

The etiology of nausea should be determined if at all possible, since proper management will depend on identifying and treating the underlying cause. The assessment of the patient with nausea should be part of the multidimensional approach to assess multiple symptoms simultaneously. It begins by taking detailed history, including the onset of the nausea, its duration, the frequency of episodes and their severity, all noted on a 0 to 10 scale of ESAS. In addition, since chronic constipation is one of the main causes of nausea, bowel function should also be assessed. The list of medications should be reviewed for possible medication side effects.

The examination of the patient should focus on life-threatening complications related to dehydration, such as hypotension and tachycardia; if present, these should be corrected promptly. It should include an abdominal examination, looking for signs of obstruction or constipation; a CNS examination to rule out raised intracranial pressure; and possibly even a cardiac examination to rule out initial symptoms of a major cardiac event.

Diagnostic tests include serum evaluation of electrolytes, serum calcium, and liver and kidney function tests. Abdominal x-rays may be obtained to gauge the degree of constipation (see the discussion of constipation above). Brain imaging may be considered if clinically appropriate.

TREATMENT

Correction of the underlying problem should be attempted if a cause can be found. Treating constipation

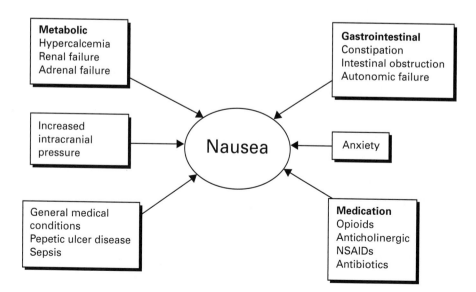

FIGURE 41-7 Causes of nausea. [*From Elsayem et al. (131). With permission.*]

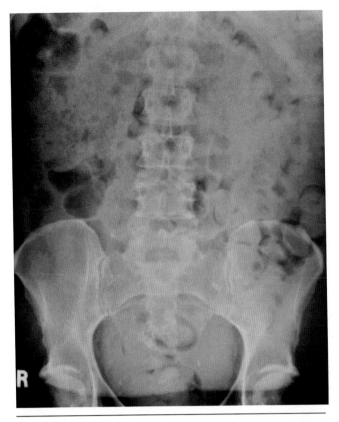

FIGURE 41-8 Constipation x-ray. [*From Elsayem et al. (131). With permission.*]

or removing the inciting medication may relieve the nausea if it was caused by any of them. Steroids or radiation may help nausea caused by increased intracranial pressure. If opioids are the cause, adding antiemetic may help; rarely, opioid rotation may be required.

Pharmacologic therapy should be directed toward the underlying problem. Table 41-9 llustrates the most commonly used antiemetics.

For most chronic, opioid-related nausea, a prokinetic agent such as metoclopramide (10 mg PO/IV/SC every 4 to 6 h) is helpful. The antidopaminergic properties of haloperidol (1 to 2 mg PO/IV/SC every 4 to 8 h) may help to relieve certain forms of refractory nausea. The $5 HT_3$ antagonists (e.g., ondansetron 4 to 8 mg PO/IV/SC) may ameliorate chemotherapy-related nausea (130, 131) but is less helpful in chronic nausea. Moreover, these agents are expensive and constipating. Octreotide, a somatostatin analog that reduces gastric motility and secretions, is helpful in nausea caused by intestinal obstruction. Benzodiazepines and other H1 antagonists may help anxiety-provoked nausea. Finally, steroids have been shown to be helpful for nausea both with a direct effect (e.g., in certain chemotherapy- or opioid-related problems with nausea) and by an indirect effect (e.g., by reducing intracranial pressure in patients with intracranial neoplasms) (132,133). Figure 41-8 is an

TABLE 41-9	\multicolumn{5}{l}{**ANTIEMETIC MEDICATIONS—DRUGS USEFUL FOR THE TREATMENT OF CHRONIC NAUSEA**}

*Drug**	*Main Receptor*	*Main Indication*	*Starting PO Dose/ Route*	*Equivalent Price[†]*	*Side Effects*
Metoclopramide	D2	Opioid-induced, gastric stasis	10 mg q4h PO, SC, IV	1	EPS (akathisia, dystonia, dyskinesia)
Prochlorperazine	D2	Opioid-induced	10 mg q6h PO, IV	3	Sedation, hypotension
Cyclizine	H1	Vestibular causes, Intestinal obstruction	25–50 mg q8h PO, SC, PR		Sedation, dry mouth, blurred vision
Promethazine	H1	Vestibular, motion sickness, obstruction	12.5 mg q4h PO, PR, IV	2	Sedation
Haloperidol	D2	Opioid, chemical, metabolic	1–2 mg bid PO, IV, SC	1	Rarely EPS
Ondansetron	$5 HT_3$	Chemotherapy	4–8 mg q8h PO, IV	84	Headache, constipation
Diphenhydramine	H1, Ach	Intestinal obstruction, vestibular, ICP	25 mg q6h PO, IV, SC	0.2	Sedation, dry mouth, blurred vision
Hyoscine	Ach	Intestinal obstruction, colic, secretions	0.2–0.4 mg q4h SL, SC, TD	0.4	Dry mouth, blurred vision, urine retention, agitation

Ach = acetylcholine; D2 = dopamine; EPS = extrapyramidal symptoms; H1 = histamine; ICP = intracranial pressure; PR = per rectum; SL = sublingual; TD = transdermal.

* Corticosteroids are not included because they vary in dosage and have limited indications (see text).

[†] Prices are compared to metoclopramide 10-mg tablets orally for 10 days based on the formulary prices at M.D. Anderson Cancer Center, November 2001.

SOURCE: Modified from Elsayem et al. (131). With permission.

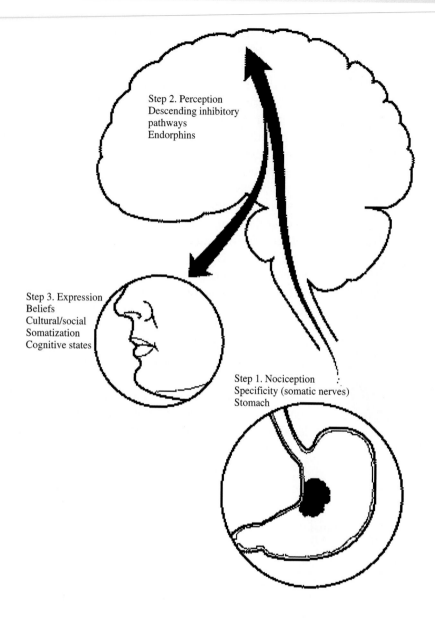

Step 2. Perception
Descending inhibitory
pathways
Endorphins

Step 3. Expression
Beliefs
Cultural/social
Somatization
Cognitive states

Step 1. Nociception
Specificity (somatic nerves)
Stomach

FIGURE 41-9 Vomiting cascade. [*From Elsayem et al. (131). With permission.*]

x-ray of a patient suffering from nausea as a result of constipation, with stool in all quadrants.

■ CACHEXIA

The cachexia syndrome, characterized by a marked weight loss, anorexia, asthenia, and anemia, is invariably associated with the growth of a tumor and leads to a malnutrition status caused by the induction of anorexia or decreased food intake. In addition, the competition for nutrients between the tumor and the host results in an accelerated catabolic state, which promotes severe metabolic disturbances. Cachexia is a complex metabolic syndrome characterized clinically by progressive involuntary weight loss, which can lead to the death of the host. The mechanism is not precisely known, but the

condition represents abnormalities of carbohydrate, fat, protein, and energy metabolism. Cachexia is found in majority of patients with advanced cancer and is a major contributing factor to death in about 50% of these patients (134). Cachexia leads to diminished appetite, weight loss, severe lethargy, fatigue, and generalized weakness known as asthenia. Patients with this syndrome are prone to have side effects and respond poorly to treatment. Cachexia commonly tends to occur in patients with solid tumors, in children, and in elderly patients. The etiology is multifactorial. It is caused mainly by tumor by-products and host cytokines, such as tumor necrosis factor, proteolysis-inducing factor, lipid-mobilizing factor, and interleukins (Fig. 41-10) (135,136).

In patients with this syndrome, the basal metabolic rate is increased. The liver produces acute-phase proteins that play a role in the inflammatory and antitumor

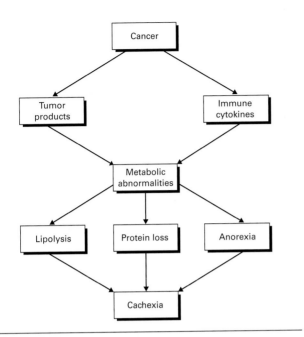

FIGURE 41-10 Mechanism of cachexia. [*From Elsayem et al. (131). With permission.*]

process but draw their energy from muscle breakdown. Glucose turnover is increased and at the same time there is a relative glucose intolerance in the muscle, with insulin resistance. There is suppression of de novo lipogenesis and peripheral activation of lipolysis, whereas central (hepatic) lipogenesis is increased. Whole-body protein turnover is increased and liver protein synthesis is directed toward an increase in the production of acute-phase proteins and lower production of albumin. Thus cachexia is characterized by an *increase* in energy expenditure, protein synthesis (largely acute-phase proteins at the expense of muscle proteins), proteolysis, lipolysis, and glucose turnover; a decrease in muscle proteins and lipogenesis; and an increase in ketone bodies (136).

Feeding of the patient with cancer cachexia was found to increase acute-phase protein production without influencing the rate of albumin synthesis (137). Other contributory factors include nausea, dysphagia, bowel obstruction, or constipation. Sometimes food aversion, depression, and apathy play a role.

ASSESSMENT

The clinical assessment includes a careful history that is focused on nutritional issues and a physical examination. A 5-lb weight loss in the previous 2 months and/or an estimated daily caloric intake of less than 70 cal/kg is a simple diagnostic indicator. Simple and inexpensive tests are available to assess body composition, such as anthropometric measurements, skinfold thickness, arm

muscle circumference and area, and weight and body mass index (BMI). Biochemical measurements are also available, such as serum albumin, transferring, and prealbumin. Careful clinical assessment and laboratory tests, especially serum sodium, are the keystones for diagnosis and effective management. Bioelectrical impedance (BEI) is an easy way to assess both nutritional status and fluid deficits in advanced cancer and should be used more often (138).

MANAGEMENT

The approach to management consists of identifying the etiology and treating the underlying cause. The nutritionist should advise on the dietary options to maximize nutritional intake. Small frequent meals are less intimidating than the usual large three meals a day.

The pharmacologic treatment consists of symptom control of the contributory factors and appetite stimulation. Chronic nausea or early satiety is treated with metoclopramide 10 mg every 4 to 6 h. Appetite stimulants include progestational agents, corticosteroids, cannabinoids, or adjuvant agents. Progestational agents include megestrol acetate; 40 to 120 mg PO qid will improve appetite in up to 80% of patients and induce weight gain in many (139,140). Symptomatic improvement in appetite occurs in less than 1 week; however, weight gain may take several weeks. Appetite stimulation with these agents lasts longer than that resulting from the use of corticosteroids. Caution must be exercised in patients with venous thrombosis, pulmonary embolism, or severe cardiac disease. Corticosteroids may stimulate appetite and decrease nausea (141,142). The effect does not last long. A cannabinoid, dronabinol, is approved for appetite stimulation and is dosed at 2.5 mg PO bid; it may produce concurrent antiemetic effects but may also produce CNS side effects (143). Antidepressants TCAs, and SSRIs may help with appetite in patients with depression. Thalidomide has been studied and has been shown to improve appetite, nausea, and well-being (144). Synthetic and semisynthetic testosterone derivatives have been studied especially in terminal AIDS patients and have been shown to be of benefit in improving appetite and reducing weight loss (145).

Enteral and parenteral forms of nutrition are inappropriate for most patients with advanced cancer (146) other than those who have a starvation component to cachexia, such as severe dysphagia or bowel obstruction. They do not enhance response to antineoplastic therapy or significantly abate its toxicity and do not improve survival or quality of life. They can be burdensome to patients and families and may obstruct transition to a hospice setting.

NONPHARMACOLOGIC THERAPY

Counseling of the patient as well as the family and loved ones is very important in assuring them that they may express their fears and needs and that their concerns will be acted on. In addition, counseling provides a venue to reframe the condition from that of "starving to death" to the more complex one of irreversible (usually) metabolic abnormalities and the futility of pushing nutrition. This reframing can decrease the distress of both patients and families and can maintain the social benefit of mealtimes. Exercise has benefit both for maintaining muscle and reducing depression; leaving the confines of the hospital room and being in sunlight have benefits for mood, depression, and overall sense of well-being.

■ HYPERCALCEMIA

Hypercalcemia is a common life-threatening complication of cancer, affecting 10 to 20% of patients; it is more common in certain cancers such as squamous cell of lung or head and neck, renal cell carcinoma, breast cancer, and multiple myeloma (82–84,147–149). The usual cause of hypercalcemia is humoral secretion of the parathyroid hormone–related protein (PTHrP), and the clinical syndrome mimics hyperparathyroidism biochemically except that the serum PTH is suppressed. Less frequent causes include ectopic production of parathyroid hormone itself. Clinically, the disorder contrasts with primary hyperparathyroidism. Hypercalcemia is abrupt in onset and is often severe; the associated neoplasm is usually obvious. It is usually unnecessary to measure the serum PTHrP levels to confirm the diagnosis; a determination of PTH will rule out intercurrent primary hyperparathyroidism. In multiple myeloma, it is caused by direct activation of bone resorption by cytokines secreted from myeloma cells in the bone marrow. Lymphomas can cause hypercalcemia by a similar local osteolytic mechanism or by conversion of vitamin D to 1,25-dihydroxyvitamin D.

CLINICAL PRESENTATION

Early symptoms are mild and include anorexia, nausea and vomiting, constipation, fatigue, weakness polydipsia, and polyuria (nephrogenic diabetes insipidus). Late symptoms are usually severe and include dehydration, altered mental status, generalized weakness, progressive gastrointestinal symptoms, and cardiac arrhythmias, especially when serum calcium levels rise rapidly. A high index of suspicion is required and the diagnosis is established by measurement of the ionized calcium or the corrected serum calcium since it is highly protein-bound.

TREATMENT

Treatment of hypercalcemia should be aimed both at lowering the serum calcium concentration and, if possible, correcting or decreasing the underlying disease (150,151). Hypercalcemia impairs both the glomerular filtration rate and urinary concentration; with the resultant azotemia and dehydration, the renal route for clearance of calcium is compromised. The mainstay of acute therapy of hypercalcemia is correction of dehydration, institution of saline diuresis to increase the renal excretion of calcium, and the use of agents to decrease bone resorption (152). Intravenous infusion of 100 to 200 mL/h can effectively replenish fluid volume and decrease serum calcium in 15 to 30% of patients.

Treatment with a bisphosphonate is usually required if the patient is symptomatic or the corrected serum calcium is above 12 mg/dL (153). Pamidronate is given in a dose of 90 mg in 500 mL of normal saline over 2 to 4 h. Pamidronate decreases bone resorption by inhibiting osteoclast activity (154). Renal function should be monitored both before and after pamidronate therapy, since this agent is relatively contraindicated in patients with renal. Zoledronic acid has emerged in some clinical trials as another bisphosphonate with results superior to those of pamidronate (155). Zoledronic acid is given at a dose of 4 mg over 15 min. The peak effect of bisphosphonates is reached after 5 to 7 days and the dose is repeated at 4-week intervals.

In severe hypercalcemia, rapid lowering of calcium levels may be achieved by subcutaneous administration of calcitonin 100 to 200 U tid for three to six doses (156). Serum calcium should be evaluated 1 day after calcitonin treatment. The other available agents for treatment of acute hypercalcemia are less useful (etidronate disodium, gallium nitrate) or toxic (plicamycin).

■ HYDRATION

"To hydrate or not" is a topic that is brought up many times in a terminal situation, both by health care providers as well as patients and family members. The traditional medical model always supported the maintenance of intravenous fluids in terminal patients (157,

158). In one study at a tertiary care teaching hospital, 73 of 106 patients died with an intravenous line running (159). This practice has been challenged by some palliative care providers (160). The negative effect of hydration in terminal patients was based mostly on anecdotal evidence rather than on scientifically tested data (161–163). Other anecdotal evidence, however, pointed to a beneficial effect of hydration in terminal patients (164). Dehydration can lead to delirium, exacerbate opioid side effects, and worsen other symptoms such as constipation, fatigue, and hypercalemia. While many patients die peacefully without parenteral fluids, there is some consensus on the need for individualized management (165,166).

ASSESSMENT

Symptoms of dehydration may include fatigue, confusion/delirium, constipation, and dry mouth. The physical examination may reveal drowsiness or confusion, poor skin turgor, decreased jugular venous pressure, dry mucous membranes, decreased urinary sodium, elevated hematocrit reflecting hemoconcentration, hypernatremia, elevated blood urea nitrogen, and normal creatinine in early dehydration.

MANAGEMENT

The decision to hydrate a patient is based on individual patient assessment and clinical presentation. Principles include the following:

1. Consider a short therapeutic trial of hydration in cases involving confusion.
2. Consider maintenance hydration in patients with obstruction of the small bowel, especially when their overall quality of life is fair.
3. Consider the disadvantages of hydration, such as maintaining IV/SC lines, issues of care at home and in rural areas, cost, worsening of symptoms in pre existing congestive heart failure.
4. Consider discontinuing hydration if the symptoms worsen.

METHODS OF HYDRATION

The option to hydrate the patient depends on the ability of the patient to take fluids orally. Oral fluid intake is the preferred route due to its ease of administration, low maintenance, and minimal cost involved. However, terminal patients may be unable to take fluids orally, especially if they are confused and drowsy. In that situation, fluids should be given intravenously (if a preexisting long intravenous line is already in place) or subcutaneously (also known as hypodermoclysis or clysis); this last is considered the better option by many palliative care specialists (167–169). Fluids may be administered via clysis as either a bolus or continuous infusion. Advantages of clysis include ease of access to site, suitability for home administration because of its ease and safety, ability to use a single site up to 7 days, and ease of disconnection for the patient's mobility. Methods of administration include normal saline at the rate of 70 to 100 mL/h via continuous infusion for rehydration. For maintenance, two-thirds dextrose and one-third normal saline at the rate of 40 to 80 mL/h, 1000 mL by gravity overnight, or 500 mL bolus twice a day, with each bolus infused over 1 h. On some occasions, hyaluronidase may facilitate fluid absorption (170).

■ COMMUNICATION IN PALLIATIVE CARE

Communication in a medical practice in general and palliative medicine in particular is the key to a successful and satisfactory experience for patients, families, and health care professionals (171,172). There is enough evidence to suggest that the emotional and psychological needs of a dying patient are of paramount importance (173,174). There are number of reasons for miscommunication between an advanced cancer patient and a health care professional (175,176). Health care professionals are typically trained to cure and therefore feel stressed when they have to break the bad news to their patients. Patients in the western world also try to avoid talk of death and dying. There are no paradigms to help us make the transition from life to death. Some of the major subjects that may call for discussion include diagnosis and prognosis, the natural history of the disease, symptom management, compliance with therapy, hopes and expectations of treatment, planning for the future, transition from curative treatment to palliative care, advance directives and do-not-resuscitate (DNR) orders, hospice care, and end-of-life issues. An honest, sensitive, and compassionate discussion about a poor prognosis sets the stage for an exploration of the emotions, fears, and spiritual needs surrounding the dying process (177). The quality of prognostic discussion has an important influence on the patient's emotional and physical well-being (173,174,178,179).

Communicating a poor prognosis is one of the most difficult ordeals faced by physicians. Multiple factors have been identified as barriers to communicating a poor prognosis. Many physicians find it stressful to give

TABLE
41-10

THE SPIKES PROTOCOL (SETUP/PATIENT'S PERCEPTION/INVITATION/KNOWLEDGE/EMOTIONS/SUPPORT)

STEP 1: SETTING UP THE INTERVIEW

Goals	*Purpose*
To prepare yourself for the interview To establish rapport with the patient and put the patient at ease To facilitate information exchange	Reflect on the task at hand. Arrange for uninterrupted time. Decide who should be present. Determine whether the patient is ready. Sit down when you speak to the patient. Have facial tissues handy. Maintain eye contact.

STEP 2: FIND OUT THE PATIENT'S PERCEPTION OF THE ILLNESS

Goals	*Purpose*
To determine what the patient understands To assess denial in the patient/family To promote rapport through listening To understand the patient's expectations and concerns	Ask open-ended questions; i.e., "Tell me what you've been told," or "I'd like to make sure you understand the reason for the tests." Correct misinformation and misunderstanding. Address denial. Address unrealistic expectation. Define your role.

STEP 3: GET AN INVITATION TO GIVE INFORMATION

Goals	*Purpose*
To determine how much information the patient wants and when he or she is ready to hear it To acknowledge that patient information needs may change over time To resolve conflicts with families regarding information disclosure	Ask "Are you the type of person who wants information in detail?" Explore sources of family concern.

STEP 4: GIVING THE PATIENT KNOWLEDGE AND INFORMATION

Goals	*Purpose*
To prepare the patient for the bad news To ensure patient understanding	"Forecast" the arrival of bad news; i.e., "I'm afraid I have some bad news…" Give the information in small parcels. Check periodically for understanding. Avoid using medical jargon. Address all questions.

STEP 5: RESPONDING TO PATIENT EMOTIONS

Goals	*Purpose*
To address emotional responses To facilitate emotional recovery To acknowledge our own emotions	Anticipate emotional reactions. Resist the temptation to try and make the bad news better than it really is. Support the patient by using emphatic response to expressions of emotion such as crying. Clarify emotions about which you are not sure. Validate the patient's feelings.

SUPPORTING THE PATIENT

Be prepared, and have a strategy (escape is not a strategy).
Have someone with you if it will be difficult.
Shift to a supportive role.
    Give the patient time to emote.
    Have facial tissue ready.
Sit down and get close if you can.
Respond to any emotions with one of the following:
    Empathic statements
    Validating statements
    Exploratory questions

SOURCE: Modified from Elsayem et al. (131). With permission.

prognostic information and wait to be asked before providing it (175,176,180,181). Physicians are often inaccurate in prognosticating and tend to be overoptimistic in their assessments 177–179,182–184). Patients in United States now want to be told of their prognosis despite such barriers (185). The myth about harming the patients with disclosure of their prognosis is ill-founded; in fact, it has been shown that patients with cancer often appreciate being told the truth (186).

Most patients who receive bad news are generally satisfied with the communication, but some have criticized the manner in which they were told of their prognosis. About 25% of the patients with advance cancer felt that the diagnosis of their disease was not communicated in a "clear and caring manner" (187). About 22 to 26% of the patients felt that they could have received more information about the poor prognosis (188,189). Patients who are informed by the telephone or in the recovery room after a diagnostic procedure are more likely to have a negative reaction to the discussion than those who are told in the office or in their hospital rooms (190). Another study of patients with cancer confirms the importance of receiving adequate information, related in a caring and hopeful way, with a supportive person present (192).

There are very few trials testing the effectiveness of different strategies in delivering bad news (193). Most recommendations on discussing bad news agree on key features (194). These recommendations can be organized into five categories: preparation, content of message, dealing with the patient's responses, and ending the encounter (Table 41-10).

■ CONCLUSION

Symptom control continues to be a challenge for oncologists, since cancer is a form of chronic disease and poses challenges at every step of treatment. Symptoms occur not only during the treatment phase from the treatment itself but also due to the complex biology of most tumors, which release a gamut of unwanted chemicals causing potentially devastating symptoms and leading to both physical and emotional turmoil. This in turn leads to loss of independence, doubts about existence and the meaning to life and connectedness to people and society. This happens while the so-called soul is slowly escaping from the body. In this difficult situation, a well-crafted team approach and dedicated members are needed to fulfill the mission of maintaining the integrity of human life and suffering. Palliative and hospice care are established models that deliver such care.

There is an urgent need for health care providers to develop a better appreciation of patients' distress beyond physical symptoms. An interdisciplinary team that is able to understand the complex symptomatology and provide compassionate and competent care to the patient and family both during active treatment as well as in advanced stages of the disease is an ideal model.

A good symptom management approach should incorporate appropriate principles to deal with complex symptoms, maintain open dialogue with patients and families, discuss various options—including treatment options, prognosis, future course, and possible symptoms during the treatment process—as well as futility of treatment whenever applicable and palliative care as a viable option. This can ideally be achieved by involving the palliative care team from the time of diagnosis.

References

1. Curtis EB, Krech R, Walsh TD. Common symptoms in patients with advanced cancer. *J Palliat Care* 1991;7:25–28.
2. Krech RL, Walsh D. Symptoms of pancreatic cancer. *J Pain Sympt Mgt* 1991;6:360–367.
3. Foley KM. Pain syndromes in patients with cancer. In: Bonica JJ, Ventafridda V (eds.), *Advances in Pain Research and Therapy.* New York: Raven Press; 1979:59–75.
4. Bonica JJ. Cancer pain. In: Bonica JJ (ed). *The Management of Pain.* Philadelphia: Lea & Febiger; 1990:400.
5. Twycross RG, Fairfield S. Pain in far-advanced cancer. *Pain* 1982;14:303–310.
6. Levin D, Cleeland CS, Dar R. Public attitudes toward cancer pain. *Cancer* 1985;56:2337–2339.
7. Foley KM. The treatment of cancer pain. *N Engl J Med* 1984;313:84–95.
8. Portenoy RK, Hagen NA. Breakthrough pain: Definition, prevalence, and characteristics. *Pain* 1990;41:273–281.
9. Bruera E, MacMillan K, Hanson J, et al. The Edmonton staging system for cancer pain: Preliminary report. *Pain* 1989; 37:203–209.
10. Bruera E, Kuehn N, Miller MJ, et al. The Edmonton symptom assessment system: A simple method for the assessment of palliative care patients. *J Palliat Care* 1991;7:6–9.
11. World Health Organization. *Cancer Pain Relief.* Geneva, Switzerland: World Health Organization; 1986.
12. Jacox A, Carr DB, Payne R, et al. *Management of Cancer Pain.* Clinical Practice Guidelines No. 9, AHCPR Publication 94-0592. Rockville, MD: US Department of Health and Human Services, Agency for Health Care Policy and Research; 1994.
13. Raja SN, Haythornthwaite JA, Pappagallo M, et al. Opioids versus antidepressants in postherpetic neuralgia. A randomized, placebo-controlled trial. *Neurology* 2002;59:1015–1021.
14. Rowbotham MC, Twilling L, Davies PS, et al. Oral opioid therapy for chronic peripheral and central neuropathic pain. *N Engl J Med* 2003;348(13):1223–1232.
15. Andersen G, Christrup L, Sjogren P. Relationships among morphine metabolism, pain and side effects during long-term treatment: An update. *J Pain Sympt Mgt* 2003;25(1):74-91.

16. Szeto HH, Inturrisi CE, Houde R, et al. Accumulation of normeperidine, an active metabolite of meperidine, in patients with renal failure of cancer. *Ann Intern Med* 1977;86(6):738–741.

17. Portenoy RK, Payne R, Coluzzi P, et al. Oral transmucosal fentanyl citrate (OTFC) for the treatment of breakthrough pain in cancer patients: A controlled dose titration study. *Pain* 1999;79(2–3):303–312.

18. Tennant F, Hermann L. Self-treatment with oral transmucosal fentanyl citrate to prevent emergency room visits for pain crises: Patient self-reports of efficacy and utility. *J Pain Palliat Care Pharmacother* 2002;16(3):37–44.

19. Davis MP, Walsh D. Methadone for relief of cancer pain: A review of pharmakokinetics, pharmacodynamics, drug interactions and protocols of administration. *Support Care Cancer* 2001;9:63–83.

20. Ripamonti C, Groff L, Brunelli C, et al. Switching from morphine to oral methadone in treating cancer pain: What is the equianalgesic dose ratio? *J Clin Oncol* 1998;16(10):3216–3221.

21. Ripamonti C, de Conno F, Groff L, et al. Equianalgesic dose/ratio between methadone and other opioid agonists in cancer pain: Comparison of two clinical experiences. *Ann Oncol* 1998;9:79–83.

22. Gorman AL, Elliott KJ, Inturrisi CE. The d-and l-isomers of methadone bind to the non-competitive site on the N-methyl-D-asparatate (NMDA) receptor in rat forebrain and spinal cord. *Neurosci Lett* 1997;223:5–8.

23. Tarumi Y, Pereira J, Watanabe S. Methadone and fluconazole: Respiratory depression by drug interaction. *J Pain Sympt Mgt* 2002;23(2):148–153.

24. Galer BS, Coyle N, Pasternak GW, Portenoy RK. Individual variation in the response to different opiods—Report of five cases. *Pain* 1992;49:87–91.

25. Hanks G, Forbes K. Opioid responsiveness. *Acta Anesthesiol Scand* 1997;41:154–158.

26. Lane NE. Pain management in osteoarthritis: The role of COX-2 inhibitors. *J Rheumatol* 1997;24:20–24.

27. Bresalier RS, Sandler RS, Quan H, et al. Cardiovascular events associated with rofecoxib in a colorectal chemoprevention trial. *N Engl J Med* 2005;352(11):1092–1102.

28. Magni G. The use of antidepressants in the treatment of chronic pain: A review of current evidence. *Drugs* 1991;42:730–748.

29. Kolke M, Hoffken K, Olbrich H, Schmidt CG. Antidepressants and anticonvulsants for the treatment of neuropathic pain syndromes in cancer patients. *Onkologie* 1999;14:40–43.

30. Rowbotham M, Harden N, Stacey B, et al. Gabapentin for the treatment of postherpetic neuralgia: A randomized controlled trial. *JAMA* 1998;280:1837–1842.

31. Backonja M, Beydoun A, Edwards KR, et al. Gabapentin for the symptomatic treatment of painful neuropathy in patients with diabetes mellitus: A randomized controlled trial. *JAMA* 1998;280:1831–1836.

32. Brietbart W. Psychotropic adjuvant analgesics for pain in cancer and AIDS. *Psychooncology* 1998;7:333–345.

33. Patt R, Propper G, Reddy S. The neuroleptics as adjuvants analgesics. *J Pain Sympt Mgt* 1994;9:446–453.

34. Reddy S, Patt RB. The benzodiazepines as adjuvant analgesics. *J Pain Sympt Mgt* 1994;9:510–514.

35. Thiebaud D, Leyvarz S, von Fliedner V, et al. Treatment of bone metastases from breast cancer and myeloma with pamidronate. *Eur J Cancer* 1991;27:37–41.

36. Berenson JR, Licherstein A, Porter L, et al. Efficacy of pamidronate in reducing skeletal events in patients with advanced multiple myeloma. *N Engl J Med* 1996;334:488–493.

37. Hortobagyi GN, Theriault RL, Porter L, et al. Efficacy of pamidronate in reducing skeletal complications in patients with breast cancer and lytic bone metastases. *N Engl J Med* 1996;335(24):178.

38. Grant R, Papadopoulos SM, Sandler HM, et al. Metastatic epidural spinal cord compression: Current concepts and treatment. *J Neurooncol* 1994;19:79–92.

39. Nagaro T, Shimizu C, Inoue H, et al. The efficacy of intravenous lidocaine on various types of neuropathic pain. *Masui* 1995;44(6):862–867.

40. Brose W, Cousins M. Subcutaneous lidocaine for the treatment of neuropathic cancer pain. *Pain* 1991;45(2):145–148.

41. Galer BS, Rowbotham MC Perander J, et al. Topical lidocaine patch relieves postherpetic neuralgia more effectively than a vehicle topical patch: Results of an enriched enrollment study. *Pain* 1999;80:533–538.

42. Mercadante S, Lodi F, Sapio M, et al. Long-term ketamine subcutaneous infusion in neuropathic cancer pain. *J Pain Sympt Mgt* 1995;10(7):564–568.

43. Yang CY, Wong CS, Chiang JY, Ho ST. Intrathecal ketamine reduces morphine requirements in patients with terminal cancer. *Can J Anaesth* 1996;43(4):379–383.

44. Ellison N, Loprinzi CL, Kugler J, et al. Phase 3 placebo-controlled trial of capsaicin cream in the management of surgical neuropathic pain in cancer patients. *J Clin Oncol* 1997;15(8):2974–2980.

45. Crawford ED, Kozlowski JM, Debruyne FM, et al. The use of strontium 89 for palliation of pain from bone metastasis associated with hormone-refractory prostate cancer. *Urology* 1994;44:481–485.

46. Serafini AN, Houston SJ, Resche I, et al. Palliation of pain associated with metastatic bone cancer using samarium-153 lexidronam: A double blind placebo-controlled clinical trial. *J Clin Oncol* 1998;16:1574–1581.

47. Arner S. The role of nerve blocks in the treatment of cancer pain. *Acta Anaesthesiol Scand* 1982;74:104–108.

48. Cousins MJ, Bridenbaug PO (eds). *Neural Blockade,* 2d ed. Philadelphia: Lippincott; 1988.

49. Brown DL, Bulley CK, Quiel EL. Neurolytic celiac plexus block for pancreatic cancer pain. *Anesth Analg* 1987;66:869–873.

50. Lillemoe KD, Cameron JL, Kaufman HS, et al. Chemical splanchnicectomy in patients with unresectable pancreatic cancer. A prospective randomized trial. *Ann Surg* 1993;217(5):447–455; discussion 456–457.

51. Wong GY, Schroeder DR, Carns PE, et al. Effect of neurolytic celiac plexus block on pain relief, quality of life, and survival in patients with unresectable pancreatic cancer. A randomized controlled trial. *JAMA.* 2004;291:1092–1099.

52. Patt RB, Payne R, Farhat GA, Reddy SK. Subarachnoid neurolytic block under general anesthesia in a 3-year-old with neuroblastoma. *Clin J Pain* 1995;11(2):143–146.

53. Smith TJ, Staats PS, Deer T, et al. Randomized clinical trial of an implantable drug delivery system compared with comprehensive medical management for refractory cancer pain:

Impact on pain, drug-related toxicity, and survival. *J Clin Oncol* 2002;20(19):4040–4049.

54. Davis MP, Walsh D, Lagman R, LeGrand SB. Randomized clinical trial of an implantable drug delivery system. *J Clin Oncol* 2003;21(14): 2800–2801.

55. Ripamonti C, Brunelli C. Randomized clinical trial of an implantable drug delivery system compared with comprehensive medical management for refractory cancer pain: Impact on pain, drug-related toxicity, and survival. *J Clin Oncol* 2003;21(14):2801–2802.

56. Meyerson BA. The role of neurosurgery in the treatment of cancer pain. *Acta Anaesthesiol Scand* 1982;74:109–113.

57. Macalusco C, Foley KM, Arbit E. Cordotomy for lumbosacral, pelvic and lower extremity pain of malignant origin: Safety and efficacy. *Neurology* 1988;38:110.

58. Weill A, Chiras J, Simon JM, et al. Spinal metastases: Indications for and results of percutaneous injection of acrylic surgical cement. *Radiology* 1996;199:241–247.

59. Cotton A, Boutry N, Cortet B, et al. Percutaneous vertebroplasty: State of the art. *Radiographics* 1998;18:311–322.

60. Goetz MP, Callstrom MR, Charboneau JW, et al. Percutaneous image-guided radiofrequency ablation of painful metastases involving bone: A multicenter study. *J Clin Oncol* 2004;22(2):300–306.

61. Stone P, Richards M, Hardy J. Fatigue in patients with cancer. *Eur J Cancer* 1998;34:1670–1676.

62. Jacobsen PB, Hann DM, Azzarello LM, et al. Fatigue in women receiving adjuvant chemotherapy for breast cancer: Characteristics, course, and correlates. *J Pain Sympt Mgt* 1999;18:233–242.

63. Cella D, Peterman A, Passik S, et al. Progress toward guidelines for the management of fatigue. *Oncology* 1998;12:369–377.

64. Portenoy RK, Itri LM. Cancer-related fatigue: Guidelines for evaluation and management. *Oncologist* 1999;4:1–10.

65. Demetri GD, Kris M, Wade J, et al. Quality of life benefit in chemotherapy patients treated with epoetin alfa is independent of disease response or tumor type: Results from a prospective community oncology study. *Oncology* 1998;16:3412–3425.

66. Bruera E, Roca E, Cedaro L, et al. Action of oral methylprednisolone in terminal cancer patients: A prospective randomized double-blind study. *Cancer Treat Rep* 1985;69:751–754.

67. Tannock I, Gospodarowicz M, Meakin W, et al. Treatment of metastatic prostate cancer with low dose prednisone: Evaluation of pain and quality of life as pragmatic indices of response. *J Clin Oncol* 1989;7:590–597.

68. Bruera E, Brenneis C, Paterson AH, MacDonald RN. Use of methylphenidate as an adjuvant to narcotic analgesics in patients with advanced cancer. *J Pain Sympt Mgt* 1989;4:3–6.

69. Breitbart W, Mermelstein H. An alternative psychostimulant for the management of depressive disorders in cancer patients. *Psychosomatics* 1992;33:352–356.

70. Katon W, Raskind M. Treatment of depression in the medically ill elderly with methylphenidate. *Am J Psychiatry* 1980;137:963–965.

71. Rajagopal A, Vassilopoulou-Sellin R, Palmer JL, et al. Symptomatic hypogonadism in male survivors of cancer with chronic exposure to opioids. *Cancer* 2004;100(4):851–858.

72. Bruera E, Driver L, Barnes EA, et al. Patient-controlled methylphenidate for the management of fatigue in patients with advanced cancer: A preliminary report. *J Clin Oncol* 2003;23:4439–4443.

73. Wasserman K, Casaburi R. Dyspnea and physiological and athophysiological mechanisms. *Annu Rev Med* 1988;39:503–515.

74. Farncombe M. Dyspnea: Assessment and treatment. *Support Care Cancer* 1997;5:94–99.

75. Hardy JR, Turner R, Saunders M, A'Hern R. Prediction of survival in a hospital-based continuing care unit. *Eur J Cancer* 1994;30:284–288.

76. Escalante CP, Martin CG, Elting LS, et al. Dyspnea in cancer patients: Etiology, resource utilization, and survival. *Cancer* 1996;78:1314–1319.

77. Anthonisen NR. Long-term oxygen therapy. *Ann Intern Med* 1983;99:519–527.

78. Nocturnal Oxygen Therapy Trial Group. Continuous or nocturnal oxygen therapy in hypoxemic chronic obstructive lung disease. *Ann Intern Med* 1980;93:391–398.

79. Bruera E, De Stoutz N, Velasco-Leiva A, et al. The effects of oxygen on the intensity of dyspnea in hypoxemic terminal cancer patients. *Lancet* 1993;342:13–14.

80. Bruera E, Scholler T, MacEachern T. Symptomatic benefit of supplemental oxygen in hypoxemic patients with terminal cancer: The use of the N of 1 randomized control trial. *J Pain Sympt Mgt* 1992;7:365–368.

81. Bruera E, MacEachern T, Ripamonti C, et al. Subcutaneous morphine for dyspnea in cancer patients. *Ann Intern Med* 1993;119:906–907.

82. Bruera E, MacMillan K, Pither J, et al. The effects of morphine on the dyspnea of terminal cancer patients. *J Pain Sympt Mgt* 1990;5:341–344.

83. Cohen MH, Johnston Anderson A, Krasnow SH, et al. Continuous intravenous infusion of morphine for severe dyspnea. *South Med J* 1991;84:229–234.

84. Davis CL, Hodder C, Love S, et al. Effect of nebulised morphine and morphine-6-glucuronide on exercise endurance in patients with chronic obstructive pulmonary disease. *Thorax* 1994;49:393.

85. Farncombe M, Chater S. Gillin A. The use of nebulized opioids for breathlessness: A chart review. *Palliat Med* 1994; 8:306–312.

86. Farncombe M, Chater S. Clinical application of nebulized opioids for treatment of dyspnea in patients with malignant disease. *Support Care Cancer* 1994;2(3):184–187.

87. Zeppetella G. Nebulized morphine in the palliation of dyspnea. *Palliat Med* 1997;11(4):267–275.

88. Coyne PJ, Viswanathan R, Smith TJ. Nebulized fentanyl citrate improves patients' perception of breathing, respiratory rate, and oxygen saturation in dyspnea. *J Pain Sympt Mgt* 2002;23(2):157–160.

89. Weir DC, Gove RI, Robertson AS, et al. Corticosteroids trials in nonasthmatic chronic airflow obstruction: A comparison of oral prednisolone and inhaled bechomethasone diproprionate. *Thorax* 1991;45:112–117.

90. Congleton J, Meurs MF. The incidence of airflow obstruction in bronchial carcinoma, its relation to breathlessness, and response to bronchodilator therapy. *Respir Med* 1995;89:291–296.

91. Neil PA, Morton PB, Stark RD. Chlorpromazine—A special effect on breathlessness? *Br J Clin Pharmacol* 1985;19:793–797.

92. Lipowski ZJ. Delirium (acute confusional states). *JAMA* 1987;258(13):1789–1792.

93. Rabins PV. Psychosocial and management aspects of delirium. *Int Psychogeriatr* 1991;3:319–324.

94. Derogatis LR, Morrow GR, Fetting J, et al. The prevalence of psychiatric disorders among cancer patients. *JAMA* 1983; 249:751–757.

95. Levine PM, Silberfarb PM, Lipowski ZJ. Mental disorders in cancer patients: A study of 100 psychiatric referrals. *Cancer* 1978;42:1385–1391.

96. Stiefel F, Finsinger R, Bruera E. Acute confusional states in patients with advanced cancer. *J Pain Sympt Mgt* 1992;7: 94–98.

97. Lipowski ZJ. Delirium in the elderly patient. *N Engl J Med* 1989;320:578–582.

98. Liptzin B, Levkoff SE. An empirical study of delirium subtypes. *Br J Psychiatry* 1992;161:843–845.

99. American Psychiatric Association. *Diagnostic and Statistical Manual of Mental Disorders,* 4th ed. Washington, DC: American Psychiatric Association; 1994.

100. Voruganti L, Cortese L, Owyeumi L, et al. Switching from conventional to novel antipsychotic drugs: Results of a prospective naturalistic study. *Schizophr Res* 2002;57(2–3): 201–208.

101. Briebart W, Marotta R, Platt MM, et al. A double-blinded trial of haloperidol, chlorazepam, and lorazepam in the treatment of delirium in the hospitalized AIDS patients. *Am J Psychiatry* 1996;153:231–237.

102. Derogatis LR, Marrow GR, Fettig J, et al. The Prevalence of psychiatric disorders among cancer patients. *JAMA* 1983: 249;751–757.

103. Wilson KG, Chochinov HM, de Faye B, et al: Diagnosis and management of depression in palliative care. In: Chochinov HM, Breitbart W (eds). *Handbook of Psychiatry in Palliative Care.* Oxford, UK: Oxford University Press; 2000:25–49, 106.

104. Green AI, Austin PV. Psychopathology of pancreatic cancer: A psychobiologic probe. *Psychosomatics* 1993;34:208.

105. Massie MJ, Holland J. The cancer patient with pain: Psychiatric complications and their management. *Med Clin North Am* 1987;71:243.

106. American Psychiatric Association. *Diagnostic and Statistical Manual of Mental Disorders,* 4th ed. Washington, DC: American Psychiatric Association; 1994.

107. Fisch MJ, Loehrer PJ, Kristeller J, et al. Fluoxetine versus placebo in advanced cancer outpatients: A double-blinded trial of the Hoosier Oncology Group. *J Clin Oncol* 2003; 21(10):1937–1943.

108. Bonsignore M, Barkow K, Jessen F, Heun R. Validity of the five item WHO Well Being Index (WHO-5) in an elderly population. *Eur Arch Psychiatry Clin Neurosci* 2001; 251(suppl 2):II27–II31.

109. Kroenke K, Spitzer RL, Williams JB. The PHQ-9: Validity of a brief depression severity measure. *J Gen Intern Med* 2001;16:606–613.

110. Hamilton M. A rating scale for depression. *J Neurol Neurosurg Psychiatry* 1960;23:56–62.

111. Montgomery S, Asberg MA. A new depression scale designed to be sensitive to change. *Br J Psychiatry* 1979;134: 382–389.

112. Massie MJ, Popkin MK. Depressive disorders. In: Holland JC (ed). *Psycho-Oncology.* New York: Oxford University Press; 1998:518–540.

113. Holland JC, Morrow G, Schmale A, et al. Reduction of anxiety and depression in cancer patients by alprazolam or by a behavioural technique (abstr). *Proc Am Soc Clin Oncol* 1988; 6:258.

114. Vickers AJ, Cassileth BR. Unconventional therapies for cancer and cancer-related symptoms (review). *Lancet Oncol* 2001;2(4):226–232.

115. Vaswani M, Linda FK, Ramesh S. Role of selective serotonin reuptake inhibitors in psychiatric disorders: A comprehensive review. *Prog Neuropsychopharmacol Biol Psychiatry* 2003;27(1):85–102.

116. Nierenberg AA, Papakostas GI, Petersen T, et al. Nortriptyline for treatment-resistant depression. *J Clin Psychiatry* 2003;64(1):35–39.

117. Pereira J, Bruera E. Depression with psychomotor retardation: Diagnostic challenges and the use of psychostimulants. *J Palliat Med* 2001;4(1):15–21.

118. Theobald DE, Kirsh KL, Holtsclaw E, et al. An open-label, crossover trial of mirtazapine (15 and 30 mg) in cancer patients with pain and other distressing symptoms. *J Pain Sympt Mgt* 2002;23(5):442–447.

119. Kast R. Mirtazapine may be useful in treating nausea and insomnia of cancer chemotherapy. *Support Care Cancer* 2001; 9(6):469–470.

120. Sykes NP. Constipation and diarrhoea. In: Doyle D, Hanks GWC, MacDonald N (eds). *Oxford Textbook of Palliative Medicine,* 2d ed. Oxford, UK: Oxford University Press; 2001: 513–526.

121. Mancini I, Bruera E. Constipation in advanced cancer patients. *Support Care Cancer* 1998;6:356–364.

122. Mercadante S. Diarrhea, malabsorption and constipation. In: Berger AM, Portenoy RK, Weismann DE (eds). *Principles and Practice of Supportive Oncology.* Philadelphia: Lippincott-Raven; 1998:191–206.

123. Mercadante S, Casuccio A, Fulfaro F, et al. The course of symptom frequency and intensity in advanced "cancer patients followed at home. *J Pain Sympt Mgt* 2000;20:104–112.

124. Bruera E, Suarez-Almazor M, et al. The assessment of constipation in terminal cancer patients admitted to a palliative care unit: A retrospective review. *J Pain Sympt Mgt* 1994; 9:515–519.

125. Sykes NP. An investigation of the ability of oral naloxone to correct opioids-related constipation in patients with advanced cancer. *Palliat Med* 1996;10:135–144.

126. Latasch L, Zimmerman M, Eberhart B, et al. Oral naloxone antagonizes morphine-induced constipation. *Anesthetist* 1997; 46:191–194.

127. Meissner W, Schimdt U, Hartman M, et al. Oral naloxone reverses opioids-associated constipation. *Pain* 2000;84:105–109.

128. Yuan CS, Foss JF, O'Connor M, et al. Methylnaltrexone for reversal of constipation due to chronic methadone use: A randomized controlled trial. *JAMA* 2000;283(3):367–372.

129. Stephenson J. Methylnaltrexone reverses opioid-induced constipation. *Lancet Oncol* 2002;3(4):202.

130. Mannix KA. Palliation of nausea and vomiting. In: Doyle D, Hanks GWC, MacDonald N (eds). *Oxford Textbook of Pal-*

liative Medicine, 2d ed. Oxford, UK: Oxford University Press; 2001:489–499.

131. Elsayem A, Driver LC, Bruera E. *The MD Anderson Palliative Care Handbook.* Houston: MD Anderson Cancer Center; 2002.

132. Bruera ED, Roca E, Cedaro L, et al. Improved control of chemotherapy-induced emesis by the addition of dexamethasone to metoclopramide in patients resistant to metoclopramide. *Cancer Treat Rep* 1983;67:381–383.

133. Mercadante S, Fulfaro F, Casuccio A. The use of corticosteroids in home palliative care. *Support Care Cancer* 2001; 9:386–389.

134. DeWys WD, Begg D, Lavin PT. Prognostic effect of weight loss prior to chemotherapy in cancer patients. *Am J Med* 1980;69:491–499.

135. Tisdale MJ. Loss of skeletal muscle in cancer: Biochemical mechanisms. *Front Biosci* 2001;6:D164–174.

136. Belizario JE, Katz M, Chenker E, Raw I. Bioactivity of skeletal muscle proteolysis-inducing factors in the plasma proteins from cancer patients with weight loss. *Br J Cancer* 1991; 63(5):705–710.

137. Barber MD, Fearon KC, McMillan DC, et al. Liver export protein synthetic rates are increased by oral meal feeding in weight losing cancer patients. *Am J Physiol Endocrinol Metab* 2000;279:E707–E714.

138. Sarhill N, Mahmoud FA, Christie R, Tahir A. Assessment of nutritional status and fluid deficits in advanced cancer. *Am J Hosp Palliat Care* 2003;20(6):465–473.

139. Loprinzi CL, Ellison NM, Schaid DJ, et al. Phase III evaluation of four doses of megestrol acetate as therapy for patients with cancer anorexia and/or cachexia. *J Clin Oncol* 1993;11: 762–767.

140. Feliu J, Gonzales-Baron M, Berrocal A, et al. Usefulness of megestrol acetate in cancer cachexia and anorexia. *Am J Clin Oncol* 1992;15:436–440.

141. Popiela T, Lucchi R, Giongo F. Methylprednisolone as an appetite stimulant in patients with cancer. *Eur J Cancer Clin Oncol* 1989;25:1823–1829.

142. Wilcox J, Corr J, Shaw J, et al. Prednisolone as an appetite stimulant in patients with cancer. *Br Med J* 1984;27:288–290.

143. Sacks N, Hutcheson JR, Watts JM, Webb RE. Case report: The effect of tetrahydrocannabinol on food intake during chemotherapy. *J Am Coll Nutr* 1990;9:630–632.

144. Bruera E, Neumann CM, Pituskin E, et al. Thalidomide in patients with cachexia due to terminal cancer: Preliminary report. *Ann Oncol* 1999;10:857–859.

145. Mulligan K, Schambelan M. Anabolic treatment with GH, IGF-I, or anabolic steroids in patients with HIV-associated wasting. *Int J Cardiol* 2002;85(1):151–159.

146. Bozzetti F, Gavazzi C, Ferrari P, et al. Effect of total parenteral nutrition on the protein kinetics of patients with cancer cachexia. *Tumori* 2000;86:408–411.

147. Mundy GR, Guise TA. Hypercalcemia of malignancy. *Am J Med* 1997;103:134–145.

148. Heys SD, Smith IC, Eremin O, et al. Hypercalcaemia in patients with cancer: Aetiology and treatment. *Eur J Surg Oncol* 1998;24:139–142.

149. Bower M, Brazil L, Coombes R. Endocrine and metabolic complications in advanced cancer. In: Doyle D, Hanks G,

MacDonald N (eds). *Oxford Textbook of Palliative Medicine,* 2d ed. Oxford, UK: Oxford University Press; 1998:709–712.

150. Bilezikian JP. Management of acute hypercalcemia. *N Engl J Med* 1992;326:1196–1203.

151. Bilezikian JP. Hypercalcemia. *Curr Ther Endocrinol Metab* 1994;5:511–514.

152. Kovacs CS, MacDonald SM, Chik CL, et al. Hypercalcemia of malignancy in the palliative care patient: A treatment strategy. *J Pain Sympt Mgt* 1995;10:224–232.

153. Riccardi A, Grasso D, Danova M. Bisphosphonates in oncology: Physiopathologic bases and clinical activity. *Tumori* 2003;89(3):223–236.

154. Gucalp R, Theriault R, Gill I, et al. Treatment of cancer-associated hypercalcemia. Double-blind comparison of rapid and slow intravenous infusion regimens of pamidronate disodium and saline alone. *Arch Intern Med* 1994;154:1935–1944.

155. Neville-Webbe H, Coleman RE.The use of zoledronic acid in the management of metastatic bone disease and hypercalcaemia. *Palliat Med* 2003;17(6):539–553.

156. Ljunghall S. Use of clodronate and calcitonin in hypercalcemia due to malignancy. *Recent Results Cancer Res* 1989; 116:40–45.

157. Micetich KC, Steinecker PH, Thomasma DC, et al. Are intravenous fluids morally required for a dying patient? *Arch Intern Med* 1983;143:975–978.

158. Siegler M, Weisbard, AJ. Against the emerging stream. Should fluids and nutritional support be discontinued? *Arch Intern Med* 1985;145:129–131.

159. Hamdy RC, Braverman AM. Ethical conflicts in long-term care of the aged. *Br Med J* 1980;280:717.

160. Burge FI. Dehydration and provision of fluids in palliative care. What is the evidence? *Can Fam Physician* 1996;42: 2383–2388.

161. Twycross RG. Symptom control: The problem areas. *Palliat Med* 1993;7:1–8.

162. Andrews M, Bell ER, Smith SA, et al. Dehydration in terminally ill patients. Is it appropriate palliative care? *Postgrad Med* 1993;93:201–208.

163. Sullivan RJ Jr. Accepting death without artificial nutrition or hydration. *J Gen Intern Med* 1993;8:220–224.

164. Yan E, Bruera E. Parenteral hydration of terminally ill cancer patients. *J Palliat Care* 1991;7:40–43.

165. Fainsinger R, Bruera E. The management of dehydration in terminally ill patients. *J Palliat Care* 1994;10:55–59.

166. Berger EY. Nutrition by hypodermoclysis. *J Am Geriatr Soc* 1984;32:199–203.

167. Bruera E, Legris MA, Kuehn N, Miller MJ. Hypodermoclysis for the administration of fluids and narcotic analgesics in patients with advanced cancer. *J Pain Sympt Mgt* 1990;5: 218–220.

168. Hays H. Hypodermaclysis for symptom control in terminal cancer. *Can Fam Physician* 1985;31:1253–1256.

169. Fainsinger RL, MacEachern T, Miller M J, et al. The use of hypodermoclysis for rehydration in terminally ill cancer patients. *J Pain Sympt Mgt* 1994;9:298–302.

170. Constans T, Dutertre JP, Froge E. Hypodermoclysis in dehydrated elderly patients: Local effects with and without hyaluronidase. *J Palliat Care* 1991;7:1012.

171. Cousins N. How patients appraise physicians. *N Engl J Med* 1985;313:1422–1424.

172. Ley P, Bradshaw PW, Kincey JA, et al. Increasing patients' satisfaction with communications. *Br J Soc Clin Psychol* 1976;15:403–413.

173. Kristjanson LJ. Quality of terminal care: Salient indicators identified by families. *J Palliat Care* 1989;5:21–30.

174. Kaplan SH, Greenfield S, Ware JE Jr, et al. Assessing the effects of physician-patient interactions on the outcomes of chronic disease. *Med Care* 1989;27:S110–S127.

175. Houts PS, Yasko JM, Harvey HA, et al. Unmet needs of persons with cancer in Pennsylvania during the period of terminal care. *Cancer* 1988;62:627–634.

176. Saunders JM, McCorkle R. Models of care for persons with progressive cancer. *Nurs Clin North Am* 1985;20:365–377.

177. Maguire P. Barriers to psychological care of the dying. *Br Med J (Clin Res Ed)* 1985;291:1711–1713.

178. Hockley JM, Dunlop R, Davies RJ, et al. Survey of distressing symptoms in dying patients and their families in hospital and the response to a symptom control team. *Br Med J (Clin Res Ed)* 1988;296:1715–1717.

179. Maguire P. Barriers to psychological care of the dying. *Br Med J (Clin Res Ed)* 1985;291:1711–1713.

180. Buckman R. Breaking bad news: Why is it still so difficult? *Br Med J (Clin Res Ed)* 1984;288:1597–1599.

181. Weissman DE. Consultation in palliative medicine. *Arch Intern Med* 1997;157:733–737.

182. McCormick TR, Conley BJ. Patients' perspectives on dying and on the care of dying patients. *West J Med* 1995;163:236–243.

183. Lind SE, DelVecchio-Good MJ, et al. Telling the diagnosis of cancer. *J Clin Oncol.*1989;7:583–589.

184. Christakis NA, Iwashyna TJ. Attitude and self-reported practice regarding prognostication in a national sample of internists. *Arch Intern Med* 1998;158:2389–2395.

185. Christakis NA. Predicting patient survival before and after hospice enrollment. *Hosp J* 1998;13:71–87.

186. Parkes CM. Accuracy of predictions of survival in later stages of cancer. *Br Med J* 1972;2:29–31.

187. Novack DH, Plumer R, et al. Changes in physicians' attitudes toward telling the cancer patient. *JAMA* 1979;241:897–900.

188. Sell L, Devlin B, et al. Communicating the diagnosis of lung cancer. *Respir Med* 1993;87:61–63.

189. Chan A, Woodruff RK. Communicating with patients with advanced cancer. *J Palliat Care* 1997;13:29–33.

190. Seale C. Communication and awareness about death: A study of a random sample of dying people. *Soc Sci Med* 1991;32:943–952.

191. Lind SE, DelVecchio-Good MJ, et al. Telling the diagnosis of cancer. *J Clin Oncol* 1989;7:583–589.

192. Peter JR, Abrams HE, Ross DM, et al. Presenting a diagnosis of cancer: Patients' views. *J Fam Pract* 1991;32:577–581.

193. Girgis A, Sanson-Fisher RW. Breaking bad news: Consensus guidelines for medical practitioners. *J Clin Oncol* 1995;13:2449–2456.

194. Ptacek JT, Eberhardt TL. Breaking bad news: A review of the literature. *JAMA* 1996;276:496–502.

Long-Term Survival

CHAPTER
42

PEDIATRIC LONG-TERM FOLLOW-UP

Nita R. Burrer
Norman Jaffe

■ LATER EFFECTS OF CHILDHOOD CANCER AND CANCER TREATMENTS—A GUIDE FOR THE COMMUNITY PROVIDER

The community health care provider will at some point be faced with caring for a survivor of childhood cancer. This may be episodic care or follow-up care for the cancer and treatment. Approximately 1 of every 350 persons living in the United States today has been diagnosed or will be diagnosed with cancer before the age of 20. Prior to 1960, nearly all children diagnosed with cancer died of their disease. Since 1960, however, due to innovative and combined treatment modalities, the rate of survival for childhood cancers has been climbing rapidly. Current estimates are that 75% of all patients diagnosed with cancer who are less than 20 years of age will now be cured (1–4). This represents a rapidly growing group of individuals who have survived both their cancer and their cancer treatment; currently it is estimated to comprise 270,000 individuals in the United States (1–4). Many of these patients are followed in one of the 26 clinics, located in 18 states, identified by Nancy Keene, well-known patient advocate and author of many books for families dealing with cancer and cancer survivorship. However, the majority of the 270,000 living survivors of childhood cancer are followed by pediatric practitioners, family practice practitioners, general practitioners, internists, or health clinics at colleges

or universities. These practitioners probably have little or no experience in managing late effects of childhood cancer and cancer treatment or in addressing cancer survivorship issues.

Patients treated up to 30 to 40 years ago, when cancer treatment was very aggressive, comprise a large group of the survivors seen in the community. In this group, radiation was used extensively and was not highly refined. The late effect could only be anticipated. Chemotherapy was in its infancy, in many cases "more was better," and the late effects on young, developing bodies were of concern but unpredictable. Surgery, while curative, was often also mutilative. Limb salvage and biotherapy were unknown.

Late effects may be defined as the result of cancer treatment that affects a survivor's health for years after the treatment has been completed and the cancer has been controlled. The late effects may be apparent at the time of the treatment or they may become only obvious at a later date.

The first intervention for the community physician when managing the long-term survivor of childhood cancer is to obtain an accurate cancer diagnosis, a complete treatment history, a family history of cancer, and information on any known existing late effects. It is often necessary to contact the physician or institution where the child received either treatment or previous late-effect surveillance. The patient and his or her family may or may not be accurate historians; therefore it is extremely important to obtain copies of the pathology report and treatment record. Communication with the attending oncologist may be invaluable. Only by being aware of the diagnosis, treatments received, and family history can proper surveillance be performed (5–8). Late effects of childhood cancer and cancer treatments will vary from patient to patient on the basis of age at time of diagnosis, treatment regimen, and the patient's underlying genetic predisposition (5). Late effects may be divided into four categories, as outlined below.

The *first* and most feared late effect is relapse of the original disease either at the primary site or as metastatic disease. The *second* and equally feared late effect is the development of a treatment-related or genetically induced second primary cancer. The *third* category of late effects comprises what is generally referred to as treatment effects that persist long after the cancer has been controlled and all treatment has been stopped. The *fourth* category of late effects is related not to the physiology or biology of the cancer or treatment but rather to the social arena of insurance, employment, adjustment, and physical or esthetic impairment.

■ OVERVIEW OF CHILDHOOD CANCERS

The peak age of cancer incidence in children occurs in infancy (at less than 1 year of age). Infantile cancer is associated with a poor survival rate of about 35% (9). During the childhood and adolescent years, survival rates improve dramatically, approaching 75%. The most common type of cancer diagnosed during infancy and childhood is leukemia, followed by lymphoma and malignancies of the central nervous system. Cancers in the adolescent are associated with a 77% survival rate, with the most common cancer being Hodgkin's disease, followed closely by germ cell tumors.

■ OVERVIEW OF SURVEILLANCE

Generally, patients off active therapy should be followed every 4 to 6 months until the risk of relapse, recurrence, or development of metastatic lesions is minimal. This is usually considered to be 2 to 5 years after treatment has been completed. Normally, the treating oncologist will provide this care. Once the risk of recurrence, relapse, or development of metastasis is minimal, the patients should be followed yearly for 5 more years and then every 1 to 2 years indefinitely. If late effects are present then, the schedule should be adjusted to accommodate the symptomatology. Should the survivor have

children, an opportunity to determine that the offspring are normal and healthy should also be provided.

During the first visit in long-term follow-up, the practitioner should obtain the following information if not already known:

1. Date of diagnosis, diagnosis, stage, grade, site, relapses, and previously diagnosed late effects
2. All treatments received for cancer, including
   a. Chemotherapy: type, route, schedule of administration, and total cumulative doses
   b. Radiation history, including type of field, total dose, and number of fractions
   c. All surgical procedures, including amputation, resection, central access line, and temporary interventions (e.g., gastrostomy)
   d. History of blood transfusions and or blood products
   e. Complication of treatment

SURVEILLANCE FOR RECURRENCE, METASTASIS, AND SECOND PRIMARY NEOPLASM

The most terrifying late effect is the possibility of recurrence of the primary tumor or the late development of a metastatic lesion. Generally, the oncologist should follow the patient until the likelihood of metastasis, relapse, or recurrence has passed. However, this is not always the case; in fact, the community physician may very well be called on to do disease surveillance during the time of high likelihood of relapse or recurrence. Surveillance during this time should continue with the same testing or diagnostic tools previously used by the oncologist to follow the disease.

Minimally in follow-up, all long-term survivors of childhood cancer who have had chemotherapy should have a yearly hemogram (complete blood count, including differential and platelet count); renal, hepatic, and metabolic profiles; and a urinalysis. For patients with a history of lymphoma, the practitioner providing surveillance should continue previously established methods of investigation for possible recurrence within the first 5 years from diagnosis. These include computed tomography, magnetic resonance imaging, positron emission tomography (currently approved for lymphomas and melanoma), or plain films. Surveillance in patients with a history of a solid tumor should include a chest x-ray to identify metastatic disease (particularly with the sarcomas). For leukemia patients, bone marrow aspiration and lumbar punctures are not generally indicated for routine surveillance unless there are symptoms of a relapse. Patients who had tumors with markers should continue to have blood drawn to test for those markers (e.g., human chorionic gonadotropin, carcinoembryonic antigen 125, erythrocyte sedimentation rate, etc.) Radiographic examination of previously radiated sites should be obtained at 2- to 3-year intervals to identify changes and detect early evidence of any second radiation-induced malignancy.

In September 2003 the Children's Oncology Group's (COG) task force for the development of Long-Term Follow-up Guidelines published its results, which are readily available from COG and on its website at http://www.childrensoncologygroup.org/disc/LE/default.htm. These guidelines should be utilized by the community provider caring for a survivor of childhood cancer when the patient's long-term follow-up care is not provided in a clinic dedicated to such surveillance.

SURVEILLANCE FOR SPECIFIC LATE EFFECTS RELATED TO TREATMENT MODALITIES

Surgery

Most of the surgical late effects are obvious; a missing limb or (known) missing organ. The practitioner should be alert to changes within the surgical site or scar that may require revision or biopsy. The practitioner may also be called on to write a prescription for a prosthesis, assist the patient in acquiring disability documentation and a handicap parking permit, provide a letter to excuse the patient from military service, or initiate an occupational intervention for special needs or other equally obvious physical needs. Prior surgical intervention may also be responsible for surgical menopause, sterility, blindness, hypothyroidism, cognitive impairment, and so on. Secondary problems related to surgical intervention (e.g., oophorectomy and premature menopause) include bone loss, osteopenia and osteoporosis, and loss of fertility.

Patients who have had a splenectomy or spleen ablative therapy should be placed on a prophylactic antibiotic, usually penicillin or erythromycin. They should receive prompt medical attention and antibiotics for suspected bacterial febrile illnesses. Pneumococcal vaccine to prevent pneumococcal pneumonia should be given routinely. The generally accepted immunizations schedule for pneumococcal vaccine is every 5 years. Patients who have no functioning spleen should also be vaccinated against hepatitis B and flu and should also receive other routine vaccinations. Finally, patients without functioning spleens should be protected from animal and mosquito bites and should wear a medical alert bracelet identifying them as "asplenic" (10).

Chemotherapy

Chemotherapy does not distinguish between cancer and noncancer cells. Generally it damages the most rapidly dividing cells (e.g., skin, gut, and mucous membranes). Long-term and late effects of chemotherapy include damage to the heart, liver, kidneys, lungs, and bone marrow.

Heart

It is widely known that anthracyclines may damage the heart. In view of this, some oncologists administer these drugs over a longer infusion period and limit the total cumulative dose (1,12). In children, cardiotoxicity increases rapidly at a cumulative dose in excess of 450 mg/m^2, but certain individual patients, exquisitely sensitive to this drug, may develop cardiotoxicity at a lower dose. Increased risk factors for anthracycline cardiotoxicity includes younger age (less than 5 years), larger dose, short infusion period, and possibly malnutrition or undernutrition with altered body habitus for age (11,12). Coadministration of other cardiotoxic drugs (e.g., cyclophosphamide or ifosfamide) may also be a factor. Pericardial radiation may also injure the heart.

The cardiotoxic effect may become apparent only in later years. Patients who are at risk of developing cardiac toxicity should be monitored yearly for heart problems, preferably with an echocardiogram. Plain chest films and electrocardiograms are also useful. Initially, patients, particularly females, may appear asymptomatic, but they can decompensate rapidly when the body is under stress, as in pregnancy. These patients should be instructed to inform the gynecologist that they may be at risk of developing complications during pregnancy. They should be monitored throughout the pregnancy and the postpartum period for cardiac decompensation. Generally a knowledgeable obstetrician is recommended for such patients.

Rigorous exercise and exercise programs that involve lifting heavy weights should be avoided. Otherwise, physical activity need not be limited unless symptoms are present or there is a decrease in the ejection fraction greater than 10% from baseline. A cardiologist experienced in cardiomyopathy related to anthracylines should be consulted for symptomatology suggestive of heart failure or a significant change in the ejection fraction (11,12).

Liver

Many chemotherapeutic agents can also place the survivor at risk of hepatic damage—specifically but not limited to methotrexate, 6 mercaptopurine, and busulfan. Concomitant oncologic therapy with administration of hepatotoxic drugs should be avoided or used minimally if possible. Yearly liver function tests and liver biopsies, if indicated, are necessary to assess the integrity of the liver. Because of blood product administration, cancer patients are also at risk for hepatitis C infection; at some point, therefore, posttreatment testing should be done. These patients should also be immunized for hepatitis B infection. Alcohol and large doses of acetaminophen should be avoided.

Lungs

Busulfan produces diffuse pulmonary fibrosis. A chest x-ray will reveal diffuse interstitial and intraalveolar infiltrates. These may appear at any time after treatment. This sequelum is associated with progressive deterioration in lung function, commonly called a "busulfan lung," it but may also be seen with cyclophosphamide.

Bleomycin may also damage lung tissue. The first indication of lung damage is inspiratory rales, followed by a decrease in oxygen diffusion capacity. Pulmonary function studies will reveal a diffuse interstitial fibrosis, restrictive pulmonary disease, and arterial hypoxemia. A chest x-ray will show a pattern of diffuse interstitial fibrosis with patchy basilar infiltrates. A lung biopsy will show an atypical alveolar cell and fibrinous exudate. A hilar membrane may be present during the acute stage. In the chronic stage, there is diffuse interstitial and intraalveolar fibrosis (11).

Gonads

Many chemotherapeutic drugs have the potential to cause gonadal failure or impairment. The aklylating agents, particularly cyclophosphamide and ifosfamide, can cause damage to the testes, resulting in sterility or lack of production of testosterone. The risk is greater in the pubescent male. There may also be damage to the ovaries in the pubescent female. This may result in infertility, lack of estrogen, and premature menopause. Patients who received cyclophosphamide or ifosfamide should be evaluated for gonadal failure, loss of testosterone or estrogen, and infertility. This may manifest itself as delayed puberty, amennorhea, absence of secondary sexual characteristics, and growth retardation in addition to infertility. Levels of follicle-stimulating hormone, luteinizing hormone, and insulin-like growth factor should be determined, semen analysis performed, and a testosterone or estrogen level obtained. In addition, the left wrist should be measured to determine bone age. If the ovaries or testes are damaged due to

lack of estrogen or testosterone, there will be impairment of the osteoblastic and osteoclastic processes in addition to infertility. Careful screening to assess osteopenia or osteoporosis may be required (11,13,14). If there is an indication of gonadal insufficiency, hormone replacement should be instituted. The community practitioner may consult an endocrinologist in managing hormone replacement.

Although cyclophosphamide and ifosfamide may result in infertility, it is never advisable to inform the long-term survivor that infertility is "absolute," since conception may occasionally still occur (13). A referral to a fertility expert is always indicated if pregnancy is desired. Several conceptions achieved by "infertile" long-term survivors, both male and female, have been reported. Contraception should always be encouraged when a pregnancy is not a desired outcome of intercourse. Brain radiation that affects the pituitary gland can also cause gonadal failure.

Kidney

Cisplatin is extremely toxic to the kidneys and may cause lifelong renal insufficiency or frank failure. Assessment of renal function should be routine in patients who have received cisplatin. (It may also cause hearing impairment.)

An outline of several frequently utilized chemotherapeutic agents and their related side effects is presented in Table 42-1. The list is not exhaustive but covers the more common important side effects as well as recommendations for investigation and guidance.

▓▓▓▓ Radiation

The younger the patient when the radiation is administered, the greater the damage (14).

Head and Neck

Radiation to the head and neck will cause growth retardation of the involved area. If radiation is administered to the eyes, the bitemporal diameter will be reduced. Radiation administered to the brain may result in a small head. If the pituitary is involved, it may cause absent or delayed sexual maturity, thyroid insufficiency, hypopituitary dwarfism, and diabetes insipidus. These patients preferably should be managed with the assistance of an endocrinologist.

With nasopharngeal radiation there may be extensive damage to the teeth, mandible and maxillary ridge, sinus cavities, and structures of the mouth and nasopharynx. Vision and hearing may also be affected. Dental radiation predisposes the patient to caries, abnormal

TABLE 42-1 | CHEMOTHERAPY FOR LATE EFFECTS

Chemotherapy Drug	Target Organ	Testing	Instruction to Patient
Actinomycin D	Liver	Chemistry profile, LFT	
Doxorubicin	Heart	Echocardiogram, ECG, CXR, cardiology consult if heart function is abnormal	Consult high-risk obstetrician for pregnancy
Daunomycin			Obtain medical clearance prior to beginning a weight-lifting program or a strenuous exercise program.
Idarubicin			Provide information on cumulative anthracycline dose prior to any surgery or during pregnancy.
Cisplatin	Kidneys	Chemistry profile, electrolytes, urinalysis	Check auditory and kidney function.
Carboplatin	Hearing	Audiogram	Patient may need hearing aid.
	Urinary bladder	Chemistry profile, electrolytes, urinalysis	Kidney function may be vulnerable.
Cyclophosphamide	Urinary bladder		
Ifosfamide	Kidneys		
	Ovaries	Pelvic exam (female) FSH, LH, estradiol	Infertility may be a problem, especially if patient is male.
	Testes	Sperm count FSH, LH, testosterone If gonadal failure, bone-density scan	
Dacarbazine	Liver	Chemistry profile, LFT	
L-Asparaginase	Liver (rare)	Chemistry profile, LFT	
Peg-asparaginase	Pancreas (rare)		
Methotrexate	Liver	Chemistry profile, LFT	
Nitrogen mustard	Ovaries	Pelvic exam (female), FSH, LH, estradiol, sperm count FSH, LF, testosterone	Infertility may be a problem, especially if patient is male.
	Testes	If gonadal failure, bone-density scan	Patient may need hormone replacement.
Procarbazine	Liver	Chemistry profile, electrolytes, urinalysis, monitor blood pressure regularly	Infertility may be a problem, especially if patient is male
	Kidneys		Patient may need hormone replacement.
	Ovaries	Pelvic exam (female) LH, FSH, estradiol	
	Testes	Sperm count, FSH, LF, testosterone If gonadal failure, bone-density scan	
6-Mercaptopurine	Liver	Chemistry profile, LFT	
6-Thioguanine			
Vincristine	Liver	Chemistry profile, LFT	
Velban/VP-16	Bone marrow	Hemagram	
Intrathecal chemotherapy	Cognitive impairment	MRI of brain, neuropsychological testing	Cognitive remediation

CXR = chest x-ray; ECG = electrocardiogram; FSH = follicle-stimulating hormone; LFT = liver function test; LH = luteinizing hormone; MRI = magnetic resonance imaging.

tooth growth, and destruction of the hard and soft palates. Dry eyes and skin damage may also occur. Sinus infections may be a major problem. Care must be taken with all dental procedures: hyperbaric oxygen pre- and post-treatment may be required.

Radiation involving the neck affects the thyroid. Careful attention must be paid to the thyroid gland throughout the lifespan looking for a secondary cancer and for hypo- or hyperthyroidism. Damage to the muscles and vascular structures of the neck may occur and patency of the carotid arteries may be affected.

Chest

Radiation to the chest may damage the heart, large vessels, and lung. Careful attention must be paid to lung function, cardiac output and electrical activity of the heart. An echocardiogram, electrocardiogram, and occasionally pulmonary function testing should be performed as follow-up for such patients.

Skin

The skin within the radiation field will be at higher risk of skin cancers and must be inspected carefully for malignant changes (11,14).

Back

Patients who have received radiation to the upper back may also experience damage to the involved area, lungs, and heart; the follow-up care should be the same as for chest radiation. The practitioner should examine adolescents and young adults who have been radiated for a unilateral Wilm's tumor and for scoliosis.

Abdomen and/or Pelvis

Radiation involving the abdomen or pelvis may damage organs within the radiation field. Secondary damage may occur from malfunctioning or nonfunctioning organs. If the ovaries are damaged, in addition to infertility, there will be impairment of the osteoblastic and osteoclastic processes because of the lack of estrogen. As described earlier, screening should be implemented for osteopenia or osteoporosis. Fibrosis of the genitourinary tract may occur. This may cause a hydronephrosis, small urinary bladder, and frank kidney damage. If the radiation port involved the femoral arteries, stenosis may develop. Radionecrosis of the femoral head and neck may also occur. Patients treated with prior radiation to the spleen must be treated similarly to those who have undergone surgical splenectomy.

Extremity

Radiation to extremities may result in deformity and growth retardation of the affected limb. All structures, including skin, in the radiation field will be affected. Follow-up care must address skin changes as well as risk of secondary bone or soft tissue cancers.

■ SUMMARY

Providing surveillance of the sequelae of disease and treatment to the survivor of childhood cancer is a complicated process optimally performed at a comprehensive cancer center by health care providers well versed in follow-up surveillance. If the community physician provides the follow-up care, either episodic or continuing, there must be a basic understanding of the natural history of the cancer and treatment. Knowledge of the late effects of the disease and the treatments will also help provide psychosocial support to the patient.

References

1. Ries LA, Percy CL, Berin GR. Introduction. In: Ries L, Smith M, Gurrey JA, et al (eds). *Cancer Incidence and Survival among Children and Adolescents: United States SEER Program, 1975–1995.* SEER pediatric monograph, NIH publication no. 99-4649. Bethesda, MD: National Cancer Institute; 1999:1–5.
2. Ries LA. In: Harris A, Edwards BK, Blot WJ, et al (eds). *Cancer Rates and Risks.* Bethesda, MD: National Cancer Institute; 1996:9–54.
3. Meadows AT, Krejmas NL, and Belasco JB. The medical costs of cure: Sequelae in survivors of childhood cancer. In: van Eys J, Sullivan MP (eds). *Status of Curability of Childhood Cancer.* New York: Raven Press; 1980.
4. Bleyer WA. The impact of childhood cancer on the United States and the world. *CA Cancer J Clin* 1990;40:355.
5. Jaffe N. Late side effects of treatment. *Pediatr Clin North Am* 1976;23:233–244.
6. Kadan-Lottick NS, Robison LL, Gurney GA, et al. Childhood cancer survivors knowledge about their past diagnosis and treatment. *JAMA* 2002;287:1832–1839.
7. Dreyer Z, Blatt J, Bleyer A. Late effects of childhood cancer and its treatment. In: Pizzo PA, Poplack DG (eds). *Principles and Practice of Pediatric Oncology,* 4th ed. Philadelphia: Lippincott, Williams & Wilkins; 2002:1431–1461.
8. Plon SE, Malkin D. Childhood cancer and heredity. In: Pizzo PA, Poplack DG (eds). *Principles and Practice of Pediatric Oncology,* 4th ed. Philadelphia: Lippincott, Williams & Wilkins; 2002:21–44.
9. Smith MA, Gloeckler LA. Childhood cancer: Incidence, survival, and mortality. In: Pizzo PA, Poplack DG (eds). *Principles and Practice of Pediatric Oncology,* 4th ed. Philadelphia: Lippincott, Williams & Wilkins; 2002:1–12.
10. American Academy of Pediatrics. Immunizations in special clinical circumstances. In: Pickering LK (ed). *2002 Red Book: Report of the Committee on Infectious Disease,* 25th ed. Elk Grove Village, IL: American Academy of Pediatrics; 2000: 56–68.
11. Von Hoff DD, Layard MW, Basa P, et al. Risk factors for doxorubicin-induced congestive heart failure. *Ann Intern Med* 1979;91:710–717.
12. Berrak S, Ewer MS, Jaffe N, et al. *Oncol Rep* 2001;8:611–614.
13. Sherins RS, DeVita VT, Effeil J. Effect of drug treatment for lymphoma on male reproductive capacity. Studies of men in remission after therapy. *Ann Intern Med* 1973;79:216–220.
14. Jaffe N. Late sequelae of cancer and cancer therapy. In: Fennbach DJ, Vietta TJ (eds). *Clinical Pediatric Oncology,* 4th ed. Boston: Mosby–Year Book; 1991.

Internet References

Adult survivors of childhood cancers. NCI The national investment in cancer research for fiscal year 2004. http://plan.cancer.gov/adult.htm

Center for Young Women's Health. Children's Hospital Boston. Premature Ovarian Failure: A Guide for Teens. Web page located at http://www.youngwomenshealth.org/pof.html

Childhood Cancer Survivor Long-Term Follow-Up Guidelines, Ver 1.1, Children's Oncology Group. Web page located at http://www.childrensoncologygroup.org/disc/LE/default.htm

Follow-up clinic for childhood cancer survivors. 2/03. http://patientcenters.com/press/clinics_2003.html

Keene N, Oeffinger K. Late Effects to the Heart: Parts I and II, Candlelighters Newsletter, Fall 2000. http://www.acor.org/disease/ped-onc/survivors/cardio/anthracyclines

Late effects from childhood cancer. ACS 4/7/2000. http://www.cancer.org/docroot/NWS/content/NWS_1_1x_Late_effects_of_Childhood_Cancer.asp

Late effects of childhood cancer. Cancer reference information. ACS 2003. http://www.cancer.org/docroot/CRI/content_2_6x_Late_effects_of_Childhood_Cancer.asp

Long-term follow-up study. University of Minnesota Cancer Center. http://www.cancer.umn.edu/ltfu

Monteleone PM, Meadows AT. Late effects of childhood cancer and treatment. DMed.com, Inc. 2003. emedicine.com/ped/topic2591.htm#section~introduction.

Outlook: Life Beyond Childhood Cancer. Web page located at http://www.outlook-life.org/index.pl?id+2002&isa+Iten&op

SEER (Surveillance, Epidemiology and End Result) at http://www.seer.cancer.gov/publications/childhood/Splenectomy fact sheet. Great Ormond Street Hospital for Children NHS.London, 2002.

ADULT LONG-TERM FOLLOW-UP

Pamela N. Schultz
Rena Vassilopoulou-Sellin

■ CANCER SURVIVOR PREVALENCE AND/OR INCIDENCE

The population of cancer survivors, which numbered 8.9 million in 1997 (1), continues to grow as "baby boomers" reach a cancer-prone age (increasing the annual incidence of new cases) and as cancer patients survive longer (increasing the prevalence of cancer survivors).

■ LITERATURE REVIEW

According to the National Institute of Health's Surveillance, Epidemiology, and End Results (SEER) *Cancer Statistics 1975–2001,* there has been an increase in 5-year relative survival rates; in 1954 the survival rate for all cancer sites was 35%, but by 2000 this figure had increased to 65.5% (2). Obviously survival rates are dependent on cancer site. Table 43-1 illustrates how cancer incidence by site does not correlate with 5-year relative survival rate.

LATE EFFECTS OF CANCER

Efforts are increasingly directed toward understanding the long-term impact of cancer and cancer therapy, es-

pecially as they might affect the quality of life of cancer survivors. There is a robust collection of literature addressing the psychosocial late effects of cancer in survivors of childhood and adult cancers. However information regarding the lasting medical late effects of cancer and cancer therapy remains limited.

Several investigators have addressed the presence and complexity of lasting medical effects of cancer throughout the adult lives of childhood cancer survivors (3–5). Stevens et al. (6) reported that 58% of survivors had at least one chronic health problem and 32% had two or more, including second primary cancers. Much less is known about the lasting medical impact of cancer treatment in survivors of adult-onset cancers. Investigators addressing the physiologic late effects of adult cancers (7,8) highlight the paucity of information but emphasize that they are aware that multiple systems are often affected. For example, pelvic surgery can impair fertility, and splenectomy increases susceptibility to bacterial infections. Certain chemotherapy agents and regimens can compromise the health of the cardiac, pulmonary, genitourinary, endocrine, and neurologic systems. Radiotherapy may potentiate these complications and also impair skeletal development and dental health in addition to contributing to the risk of second primary cancers. Com-

TABLE 43-1	INCIDENCE AND 5-YEAR SURVIVAL RATE BY SPECIFIC CANCER SITE	
Cancer Site	*Incidence per 100,000 U.S. Population*	*Survival (%)*
Hodgkin's lymphoma	2.7	85.2
Testis	2.6	95.9
Cervix	4.8	72.7
Lymphocytic leukemia	5.5	70.4
Brain	6.0	30.3
Oral cavity and pharynx	10.7	58.7
Exocrine pancreas	11	4.4
Kidney	11.3	63.9
Non-Hodgkin's lymphoma	2.7	85.2
Colorectal	53.7	63.4
Lung	61.7	15.2
Breast	73.9	87.6
Prostate	75	99.3

bined treatments can increase the number and severity of medical late effects.

Recently attention has been directed toward the impact of cancer treatment on long-term survivors, particularly as it concerns quality of life. Several investigators have begun to characterize the physiologic and psychosocial health profiles of survivors of childhood cancers and the psychosocial profiles of survivors of adult cancers. However, there remains a stark paucity of data regarding the physiologic health profile of survivors of adult cancers.

DEFINITION OF *SURVIVOR*

Further complicating the understanding of the impact of cancer treatment on long-term survivors is how one defines the term *survivor*. Survivors groups have emphasized that one who is diagnosed with cancer is a "survivor" from the onset of the diagnosis. How does one differentiate the cancer survivor being treated for active disease from the survivor who has been treated and is free of disease? Traditionally, one's 5-year anniversary after a diagnosis of cancer has been designated an important milestone in survival.

■ "LIFE AFTER CANCER CARE" PROGRAM

Cancer survivors have unique health needs; however, their antecedent malignancy and/or the often intensive

treatments required to achieve cure may affect their long-term health status. At M.D. Anderson Cancer Center (MDACC), we have developed the Life after Cancer Care (LACC) program, which focuses on the health of cancer survivors. The LACC clinic was established to give long-term cancer survivors the opportunity to have follow-up medical care targeting diagnosis, appropriate referral and consultation, and treatment of possible long-term effects of previously treated disease. After successful cancer treatment, survivors would inevitably experience other medical conditions that were going untreated or inadequately treated because of the uncertainty of the origin or etiology of subsequent medical conditions. Primary care providers have been reluctant to treat such patients because of concerns about how distant cancer treatment might have affected new medical conditions.

■ TEN THOUSAND CANCER SURVIVORS

Recently there has been increased interest in understanding the long-term effects of cancer and cancer therapy, especially as they may affect the quality of life of cancer survivors. However, information regarding the lasting late effects of cancer and cancer therapy in long-term adult cancer survivors remains limited. Because of this lack of information, the LACC program began a systematic search for living cancer survivors who had been treated at MDACC. The inclusion criteria were that they had been diagnosed with cancer, were at least 5 years from their cancer diagnosis, were 18 years or older at diagnosis, had a U.S. address, and at their last contact were free of malignant disease. Surveys were developed to systematically collect health information from such survivors, and the resulting questionnaires were sent out to over 20,000 individuals who met the above criteria. Simultaneously, the survey was made available through the Internet at www.mdanderson.org/Departments/LACC.

Preliminary analyses were initiated after the receipt of the first 6000 entries, 5209 of which included complete information. These responders included 3344 women (64.2%) and 1865 men (35.8%). The response rates were evaluable for the mailed surveys and were reassuringly robust independent of gender (50.8% for women and 50.9% for men) but are possibly underestimated (we could not confirm, for example, that all mailed surveys were received). Cancer survivors therefore appear willing to provide information about their health. Almost one-third of the survivors also provided additional contact information (addresses, telephone numbers), and often voluminous unsolicited comments about their cancer, their health, and their opinions. Additional contact information can be used to update or provide additional information for those willing to participate in that manner.

Data from more than 10,000 survivors are now available for analysis. Complete data are available on 8739 survivors who meet the criteria outlined above. Of the entire sample, 62% are female and 92% are white. The distribution by age at diagnosis is illustrated in Fig. 43-1 and the mean ± standard deviation (SD) of age at diagnosis was 47.9 ± 14.2 years.

Fifty percent of the survivors were diagnosed between the ages of 18 and 48 years and 25% were diagnosed after the age of 59 years. Male survivors were significantly older at diagnosis than female survivors (50.6 ± 15.1 versus 46.3 ± 13.3 years, $p < 0.00001$), and Hispanic survivors were significantly younger at diagnosis than white and black survivors (42.9 ± 14.3 versus 48.2 ± 14.1 and 46.9 ± 14.2 years, $p = 0.00002$).

Approximately 25% of the survivors in our database have lived more than 20 years since their original diagnosis. Fig. 43-2 shows the distribution of survivors by time from diagnosis. Ten percent of survivors are at least 30 years from diagnosis.

Breast cancer patients are the most common long-term survivors in our database (1987, or 23%). Figure 43-3 illustrates the distribution of survivors by cancer type.

The gender distribution of cancers—other than breast, gynecologic, prostate, or testicular—is illustrated in Fig.

43-4. This figure illustrates that long-term survivors have similar representation in our database as in the incidence patterns by cancer type.

For instance, the incidence of thyroid cancer is predominantly female and cancer of the head and neck is predominantly male; this is congruent with our database of long-term survivors. Naturally, the distribution of the diagnoses reflects the likelihood of long-term survival with different cancers and patterns that may be unique to MDACC referral.

AGE AT DIAGNOSIS AND HEALTH EFFECTS

Survivors were asked to respond to the question "Has cancer affected your overall health?" Interestingly, only 37.4% replied yes to that question, and there were no gender or ethnic differences in their replies. Previously we had reported gender differences in a smaller cohort of survivors (5836) (10). In the larger cohort, univariate analysis indicated that age at diagnosis accounted for the gender variance: females tended to be younger at diagnosis and those who reported that cancer affected their overall health were younger at diagnosis than those who did not report health effects (Fig. 43-5). However when the response to that question was analyzed according to cancer type, it was clear that cancer type affected the survivors' responses. Likewise, those survivors who were most likely to report health effects tended to be younger at diagnosis. Table 43-2 illustrates those findings.

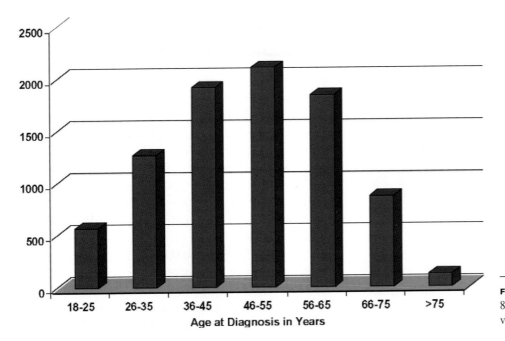

FIGURE 43-1 Age at diagnosis in 8739 adult long-term cancer survivors.

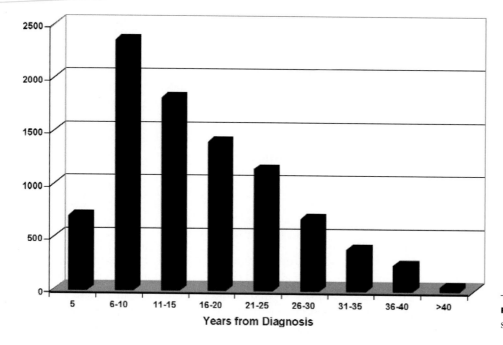

FIGURE 43-2 Distribution of cancer survivors by years from diagnosis.

Age at diagnosis seems to be an extremely good predictor of how the survivor experiences long-term survival. When the survivors are grouped according to age at diagnosis, there is the tendency for the survivor to attribute fewer overall health effects from the cancer as they age. Of survivors diagnosed between 18 and 40 years of age, 41% report overall health effects from cancer; of those diagnosed between 41 and 65 years of age, 36% reported overall health effects; and of those diagnosed after 65 years of age, 28% reported overall health effects. Perhaps health effects in the older person

were less likely to be attributable to cancer effects. It is obvious that aging would have a considerable impact of an individual's perception of his or her health, and this would possibly allow the sequelae of a distant diagnosis and treatment for cancer to be overlooked.

Previously we have reported that specific health effects reported by long-term cancer survivors illustrate a complex interplay between age, gender, cancer type, and cancer treatment as well as ethnicity, race, and social and cultural factors (9–11,27). For instance the most frequently reported health effect was arthritis/osteoporosis (1541 survivors, or 26.4%).

Gender was an important variable, as men generally reported fewer specific problems; the most frequently mentioned were heart problems (17.2% of responding men), hearing loss (14.9%), and arthritis/osteoporosis (15.5%). Women generally reported more specific problems; the most frequently mentioned were arthritis/osteoporosis (32.9% of responding women), heart problems (13.9%), and thyroid problems (12.1%). There was a gender difference in the likelihood of reporting any of the specific health problems; for example, women were more likely to report thyroid problems (12.1% versus 6.2%, $p < 0.00001$) or arthritis/osteoporosis (32.9% versus 15.5, $p < 0.00001$). Men, on the other hand, were more likely to report kidney/bladder problems (14.2% versus 9.8%, $p < 0.00001$) or hearing loss (14.9% versus 9.9%, $p < 0.00001$). These patterns likely reflect a complex interaction of gender-related cancer diagnoses and comorbidities.

Arthritis/osteoporosis and heart problems were among the most frequently mentioned health problems. The

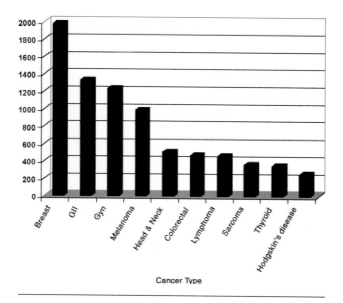

FIGURE 43-3 Distribution of cancer survivors by the 10 most frequent cancer types within the sample of adult survivors.

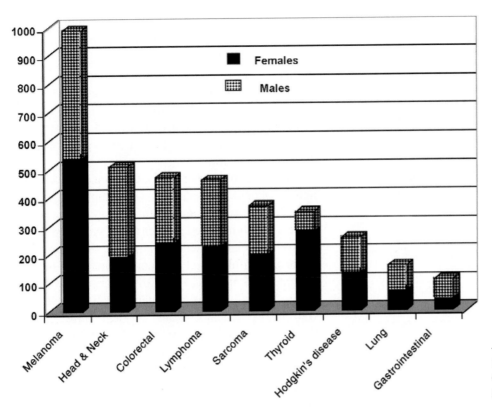

FIGURE 43-4 Distribution of cancer survivors by cancer types and gender.

pattern of perceived and reported health problems was different among the cancer types. For example, survivors of Hodgkin's disease prominently reported thyroid and lung problems (33.8% of responders with the diagnosis), while a prior diagnosis of lymphoma was associated with frequent mentions of memory loss (14.7%).

NATIONAL HEALTH INTERVIEW SURVEY

A large number of health conditions are reported by the National Health Interview Survey and categorized by age, ethnicity/race, and gender (11a). Five of these health conditions were comparable with health conditions reported by our cancer survivor cohort: arthritis symp-

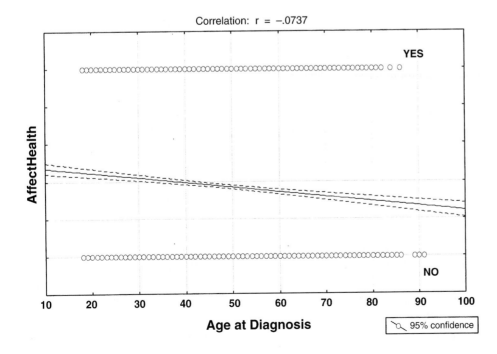

FIGURE 43-5 Inverse correlation between age at diagnosis and self-reported health effects.

TABLE 43-2	PERCENTAGE OF SURVIVORS WHO RESPONDED "YES" TO "HAS CANCER AFFECTED YOUR HEALTH?"	
Cancer Type	**Affected Health**	**Mean Age at Diagnosis in Years**
Melanoma	16.7	43.4
Colorectal	31.3	50.2
Gynecologic	31.4	44.5
Breast	35.9	46.5
Genitourinary	36.4	55.5
Sarcoma	39.5	40.5
Head and neck	39.8	50.8
Acute leukemia	45.3	39.8
Thyroid	50.3	35.4
Lung	53.3	55.9
Lymphoma	56.9	46.3
Gastrointestinal	57.0	56.0
Chronic leukemia	60.2	49.3
Hodgkin's disease	61.7	30.3

toms, diabetes, migraine or severe headaches, heart disease, and hearing loss. The frequencies of these conditions in the general population (computed as affected individuals per 1000 people) were compared with their frequencies in our cancer survivor cohort relative to patient age, ethnicity/race, and gender. There were significant differences in the frequencies of the five health conditions between men and women and among ethnic/racial groups. The most common difference in our cancer survivor cohort for all groups analyzed was a statistically significant loss of hearing. Hispanic-American women had significantly more reports of diabetes and African-American men had significantly more reports of heart disease than the race-adjusted national prevalence rates. Whereas apparent differences in the frequency of these health conditions may be the result of the methodology of the questionnaires, prior cancer or cancer therapy may also play a role in the survivors' health profile. For example, the consistent overreporting of hearing loss may be related to ototoxic chemotherapy. Clearly, further detailed analysis is needed in this area. Further research about health comorbidities may provide information about health effects from a past cancer diagnosis.

The importance of the uniqueness of the cancer type was made obvious in two studies from our survey cohort of thyroid cancer survivors and breast cancer survivors. We previously published the thyroid cohort and noted several distinctions (9). Thyroid cancer survivors tended to be significantly younger at diagnosis, were significantly closer to their diagnosis, were significantly more likely to be women, and reported significantly more spe-

cific health effects. However we were impressed by the frequent complaints of symptoms that were reminiscent of thyroid hormone imbalance, and we described these effects as "thyroid dysregulation." Most of the patients in the thyroid cohort usually survive for many years. However, we found that lifetime supplementation of thyroid hormone carried unique problems that compromised the patients' perception of their overall health.

Likewise in another study, 291 breast cancer patients (not randomly selected) who completed the original survivor survey agreed to participate in another survey, which included queries about symptoms commonly associated with menopause, including hot flushes, painful sexual intercourse, inability to concentrate, fatigue, and sleep disturbance. Two other items, which pertained to quality of life (QOL) but were not specifically related to menopause, queried the participants about unhappiness and lymphedema (29). Forty-six percent of these breast cancer survivors indicated that breast cancer had affected their overall health. The number of survivors reporting this was highest among those who had received chemotherapy alone or in combination with radiotherapy. In addition, there were 19 self-reported specific health conditions analyzed by treatment. We thought that increased menopausal symptoms caused by breast cancer might account for the difference in the survivors' QOL compared with that of women in the general population. However, we encountered a problem in differentiating between naturally occurring menopausal symptoms and other physical health problems that affect QOL. In our sample, hot flushes and painful sexual intercourse were obviously related to menopause. Because of the close relationship between these symptoms and the ability to concentrate, fatigue, sleep problems, and general unhappiness, it is difficult to determine whether these represent normal menopausal symptoms or long-term sequelae of cancer treatment. No one would argue that long-term effects of cancer treatment might include cognitive impairment, sleep disturbances, and general unhappiness; however, these conditions are also characteristic of normal menopause, whether or not the patient experiences breast cancer. The relationship among menopausal symptoms, QOL and health effects of cancer treatment is complex. Our study has shown that QOL parameters need to be rigidly defined and that they are time-sensitive or, more specifically, age-specific. There is indication that there are complex interactions between QOL indicators and specific physiologic consequences of treatment. It is important for menopausal symptoms to be understood within the context of the breast cancer survival and not lost among the QOL/psychosocial issues faced by the cancer survivor. This study reminds us that breast cancer and menopause are independent issues. Further study is necessary to understand these complicated interactions and how to better integrate the issues of aging, long-term cancer survival, and QOL as they relate to the consequences of cancer treatment.

These findings emphasize that cancer survivors should not be lumped into one cohort and that generalizations should not be made about their cancer experience. Cancer type is a major determinant of survival potential. If we are to understand how cancer affects long-term survivors, we should develop studies in which cancer type is matched. Thyroid and breast cancer survivors have unique problems as a result of cancer treatment. Some health effects are clearly related to their cancer, but others are not so clear. Is the fatigue and cognitive impairment a result of too little thyroid hormone replacement, a consequence of normal menopause, or due to their cancer treatment? These questions need further clarification.

ETHNIC AND RACIAL INFLUENCES ON CANCER SURVIVORSHIP

We have previously reported (11) that ethnicity did not appear to be a factor in the self-reporting of health effects overall. However, caution should be exercised, in that ethnic minorities are markedly underrepresented in our database of survivors. In the larger cohort, Asians and Native Americans make up <1% of the survivors, but 48 and 56%, respectively, reported that cancer had affected their overall health.

Previously we have reported that there were significant differences among Caucasians, Hispanics, and blacks in the types of specific health effects they experienced as long-term survivors of cancer (11). We found significant ethnic/racial differences with respect to age at diagnosis, interval since diagnosis, marital status, educational level, insurability, regular medical care, and the effects on family relationships. Differences in health effects probably reflected not only ethnicity/race but also cancer type, gender, type of treatment, and disease stage, to name a few. There was a complex relationship between ethnicity/racial group, family and intimate relationships, and treatment types for survivors of cervical cancer.

Published literature specifically focusing on the impact of ethnic/racial factors in long-term cancer survivors (>5 years from diagnosis) is scarce at best. There are ethnic/racial differences in the incidence and

mortality of various cancers (1); these are generally considered to be due to disparities in access to health care and/or the inequities of health care for the poor, resulting in more advanced disease at the time of diagnosis (12); however, other intrinsic factors may also play a role.

It is generally accepted that ethnic/racial factors can (and do) contribute to important disparities in health care access and health outcomes (13–15). A study examining information from the National Survey of Functional Health, Ren et al. (16) reported that race and class discrimination were pervasive and adversely affected the health status of ethnic/racial minorities. Although studies addressing the impact of ethnic/racial differences on health generally relate to diagnosis and treatment-related outcomes (17–22), it is plausible that they may also influence other physiologic and psychosocial aspects of health. In examining the information provided by cancer survivors in our review, we found that, for the most part, cancer survivors had a similar view of the impact or lack thereof of their cancer experience on their physiologic health overall. There were, however, differences with respect to specific health items. For example, African Americans were more likely to report arthritis/osteoporosis than were Caucasian Americans or Hispanic Americans, whereas Hispanic Americans were more likely to report abdominal pain and diabetes mellitus. Such differences in health profile and patterns may be partially related to other ethnic/racial propensities, as demonstrated by Brooks et al. (17) in a study showing that the poor outcomes of African-American women with cervical cancer were associated with preexisting comorbidities. Care must be taken in interpreting these ethnic/racial differences, since race is largely a social and political construct (23).

Grenier and Lipschultz (24) found that African-American childhood cancer patients treated with anthracyclines might be at higher risk for cardiotoxicity; they suggested that this could be true also of adult cancer survivors. We also found a higher incidence of self-reported heart disease in African-American cancer survivors when compared with Caucasian American or Hispanic American cancer survivors. Whereas such differences may have a biological basis, socioeconomic parameters may also play a role. It is not clear how powerful one parameter is over the other in influencing these differences. For example, does education and family support have a greater impact on the health of cancer survivors than cancer type and treatment, or vice versa? Which of these factors is most influenced by ethnicity or race? Clearly, further research in socioeconomically diverse populations is needed.

Ren et al. (16) showed that education was another factor adversely affecting health in Hispanic Americans. Although we found some difference in education among the ethnic/racial groups, this factor did not appear to affect the cancer survivors' perceptions of their overall health except in the Hispanic-American survivor group. Overall, however, the groups were well educated; referral patterns at MDACC may have affected these results in our cohort of survivors.

It is generally thought that marital status is closely related to health conditions (25). Unmarried people tend to have higher mortality from all causes, they use more health services, they have more psychological distress, and their perceptions of their own general health are poorer compared with those of married people. In a study of marriage in survivors of childhood cancers, Rauck et al. (26) found that Caucasian Americans had the lowest divorce rates and that African Americans had the highest ones; Hispanic Americans fell in between. We found differences in health perception among the ethnic/racial groups according to marital status at the time of the survey. We did not consistently find a protective effect of marriage; however, our results suggest that there is a positive correlation between the perception of overall health and the perceived positive impact of the cancer experience on family relationships.

It is clear that socioeconomic, psychological, and cultural factors interact with the physiologic factors. To better understand these interactions, further research is needed with larger populations that are racially and ethnically diverse.

We reported previously that effects on physiologic health in survivors of cervical cancer appeared to be related to treatment rather than histologic type or ethnic/racial group (11). A consistent finding in analyzing the effect of cancer on family relationships was the differences among the ethnic/racial groups. Hispanic-American survivors were more likely to report that having cancer (especially cervical cancer) had improved their family relationships; clearly, the families of Hispanic-American cancer survivors are affected differently from African-American and Caucasian-American families.

It is clear that ethnicity and race influence the cancer survivor experience. In order to understand these differences, multiculturalism must be incorporated into cancer survivor research. Our present findings point to a significant impact of ethnic/racial influences in the health profiles of cancer survivors. However, non–Caucasian Americans constitute a small minority of the overall cohort. Accordingly, any observations and conclusions must be interpreted with caution and configured with additional research involving much larger populations.

WORK-RELATED ISSUES FOR CANCER SURVIVORS

We analyzed survey information from 4264 long-term survivors of cancer in which survivors were asked to respond to items describing their ability to work, their experience of job discrimination, and their QOL (27). Thirty-five percent of the respondents were working at the time of the survey; significantly more of these individuals were men rather than women and proportionately more were Hispanic Americans than white Americans or African Americans. According to the correlation coefficient ($r = -0.49, p < 0.05$), the younger the survivors were at the time of diagnosis, the more likely they were to be working. Univariate analysis indicated a significant effect of age and cancer type on whether or not the participant was working ($p = 0.0008$). For most cancer types, workers were significantly younger at diagnosis than individuals who were not working, and they had a significantly higher QOL score than those who were not working. Further correlations regarding the potential influence of other medical and social factors on employment are needed.

Of the survivors working at the time of the survey 7.3% indicated they had experienced job discrimination; this finding was independent of age, gender, and ethnic/racial group. One participant characterized the job discrimination as originating from coworkers' attitudes toward him as a cancer survivor, whereas another individual indicated that the job discrimination was more age-related than cancer-related. Two survivors described their job experiences in detail. One indicated that the employer in this instance was unsympathetic and resistant to adjusting job responsibilities to accommodate the employee's chronic fatigue. This employee had used all of his "sick time" and "vacation time" over an 8-year period while continuing to work. Another participant reported being suspended from the job on three separate occasions as a result of absences from work during treatment for cancer recurrences. This participant indicated that the employer expressed disbelief over the necessity of taking sick leave.

There were 371 (8.5%) participants who indicated that they were unable to work as a result of the effects of cancer, cancer treatment, or both. Significantly more women reported being unable to work than did men (9.2% versus 7.2%, $p = 0.02$), and significantly more African Americans reported being unable to work than did white Americans or Hispanic Americans (23.2, 9.7, and 4.3%, respectively). The role of socioeconomic factors in these findings is not clear. The mean age at diagnosis for this group of survivors was 46.3 ± 14.1 years, with a mean time from diagnosis of 19.6 ±

8.6 years. The cancer type did influence the survivors' ability to work. Survivors of melanoma were least likely to report inability to work (3.7%), whereas survivors of gastrointestinal cancers were most likely to be unable to work (20%).

Those who considered themselves unable to work were significantly older at diagnosis. Proportionately, more men were working than unable to work, and proportionately more African Americans were likely to be unable to work than to be working. The distribution of cancer types among those working and the unable-to-work was also different. Cancer types most associated with working status were genitourinary, melanoma, and Hodgkin's disease. Cancer types most associated with inability to work were gynecologic, lung, head and neck, gastrointestinal, and colon cancers. Cancer types that were similar proportionately in their association with the ability to work were breast, lymphoma, thyroid, sarcoma, and leukemia.

A reassuring finding is that most cancer survivors do not perceive employment-related problems. Most survivors assimilate back into the workforce with few cancer-related issues. However, for those who do have such issues, little is known about their experiences, because research data for this group is scanty and heterogeneous. Nevertheless, the physical and psychological impact of cancer as a life-threatening illness is widely accepted, but its impact on society, other than economic, is not well studied or understood. From these results, we know that cancer by type, age, gender, and possibly ethnic/racial group may interact to affect the survivor's ability to work.

INTERNET MESSAGE BOARD FOR CANCER SURVIVORS AND THEIR FAMILIES

As a component of LACC, a message board was created whereby cancer patients and their family members or other loved ones could communicate with and provide support for other patients and families. The message board was accessible to anyone who visited the MDACC web page. It was also monitored, and findings from the postings were used to further clarify the cancer experience and to facilitate support for cancer patients (28). During the initial 16 months of its creation, 972 individuals logged onto the message board (users) and 284 persons posted 619 messages (posters). The majority of the posters posted only one message (64%), 59 posted two messages (21%), and the rest posted multiple messages. Sixty percent of the posters had cancer and (40%) did not. Of those who did not have cancer, 22% identified themselves as spouses of a cancer patient, 69% as other family members, and 9% as non–

family members. The majority of the message posters were women (74%); the majority of the posters who identified themselves as cancer patients were also women (72%).

Messages were read and analyzed for content. The most common cancer types represented by the posted messages were breast cancer, gastrointestinal cancer, lung cancer, gynecologic cancer, head and neck cancer, and colon cancer. Forty-seven messages did not indicate a specific cancer type. The most frequent themes were questions about treatment, support, and long-term effects. The pattern of message themes differed between posters who had cancer and those who were posting a message for another person with cancer. For example, whereas the most frequent queries for all posters were about treatment, such queries more frequently came from those without cancer. Of interest, posters posed questions about the long-term effects of cancer significantly more often than did those without cancer. Questions about support and diagnosis appeared to be of similar interest to both groups of posters.

Posters dealing with breast cancer were more likely to post messages about treatment than posters dealing with head and neck cancer. On the other hand, posters dealing with lung cancer were more likely to post messages about support than posters dealing with colon cancer. In general, treatment was the most prominent message theme.

Message board entries reflect yet another aspect of cancer survivors' experience. In general, literature pertaining to health care and the Internet highlights the significance of this resource. However few data are available about the types of information on which Internet users tend to concentrate. Such information would allow health care providers and educators to develop materials better suited to respond to the needs of consumers and patients.

The concept of using the Internet and message boards for data collection and research has not yet received a great deal of attention within the health care arena. We suggest that continued, systematic analysis of website traffic, message content, and utilization patterns may prove promising in clarifying the interests and information needs of patients and their families.

■ CANCER SURVIVORSHIP AND THE FUTURE

The successfully treated cancer patient has much to teach us. Traditionally cancer research has focused on the diagnosis and treatment of cancer, and appropriately so. We have studied those who have not responded to treatment seeking answers in order to develop better treatments. We should, in our quest to eradicate cancer, look not only to those patients who have succumbed to the disease but also to those who have survived. They provide a living laboratory for the understanding of cancer. We have only scratched the surface in understanding how the survivor of cancer has arrived at long-term survivorship. We have accumulated over 10,000 individual cancer survivors' responses to a survey designed to shed some understanding of the cancer survivors' long-term sequelae of cancer treatment. This survivorship project has raised many questions that need further research. This work requires longitudinal and prospective studies of large numbers of survivors. MDACC is poised through programs like LACC to lead the cancer survivorship initiative.

References

1. American Cancer Society. *Cancer Facts & Figures: SEER Cancer Statistics Review, 1973–1998.* Bethesda, MD: National Cancer Institute; 2002.

2. Ries LAG, Kosary CL, Hankey BF, et al (eds). *SEER Cancer Statistics Review, 1975–2001.* Bethesda, MD: National Cancer Institute; 2004. http://seer.cancer.gov/csr/1975_2001/, 2004.

3. Meadows AT, Hobbie WL. The medical consequences of cure. *Cancer* 1986;15(suppl 2):524–528.

4. Ried H, Zietz H, Jaffe N. Late effects of cancer treatment in children. *Pediatr Dent* 1995;17:273–284.

5. Marina N. Long-term survivors of childhood cancer. The medical consequences of cure. *Pediatr Clin North Am* 1997; 44:1021–1042.

6. Stevens MC, Mahler H, Parkes S. The health status of adult survivors of cancer in childhood. *Eur J Cancer* 1998;34:694–698.

7. Loescher LJ, Welch-McCaffrey D, Leigh SA, et al. Surviving adult cancers. Part 1: Physiologic effects. *Ann Intern Med* 1989;111:411–432.

8. Ganz PA. Late effects of cancer and its treatment. *Semin Oncol Nurs* 2001;17:241–248.

9. Schultz PN, Stava C, Vassilopoulou-Sellin R. Health profiles and quality of life of 518 survivors of thyroid cancer. *Head Neck* 2002;5:349–356.

10. Schultz PN, Beck ML, Stava C, Vassilopoulou-Sellin R. Health profiles in 5836 long-term cancer survivors. *Int J Cancer* 2003;104:488–495.

11. Schultz PN, Stava C, Beck ML, Vassilopoulou-Sellin R. Ethnic/racial influences on the physiologic health of cancer survivors. *Cancer* 2004;100:156–164.

11a. Blackwell DL, Collins JG, Coles R. Summary health statistics for U.S. adults: National Health Interview Survey, 1997. *Vital Health Stat 10* 2002;(205):1–109.

12. President's Cancer Panel. *Voices of a Broken System: Real People, Real Problems.* Bethesda, MD. National Cancer Institute, 2000–2001.

13. Ross H. Lifting the unequal burden of cancer on minorities and the underserved. Office of Minority Health. US Department of Health and Human Services. Closing the gap. August issue, 2000.

14. Shavers VL, Brown ML. Racial and ethnic disparities in the receipt of cancer treatment. *J Natl Cancer Inst* 2002;94:334–357.

15. Rodney P, Rodney ZK, Nu S, Hemans-Richards JE. Cervical cancer and black women: An analysis of the disparity in prevalence of cervical cancer. *J Health Care Poor Underserved* 2002;13:24–37.

16. Ren XS, Amick BC, Williams DR. Racial/ethnic disparities in health: The interplay between discrimination and socioeconomic status. *Ethnicity Dis* 1999;9:151–165.

17. Brooks SE, Baquet CR, Gardner JF, et al. Cervical cancer—The impact of clinical presentation, health and race on survival. *J Assoc Acad Minor Phys* 2000;11:55–59.

18. Flores-Luna L, Salazar-Martinez E, Escudero-De Los Rios P, et al. Prognostic factors related to cervical cancer survival in Mexican women. *Int J Gynaecol Obstet* 2001;75:33–42.

19. Grenier MA, Lipshultz SE. Epidemiology of anthracycline cardiotoxicity in children and adults. *Semin Oncol* 1998;24: 72–85.

20. Grigsby PW, Hall-Daniels L, Baker S, Perez CA. Comparison of clinical outcome in black and white women treated with radiotherapy for cervical carcinoma. *Gynecol Oncol* 2000;79:357–361.

21. Hamilton AS, Stanford JL, Gilliland FD, et al. Health outcomes after external-beam radiation therapy for clinically localized prostate cancer: Results from the Prostate Cancer Outcomes Study. *J Clin Oncol* 2001;19:2517–2526.

22. Potosky AL, Harlan LC, Stanford JL, et al. Prostate cancer practice patterns and quality of life: The Prostate Cancer Outcomes Study. *J Natl Cancer Inst* 1999;91:1719–1724.

23. Graves JL Jr. *The Emperor's New Clothes.* Piscataway, NJ: Rutgers University Press, 2001.

24. Grenier MA, Lipshultz SE. Epidemiology of anthracycline cardiotoxicity in children and adults. *Semin Oncol* 1998;24: 72–85.

25. Ren XS. Marital status and quality of relationships: The impact on health perception. *Soc Sci Med* 1997;44:241–249.

26. Rauck AM, Green DM, Yasui Y, et al. Marriage in the survivors of childhood cancer: A preliminary description from the childhood cancer survivor study. *Med Pediatr Oncol* 1999;33:60–63.

27. Schultz PN, Beck ML, Stava C, Vassiloupoulou-Sellin R. Cancer survivors: Work related issues. *Am Assoc Occup Health Nurs J* 2002;50:220–226.

28. Schultz PN, Stava C, Beck ML, Sellin RV. Internet message board use by patients with cancer and their families. *J Clin Oncol Nurs* 2003;7(6):663–667.

29. Schultz PN, Klein MJ, Beck ML, et al. Breast cancer: Relationship between menopausal symptoms, physiologic health effects of cancer treatment and physical constraints on quality of life in long-term survivors. *J Clin Nurs* 2005;14(2):204–211.

CHAPTER 22

REHABILITATION

Naveen Ramineni
Ki Y. Shin

■ GENERAL PRINCIPLES

Continued advances in cancer diagnosis and treatment are allowing people to live longer with cancer. These patients are often left with impairments that can cause significant disability. The major goal of cancer rehabilitation is to improve quality of life by minimizing the disability caused by cancer and its treatments and decreasing the "burden of care" needed by cancer patients and their caregivers. The more patients can do for themselves, the more personal dignity they are able to maintain and the less help they require from those around them.

In 1972, Justus Lehmann, supported by the National Cancer Institute (NCI) screened 805 randomly selected cancer patients, identifying multiple problems in the cancer patient population that could be improved by rehabilitation intervention and also multiple barriers limiting the delivery of cancer rehabilitation care (1). More than 20 years later, many of Lehmann's remediable cancer rehabilitation problems as well as barriers to rehab care remain the same (Table 44-1).

Cancer rehabilitation is appropriate for patients across the spectrum of their disease. Patients who are cured of disease, patients who are undergoing active treatment, and those who are at the end of life can all benefit from rehabilitation interventions.

Stages of cancer rehabilitation have been described as preventative, restorative, supportive, and palliative (2). Preventive therapies are begun before or immediately after a treatment to prevent loss of function or disability. Restorative therapies include comprehensive restoration of function in a cured or controlled patient with disability.

Supportive rehabilitation efforts are directed toward increasing self-care and mobility in patients with progressive cancer and disability. Finally, palliative rehabilitation efforts are used to maintain comfort or function in patients with terminal cancer.

Examples of rehabilitation interventions for cured patients can include return-to-work training, return-to-driving training, or lymphedema management.

Rehabilitation for patients receiving active treatment will often depend on the extent of their disease and the side effects and timing of treatment. With the generalized asthenia associated with some combination chemotherapy regimens, endurance and gait training may be necessary prior to, during, and following treatment. With anatomic or neurologic deficits from tumor involvement or surgical resection, specific strengthening combined with adaptive rehabilitation techniques may be necessary to achieve rehabilitation goals.

For patients at the end of life, directed rehab efforts in family training, pain management, bowel and blad-

SOURCE: Data from Lehmann et al. (1). With permission.

TABLE 44-1	REMEDIABLE REHABILITATION PROBLEMS AND BARRIERS TO DELIVERY OF REHABILITATION CARE		
Remediable Rehabilitation Problems			*Barriers to Delivery of Rehabilitation Care*
Psychological/psychiatric impairments	Lymphedema management		Lack of identification of patient problems
Generalized weakness	Musculoskeletal difficulties		Lack of appropriate referral by physicians
Impairments in activities of daily living	Swallowing dysfunction		unfamiliar with the concept of
Pain	Impaired communication		rehabilitation
Impaired gait/ambulation	Skin management		Patient too ill to participate
Disposition/housing issues	Vocational assessments		Patient denies need
Neurologic impairments	Impaired nutrition		Cancer prognosis too limited
Vocational assessments	Lymphedema management		Rehabilitation unavailable
Impaired nutrition			No financial resources

der training, and transfer techniques may be required for safe care of the patient at home.

Cancer rehabilitation occurs in various settings including acute inpatient rehabilitation in a hospital, in outpatient clinics, with professionals in the home, or in a skilled nursing facility, nursing home, palliative care unit, or hospice.

Acute inpatient cancer rehabilitation can directly follow cancer treatment requiring hospitalization, such as surgery or chemotherapy, attempting to improve mobility and self-care function for safe discharge. Marciniak described functional improvements after acute inpatient rehabilitation at a free-standing rehabilitation facility (3). Functional improvements after rehabilitation recommendations from an inpatient consultation service have also been described. In addition, outpatient rehabilitation can occur for patients who do not require hospitalization and after inpatient rehabilitation to reinforce concepts and techniques taught during inpatient rehabilitation.

Rehabilitation goals are accomplished by the efforts of a comprehensive interdisciplinary team of health care professionals, including the rehabilitation physician, rehabilitation nurse, physical therapist, occupational therapist, speech therapist, dietitian, pharmacist, chaplain, social worker, and case manager. Each member of the team has specific expertise in assisting the patient with a care plan of maximizing medical stability, function, financial resources, and caregiver involvement for a discharge that is as safe and meaningful as possible (Fig. 44-1).

Also crucial to rehabilitation success is the active involvement of oncologists, surgeons, and other medical specialists to assist in managing the ever-present and complex medical issues with which these patients present.

At the University of Texas M.D. Anderson Cancer Center (MDACC), our cancer rehabilitation practice includes five physical medicine and rehabilitation physicians, a rehabilitation therapy staff of over 50 physical therapy and occupational therapy clinicians, and 8 speech pathologists. Rehabilitation therapists see over 150 inpatients and 50 outpatients per day. The inpatient rehabilitation unit at MDACC had 403 admissions from September 2002 to August 2003. A total of 865 inpatient physical medicine and rehabilitation consultations were performed. Patients included most of the different tumor types seen in the institution, the most common being brain, spine, lung, breast, hematologic, genitourinary, gastrointestinal, and head and neck tumors. The most common inpatient rehabilitation diagnoses included asthenia, gait abnormality, dyspnea, hemiparesis, spinal cord injury, and neurogenic bowel and bladder. Common outpatient rehabilitation diagnoses included lymphedema, myofascial pain, rotator cuff dysfunc-

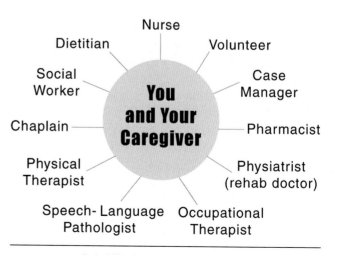

FIGURE 44-1 Rehabilitation team.

tion, peripheral neuropathy, and low back pain. Inpatient and outpatient electromyograms were performed for neuropathic and myopathic diagnoses and spasticity management.

Like other supportive care specialties such as pain management and palliative care, cancer rehabilitation is appropriate for all cancer patients, not only medical oncology patients but also surgical and radiation patients with cancer-related disability issues. Our practice at MDACC works very closely with the palliative care and pain services in providing assessments and treatment plans.

PRACTICAL ASPECTS OF CANCER REHABILITATION

One of the most practical and simple rehabilitation techniques that an inpatient must learn is to transfer. A transfer is a change in station or position from sitting in bed to standing or from sitting in bed to sitting in a chair. A person must transfer to get into a wheelchair or into a car seat. Patients cannot effectively mobilize until this is accomplished. Depending on the patient's level of disability, a transfer may be done sit to stand, stand and pivot, with sliding board requiring some physical assistance, or with a lift requiring total assistance. After basic transfers are mastered, ambulation may be the next goal to increase mobility. Weakness from paresis, deconditioning, neuropathy, or brain injury can also make self-care difficult. Practical skills such as feeding, grooming, bathing, and dressing are taught or relearned to improve independence (Figs. 44-2, 44-3, and 44-4).

A frequent reason for cancer rehabilitation consultation is to assess the patient's functional status for safe

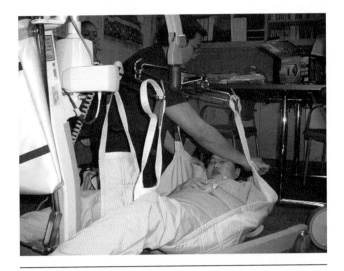

FIGURE 44-3 Lift transfer.

discharge. Important factors in this assessment include the patient's physical abilities, cognitive status, amount of family or caregiver support, and financial resources. A safe discharge usually requires some combination of these factors.

Many inpatient cancer rehabilitation patients require supervision and assistance at discharge both physically and cognitively. These patients were often independent prior to their most recent hospital admission. They must now make a choice to give up a large portion of their autonomy in exchange for personal safety. This may also require time and or financial resources from the patient and family.

It is at this important time of potential discharge that previous family tensions and dynamics can surface.

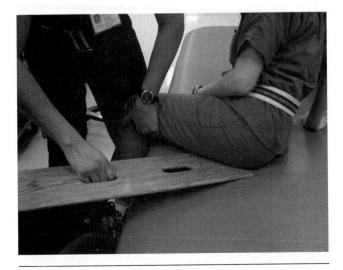

FIGURE 44-2 Sliding-board transfer.

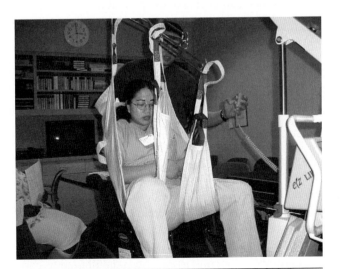

FIGURE 44-4 Lift transfer.

Who will help the patient? Who will take care of the patient? Who will help pay for the patient's needs? Many times it is not feasible to give up one's vocation or job due to additional fiscal and family responsibilities. Furthermore, sometimes people need to continue to work just to keep up the medical insurance needed to pay for the patient's medical treatments. What is done in this situation? Attention is directed to community resources, the church, and friends to assist in whatever way possible.

In the case of patients receiving palliative rehabilitation, the patient may have limited energy to pursue daily activities. Physical therapies and exercise may lead to early fatigue, preventing the patient from spending quality time on desired activities. Finally, rehabilitation professionals can give a functional perspective of the patient, providing important information to treating oncologists for palliative care–directed decisions.

For many professionals in the cancer rehabilitation team, a close bond is formed with patients after motivating and pushing them to improve functionally. The emotional and physical investment of maximizing a patient's abilities can often be great. The eventual functional decline of patients with advanced disease can be frustrating and disappointing to the team. The traditional noncancer rehab patient does not have a fluctuating clinical and rehabilitation course, with treatment of disease followed by recurrence or relapse. It is the morbidity and mortality associated with cancer that most challenges the cancer rehabilitation process. The patient's and family's new appreciation of everyday activities and their comfort level with them makes the process worthwhile for both patient and team. One of the most important things accomplished in cancer rehabilitation is the alleviation of fear in patients and caregivers, which can decrease the patient's concern about being a burden (4). Also, seeing what cancer patients have to deal with on a daily basis helps clinicians to prioritize what is important in their lives.

TOPICS IN CANCER REHABILITATION

The basic foundations and principles of cancer rehabilitation have been delineated; specific subjects in cancer rehabilitation are presented below. This includes the rehabilitation of patients with brain tumors, patients with spinal cord injuries related to cancer, and cancer-related deconditioning.

Thrombocytopenia, a specific issue unique to cancer rehabilitation, is also described.

REHABILITATION OF BRAIN TUMORS

Primary brain tumors are classified by cell of origin; the primary system of classification is that of the World Health Organization, which divides tumors into nine categories. The most common categories include tumors that displace brain parenchyma of the intracranial supratentorial compartment. Of these tumors, the most common are the gliomas, particularly the astrocytic gliomas (5).

In addition to primary brain tumors, brain metastases are estimated to occur in 20 to 40% of cancer patients. The most common mechanism of metastasis to the brain is through hematogenous spread. Most of the metastases are located in the cerebral hemispheres, followed by the cerebellum and then the brainstem.

Normal brain parenchyma can be destroyed or compressed by the tumor, and the location of the tumor determines the resultant neurologic deficit. In rehabilitation medicine, the physical impairments that could result in functional deficits are primarily addressed. These include neurologic muscle weakness, ataxia, aphasias, cognitive impairments, dysphagias, bowel or bladder dysfunctions, and spasticity.

Patients who have impairments resulting in functional decline that could affect bed mobility, ambulation, transferring from sitting or lying to a standing position, and/or activities of daily living (ADL) (such as eating, grooming, dressing, bathing, and toileting) can benefit from comprehensive inpatient rehabilitation. Brain tumor patients can achieve functional outcomes and rates of discharge comparable to those of patients with stroke, and they have a shorter length of stay than stroke patients (6).

Neurologic Muscle Weakness

Patients with hemiparesis or muscle weakness that results in an unsafe gait pattern, placing the patient at high risk for falls, may require admission to a comprehensive inpatient rehabilitation unit. There, with coordinated efforts from physical and occupational therapists, the patient will undergo gait training, using an appropriate assistive device such as a rolling walker or quad cane. Furthermore, training in the safe transfer from bed to a standing position is instituted, along with ADL evaluations and adaptations. Once a patient is functionally safe using an assistive device such as a rolling walker he or she can be discharged home. Then the patient can continue with outpatient rehabilitation, gradually improving his or her ambulation with an assistive device and further strengthening weakened muscles by way of a progressive resistance exercise program.

The pattern of recovery of muscle strength and function does not always follow the pattern of recovery observed in stroke patients. However, the stroke recovery pattern is often used as a guideline for patients with brain tumors. In patients who have had a stroke, lower extremity function often recovers earliest and most completely, followed by upper extremity function. The recovery of strength occurs in a proximal-to-distal direction, with flaccidity and decreased muscle tone progressing to spasticity and increased muscle tone. The spasticity in the affected limbs can evolve into flexor or extensor synergy patterns. Recovery of muscle movement may plateau at any stage or may progress to isolated coordinated volitional motor movement (7,8).

Several techniques and exercises are used for neuromuscular facilitation in stroke patients. Often a combination of procedures and techniques from the various programs are used in cancer patients with neuromuscular weakness. Proprioceptive neuromuscular facilitation developed by Kabat, Knott, and Voss relies on several mechanisms such as spiral diagonal movement patterns of the extremities and quick stretch. Brunnstrom movement therapy facilitates the use of the synergy patterns mentioned above as a means of developing voluntary control. Rood proposed that cutaneous sensory stimulation in the form of superficial stroking, tapping, brushing, vibrating, or icing provides facilitatory or inhibitory inputs (9).

In addition to the traditional range-of-motion and strengthening exercises as well as neuromuscular facilitation techniques, functional electrical stimulation can also be incorporated into the rehabilitation program for neuromuscular weakness. It uses a low-level electrical current that stimulates motor nerves or reflex sensory nerves to produce muscle contraction. The goal of functional electric stimulation is to produce purposeful, functional movements in paretic or paralytic muscles (10).

Sometimes, owing to weakness of the ankle dorsiflexors, it is necessary to use an ankle-foot orthosis (AFO) to improve hemiparetic gait. There are two major types of AFOs: the double metal upright AFO attached to an orthopedic shoe and the molded plastic AFO, which is more commonly used. With the plastic AFO, the footplate sits within the shoe and extends upward behind the calf. The advantages of a plastic AFO over a double metal upright AFO include better cosmesis, lighter weight, and the freedom to wear different shoes.

Shoulder subluxation, predominantly inferior, which is caused by the loss of normal motor control of the shoulder stabilizers, especially of the supraspinatus muscle, is often seen in the hemiparetic patient (11). It can often be the cause of shoulder pain in hemiplegic

patients (12,13). Other possible causes of shoulder pain in this patient population include complex regional pain syndrome, traction injury of the brachial plexus, rotator cuff tendinitis or tear, subacromial or subdeltoid bursitis, adhesive capsulitis, or heterotopic ossification. Diagnosis of glenohumeral subluxation is made through physical examination and radiographic evaluation. The acromiohumeral interval is compared on each side with the arms in an unsupported position during physical examination, and radiographic evaluation is used to quantify the amount of subluxation. Radiographic studies can provide an early evaluation for subluxation with slight gapping of the superior aspect of the glenohumeral joint (14).

Treatment of hemiparetic shoulder subluxation involves proper positioning of the arm, physical modalities, and exercise. The use of an arm sling can help maintain proper positioning and posture during ambulation. However, this is discouraged when the patient is seated, and its overuse may contribute to compromise of superficial blood flow as well as to joint contracture. Arm troughs and lapboards are used while patients are seated (15). Other interventions include biofeedback and functional electrical stimulation.

Hemisensory deficit and homonymous hemianopsia may be seen with hemiparesis. Visual or somatic hemineglect is more frequently seen when the nondominant cerebral hemisphere is affected. Hemispatial neglect has a negative effect on sitting balance, visual perception, wheelchair mobility safety awareness, and risk of falling (9). Patients with neglect have difficulty with hygiene and self-care activities on the affected side. Rehabilitation programs must address the issue of hemispatial neglect through focused measures led by speech therapists, occupational therapists, and physical therapists. Family training and education are important in this setting as well.

Ataxia

Cerebellar ataxia may be seen with mass effect within the posterior fossa. Of note, cerebellar ataxia can also be seen in paraneoplastic cerebellar degeneration and with high-dose administration of cytarabine (ara-C) or 5-fluorouracil (5-FU) (16,17). Involvement of the cerebellum can produce intention tremors, dysmetria, and dysdiadochokinesis as patients lose the ability to coordinate the agonist and antagonist muscle groups (18).

The response to pharmaceutical management has been poor; consequently physical and occupational therapy has been the mainstay of treatment for ataxia. This includes the teaching of compensatory techniques for performing basic self-care and occupational activities and the possible use of weighted bracelets or similar devices to help decrease the oscillations. Physical therapy directed at gait training with the use of assistive devices can help improve mobility in ataxic individuals (19).

Aphasia

Depending on its location, a tumor may be associated with deficits in speech, which can vary in severity and type. Often one can diagnose the type of aphasia from a comprehensive neurologic examination including speech comprehension, fluency, and repetition. These include Broca's aphasia, Wernicke's aphasia, anomic aphasia, global aphasia, conduction aphasia, and the transcortical motor and sensory aphasias.

A speech pathologist will implement treatment approaches including melodic intonation therapy, Amer-Ind Code treatment, functional communication treatment, stimulation approach, and PACE therapy (20).

Cognitive Deficits

Cognitive deficits can arise from direct injury to the brain tissue due to the tumor itself, from surgical resection, and/or the effects of radiation and chemotherapy. Steroid medications and anticonvulsant therapy can affect cognitive functioning. Additionally, common emotional sequelae such as anxiety and depression may worsen cognitive function or may be overlooked in the presence of cognitive deficits (21). The most often seen deficits include impairments in memory and attention, decreased initiation, and psychomotor retardation (21).

The rehabilitation physician will assess the patient's cognitive status as part of the physical examination. This assessment is needed in order to formulate a rehabilitation program involving speech pathologists. Specific deficits in language and cognition can further be delineated through specific testing performed by a speech pathologist. However, it is sometimes necessary to have formal neuropsychological testing done, especially in cases where the patient wishes to return to work.

Treatment involves the coordinated efforts from the speech pathologist and neuropsychologist as well as possible pharmacologic interventions. Methylphenidate, which promotes the release of dopamine and norepinephrine and blocks the reuptake of catecholamines, can be used for hypoarousal and inattention. Typically, the starting dose is 5 mg twice a day, preferably at 8 a.m. and 12 noon. In addition, stabilization of the patient's sleep-wake cycle can help decrease daytime drowsiness, which may improve attention.

DYSPHAGIA

A disruption in the swallowing process can also occur in patients with brain tumors or following craniotomies. It is important to determine, through clinical assessment, whether dysphagia is present, because there is the potential for serious complications such as malnutrition and aspiration pneumonia if dysphagia remains undetected. Often its presence can be established from a history and neurologic examination. If dysphagia is suspected, a speech pathologist is consulted; then daily swallowing therapy and exercises are incorporated into the therapeutic milieu.

Treatments include dietary modifications and dysphagia exercise and facilitation techniques (22). Depending on the results from a clinical swallowing evaluation or videofluoroscopic evaluation, food can be modified to different consistencies, including puree, semisolid, or solid. Liquids may also have to be thickened by using various thickening agents (22).

Exercises and facilitation techniques are employed to aid and strengthen various components of the swallowing process. These include exercises employed for treatment for the lips to facilitate the ability to prevent food or liquid from leaking out of the oral cavity. There are exercises to assist the pharyngeal swallow by improving tongue base retraction. Vocal cord adduction exercises are instituted to strengthen weak cords to prevent aspiration.

Compensatory strategies include proper head and trunk positioning, which for most patients is to be seated upright with head midline, trunk erect, and the neck slightly flexed forward. Other techniques include the chin-tuck method and head turning and tilting during swallowing.

After dysphagia has been identified and measures are implemented for its treatment, regular follow-up to assess for improvement is required. This again can be done through clinical examination or radiographically. If improvement is noted, the diet may be advanced appropriately.

Spasticity

Spasticity is defined as velocity-dependent resistance to passive movement across a joint. It is an abnormality involving increased muscle tone and is one of the positive findings of the upper motor neuron syndrome.

Often brain tumors can cause muscle spasticity. This can affect the gait pattern, ADL, and, in severe cases, can cause pain and joint contractures as well as being a detriment to hygiene of the involved areas. Sometimes spasticity may be beneficial, as when a patient may use knee extensor spasticity to assist in transferring from a sitting to a standing position. Indications for the treatment of spasticity include the need to decrease pain, improve hygiene, improve gait and transfers, minimize contractures, and improve self-care.

Treatment measures for spasticity include physical and medical interventions. Proper positioning, passive range-of-motion exercises, serial casting, splints, and braces are some of the physical interventions used in treating spasticity. In addition, pharmacologic therapy may be instituted with medications such as tizanidine, dantrolene sodium, and baclofen. Tizanidine or dantrolene is recommended by most clinicians for treating spasticity stemming from primary brain pathology (23). Tizanidine, a centrally acting alpha-2 agonist, is usually the first-line agent because it is least likely to be associated with muscle weakness, like dantrolene sodium (23). The use of baclofen in patients with spasticity secondary to brain pathology is limited owing to its potential side effect of drowsiness. For more severe cases, the use of botulinum toxin or an intrathecal baclofen pump may be indicated.

Bladder Dysfunction

As in stroke patients, bladder incontinence may be present in patients with brain tumors. The causes of bladder incontinence can be multifactorial and include an untreated urinary tract infection, inability to ambulate to the bathroom, and altered cognitive status. If the pontine micturition center is preserved, patients with brain tumors can have upper motor neuron bladder dysfunction, which is characterized by bladder hyperreflexia with reflex or urge incontinence and complete emptying (24). Postvoid residual volumes are generally low in the absence of bladder outlet obstruction. Persistent areflexia and retention may occur with bilateral lesions (24).

Treatment first involves identifying the cause of the bladder dysfunction. Obtaining a urinalysis with cultures and sensitivities and then starting appropriate antibiotics is the treatment for urinary tract infections. Using a bedside commode or a urinal is of benefit for patients who have weakness or inability to safely ambulate to the bathroom. A timed voiding program that has the patient urinate at set times throughout the day, before the bladder can contract, can be of help for patients with hyperreflexic urgency. Anticholinergic medications such as oxybutynin (Ditropan) or tolterodine tartrate (Detrol) can be used for persistent incontinence in this setting of a hyperreflexic detrusor (25).

REHABILITATION OF CANCER-RELATED SPINAL CORD INJURY

Traditionally, traumatic spinal cord injury is one of the mainstays of comprehensive inpatient rehabilitation. In the cancer patient, spinal cord injury has several etiologies. These involve primary spinal cord tumor or metastatic lesions. Primary tumors such as meningiomas, neurofibromas, and gliomas are relatively rare, and the majority of tumors involving the spinal cord are metastatic. The metastatic lesions that cause nerve root or spinal cord compression can be paravertebral, extradural, intradural, or intramedullary; however, 95% of metastatic lesions are extradural. These lesions most often originate from primary tumors of the breast, lung, and prostate. Most extradural metastases arise from the vertebral body and result in compression of the anterior spinal cord. Approximately 70% of spinal metastases occur in the thoracic spine, which has a smaller ratio of canal-to-cord diameter than the other two spinal segments (26).

Pain that is worse at night and in the supine position is a common clinical presentation. Weakness and sensory loss and the development of bowel or bladder incontinence may indicate spinal cord compromise. Rapid progression of paraparesis over only a few hours indicates arterial compromise by tumor invasion or pressure; slowly evolving symptoms suggest gradual cord impingement and may respond to steroids and radiotherapy (27).

Corticosteroids can alleviate pain and improve neurologic function, and radiation therapy is the treatment of choice with most cases of cord compression. If the tumor involves two or three columns of the spine, spinal stability is of concern; consequently, treatment is aimed toward stabilization of the spinal column. This can be done with cervical orthoses. Sternal occipital mandibular immobilization (SOMI) is well tolerated and provides adequate flexion and extension as well as stability to the lower cervical segments. Philadelphia collars provide stability in flexion and extension for higher levels but do not restrict rotation and lateral bending in the lower cervical segments. The "clamshell" thoracic lumbar-spinal orthosis is used to provide thoracic and lumbar support but may not be an option in patients with friable or intolerant skin following chemotherapy or steroid use. Therefore the Taylor-Knight brace, which limits spinal extension, and the Jewitt brace, which limits spinal flexion, can be used to provide thoracic and lumbar support (27).

Surgery is also indicated sometimes with instability and neurologic compromise; indications include pathologic fracture and dislocation, failure of radiation therapy, and rapidly progressing myelopathic signs and symptoms.

As with traumatic spinal cord injury, once spinal stabilization is achieved, comprehensive inpatient rehabilitation can address the impairments, functional limitations, and disabilities associated with spinal cord compression and injury due to cancer. Individuals with nontraumatic spinal cord injuries can achieve significant gains in functional independence measurements during inpatient rehabilitation (28).

Classification

The American Spinal Cord Injury Association (ASIA) produced the international standards for neurologic and functional classification of spinal cord injury, which classifies patients based on clinical examination and not on radiologic or anatomic abnormalities. This is essentially a scoring system based on comprehensive muscle strength testing and sensory evaluation; it classifies injuries into neurologic levels and injuries that are complete or incomplete to various degrees. Once an ASIA level is scored, functional expectations for patients can be predicted on the basis of the neurologic level of injury.

Bladder Management

Tumors involving the spinal cord cause suprasacral neurogenic bladder problems, which typically result in a hyperreflexic detrusor; this is characterized by low urinary volumes, high bladder pressures, and diminished bladder compliance. Incomplete lesions may produce the supraspinal pattern, with urgency and adequate emptying, while patients with complete lesions have reflex incontinence and incomplete voiding due to detrusor-sphincter dyssynergia (24). Some patients have hypocontractile or areflexic bladders, with urinary retention and associated overflow incontinence if the lesion involves the sacral micturition center. Sometimes there is a mixed picture of upper motor neuron dysfunction, hyperreflexic bladder and lower motor neuron dysfunction, and areflexic bladder.

Management of lower motor neuron bladder dysfunction involves the use of a condom catheter for men or an indwelling catheter for women in the situation where sphincter tone is diminished with normal or compromised detrusor tone. When the sphincter tone is competent but the bladder tone diminished, an intermittent catheterization program is instituted.

The management of upper motor neuron bladder dysfunction involves the use of an anticholinergic medication such as oxybutynin to decrease detrusor tone and allow for greater capacity; then an intermittent catheterization program can be instituted.

An intermittent catheterization program first involves daily measurements of postvoid residuals, or the volume of urine left in the bladder after a void. This can be performed noninvasively by an ultrasound-mediated bladder scanner or, more accurately, by straight catheterization and measurement postvoid. If the postvoid volumes are 100 to 150 mL or greater, an intermittent catheterization program is initiated. The patient is catheterized initially every 4 h. The goal is to have the catheterized volumes not exceed 400 to 500 mL. If the volumes remain consistently below those numbers, the frequency of catheterization can be decreased to every 6 h.

In addition, management of bladder dysfunction in this population involves assessing for urinary tract infections, which can be common. Appropriate antibiotics should be started based on urinalysis, cultures, and sensitivities.

It is important to note that in the cancer population, life expectancy often plays a part in rehabilitation management. Intermittent catheterization is the preferred method of management for the scenarios mentioned above; however, a Foley catheter is sometimes used instead for ease and comfort.

Bowel Management

Typically, with lesions above the conus medullaris, an upper-motor-neuron bowel dysfunction is present, with the muscles of the external anal sphincter and pelvic floor becoming spastic. The connection between the spinal cord and the colon remain intact and bowel and stool can be propelled by reflex activity. With lesions below the conus medullaris, an areflexic lower-motor-neuron bowel dysfunction is present, with the myenteric plexus intrinsically moving stool slowly (29).

A complicating matter with cancer patients is opioid-induced constipation. This and other premorbid factors and current bowel function must be ascertained before instituting a bowel program. Often a plain x-ray of the abdomen is obtained to assess for obstipation before beginning a bowel program. If obstipation is present, an enema is given to clean out the bowels and especially to evacuate the rectal vault.

The goal of a bowel management program is to prevent fecal impaction. This is a logical, structured program based initially on evaluation of the current bowel pattern. A bowel management program begins with a proper diet, which should contain adequate amounts of fluid and fiber in order to create soft bulky stools, which can decrease bowel transit time. Fatty foods can increase transit time. Medication management involves the introduction of a stool softener such as docusate sodium or a stimulant such as senna. A bisacodyl suppository can be used as an adjunct.

To summarize: in stepwise fashion, a bowel program begins with an x-ray in order to determine whether evacuation by enemas is necessary; then an appropriate diet is begun, along with stool softeners and/or stimulants. To take advantage of the gastrocolic reflex, the patient is placed on the commode approximately 30 min after a meal, preceded by a bisacodyl suppository ten minutes before the patient is placed on the commode. In addition, manual digital stimulation 20 min after suppository insertion can induce the rectocolic reflex (24).

Spasticity

Many patients with spinal cord injury suffer from spasticity, which is an abnormality of muscle tone and is velocity-dependent resistance to passive movement across a joint. In addition they experience muscle flexor spasms, which also respond to the same treatment strategies as those used for spasticity.

Treatment begins with proper positioning and can also involve splinting, casting, stretching, range-of-motion exercises, and the use of medications. In contrast to spasticity originating from brain pathology, spasticity associated with spinal cord injury is treated medically, primarily with baclofen. Tizanidine is also an appropriate choice. In addition, chemical neurolysis, botulinum toxin, and—for severe cases—an intrathecal baclofen pump may be used.

REHABILITATION OF GENERALIZED DECONDITIONING

A common problem in patients with cancer is generalized weakness and deconditioning, which simply means a loss of or decrease in a prior state of conditioning. Often this results from prolonged bed rest. It was stated earlier that many patients admitted to the hospital with cancer develop asthenic symptoms. This is due to the severity of their disease process or prolonged bed rest, which results in a deconditioned state. The role of rehabilitation in this setting is to either help prevent a deconditioned or to "recondition" a deconditioned patient.

There are three types of muscle fibers. Type I muscle fibers are the slow-twitch oxidative metabolism fibers, which have slow fatigability and are used for prolonged activity. Type IIB fibers are the fast-twitch fibers, which use glycolytic anaerobic metabolism and have rapid fatigability. Type IIA is an intermediate fiber.

Prolonged bed rest can result in muscle weakness. In a classic study by Mueller, the muscles of a person on strict bed rest can decrease approximately 1.0 to 1.5% of their initial strength per day, corresponding to approximately a 10 to 20% loss of strength per week (30). Antigravity muscles like the gastrocnemius and back extensor muscles tend to lose strength disproportionately, with larger muscles losing strength more quickly than smaller muscles; handgrip strength is unaffected (31,32). Type I fibers are more affected than type II fibers (33).

These effects on muscles can be counteracted by a daily stretching program, which delays muscle atrophy (34). In addition, daily isometric muscle contractions of 10 to 20% of maximal tension for 10 s can help maintain muscle strength (30). Electrical stimulation of muscles can also be used. In general, it may take two or more times as long as the period of immobilization to recover muscle strength (35).

Joint contracture is an abnormal limitation of passive joint range of motion and can be caused by prolonged immobilization. Typical contractures from immobilization include hip flexion, knee flexion, elbow flexion, and internally rotated shoulder contractures as well as ankle plantarflexion contractures. Once they have developed, contractures are treated with range-of-motion exercises. For more severe cases, deep heating followed by range-of-motion exercises and serial casting may be necessary. In addition the avoidance of an overly soft mattress and lying occasionally in a prone position can help prevent hip flexion contractures. Dorsiflexion exercises and footboards can prevent ankle plantarflexion contractures.

Immobilization affects the bones. Wolff's law states that the ratio of formation to resorption is influenced by the stresses to which bones are subjected. The primary stress on most bones is weight bearing, which causes a buildup of bone; a lack of stress on bones leads to a predominance of bone resorption. Weight bearing is eliminated when lying in bed in a supine position and can lead to disuse osteoporosis. This is best treated with preventive measures such as active muscle contraction and active weight-bearing exercises. Exercises conducted in bed are not particularly effective (36).

There are cardiovascular effects from prolonged bed rest. The first such form of cardiac deconditioning is resting tachycardia. After a period of bed rest, the heart rate can increase by about one-half beat per minute each day for the first 3 to 4 weeks of immobilization (37). In addition, there are decreased diastolic filling times, with resultant decreased myocardial perfusion, decreased stroke volume with submaximal and maximal exercises, decline in cardiac output at submaximal exercise, and deleterious hemodynamic and orthostatic changes (36).

Thrombotic complications, such as the development of deep venous thrombosis, are a risk from immobility.

Virchow's triad states that hypercoagability, endothelial injury, and stasis of blood flow are factors that can contribute to clot formation.

The treatment of the cardiovascular effects is mainly aimed at prevention. Sitting in a chair prevents deterioration of $\dot{V}_{O_2max}$ and orthostatic intolerance. Isometric exercise minimizes decreases in $\dot{V}_{O_2max}$ (38). Cardiovascular deconditioning can be reversed by a progressive increase in activity and regaining an upright posture. Orthostatic intolerance can be helped by range-of-motion exercises, progressive ambulation, abdominal strengthening, and leg exercises to reverse venous stasis. In addition, supportive treatments for orthostatic intolerance include the use of a tilt table, supportive garments, leg stockings, abdominal binders, and medications such as ephedrine and fludrocortisone acetate (Florinef Acetate). Finally, it is essential to prevent deep venous thrombosis. This is done by mobilizing the patient, encouraging ambulation on a continual basis, using external intermittent leg compression devices, and administering low-dose anticoagulation (36).

THROMBOCYTOPENIA

In the cancer population, thrombocytopenia is often seen, especially in patients receiving chemotherapy and/or extensive irradiation, with resulting myelosuppression, bone marrow infiltration, and splenomegaly as well as leukemias and lymphomas. A rehabilitation program or exercise in a thrombocytopenic patient is controversial. The major concern in this situation is the development of an intercranial hemorrhage. With platelet counts over $5000/mm^3$, one study found fatal intercranial hemorrhage in only 1 of 92 patients receiving chemotherapy (39).

Hematologic guidelines in the University of Michigan Hospitals allow nonresistive activities at platelet counts between 5000 and $10,000/mm^3$ and light resistive exercises with counts above $10,000/mm^3$, with ambulation allowed with counts above $5000/mm^3$. Clinicians must use their own judgment with individual patients. In addition, platelet transfusions with counts below 10,000 should be performed in patients undergoing comprehensive rehabilitation.

References

1. Lehmann JF, DeLisa JA, Warren CG. Cancer rehabilitation: Assessment of need, development, and evaluation of a model of care. *Arch Phys Med Rehabil* 1978;59(9):410–419.
2. Dietz JH. *Rehabilitation Oncology.* New York: Wiley; 1981.
3. Marciniak CM, Sliwa JA, Spill G. Functional outcome following rehabilitation of the cancer patient. *Arch Phys Med Rehabil* 1996;77(1):54–57.
4. Mackey KC, Sparling JW. Experiences of older women with cancer receiving hospice care: Significance for physical therapy. *Phy Ther* 2000:80(5):459–468.
5. Berger MS, Leibel SA, Bruner JM, et al. Primary cerebral tumors. In: Levin VA (ed): *Cancer in the Nervous System,* 2d ed. New York: Oxford University Press; 2002:75–134.
6. Huang ME, Cifu DX, Keyser-Marcus L. Functional outcome after brain tumor and acute stroke: A comparative analysis. *Arch Phys Med Rehabil* 1998;79(11):1386–1390.
7. Twitchell TE. The restoration of motor function following hemiplegia in man. *Brain* 1951;64:443–480.
8. Sawner K, LaVigne J. *Brunstromm's Movement Therapy in Hemiplegia: A Neurophysiological Approach,* 2d ed. Philadelphia: Lippincott; 1992.
9. Roth EJ, Harvey RL. Rehabilitation of stroke syndromes. In: Braddom RL (ed): *Physical Medicine and Rehabilitation.* Philadelphia: Saunders; 1996:1053–1099.
10. Kraft GH. New methods for the assessment and treatment of the hemiplegic arm and hand. *Phys Med Rehabil Clin North Am* 1991;2:579.
11. Chaco J, Wolf E. Subluxation of the glenohumeral joint in hemiplegia. *Am J Phys Med Rehabil* 1971;50:139.
12. Calliet R. The shoulder in hemiplegia. Philadelphia: Davis; 1980.
13. Van Ouwenaller C, Laplace PM, Chantraine A. Painful shoulder in hemiplegia. *Arch Phys Med Rehabil* 1986;67:23.
14. Shai G, Ring H, Costeff H, Sozi P. Glenohumeral malalignment in the hemiplegic shoulder. An early radiological sign. *Scand J Rehabil Med* 1984;16:133.
15. Garrison SJ, Rolak LA. Rehabilitation of patients with completed stroke. In: DeLisa JA (ed): *Rehabilitation Medicine, Principles and Practice,* 2d ed. Philadelphia: Lippincott; 1993:801.
16. Macdonald DR. Neurologic complications of chemotherapy. *Neurol Clin* 1991;9:955.
17. Posner JB: Paraneoplastic syndromes. *Neur Clin* 1991;9:919.
18. Diener HC, Dichgans J. Pathophysiology of cerebellar ataxia. *Mov Disord* 1992;7:95.
19. Silver, KH, Fishman P, Speed J. Movement disorders. In: O'Young BJ, Young MA, Steins SA (eds): *Physical Medicine and Rehabilitation Secrets,* 2d ed. Philadelphia: Hanley & Belfus, 2002:182–193.
20. Rao PR. Adult communication disorders. In: Braddom RL (ed): *Physical Medicine and Rehabilitation.* Philadelphia: Saunders; 1996:43–65.
21. Gillis TA, Yadav R, Guo Y. Rehabilitation of patients with neurologic tumors and cancer-related central nervous system disabilities. In: Levin VA (ed): *Cancer in the Nervous System,* 2d ed. New York: Oxford University Press; 2002:470–492.
22. Noll S, et al. Rehabilitation of patients with swallowing disorders. In: Braddom RL (ed): *Physical Medicine and Rehabilitation,* 2d ed. Philadelphia: Saunders; 2000:535–557.
23. Kaplan M. Upper motor neuron syndrome and spasticity. In: Woo BH, Nesathurai S (eds): *The Rehabilitation of People with Traumatic Brain Injury.* Malden, MA: Blackwell Science; 2000:85–99.
24. Cardenas DD, Mayo ME, King JC. Urinary tract and bowel management in the rehabilitation setting. In: Braddom RL

(ed): *Physical Medicine and Rehabilitation.* Philadelphia: Saunders; 1996:555–579.

25. Abbott K, Blaustein D. Stroke rehabilitation. In: Nesathurai S, Blaustein D (eds): *Essentials of Inpatient Rehabilitation.* Malden, MA: Blackwell Science; 2000:117–126.

26. Gilbert RW, Kim JH, Posner JB. Epidural spinal cord compression from metastatic tumor: Diagnosis and treatment. *Ann Neurol* 1978;3:40–51.

27. Garden FH, Gillis TA. Principles of cancer rehabilitation. In: Braddom RL (ed): *Physical Medicine and Rehabilitation.* Philadelphia: Saunders; 1996:1199–1214.

28. McKinley WO, Conti-Wyneken AR, Vokac CW. Rehabilitative functional outcome of patients with neoplastic spinal cord compressions. *Arch Phys Med Rehabil* 1996;77(9):892–895.

29. Bergman, SB. Bowel management. In: Nesathurai S (ed): *The Rehabilitation of People with Spinal Cord Injury,* 2d ed. Malden, MA: Blackwell Science; 2000:53–58.

30. Mueller EA. Influence of training and of inactivity on muscle strength. *Arch Phys Med Rehabil* 1970;51:449–462.

31. Dietrick JE, Whedon GD, Shorr E. Effects of immobilization upon various metabolic and physiologic functions in normal men. *Am J Med* 1948;4:3–36.

32. Greenleaf JE, Wade CE, Leftheriotis G. Handgrip and general muscular strength and endurance during prolonged bed rest with isometric and isotonic leg exercise training. *Aviat Space Environ Med* 1983;54:696–700.

33. Appell H. Muscular atrophy following immobilization. *Sports Med* 1990;10:42–48.

34. Baker JH, Matsumoto DE. Adaptation of skeletal muscle to immobilization in a shortened position. *Muscle Nerve* 1988; 231–244.

35. Houston ME, Bentzen H, Larsen H. Interrelationships between skeletal muscle adaptations and performance as studied by detraining and retraining. *Acta Physiol Scand* 1979; 105:163–170.

36. Buschbacher RM. Deconditioning, conditioning, and the benefits of exercise. In: Braddom RL (ed): *Physical Medicine and Rehabilitation.* Philadelphia: Saunders; 1996:687–707.

37. Taylor HL, Henschel A, Brozek J, Keys A. Effects of bed rest on cardiovascular function and work performance. *J Appl Physiol* 1949;2:223–239.

38. Stremel RW, Convertino VA, Bernauer EM, Greenleaf JE. Cardiorespiratory deconditioning with static and dynamic leg exercise during bedrest. *J Appl Physiol* 1976;41:905–909.

39. Gaydos LA, Freineich EJ, Mantel N. The quantitative relation between platelet count and hemorrhage in patients with acute leukemia. *N Engl J Med* 1962;266:905.

INDEX

Cyclophosphamide
acute lymphoblastic leukemia, 9t
aggressive NHL, 126t, 128t, 130t
breast cancer, 472
chronic lymphocytic leukemia, 47
endometrial cancer, 674t
gestational trophoblastic disease, 594t
indolent lymphoma, 84
preoperative allogeneic transplantation preparation, 199–200
small cell lung cancer, 242
Cyclosporine for graft-versus-host disease, 203
Cytarabine
acute lymphoblastic leukemia, 9t
aggressive NHL, 126t, 130t
Cytochrome P-450 3A4-inducing agents, 808, 808t
Cytokines for fungal infections, 979
Cytomegalovirus (CMV)
diagnosis, 982–983, 983f
overview, 982
therapy, 983–984

D

Dacarbazine
melanoma, 871
uterine sarcomas, 681t
Dactinomycin for gestational trophoblastic disease, 593t–594t
Dartmouth regimen for melanoma, 872
Decitabine, 70
Delirium
assessment, 1069
clinical features, 1068
overview, 1068, 1069f
treatment, 1069–1070
Depression
assessment, 1071
overview, 1070, 1070f
pharmacotherapy, 1071, 1072t
treatment, 1071
Dexamethasone
acute lymphoblastic leukemia, 9t
aggressive NHL, 126t, 128t, 130t
indolent lymphoma, 84
DHAP regimen for aggressive NHL, 130t
Diabetes insipidus, as endocrine manifestation of nonendocrine tumors, 996
Diabetes mellitus, as endocrine manifestation of nonendocrine tumors
interferon alpha, 995
L-asparaginase, 994
overview, 994
streptozocin, 994–995
DICE regimen for aggressive NHL, 130t
Differentiated thyroid carcinoma. *See* Thyroid carcinoma, differentiated
Diffuse large B-cell lymphoma, 104–106, 104f–106f
Disseminated intravascular coagulation (DIC), 24
DNA ploidy analysis, 548
Docetaxel
head and neck cancer, 299
metastatic breast cancer, 511–512
non–small cell lung cancer, 279t

ovarian cancer, 563
small cell lung cancer, 242, 245
Doxorubicin
acute lymphoblastic leukemia, 9t
aggressive NHL, 126t, 128t, 130t
endometrial cancer, 673, 674t
indolent lymphoma, 84
Kaposi's sarcoma, 909
leiomyosarcoma, 680, 680t–681t
mixed Müllerian tumor, 682t
small cell lung cancer, 242
soft-tissue sarcomas, 886–887, 887f
uterine sarcomas, 681t
Ductal carcinoma in situ, 465
epidemiology, 533
pathologic features, 534
treatment
local therapy, 534
systemic therapy, 534–535
Durie-Salmon staging system for multiple myeloma, 181t
Dysgerminoma, 568
Dysphagia
bladder dysfunction, 1113
overview, 1112
spasticity, 1112–1113
Dyspnea
assessment, 1067
overview, 1067, 1067t
treatment
of the cause, 1068
overview, 1067
symptomatic
drug therapy, 1068
general supportive measures, 1068
oxygen therapy, 1068

E

Electrolyte and water disorders, as endocrine manifestations of nonendocrine tumors
diabetes insipidus and hypernatremia, 996
overview, 996
syndrome of inappropriate antidiuretic hormone secretion (SIADH) and hyponatremia, 996
Emergencies, oncologic. *See* Oncologic emergencies
Endocrine malignancies
anaplastic thyroid carcinoma
overview, 833–834
pathology, 834, 834f
therapy, 834
differentiated thyroid carcinoma
children, 830
diagnostic evaluation of solitary thyroid nodule, 820, 821f, 821t
etiology, 820–822
long-term follow-up
imaging, 826–827, 827f–828f
monitoring serum thyroglobulin, 827
recombinant human TSH, 828
metastatic disease, 828–830, 829f–830f
overview, 820
pathology, 822–823, 822f–823f